W9-BPL-232

ENCYCLOPEDIA OF HEALING THERAPIES

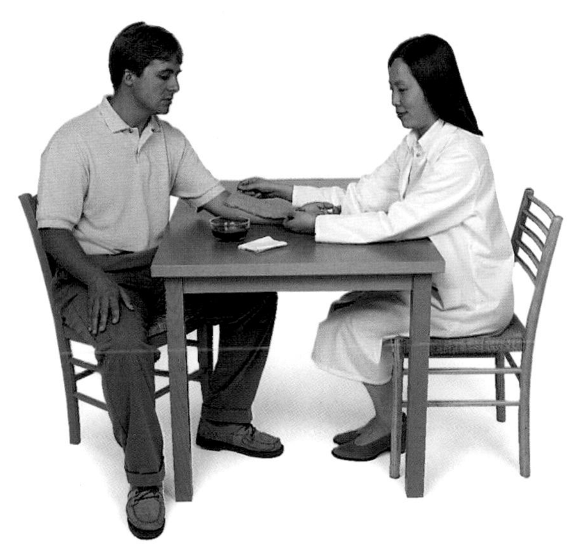

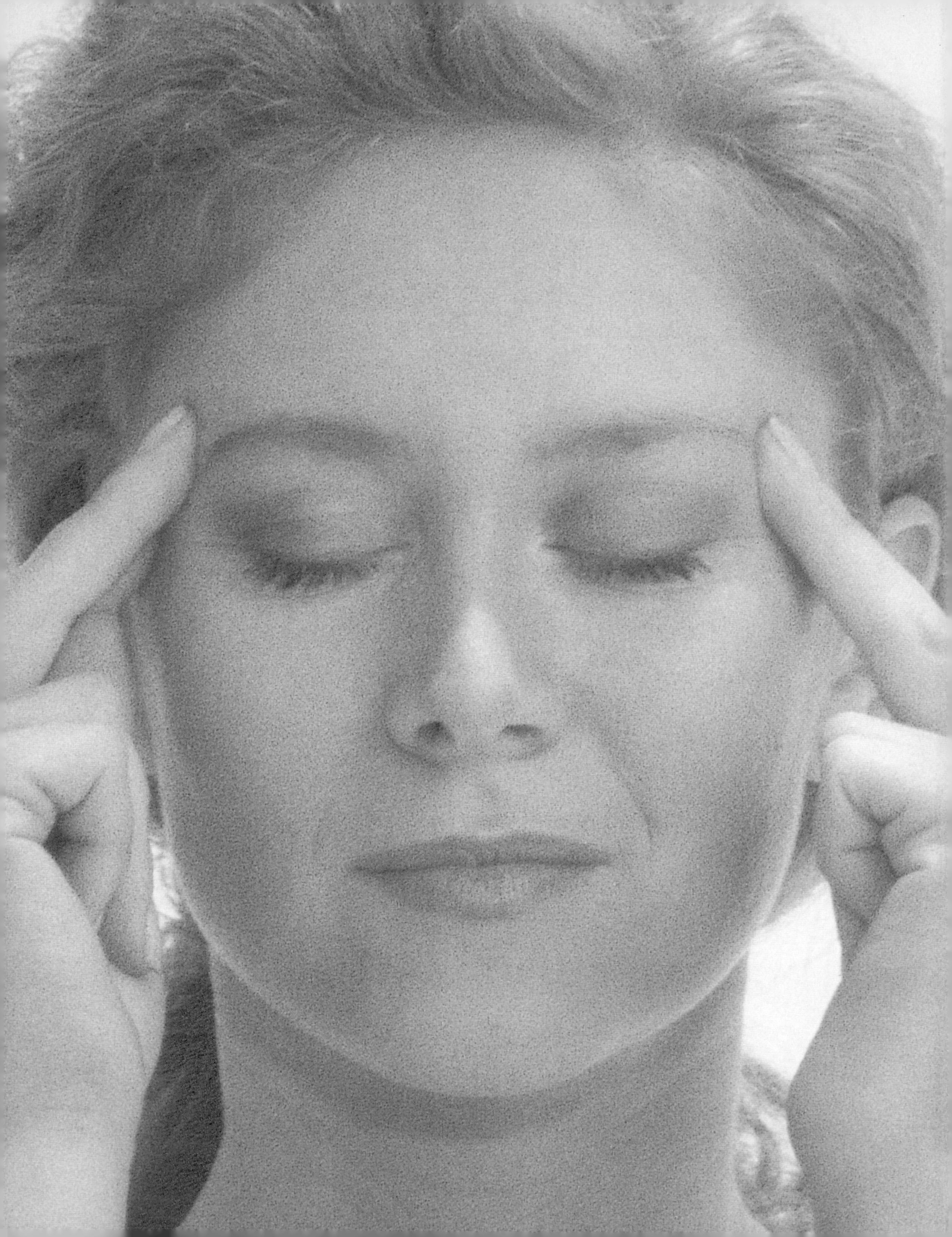

ENCYCLOPEDIA OF HEALING THERAPIES

ANNE WOODHAM AND DR. DAVID PETERS

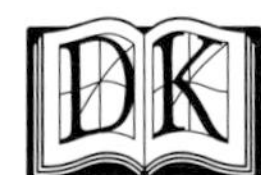

DORLING KINDERSLEY
LONDON • NEW YORK • SYDNEY • MOSCOW

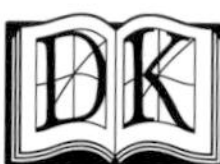

A DK PUBLISHING BOOK

Project Editor Stephanie Farrow

Art Editor Carmel O'Neill

Editors Claire Benson, Tracey Beresford, Christa Weil, Nell Graville, Constance Novis, Monica Chakraverty, Annabel Martin

Editorial assistants Nicola Nieburg, David Summers

Designers Rachana Shah, Maxine Chung, Claudia Norris, Judith Robertson, Robert Ford

Senior Editor (Ailments) Penny Warren

Senior Editor Rosie Pearson

Senior Art Editor (Ailments) John Dinsdale

Senior Art Editors Jo Grey, Kelly Flynn

DTP Designers Karen Ruane, Harvey de Roemer

Managing Editor Susannah Marriott

Managing Art Editor Toni Kay

Main Photographer Andy Crawford

Production Manager Maryann Rogers

US Editor Constance M. Robinson

US Consultant David Riley, M.D.

To our long-suffering and supportive partners, Stephen and Mary

AUTHORS' NOTE

The authors strongly recommend that you consult a conventional medical practitioner before following any complementary therapies if you have any symptoms of illness, any diagnosed ailment, or are receiving conventional medication or treatment for any condition. Do not cease conventional treatment or medication for any reason without consulting a doctor. Always inform both your doctor and your complementary practitioner of any treatments, medication, or remedies, both conventional and nonconventional, that you are taking or intend to take. The safety and efficacy of many of the therapies described in this book are unproved and they may conflict with conventional treatment.

PUBLISHER'S NOTE

Part of the information for this book was provided by the Research Council for Complementary Medicine, an independent charity founded in 1983 to promote rigorous research into complementary therapies that is linked with the US National Institutes of Health Office of Alternative Medicine. However, the opinions expressed are the responsibility of the authors and are not necessarily those of the RCCM and OAM.

First American edition, 1997
2 4 6 8 1 0 9 7 5 3 1
Published in the United States by
DK Publishing, Inc., 95 Madison Avenue
New York, NY 10016

Visit us on the World Wide Web at http://www.dk.com

Published in Great Britain by Dorling Kindersley Limited.

Library of Congress Cataloging-in-Publication Data
Woodham, Anne
The encyclopedia of healing therapies / by Anne Woodham and David Peters.
p. cm.
ISBN (hardback) 0–7894–1984–X
(paperback) 0–7894–2993–4
1. Alternative medicine. 2. Medicine, Popular. I. Peters, David, 1984– II. Title
R733.W65 1997
615.5--dc21. 97–16171
CIP

Reproduced in Italy by GRB Editrice, Verona
Printed and bound in Italy by New Interlitho, Milan

Consultants

The following practitioners have greatly contributed to this book by acting as consultants, supplying information to the authors and publishers, and checking the factual accuracy of text, excluding the medical opinion. Their assistance in the preparation of this encyclopedia is most appreciated.

General Consultant
Professor Patrick Pietroni
FRCGP, MRCP, DCH

Acupuncture
Gerry Harris BA, BAcC

The Alexander Technique
Kate Kelly MSTAT
Joe Searby MSTAT

Anthroposophical Medicine
Dr. Michael Evans

Applied Kinesiology
Clive Lindley-Jones DO, MRO, DipICAK

Aromatherapy
Shirley Price
Robert Tisserand

Art Therapy
Bruce Currie
BA(Hons), DipAT, AdvDipAT, RATh

Autogenic Training
Jane Bird RN, MemBAFATT

Ayurveda
Dr. N. Sathiya Moorthy
BAMS, PhD, MAMA

Bioenergetics
John Miller PhD

Biofeedback
Elizabeth L. Stroebel MEd, PhD

Chinese Herbalism
Dr. Guang Xu MATCM, MRTCM

Chiropractic
Chris Turner DC, CCSP

Clinical Ecology
Dr. Michael Tettenborn

Color Therapy
Pauline Wills HDipCTh, MIACT

Cranial Osteopathy
Carina A. Petter DO, MRO

Dance Movement Therapy
Bodhi Shaw MA(DMT)

The Feldenkrais Method
Allan Rudolf PhD
Certified Feldenkrais Practitioner

Healing
Dr. Daniel Benor

Hellerwork
Ms. Terry Petersen MA
Certified Hellerworker

Homeopathy & Biochemic Tissue Salts
Dr. Nicola Geddes MFHom

Hypnotherapy
Vera Peiffer BA(Psych), FAAT

Light Therapy
Natalie Handley MBSR

Massage
Clare Maxwell-Hudson

Music Therapy
John Strange DipMTh, RMTh, DipEd

Naturopathy & Hydrotherapy
Roger Newman Turner
BAc, ND, MRO, MRN, FBAcC
Leon Chaitow DO, MRO

Nutritional Therapies & Orthomolecular Therapy
Dr. Damien Downing

Osteopathy
Jonathan Le Bon DO, MRO

Polarity Therapy
Rosamund Webster MFPTR

Psychotherapy & Counseling
Jenny Corrigall PhD

Qigong & T'ai Chi Ch'uan
Michael Tse

Reflexology
Claire Parker MBSR

Reiki
Chris Parkes
Reiki Master

Rolfing
Prue Rankin-Smith
Certified Rolfer

Shiatsu & Do-in
Paul Lundberg
BAc, BAcC, MRSS

Therapeutic Touch
Jean Sayre-Adams RN, MA

Tragerwork
Bill Scholl

Western Herbalism
Anne McIntyre MNIMH

Yoga
Ruth White

Contents

Introduction 8

What is Complementary Medicine? 10

An Explanation of Holistic Medicine 12
The Rise in Popularity 14 ◆ The State of Research 16
Mind/Body Medicine 18 ◆ The Future of Medicine 20

A Guide to Well-Being 22

What is Illness? 24
The Balanced Body 26
Well-Being Questionnaire 28
A Balanced Diet 34 ◆ Healthy Eating 36
Dealing with Stress 38 ◆ The Value of Sleep 39
The Benefits of Exercise 40 ◆ Choosing an Activity 42
Coping with Difficult Emotions 44
The Power of Positive Emotions 46

Key Healing Therapies 48

A visual guide to over 90 widely used complementary therapies with information on their history, how they work, what to expect at a consultation, research and evidence, self-help techniques, and compatibility with conventional medicine

How to Choose a Therapy 50
How to Use this Section 52

Touch & Movement Therapies 54

Massage 56 ◆ Biodynamic Massage 61 ◆ Aromatherapy 62
Medical Aromatherapy 65 ◆ Reflexology 66 ◆ The Metamorphic Technique 69
Chiropractic 70 ◆ Network Chiropractic 75
Osteopathy 76 ◆ CranioSacral Therapy 81 ◆ Rolfing 82
Aston-Patterning 83 ◆ Hellerwork 84 ◆ The Feldenkrais Method 85
The Alexander Technique 86 ◆ Tragerwork 88 ◆ Bioenergetics 89
Acupuncture 90 ◆ Auricular Acupuncture 94 ◆ Acupressure 95 ◆ Shiatsu 96
Do-in 98 ◆ Thai Massage 98 ◆ Qigong 99 ◆ T'ai Chi Ch'uan 100
Polarity Therapy 102 ◆ Healing 104 ◆ Therapeutic Touch 106
Reiki 107 ◆ Yoga 108 ◆ Dance Movement Therapy 112
The Bates Method 114 ◆ Other Therapies 115

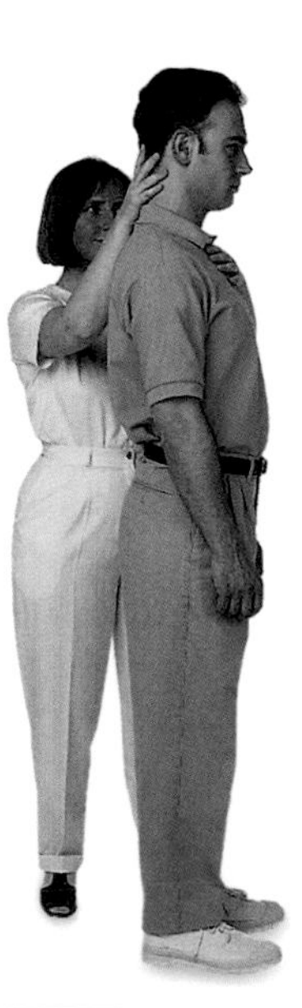

Medicinal Therapies 116

Naturopathy 118 ◆ Hydrotherapy 122
Anthroposophical Medicine 124 ◆ Homeopathy 126
Biochemic Tissue Salts 131 ◆ Bach Flower Remedies 132
Crystal Therapy 133 ◆ Western Herbalism 134
Chinese Herbalism 140 ◆ Ayurveda 144
Nutritional Therapies 148 ◆ Orthomolecular Therapy 153
Clinical Ecology 154 ◆ Magnetic Therapy 156 ◆ Other Therapies 157

Mind & Emotion Therapies 158

Psychotherapy & Counseling 160 ◆ Hypnotherapy 166
Autogenic Training 168 ◆ Biofeedback 169 ◆ Relaxation & Breathing 170
Meditation 174 ◆ Flotation Therapy 177 ◆ Visualization 178
Sound Therapy 180 ◆ Music Therapy 181 ◆ Art Therapy 182
Feng Shui 184 ◆ Geomancy 185 ◆ Color Therapy 186
Light Therapy 188 ◆ Biorhythms 189 ◆ Other Therapies 190

Diagnostic Techniques 191

An illustrated explanation of the various methods of diagnosis used within different complementary therapies

Pulse Diagnosis 192 ◆ Tongue Diagnosis 193 ◆ *Hara* Diagnosis 194
Hair Analysis 194 ◆ Iridology 195 ◆ Applied Kinesiology 196
Touch for Health 197 ◆ Dowsing 198 ◆ Nutritional Testing 199
Energy Medicine 200 ◆ Kirlian Photography 201

Treating Ailments 202

An extensive index of treatment options for over 200 mental, physical, and emotional health problems

How to Use this Section 204
The Brain & Nervous System 206
Skin 214 ◆ Eyes 220 ◆ Ears 222
The Respiratory System 224
Mouth & Throat 228 ◆ Digestion 230
The Urinary System 240 ◆ Heart & Circulation 242
Muscles, Bones & Joints 250 ◆ Hormones 262
Women's Health 264 ◆ Men's Health 276 ◆ Children's Health 278
Mind & Emotions 286 ◆ Allergies 298 ◆ Cancer 304
The Immune System 308 ◆ Pain 314 ◆ First Aid 316

Finding a Practitioner 318 ◆ Useful Addresses 319 ◆ Glossary 324
Bibliography 326 ◆ Index 328 ◆ Acknowledgments 336

INTRODUCTION

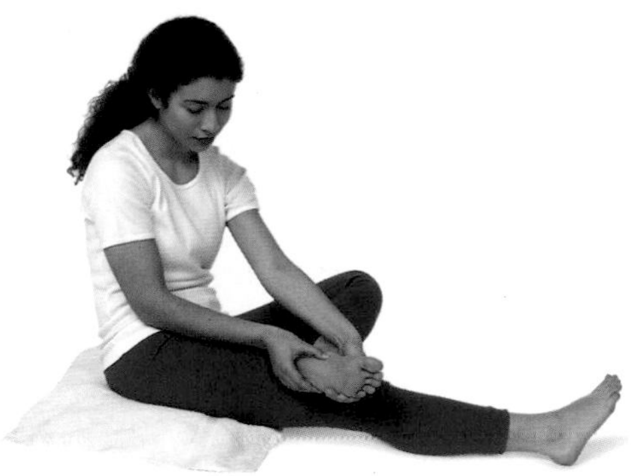

AT A TIME WHEN HIGH-TECHNOLOGY MEDICINE is pushing back barriers in areas such as gene therapy, laser surgery and high-resolution body scanning, it seems paradoxical that natural medicine is also enjoying a remarkable renaissance. While traditional folk remedies are the first and often the only health care option for most of the world's population in developing countries, surveys show that between one-third and half of those in affluent Western nations, where science-based medicine is readily available, are willing to use complementary therapies. And as pharmaceutical companies pour money into isolating and synthesizing chemical components found in plants, sales of herbal remedies containing these substances in natural form are among the fastest-growing health markets in North America, Europe, and Australia.

CHANGING PROFESSIONAL ATTITUDES

The popularity of complementary medicine has obliged the medical profession to take nonconventional therapies more seriously, and their use alongside – rather than instead of – mainstream medicine is growing. Many health professionals are more willing to subscribe to a "holistic" approach to health care that takes into account not only the individual's physiological condition, but psychological, social, environmental, and even spiritual dimensions that may reveal underlying factors contributing to illness. More doctors than ever are training in complementary therapies so that they can offer nonconventional as well as orthodox treatment options. "Integrated" medicine, which draws on both conventional and complementary methods, is seen as a real way forward.

GRASS ROOTS OPINION

Half a century ago the public placed enormous faith in the miracles of science. The discovery of "wonder drugs" such as penicillin elbowed aside less exciting, common sense principles of health (a low-fat diet rich in fruits, vegetables, and cereal grains, plenty of water, fresh air, exercise, and rest) that had always been at the heart of naturopathy and other traditional systems, and that medical research is now vindicating. Meanwhile, the failure of drug-centered medicine to cure stress-related, environmental, and psychological illness as well as long-term or recurring disease, plus a history of surgical accidents, negative side effects of drugs and a growing resistance to antibiotics, have driven some doctors and medical researchers to look again at traditional folk medicine. People generally are also better informed than previous generations and, as a result, more interested in taking greater responsibility for their own health. Add to this the ever-increasing cost of high-tech, intensive medical care, and the lively interest in preventive medicine and self-healing is all the more understandable.

The holistic approach of complementary medicine has much to offer. Health and well-being are often compared to a three-legged stool: one leg is pharmaceuticals; the second is surgery and procedures; and the third leg is self-care. To date, self-care, one of the cornerstones of complementary medicine, has been the poor relation. Good nutrition and exercise are undeniably important, but attention is now being paid to the inner world of the emotions and spirit, and the way the interaction of these and other elements contributes to well-being. The mind can play an influential role in self-healing – witness the power of expectation and the "placebo response" (see page 17). Today, scientists working in the new field of psychoneuroimmunology (mind/body medicine) are finding that the health of mind and body are indeed inextricably linked, the state of one influencing the other.

New Imperatives

In this book, we look at what is happening in complementary medicine today, and consider its development in reaction to the dominance of science, which often outlawed traditional folk medicine and paid scant attention to the part played by an individual's beliefs, attitudes, and feelings in becoming ill and getting better. An uncritical acceptance of all things "alternative," however, is as irrational as a slavish dependence on technology. Many alternative therapies claim therapeutic benefits due to "energies" as yet indefinable by science, or allege results that are backed only by anecdote. The same questions that are asked of conventional treatments must now be applied to complementary treatments. Do they work? Are they safe? Is there proof?

Using Complementary Therapies

Complementary therapies aim to mobilize self-healing processes to restore the harmonious working of the physical and biochemical elements of the body, and of the mind and emotions. In this book, we explain the various causes of imbalance using a self-assessment questionnaire designed to help you evaluate your state of well-being, followed by advice on how to improve your health.

In the 1980s and 1990s, the popularity of complementary therapies soared, and it is now more important than ever that the benefits claimed for these therapies are closely analyzed. This book shows how to identify the therapies that might suit you best, and gives guidance on choosing a competent practitioner. More than 90 therapies are explained and evaluated: expert practitioners demonstrate key techniques, and a ratings system, incorporating research data and information on the therapy's credibility among conventional doctors, provides a straightforward appraisal. In the final section, complementary treatment options are considered for over 200 conditions, including everyday complaints, emotional problems, and serious illnesses. We also note any clinical research that substantiates the use of a therapy for a particular disorder.

The Aims of this Book

Complementary medicine is now a formidable force in health care, but because it has been driven from the grass roots and shaped by idiosyncratic and personal interests, there is as yet relatively little coherence, organization, or validation. This book, we hope, will help demystify the complexities and ambiguities of complementary medicine, and encourage you to ask the questions that will lead to the safest, most effective, and most beneficial therapy for you.

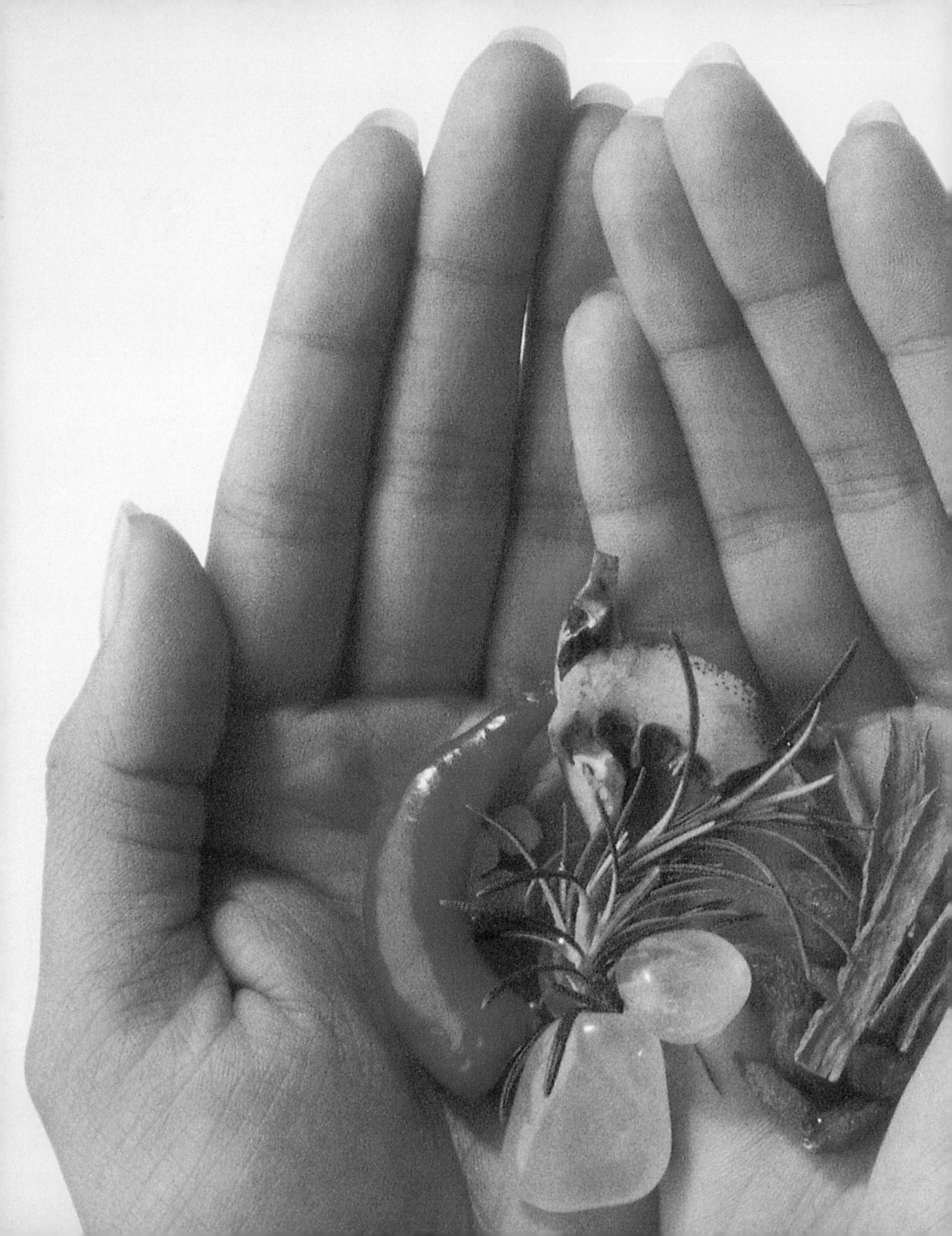

WHAT IS COMPLEMENTARY MEDICINE?

1

Complementary and conventional medicine adopt very different approaches toward the definition and treatment of disease. Conventional medicine is diagnosis-led: doctors use symptoms and medical tests to assess the problem, and prescribe treatment accordingly. Complementary practitioners aim to deal with the patient as a whole: for them, illness signifies a disruption of physical and mental well-being. Treatment attempts to stimulate the body's natural self-healing and self-regulating abilities.

This section looks at the "holistic" approach to health – the central tenet of which is that mind and body are inextricably linked. It also assesses scientific investigations into the effect of the mind on the body. As complementary medicine grows in popularity, issues of efficacy and safety become increasingly important. Given the valuable contributions of both traditions, the most positive way forward for medicine as a whole promises to be an integration of the best aspects of conventional medicine and complementary therapies.

AN EXPLANATION OF HOLISTIC MEDICINE

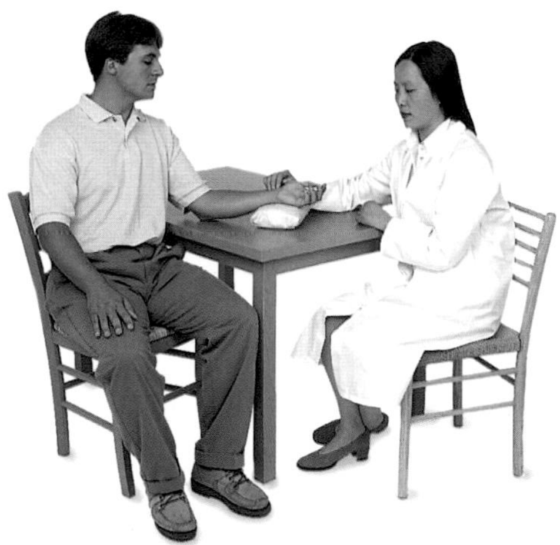

***Most complementary practitioners** look not only at the physical symptoms of illness, but also work closely with the patient to explore emotional and spiritual concerns. This holistic approach to health encourages the patient's powers of self-healing.*

HOLISM (the word is derived from the Greek *holos*, meaning "whole") is the idea that everything in the universe is greater than, and different from, the sum of its parts. Holistic medicine is an approach to health that aims to deal with the patient as a whole and not merely with physical symptoms. It takes into account the psychological state of an individual, social and environmental factors, and an indefinable dimension known as "spirit."

TREATING THE WHOLE PERSON

According to many of the world's holistic health systems, such as naturopathy, homeopathy, and Traditional Chinese Medicine, the body has a natural tendency toward equilibrium, or "homeostasis" (see box, opposite), the maintenance of which is the key to good health. When equilibrium is disrupted, holistic practitioners work in partnership with the patient, focusing on all aspects of his or her life, to promote self-healing.

A common misconception is that holistic healing is the sole preserve of complementary practitioners. In fact, many conventional doctors have a holistic approach, considering patients in the context of their lifestyle and emphasizing health education and self-care. Psychiatrists and psychologists also give a distinct nod to holistic principles.

On the other hand, not all complementary therapies are inherently "holistic" or "spiritual" – terms often used to distinguish them from "uncaring" medical science – nor are they necessarily "antiscientific" or "anti-intellectual." Some complementary practitioners, for example, might focus on certain physical symptoms in a similar way to conventional doctors, and therapies such as osteopathy and chiropractic are in many ways as practical and grounded in anatomy and pathology as conventional medicine. Because of this confusion of meaning, conventional and complementary practitioners interested in holistic principles often prefer to talk of "integrated" medicine.

An integrated approach can – and often does – combine the best in mainstream medicine and complementary therapy. While a nonholistic conventional doctor would treat only asthma symptoms, prescribing drugs to suppress them, a doctor with an integrated approach would treat the symptoms with medication but also address underlying causes, such as an allergic reaction or anxiety, and investigate the patient's emotional makeup. Cognitive behavioral therapy might be suggested as a strategy for coping with asthma attacks, hypnosis to relieve stress, or the purchase of special bedding and vacuum cleaners to minimize house dust mites if they trigger attacks. A complementary practitioner might prescribe an herbal remedy to relax bronchial muscles, a diet to eliminate food intolerances, acupuncture to restore the flow of *qi*, or essential oil massages to ease tension and induce relaxation.

Caduceus

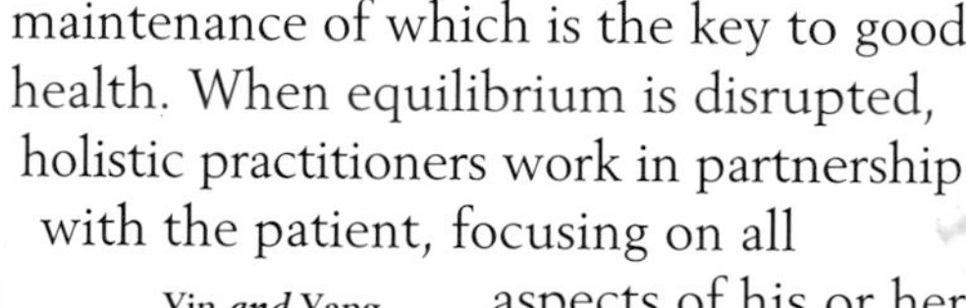

Yin *and* Yang

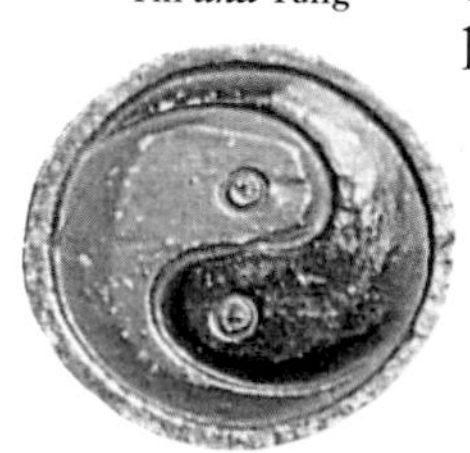

***Ancient symbols** of the equilibrium between opposing but interdependent forces can be found in both Western and Eastern cultures. The Western emblem of medicine, the caduceus, and the Chinese symbol for* yin *and* yang *both represent opposites held in a healing balance.*

THE POWER OF THE MIND

Modern epidemics of long-term and stress-related diseases that only seem to be partially alleviated by conventional medicine have led many medical practitioners to question 20th-century science's distinction between mind and body (see page 18). The origins of this schism are often ascribed to the 17th-century French philosopher Descartes, who sought to accommodate tensions between the Catholic church and the emerging science of medicine by allotting the intangible soul to the care of priests and the physical, "measurable" body to that of physicians. From here it was an easy step for the medical establishment to regard illness as purely a mechanical breakdown in the body's machinery.

But can our emotions affect our physical health? After all, we talk about "butterflies in the stomach" before an important event, and traffic jams as a "pain in the neck." At the very heart of science lies a phenomenon that supports the theory of holistic medicine – the placebo response (see page 17), in which an inactive treatment has a positive effect, providing intriguing evidence of the power of the mind over the body. Belief in a treatment, whether on the part of the patient or practitioner, or simply faith in the practitioner, can be so powerful that the patient actually gets better. The placebo response has reduced blood pressure, healed ulcers, eased swelling, overridden the effects of stimulants, and relieved arthritis, hay fever, and depression. In actively encouraging patients to participate in their own healing, practitioners may be able to exploit the power of this mind/body response.

Professor Herbert Benson of the Mind/Body Medical Institute of Harvard Medical School reports that, when actual patient cases are studied, the success rate of the placebo response can be as high as 90%. The power of belief and expectation, he believes, may be harnessed by eliciting the "relaxation response," a mental state that triggers significant physiological changes, including lowered blood pressure, slower breathing, reduced muscle tension, and diminished stress hormone levels (see page 171). Any technique in which the mind is quietly focused, such as meditation, visualization, diaphragmatic breathing, biofeedback, hypnosis, qigong, or yoga, can induce the relaxation response, and conventional practitioners at medical centers in the US and UK now employ these methods to improve the well-being of their patients.

The Spiritual Dimension

In holistic medicine, spiritual concerns rank with those of the mind and body. We are creatures that puzzle over what life means, where we come from, and where we are bound. To be anxious and bewildered at times is to be human. For many of us, the past has been painful, the present is insecure, and the future uncertain. In the struggle to make sense of life, certain activities create a supportive framework that connects us to our "inner selves," to each other, and to the world. These activities include art, literature, music, community, family, worship, and play, and they are especially important when illness presents us with the reality of our vulnerability, limitations, and dependency. Broadly speaking, this is the realm of spirituality.

In his studies, Professor Benson found that 23% of his patients reported feeling "more spiritual" after relaxation exercises and experienced fewer medical symptoms than those reporting no increase in spirituality. In 1995, US researchers at the Dartmouth Medical School found that patients who derived strength and comfort from religious faith were three times more likely to survive the six months after open-heart surgery than those with no religious beliefs. The same study also reported that people who never crossed the threshold of a church, yet nonetheless held deep spiritual beliefs, were equally likely to survive. Being actively involved with some sort of organization, whether a choir or political party, conferred the same protection, and the combination of faith and participation in any kind of group increased the likelihood of postoperative survival ninefold. More relevant to our well-being than organized religion and church membership, it seems, is a spiritual awareness and "connectedness" with fellow human beings.

Homeostasis

Holistic practitioners believe that the mind and body tend toward a state of balance, or homeostasis, and have a natural capacity for self-regulation. The ability to maintain equilibrium, however, can be overwhelmed when we are under strain physically or emotionally (see page 26). Demands on one part of the "whole" affect other parts – constant emotional tension, for example, may cause physical fatigue. Optimum health, therefore, is achieved by attending to all parts of the whole.

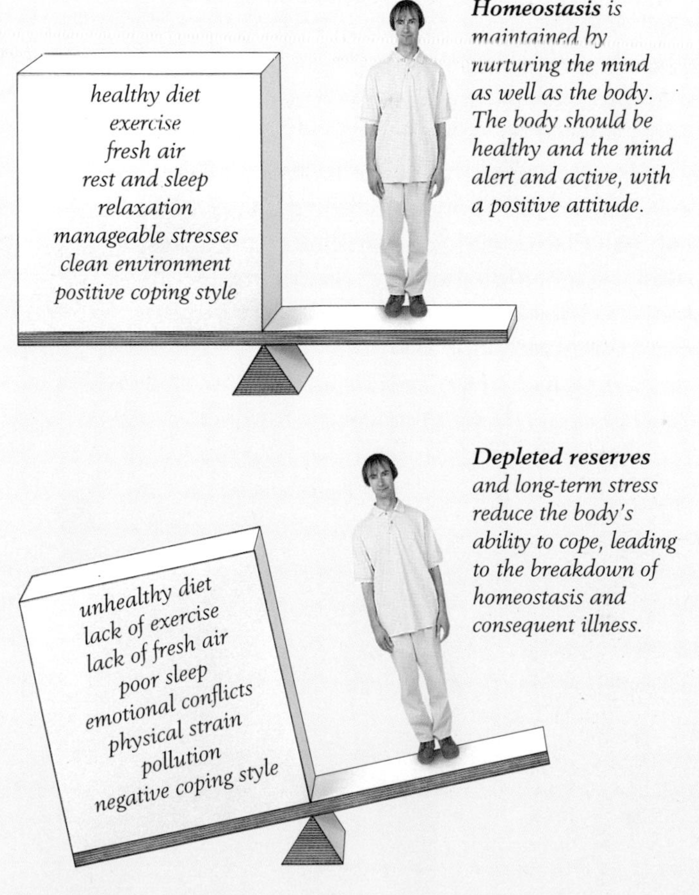

***Homeostasis** is maintained by nurturing the mind as well as the body. The body should be healthy and the mind alert and active, with a positive attitude.*

***Depleted reserves** and long-term stress reduce the body's ability to cope, leading to the breakdown of homeostasis and consequent illness.*

THE RISE IN POPULARITY

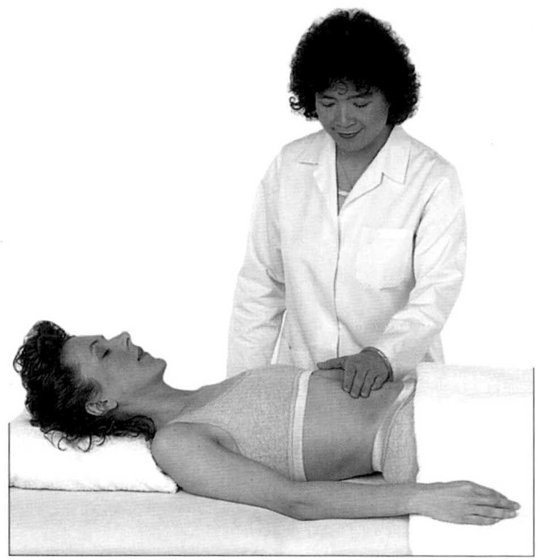

***Close partnership** between the patient and practitioner in many complementary therapies encourages the active participation of the patient in the healing process and is one of the main reasons for the growing popularity of complementary therapies.*

TODAY'S INTEREST IN COMPLEMENTARY medicine appears to be worldwide. Popularity in the West has grown steadily since the 1970s, accelerating in the 1980s and 1990s. A survey in 1993 showed that one in three American adults used some form of nonconventional therapy, and it has been predicted that the number will rise to one in two by the year 2000. The survey also revealed that more visits were made to complementary practitioners than to conventional doctors. Traditional Chinese Medicine, Ayurveda, and chiropractic attract an enthusiastic following in the US, but therapies widely used in Europe, such as homeopathy and aromatherapy, have been slower to gain ground. Following public demand and suspecting cost benefits, several American health insurers now cover some complementary treatments. In Australia complementary medicine is even more popular than it is in the US. Nearly half the population is said to use at least one remedy not prescribed by a doctor; over one-fifth have visited a complementary practitioner.

In Europe, studies suggest that between one-third and one-half of the adult population has used some form of complementary medicine at some time, although the popularity of different therapies and regulations concerning their practice vary from one country to another. In 1995, a Consumers' Association survey in the UK revealed that osteopathy, chiropractic, homeopathy, aromatherapy, and acupuncture were the most popular therapies. In the UK, a nationwide survey in 1991 suggested that 20–30% of the 30,000 general practitioners in the National Health Service would like complementary therapies to be more accessible within the state system. As yet most are privately funded.

In India, China, and Africa, traditional healing systems are in common use and may receive government backing. Cynics point out that "folk" medicine is cheaper to provide, but others detect strengths that complement "high-tech" medical science. Universities in India, for example, offer degrees in Ayurveda that incorporate Western pathology, proving that the two systems can work well side by side.

DISENCHANTMENT WITH MEDICAL SCIENCE

In some ways, the very success of conventional medicine is partly responsible for the rising popularity of complementary therapies. Improvements in living standards, and medical and scientific progress, have raised people's expectations of health and health care. The discovery of drugs such as penicillin and mass inoculation programs have diminished the terror of once-fatal infectious diseases. Medical technology in the form of X rays, brain scans, and keyhole surgery, and scientific miracles such as heart transplants and the saving of premature babies, seemed to give doctors godlike power over life and death. But the blind faith many people placed in medicine was shaken when

***Many complementary therapies**, which have been an integral part of health care in other societies for centuries, are relatively new to the developed world. Modern medicine in the West has been dominated by pharmaceutical drugs and medical technology, but there is now growing interest in therapies that treat the patient as a whole.*

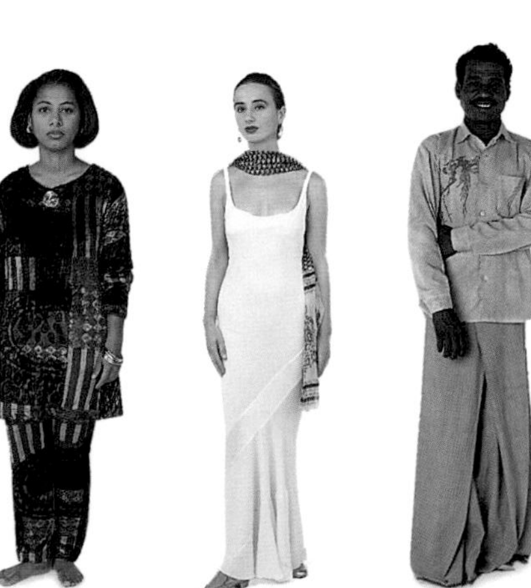

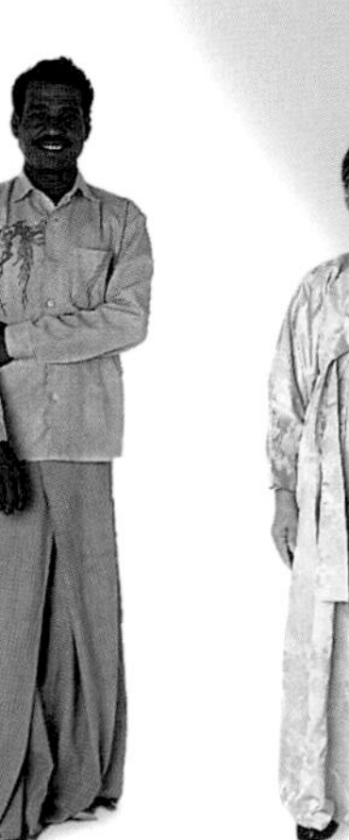

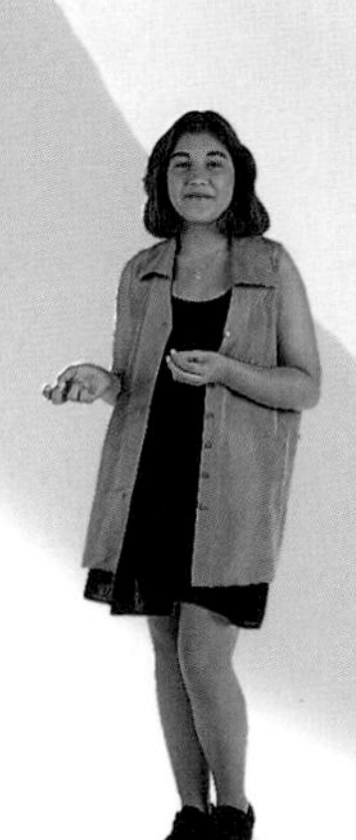

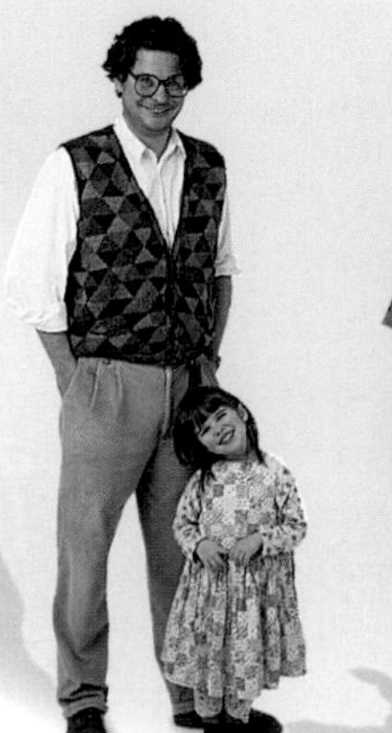

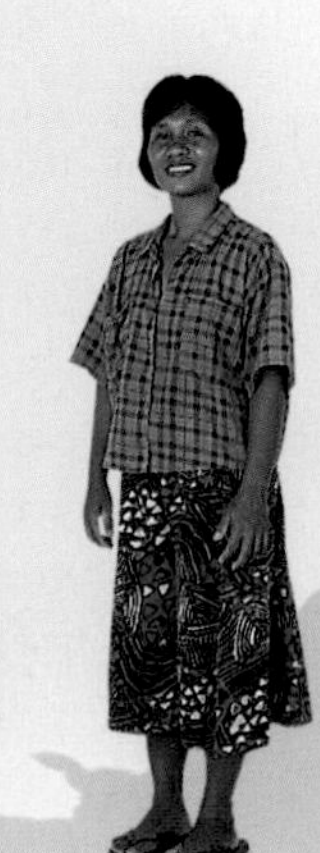

so-called wonder drugs revealed unpleasant or dangerous side effects, bacteria and viruses developed resistance to many of the drugs that once annihilated them, and pharmaceutical drugs and invasive surgical procedures failed to deliver the complete cures that were, perhaps unrealistically, expected of them. Despite some progress, cures for cancer and AIDS remain elusive, and long-term diseases such as asthma and arthritis are still difficult to treat and can be just as painful.

Disenchantment with medical science has certainly prompted a number of people to use complementary therapies, but not everyone is motivated by a flight from technology. Studies show that it is relatively rare for people to abandon conventional medicine completely, and many continue to hold it in high regard. Complementary medicine can sometimes simply seem more appealing.

WHAT COMPLEMENTARY MEDICINE CAN OFFER

A 1995 survey in the *British Journal of Clinical Psychology* revealed that many people turn to complementary therapies because they believe them to be more effective for their condition than conventional medicine. The emphasis on treating the whole person and allowing patients to play an active part in maintaining health is also attractive. The attention paid by health professionals and the media to health promotion and preventive medicine – a healthy diet, regular exercise, stress management techniques, and self-monitoring for symptoms of illness – encourages us to take responsibility for our well-being and to be involved in discussions about treatment. The length of time and amount of consultation that this requires may not, with the best will in the world, be within the scope of the average hard-pressed doctor. Complementary medicine, with its focus on partnership, holism, and self-healing, can therefore seem like the more natural approach, in every sense. Even the fact of paying for treatment, in commitment as well as money, can add to its value.

Many patients do not need to choose between approaches to treatment, since complementary therapies can often be followed alongside conventional procedures and medication. So far, people using complementary medicine have asked remarkably few questions about efficacy or safety – presumably grateful to have escaped what they see as the drawbacks of conventional medicine, or pleased to have found a treatment that relieves symptoms. In 1993, the British Medical Association urged its members to find out more about complementary therapies in order to advise their patients. As complementary medicine moves toward the mainstream and growing numbers of conventional doctors do become interested, therapists must be prepared for more critical and discriminating questions, such as "Does this treatment work?" and "What is the evidence?" People are hungry for a new kind of medicine, but not at any price. Just as the popularity of non-conventional therapies is making the medical profession examine its own practices, so complementary practitioners must account for their own claims and competence.

WHO USES COMPLEMENTARY MEDICINE?

International surveys have shown that people in developed countries using complementary therapies tend to be better educated and enjoy higher incomes than average.

UK research has shown that users fall into two categories: those with a specific problem, and those who sympathize with complementary medicine's "approach to life." On the whole, men are most likely to consult practitioners of therapies such as osteopathy or chiropractic, not because they are concerned about any toxic side effects but, more pragmatically, because conventional medicine did not help their specific problem. Women, however, tend to be more interested in easing stress and maintaining well-being, and are drawn to gentler therapies, such as reflexology and aromatherapy. Often those who turn to therapies for a specific problem experience other positive benefits, thus encouraging an interest in the approach to life offered by complementary medicine.

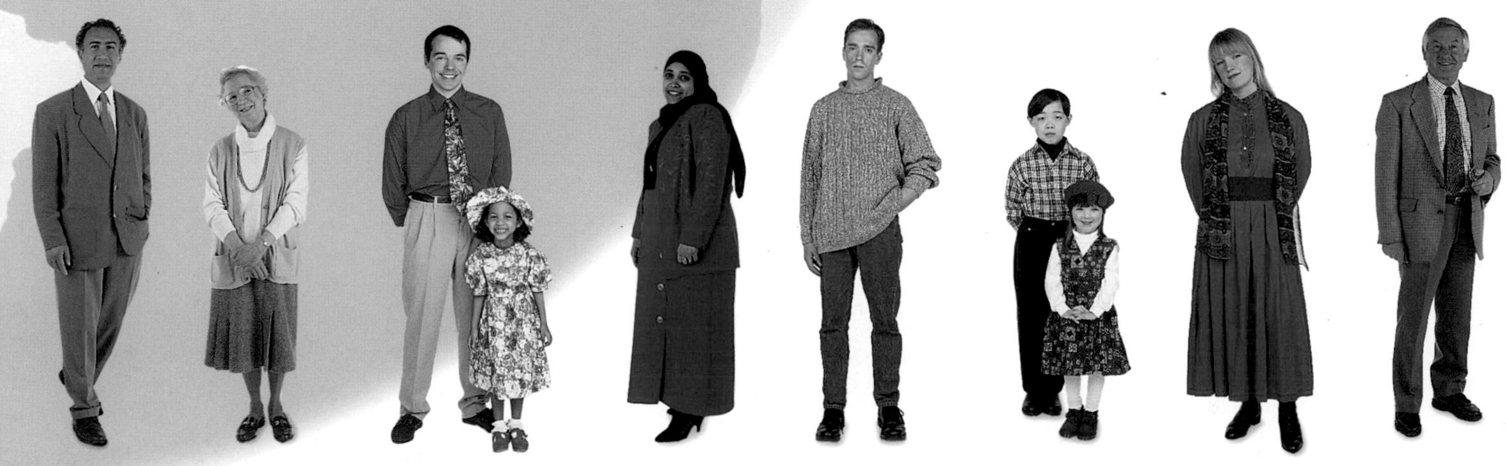

THE STATE OF RESEARCH

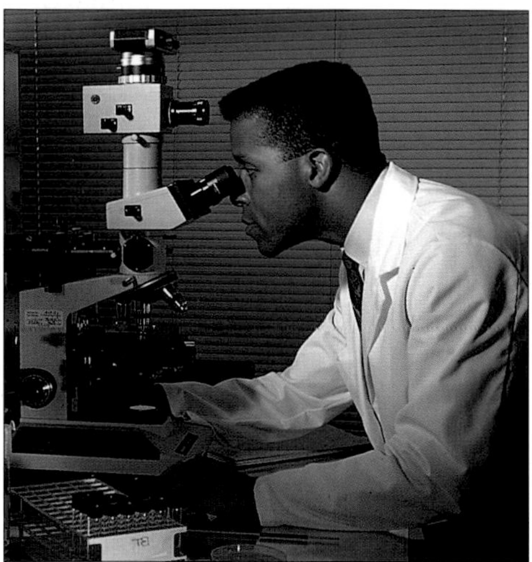

Much more research *into complementary therapies is needed. Some conventional research methods, however, are not ideally suited to evaluating the benefits of these therapies because they do not take into account the patient's participation in the healing process.*

ALTHOUGH THE POPULARITY of many complementary therapies may be widespread, it is not generally based on a broad understanding of what these therapies can offer. Complementary medicine seems to be largely taken on trust. Given its popular status, there is a somewhat surprising and troubling lack of research on the subject. To a large extent even the most basic questions remain unanswered. Which complementary therapies are effective? Are they as safe and natural as claimed? More complex issues are even more difficult to resolve. Do complementary therapies promote health or prevent illness? Could they reduce medical expenditure? Is there a "scientific basis" for their action?

TYPES OF CLINICAL TRIALS

Different types of clinical trials, originally devised to test pharmaceutical drugs and treatments in conventional medicine, are now being used to investigate complementary therapies. A *controlled* clinical trial compares at least two groups of patients: an experimental group that receives the treatment, and a control group that does not. This does not necessarily determine whether a procedure or medication "works," however, since any treatment, even taking a medical history, tends to have a therapeutic effect. To take this into account, the *placebo controlled* clinical trial was devised, in which both groups are given seemingly identical treatments, but the treatment of the control group is inactive (see box, opposite). For the treatment to be deemed to have worked, patients in the experimental group must perform significantly better than those taking the placebo. Researchers also try to include as many people as possible in the trial to balance out any personal factors, such as one patient being more ill than another, and to reduce the likelihood of therapeutic benefits being attributable to chance.

There is little incentive *for commercial funding of research into herbal medicine due to the lack of profitable patents to acquire, since many plant remedies have been used for hundreds of years and are widely available.*

Further risks of bias are ruled out by assigning patients at random into both groups, and the *randomized controlled* trial has been the gold standard in scientific research since the 1950s. Taking this one step further, the ultimate type of research trial is the *randomized double-blind* study, in which neither the patient nor the practitioner knows if the treatment is real or a placebo. The aim of this method is to ensure that any improvement in the treated group has not been influenced by individual attitudes, such as a practitioner's strong belief in the efficacy of a treatment.

Clinical trials are sometimes evaluated with what is known as a *systematic review* or *meta-analysis*, in which the results of a number of trials are combined. Small trials that remain inconclusive themselves may, when linked with trials that are designed better, yield more significant results. In complementary medicine, there are few possibilities for meta-analyses until more trials of therapies are available, but in the 1990s several reviews of this type did produce evidence that homeopathic treatments, acupuncture, and manipulative therapies have clinical benefits.

PROBLEMS WITH CLINICAL TRIALS

The use of randomized controlled trials to investigate complementary therapies can be problematic. Critics point out that randomization neglects a patient's right to choose, and that the success of complementary therapies depends to a great degree on the knowledge, skills, and attitude of practitioners. In many cases – particularly for mind-, body-, and movement-oriented therapies – treatment is more complex than a simple administration of pills, and it can be hard to select a "blinded" control treatment. How do you give a placebo massage, or even placebo acupuncture, not to mention placebo psychotherapy? Clinical trials also contradict the desire of many patients to participate in the healing process, a vital factor in many complementary therapies.

The *Evidence & Research* cited in the therapies and diagnostic sections (see pages 48–201) is based on the best scientific research available: the 1,500 randomized controlled trials (not all double-blind) on the database of the Research Council for Complementary Medicine in the UK, which has worked with the Office of Alternative and Complementary Medicine of the National Institutes of Health in the US. Our findings suggest that some complementary therapies can be analyzed in this way and may be clinically effective, but there is a lack of research. Researchers in conventional medicine have yet to show great interest in complementary medicine, nor have complementary practitioners had much interest in research. Much of the research so far has been by doctors practicing complementary therapies.

WHY IS THERE SO LITTLE RESEARCH?

Unlike drug trials, funding for complementary medicine research is scant. Drug companies are not likely to invest, since there are few financially attractive patents to acquire; most herbal remedies, for example, have been in use for centuries. Nor do complementary practitioners wanting to carry out research have the backing of universities, hospitals, statisticians, and full-time research staff – all elements that create a research environment for conventional medicine. As complementary therapies develop their own professional bodies and academic groups, the facilities to carry out research will grow and coherent programs will develop.

Ailments studied in conventional research may not be representative of those commonly treated by complementary medicine. Postoperative nausea, for example, has been studied because it can be easily gauged and a hospital-based researcher has access to a large number of patients, but it is not a condition for which complementary therapies are often used. Chronic fatigue syndrome, on the other hand, is often helped by complementary medicine, but is unlikely to be treated in hospitals and cannot be quantified easily.

It will always be difficult to make general statements about the efficacy of complementary medicine, because therapies differ so much, and because so much depends on the approach and skill of the practitioner. Even if a definite statement could be made about one therapy, it might only apply to one condition; for example, a therapy shown to be effective for irritable bowel syndrome may not be proved to work for any other ailment.

Adapting research conclusions into practical knowledge is also far from simple. For example, a placebo controlled trial of homeopathy might find this therapy more effective than a placebo for migraines, but it fails to indicate whether homeopathy would be more effective than another approach for the same condition. There *are* scientifically rigorous ways of researching complementary therapies that take account of individuality and relationships, but they are often more complex than randomized controlled trials.

THE WAY FORWARD

It is important to note that many conventional treatments – most surgery and physiotherapy, for example – have never been subjected to clinical trials. Moreover, only a quarter of studies reported in leading medical journals are estimated to be based on randomized controlled trials. If complementary and mainstream medicine are to integrate more closely, and new approaches are to be evaluated, thorough research is needed, and a way to apply clinical trials must be found.

Finding a scientific explanation for the principles behind many complementary therapies is one of the most difficult issues. For example, there is no anatomical basis for the existence of acupuncture meridians, nor a biochemical explanation of how homeopathic remedies could work. Although the use of acupuncture in conventional pain management took a great leap forward when it was discovered that endorphins (see glossary) could be released during treatment, this kind of research depends on high technology, and there is limited funding.

The way forward can be summarized by Professor Edzard Ernst of the University of Exeter, UK, in his book *Complementary Medicine: An Objective Appraisal*: "If the present popularity of complementary medicine is to be more than yet another passing fashion, it is essential to cultivate an atmosphere of constructive criticism, informed debate, and balanced views … those who are inspired by an attitude of constructive criticism will surely turn out to be the true champions of complementary medicine."

THE PLACEBO RESPONSE

A placebo (from the Latin for "I will please") is an inactive medication or treatment given to a patient in place of a genuine drug or medical technique. In clinical trials, new treatments are tested against a placebo, which may be a sugar pill or meaningless procedure. Because patients expect it to work, the placebo may have a therapeutic effect. This is in fact the self-healing response, which conventional doctors often dismiss because placebos are not an intervention. However, it is highly significant that, when given a placebo, around 30% of people in clinical trials feel much improvement; some researchers say this can rise to as much as 90% (see page 13). The opposite also appears to be true – patients receiving insensitive treatment from practitioners often feel worse – a "nocebo" effect. How a treatment is given, by whom, and in what setting, is clearly important, but little is understood about the physical and psychological processes involved. All treatments, however, particularly surgical procedures, do have a large placebo component. Immune system research has shown how patients' expectations and feelings can influence healing processes, and the mind/body relationship in all illness, especially long-term disease, has a major effect on the outcome of health problems (see pages 18 and 26).

MIND/BODY MEDICINE

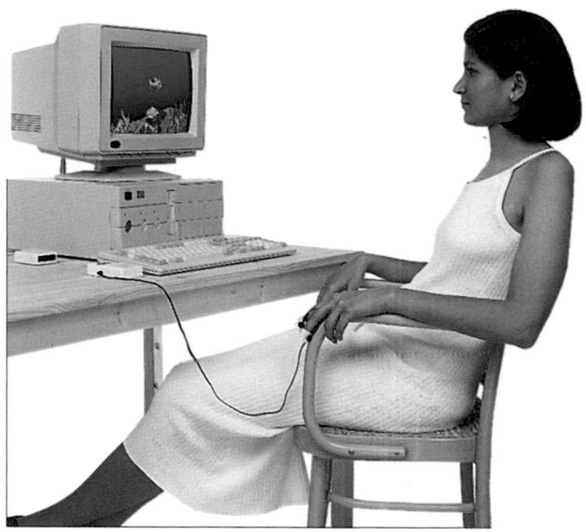

Biofeedback *(see page 169) demonstrates how the mind is able to influence the body. By monitoring unconscious biological responses with electronic equipment, you can learn to regulate physiological processes, such as heart rate and brain-wave patterns.*

AS RECENTLY AS the early 1980s, conventional medicine tended to treat body and mind as separate entities and saw them as the concern of distinct medical specialties. However, scientific evidence is now accumulating to support the underlying theory of holistic medicine, which is that the mind and body are inextricably linked, and that the health of one influences the other. This area of research and practice is known as mind/body medicine.

The possibility that something as intangible as emotion might modify the behavior of cells in the body raises the question of whether psychological factors can actually cause, prevent, or even treat disease. And if so, by what means?

PSYCHONEUROIMMUNOLOGY

Psychoneuroimmunology (PNI) is the scientific study of the interrelations between the mind ("psycho"), nervous and hormone systems ("neuro"), and the immune system ("immunology"). Interest in mind/body research was aroused in 1974, when psychologist Robert Ader and immunologist Nicholas Cohen, both Americans, conditioned laboratory rats to decrease their number of natural killer cells in response to a cue of sweetened water – evidence that a connection exists between the brain and the immune system, the body's defense against infection and disease.

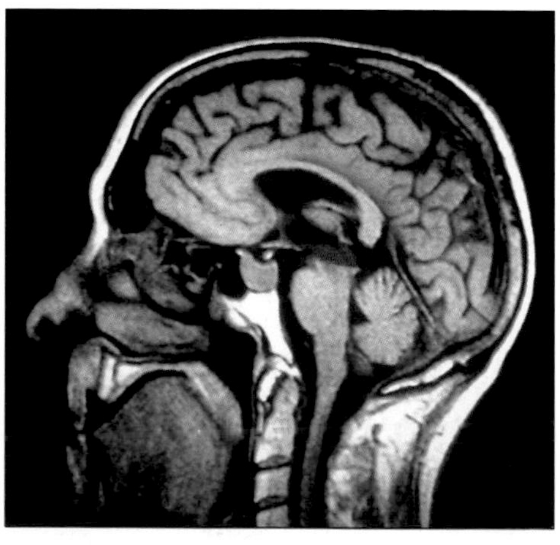

The brain *constantly monitors and regulates billions of electrical and chemical impulses. Neurotransmitters, released from nerve endings, transmit impulses to other nerves and muscles in the body. Research has indicated that emotions may affect this network of communication and help to trigger physical reactions.*

When scientists from different disciplines – psychology, immunology, and endocrinology (the study of hormones) – began to work together, they learned more about hormones and neurotransmitters, chemical messengers from nerve endings that "lock on" to cells in other body systems. They were able to track the pathways linking stress, the brain, and physiological processes such as breathing and digestion. The hormones epinephrine and cortisol, for example, which are produced by the body in stressful situations, were shown to suppress the immune response, the body's defensive reaction to antigens, or foreign substances.

CHEMICAL MESSENGERS

How exactly does the brain communicate with the immune system? The answer may be provided by research into a group of neurotransmitters, known as neuropeptides, by Dr. Candace Pert, at Rutgers University. Neuropeptides are chemicals found everywhere that act as messengers within the nervous system. They enable different body systems, such as the endocrine system, which regulates hormones, the digestive system, the reproductive system, and the immune system, to send signals to one another, propelled through tissues as well as through the nerves between them.

On the surfaces of cells in all these systems are receptors. Each receptor acts as a "lock" for a particular neuropeptide, which slips in like a key and turns on the relevant body process. For example, when laboratory rats are injected with a neuropeptide linked with thirst, they drink continuously, even when sated with fluid. Their kidneys retain urine because the message to the body is "want water, save water."

According to Dr. Pert, emotions may be the trigger that sends a surge of neuropeptides through the body. In 1975, the discovery of a type of neuropeptide called endorphins – natural opiates in the brain that generate pleasurable responses – showed that the brain could actually produce chemicals that change physical reactions. Further research in the 1980s discovered endorphins not only in the brain, but throughout the body, even in the immune system. Dr. Pert has speculated that as emotions fluctuate – for example, from anger to pleasure – neuropeptides sweep through the body systems in response, signaling physical changes such as a rise in blood pressure or relaxation of muscles.

Viruses use the same receptors as neuropeptides, so whether or not a virus can enter a cell may depend on how much of the appropriate type of neuropeptide is around to block it. In Dr. Pert's opinion, the challenge lies in identifying which emotions are linked to which neuropeptides so that, theoretically, it may one day be possible to evoke a specific feeling to fight a related viral infection.

EMOTIONS & STRESS

Emotions, such as anxiety, stress, depression, and loneliness, have been shown to affect the immune system, reducing natural killer cell activity and antibody production (see pages 44 and 308). In experiments between 1984 and 1991 by psychologist Janice Kiecolt-Glaser and her husband, immunologist Ronald Glaser, of Ohio State University, blood samples taken from students before and during stressful events, such as exams, showed that the fighting power of natural killer cells slumped during these periods. Other studies have linked stress with a greater susceptibility to colds, cold sores, and other viral infections. Indeed, traumatic life events, such as divorce or bereavement, have been shown to double the risk of catching a cold.

According to research in 1987 at the State University of New York at Stony Brook, the antibody levels of students were higher on days when they felt buoyant and positive and lower on days when they felt depressed and negative. Even allowing for the effects of unhealthy living on the immune system, depression has been associated with suppressed immune responses (depressed people have a greater tendency to smoke, drink alcohol, take drugs, and eat an inadequate diet than those who have a positive attitude, and they also sleep and exercise less).

Stressful events can also have a long-term impact. Almost ten years after the Three Mile Island nuclear power plant threatened meltdown in 1979, people living in the area showed suppressed immune responses.

THE VALUE OF RELATIONSHIPS

Emotional support from other people may help protect against stress and disease (see page 46). In further studies by the Glasers, people showing evidence of suppressed immune response included separated or divorced couples and sparring newlyweds. Medical students with plenty of friends produced more antibodies in response to a hepatitis B vaccination than those who described themselves as lonely.

Epidemiological research, which studies the connection between certain diseases and the population at large, bears out these findings. In 1992, a study of heart patients at Duke University showed that those without a spouse or confidant were three times as likely to die within five years of diagnosis as those who were married or had a close friend. At Stanford University, in California, Dr. David Spiegel found that women with late-stage breast cancer who participated in weekly support groups reported less pain and doubled their survival times. A study at the University of California published in 1993 found that when patients with malignant melanoma had weekly support sessions that included education, stress management, coping skills, and discussion, they felt better and were more positive, although their defenses showed little change. Six months later, when support groups had discontinued, two-thirds of the group showed a rise in natural killer cell activity and enhanced immune response. Six years later, there were fewer cases of recurrence and higher rates of survival than for other patients. More than any research to date, this indicates that psychological factors may have a role in actually treating disease.

The mind seems to play a part in autoimmune diseases (see glossary), including rheumatoid arthritis, multiple sclerosis, and inflammatory bowel disease. While stress and a lack of emotional support may precipitate and exacerbate these conditions, cognitive behavioral therapy, which changes ways of thinking and behaving (see page 164), can relieve symptoms, including pain and joint inflammation in rheumatoid arthritis. In 1964, American psychiatrists Dr. George Solomon and Dr. Rudolf Moos found that people with an inherited disposition to rheumatoid arthritis, but who were optimistic and positive, did not become ill.

CAN THE MIND CAUSE DISEASE?

Can a negative emotional state actually cause disease? Could certain kinds of personality invite illness? A 15-year study by Dr. Stephen Greer at King's College Hospital, London, suggests that women who respond to early-stage breast cancer either with a fighting spirit, or with the kind of denial that gives them space to cope, have less recurrence and longer lives than those who react fatalistically or helplessly. It is less clear whether repeated negative experiences or the repression of anger, frustration, or other strong emotions can contribute to the onset of malignancy. The possibility that individuals may be able to "give" themselves a disease – that conditions such as cancer or diabetes may be due to something they said, did, or didn't do, years beforehand – has generated feelings of guilt in patients. So far, there is no convincing evidence to link any ailment a patient may currently have with any changes in the immune system that resulted from a specific event in the past. Diseases such as cancer are more likely to result from a complex interaction of genetic and environmental factors, including nutrition. Emotions probably play only a small part in determining susceptibility to serious diseases. Psychological factors can affect survival, but their effect seems relatively small, especially in later and serious stages of disease, or when the immune system is severely compromised, as in AIDS. However, these factors could have a crucial impact on the quality of life and the severity of many chronic diseases. Given a particular set of circumstances, how a patient copes mentally with the stress of these conditions may be significant.

THE FUTURE OF MEDICINE

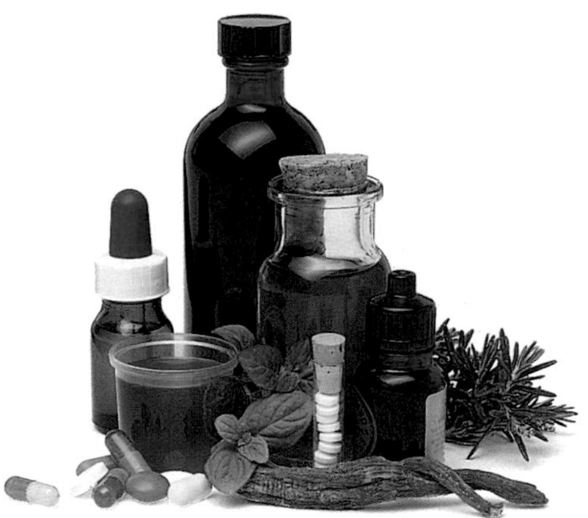

***Conventional and complementary** practitioners need to exchange ideas and cooperate to combine the best drugs, herbs, and other treatment approaches to improve the well-being of their patients. Integration is the key to the best possible health care for the future.*

THE MEDICAL ESTABLISHMENT is beginning to show increasing interest in complementary medicine, as rising health care costs and the alarming side effects of some conventional treatments take their toll on the popularity of standard methods. Already complementary therapies and mind/body approaches are included in some managed care programs. Hope lies in finding new methods of treatment for those conditions where current methods are expensive, intolerable (as in the case of cancer), or ineffective (as in the developed world's epidemic of stress-related diseases). But will complementary medicine be able to contribute?

Health is more than just a medical issue; other factors in its breakdown include basic needs, such as adequate food and shelter, and strong relationships and communities. It is when body and mind fail to adapt to difficult personal and social circumstances that we become more susceptible to disease (see pages 18 and 26). Conventional medicine is starting to recognize that these wider issues have a role to play, and that the search for effective therapies, whether conventional or not, will always take place within this larger context. The incorporation of mind/body techniques, such as biofeedback and yoga, into mainstream medicine could be part of the solution to improved health care, but education, supportive relationships, and stable communities will play the greater part.

***Mind/body techniques** such as yoga have already been incorporated into some innovative health regimes, such as the Ornish program for reversing heart disease (see page 152).*

It remains to be seen whether the medicine of the 21st century will include more complementary therapies, and whether these therapies can deal with certain problems more effectively, less expensively, and with fewer side effects than conventional medicine.

HEALTH & ADAPTATION

There is a tendency today to worship the idea of health and to denigrate the failure to be well, as if being ill is a sin. The concept of "mind/body connectedness" is a core tenet of complementary medicine from which has arisen the notion that we should assume responsibility for somehow causing our illness. Although the way in which conventional doctors can treat disease as if it were a self-contained problem, rather than part of a human being, may depersonalize patients, at least it avoids this peculiar new potential for victim-blaming promoted by some "holistic" practitioners.

However, there are many ways in which conventional health care does have to improve. New ways of triggering the body's ability to maintain health ("homeostasis"; see page 13) may be the key. Complementary therapists have a good reputation for this, even if scientific research has yet to validate it. The challenge for future health care is to find the middle ground between placing too much onus on the patient and conventional medicine's tendency toward technological disempowerment. Health is, after all, about the ability to adapt, which might mean coming to terms with less than perfect functioning of the mind or body. Healthy adaptation can occur even in the face of chronic or terminal disease, but its success is usually dependent on profoundly human factors, such as supportive friends or a loving partner, rather than medicines or treatments. We should avoid the trap of expecting complementary medicine to provide magical cures.

NEW MAGIC BULLETS

All forms of medicine search for causes of illness, and devise treatments accordingly, but it is only Western medicine that has focused almost exclusively on chemical or cellular causes. With military-style precision, it attempts to combat invading pathogens, destroy malignant cells, and overcome tissue degeneration. To wage this techno-war there must be an identifiable enemy – a germ or virus, a tumor, or a blocked artery. If tests and X rays reveal the adversary, treatment can do battle, and anesthesia, life support techniques, and joint replacement are examples of conventional medicine's almost miraculous achievements. Against tumor cells, however, there has been less success, and the use of drugs for cancer, heart disease, and mental disorders is problematical. Nor has much changed in the treatment of certain diseases, such as arthritis or eczema, in the last 15 years. With all this in mind, the medicine of the future will be increasingly concerned with finding ways to optimize the body's resilience and ability to maintain homeostasis.

The quest for new and more effective "magic bullets" in conventional medicine now seems less adventurous as the costs become clearer, both financially and in terms of potential side effects of a drug or treatment. As a result, medical science is more willing to turn to traditional sources of treatment, such as plants, in the search for new, cheaper, and safer medicines. Since many doctors also realize that current treatments are often expensive or unsatisfactory, they are beginning to look toward nonconventional approaches for clues to better methods. If research shows which complementary therapies can fulfill their promises, future medicine will undoubtedly make use of them.

Integrating Ideas & Methods

Conventional medicine has always adapted to new ideas and methods, and it will certainly continue to change and develop. It is already taking account of new insights into the connections between body, mind, and society. In areas where some of the most difficult problems are encountered, such as persistent-pain clinics, cancer centers, hospices, or psychiatric and rehabilitation units, groups of practitioners with different specialties are trying to integrate the best of medicine, nursing, and counseling to support patients in their ability to cope with and adapt to their health problems. Complementary therapies will almost certainly play a part in the future moves toward integrated health care.

The opportunity for conventional medicine to learn from different complementary therapies will largely depend on the willingness of both complementary and conventional practitioners to explore this potential together. This co-operation and dialogue will demand open-mindedness. The current popular attitude of uncritical acceptance of all things complementary, and the pervasive sense that "natural" and "holistic" therapies have the moral high ground, encourages complacency. This may not seem to be a problem for those who regard the future of complementary medicine as an alternative to mainstream medicine, but an attitude of constructive criticism would actually be more helpful where cooperation and innovation are on the agenda.

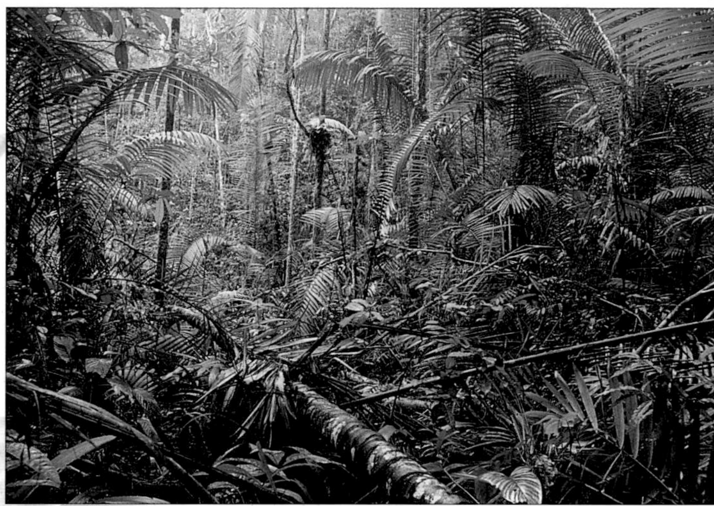

Natural environments *such as the Amazonian rain forests are being explored in the search for medicines that it is hoped may be less expensive and safer than some costly pharmaceutical drugs with harmful side effects.*

If conventional and nonconventional systems are to integrate what is best in each and thereby truly complement one another, it is important to aim for high standards in education, practice, and research. This process of sharing ideas about health has already begun in universities and on government committees. In modern health care programs, where doctors, psychotherapists, and complementary practitioners work together, the theoretical and practical groundwork is being created for a new style of medicine.

Ideals & the "Whole Person"

Complementary medicine appeals not only for practical reasons, but for its associations with gentle, natural methods, and its aim to prevent disease and integrate mental, physical, and spiritual concerns. Conventional medicine can be dehumanizing, viewing a person as a collection of fragments, each to be treated by a different specialist. The desire to be "made whole" has a particular attraction at a time when many communities, families, and even religions seem to be falling apart. But there is a limit to what even the most comprehensive health care system can do: the cure of souls and societies is certainly beyond it.

One danger is that admirable holistic intentions do not necessarily take into account the fact that human beings are vulnerable – they do face limitations and they are not always independent. When health fails to improve miraculously, it can be a small step from open enthusiasm to anger or guilt. At one extreme, the search for well-being becomes a kind of tyranny of the fit – all in pursuit of a beautiful body, psychological balance, and spiritual enlightenment. We should treat these ideals with caution; few of us could achieve such sublime heights, even if we wanted to. The "whole person" is not a superhuman machine, but a balanced individual who has the ability to adjust and cope with life.

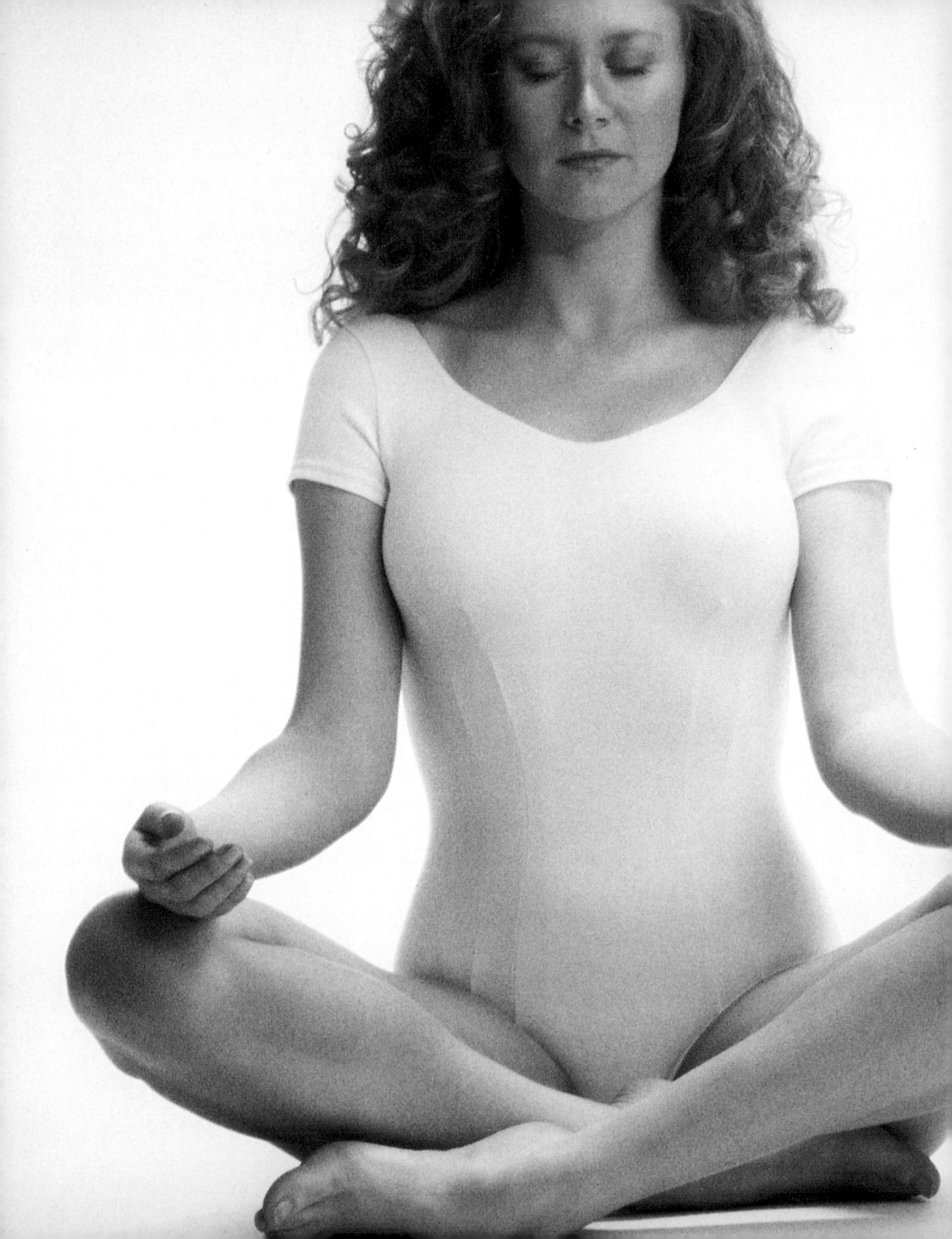

A Guide to Well-Being

Well-being occurs when the mind and body work in harmony: energy and enthusiasm are abundant, the body functions efficiently, the mind is alert, and there is a feeling of being emotionally supported by family and friends, of being able to deal with most of life's challenges. But good health can never be taken for granted: stress, age, responsibilities, poor diet, and a sedentary way of life will almost inevitably have an adverse effect.

Definite symptoms – pain, indigestion, fever – may prompt us to seek medical advice, but often there is simply a nagging sense of feeling not quite right. Complementary practitioners emphasize that optimum health is dependent on the interaction of a number of factors, including lifestyle, environment, relationships, and ability to cope. They believe that by learning to understand and recognize what makes us susceptible or resilient, we can make lifestyle adjustments that will restore and enhance well-being.

The well-being questionnaire in this section of the book is designed to help you evaluate the different aspects of your life, from diet to relationships, and pinpoint areas for improvement. It is followed by advice on nutrition, exercise, sleep, emotions, and stress, to help you protect and reinforce your own well-being.

What is Illness?

Illness and disease are not the same thing. It is quite possible to feel ill without a doctor being able to diagnose a recognizable disease from physical symptoms, but without a diagnosis it is often difficult for conventionally trained doctors to prescribe treatment. Complementary practitioners, on the other hand, work on the principle that health depends on the interaction of body and mind. They consider personality, lifestyle, and emotional state, as well as physical symptoms, and this can enable them to tailor treatment to restore the body's self-healing ability and enhance its natural resilience.

***Conventional doctors** examine the body for a pattern of physical changes that helps to identify a recognized disease.*

Conventional Diagnosis

Conventional doctors look for recognizable symptoms and clinical signs to enable a specific disease to be identified and treatment prescribed, for example:

Illness	Clinical Signs	Test	Disease	Treatment
Sore throat and chills	*Red throat, raised temperature, swollen lymph nodes in neck*	*Blood count shows increased white cells*	*Streptococcal infection*	*Antibiotics*

Diagnosing Disease

When we feel ill we describe the physical symptoms we have noticed to the doctor, who looks for clinical signs, such as a raised temperature, unusual sounds in the lungs, or an alteration in heart rhythm, which we may not have noticed. Blood tests and X rays may be arranged to confirm that the body is working abnormally, and the doctor then tries to relate these observations and test results to recognized patterns known to occur in certain named diseases. If a specific disease can be identified, there may be an appropriate treatment.

Some problems may have no obvious clinical signs, but are still diagnosable diseases; for example, a withdrawn patient complaining of no energy, loss of appetite, and early waking might be diagnosed as having clinical depression and treated with antidepressants. Other diseases, such as high blood pressure, can be revealed by tests despite the patient feeling well and having few or no symptoms.

Treatment becomes more difficult when people feel ill without having a disease with an identifiable cause. In cases of

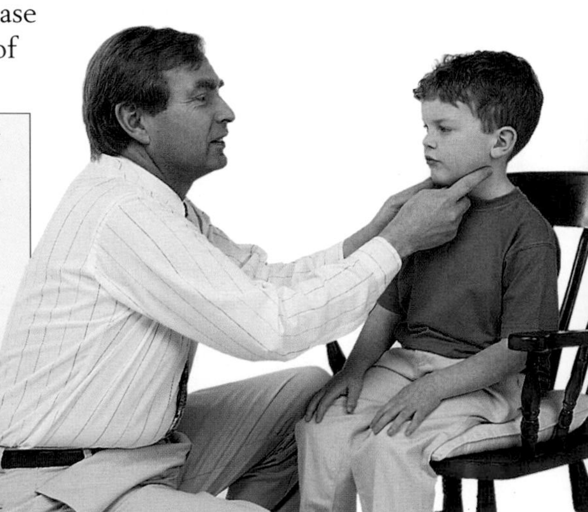

***Physical examination** plays a part in complementary diagnosis, but a wide range of other factors are also considered.*

Complementary Diagnosis

Complementary practitioners use a wide range of diagnostic techniques, assessing factors such as physical and emotional health, lifestyle, and personality. A clinical ecologist, for example, might approach symptoms and illness in the following way:

Illness	Clinical Signs	Test	Condition	Treatment
Frequent colds and sore throat	*Looks exhausted, poor circulation in skin, swollen glands in neck, bloated abdomen*	*A diary of dietary intake, and an exclusion diet to establish any food intolerances*	*Poor ability to absorb nutrients due to food intolerance*	*Restore energy with diet and supplements, and exclude irritant foods*

chronic fatigue or persistent pain syndromes, for example, the patient's body tissues are normal, and tests reveal nothing unusual. Feelings of unwellness with no named cause are frustrating for conventional doctors and also for the patient. A wise doctor faced with such "undifferentiated illness" will generally wait for the patient to get over his or her symptoms, such as fatigue, indigestion, or vague headaches. If the patient does not get better, the doctor may ask what factors, such as stress or poor diet, are obstructing the normal processes of self-restoration. However, a string of investigations may still reveal little basis for treatment. For conventional medicine, the treatment of such illnesses is a great challenge because drugs usually have no place, psychotherapy is probably irrelevant, and yet patients feel unwell in their body and often expect the doctor to *do* something.

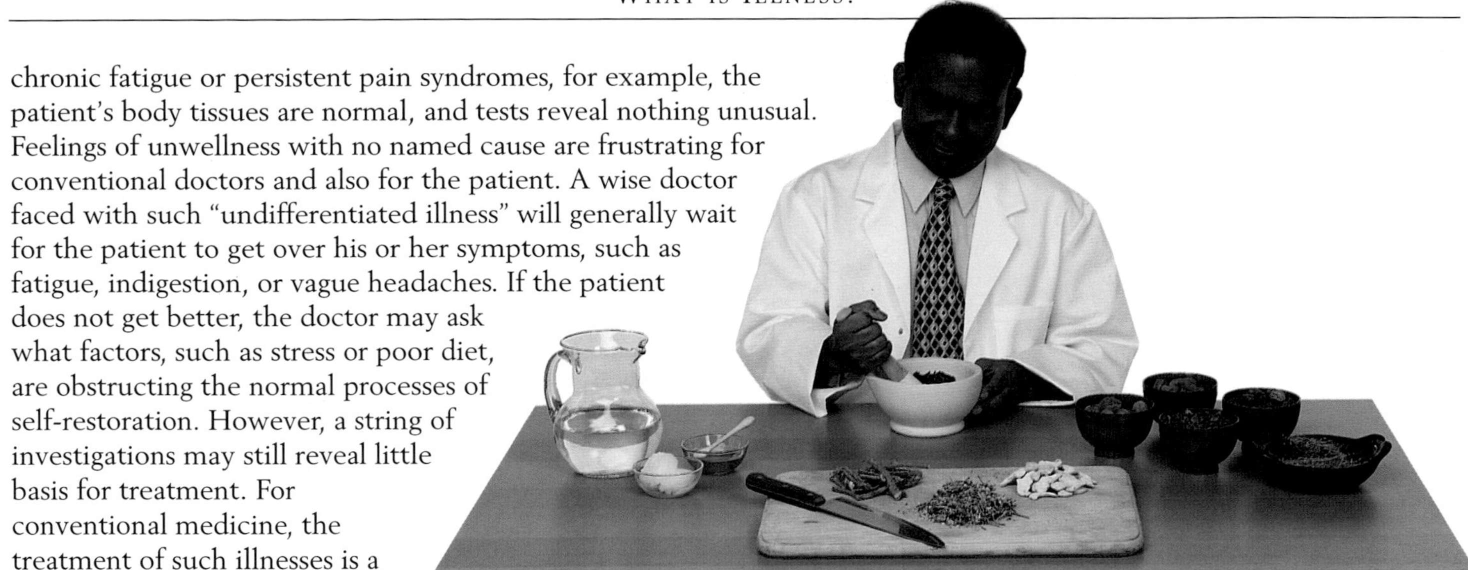

***Each major traditional health system** classifies illness differently. An Ayurvedic practitioner bases diagnosis on an assessment of the patient's* doshas, *or "vital energies." His diagnosis may use terms not familiar to conventional medicine, such as "excess* pitta,*" and he may prescribe a remedy of ten or more herbs to pacify any* doshic *excesses that are causing illness (see page 144).*

A DIFFERENT VIEW

It is in such cases of "undifferentiated illness" that the strength of complementary medicine lies – conditions treated the most are painful and stress-related illnesses that have not responded to conventional medicine. In traditional systems of medicine, such as Chinese or Western herbal medicine, the presence of a recognizable set of physical symptoms is less of a problem, since diagnoses are based more on what practitioners see or feel and how they interpret the patient's story. Each type of complementary therapy has its own diagnostic labels, such as "food intolerance," "stuck Liver *qi*," "geopathic stress," or "sacroiliac torsion," that conventional medicine does not recognize. However, if it can be shown that the diagnosis leads to effective treatments that relieve pain and enable people to cope, especially if these treatments are more tolerable and less expensive than conventional ones, then mainstream medicine may eventually incorporate them.

RED LIGHT SYMPTOMS

The symptoms below can be a sign of serious disease: check them with a doctor as soon as possible. Some complementary practitioners are not trained to detect the signs and symptoms of the diseases recognized by conventional medicine. This may not matter, given the problems they usually deal with, but certainly would if a life-threatening disease were to go untreated. When seeking complementary advice, always tell the practitioner of any symptoms, medical diagnoses, or prescribed drugs you are taking.

- Chest pain or discomfort
- Unusual shortness of breath; if accompanied by acute pain in the chest, arms, throat, or jaw, call an ambulance at once
- Unexplained dizziness
- Persistent hoarseness or cough; persistent sore throat
- Difficulty in swallowing
- Persistent abdominal pain or indigestion
- Coughing up blood
- Persistent unexplained weight loss
- Persistent and unexplained fatigue
- Changes in shape, size, color, or itching and bleeding in a mole
- Unexplained change in bowel or bladder habits
- Passing blood, either bright red or black, in the stool
- Vaginal bleeding between periods, after sex or after the menopause, or unusual vaginal discharge
- Thickening or lump in a breast; discharge or bleeding from the nipple; flattening of the nipple; change in shape or size of a breast; dimpling or puckering of the skin
- Change in shape or size of testicles; lump or swelling in a testicle; total and persistent failure to get an erection
- Unusual onset of severe headaches; persistent one-sided headaches; blurring or disturbance in vision
- Any sore that does not heal
- Persistent and unexplained lumps or swellings
- Frequent back pain that persists even when resting
- Unexplained leg pain and swelling

THE BALANCED BODY

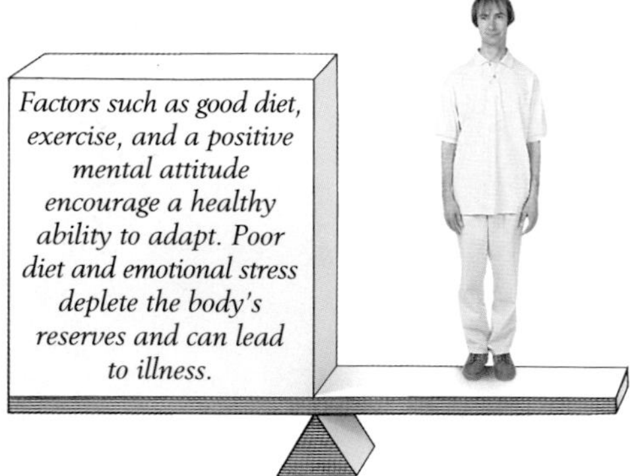

Factors such as good diet, exercise, and a positive mental attitude encourage a healthy ability to adapt. Poor diet and emotional stress deplete the body's reserves and can lead to illness.

"Homeostasis" *is the process of achieving mental and physical harmony and well-being (see page 13). To maintain it requires caring for both mind and body.*

WE ALL EXPERIENCE TIMES when we feel sick, and generally we recover, though sometimes it is clear that our body's resilience has been worn down by life events, inner conflict, or poor diet. However, the specific pressures and stresses that led to the breakdown of our defenses are not always so obvious.

CAUSES OF IMBALANCE

The body consists of three interdependent realms, the biochemical, the structural, and the psychological, which work together to maintain "homeostasis" – the stable internal environment that sustains life. When faced with a physical or mental challenge, the body adapts to this stress by drawing on its resources in each realm. Generally, the body adapts well to infrequent bouts of stress, but adaptation to persistent stress requires so much energy that it steadily depletes the ability to maintain homeostasis. Long-term adaptation and strain can cause health problems in any of the three realms. For example, a biochemical disorder such as nutritional deficiency or food intolerance may lead to a psychological effect such as depression. A psychological problem could cause loss of appetite and nutritional problems, while a structural problem might cause physical pain that leads to relationship difficulties. In the 1950s, Dr. Hans Selye, one of the first researchers of stress, described three stages of adaptation as the body copes with stress over a sustained period (see opposite).

REALMS OF THE BODY

The body consists *of three interdependent realms: biochemical, structural, and psychological. An imbalance in one realm can cause health problems and affect the working of the other two realms.*

PSYCHOLOGICAL
How thoughts, feelings, actions, or relationships can help or hinder the body's ability to cope with life.

Psychological problems such as depression can cause loss of appetite and impair biochemical processes

Psychological strain, such as anger or fear, can lead to muscular tension and poor posture, inhibiting structural function

If biochemical processes, such as diet or elimination of toxins, are poor, psychological problems like fatigue and depression can follow

Structural upper body tension can increase anxiety and psychological strain

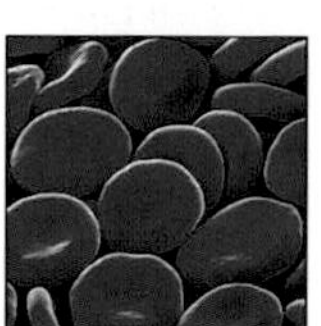

BIOCHEMICAL
How cells, organs, and body systems, such as respiration, digestion, and the lymphatic system, work to keep the body's processes balanced.

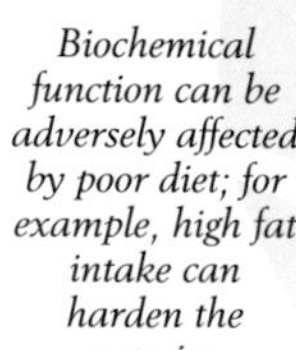

Biochemical function can be adversely affected by poor diet; for example, high fat intake can harden the arteries

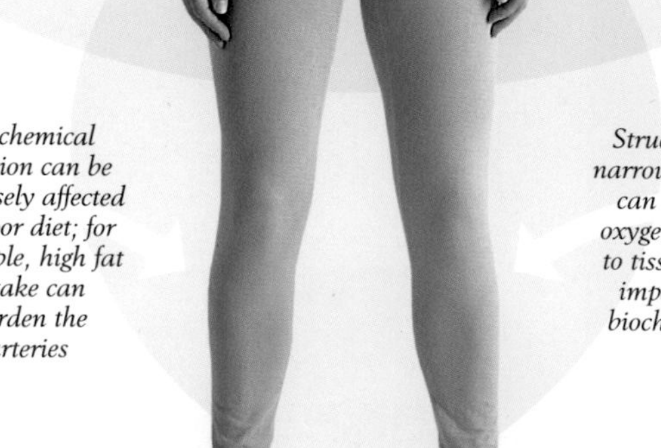

Structurally narrow arteries can restrict oxygen supply to tissues and impair cell biochemistry

STRUCTURAL
How structural elements, such as muscles, bones, nerves, and blood vessels, support body systems such as circulation and digestion.

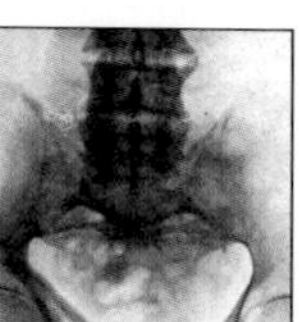

Helping the Body Cope with Stress

It is evident that the body has some ability to heal itself: wound repair and the renewal of cells are examples of the continual process of breakdown and buildup in the body. For complementary practitioners, all recovery and cure is self-healing – treatment simply mobilizes the body's own resources. A complementary practitioner will treat the realm he believes to be the most important in order to sustain the body's capability to cope. However, more research is needed into the self-healing process to determine whether and how complementary therapies can increase the body's adaptive energy and prevent the breakdown of well-being.

Holistic medical systems, such as Traditional Chinese Medicine and Ayurveda, share similarities with Dr. Selye's view of how we become exhausted. Through centuries of observation, these systems have recorded the changes that occur as the body and mind struggle to adapt to prolonged stress. These insights can help practitioners determine which physical and psychological processes are undermined and need to be supported to restore health. In Eastern systems of medicine, especially Chinese and Indian, these theories and treatments are highly developed; in Western systems, such as herbalism or naturopathy, they are less complex but are based on similar principles.

The most common method of conventional medicine is to target specific drugs at the biochemical aspects of a disease once the damage has been done, rather than to build up the patient's ability to adapt and maintain well-being. But a new approach may be possible as mainstream medicine learns more about how to trigger the restoration of good health or how to build up resilience and resistance. It is worth noting that the sort of advice doctors now give, about coping with stress and the importance of diet and exercise, closely resembles the approach naturopaths were promoting at the turn of the century.

Challenges to the Body

Small, moderate, and big challenges affect the coping capacity of the three realms of the body in different ways.	PSYCHOLOGICAL	BIOCHEMICAL	STRUCTURAL
Challenges	**Example**	**Example**	**Example**
Small: *May be within the body's ability to adapt, but still accumulate to affect its capacity to cope*	*Job stress*	*Air pollution*	*Minor injury*
Moderate: *May accumulate beyond the body's capacity to cope and impair the body's functioning*	*Bereavement*	*Poor diet*	*Repetitive occupational injury*
Big: *Can be too great for the body's capacity to cope and may even cause death*	*Suicidal depression*	*Poisoning*	*Severe injury*

The Stages of Adaptation

Dr. Hans Selye researched *the effects of stress on health in the 1950s and identified three stages of adaptation to describe how the body copes with short-, medium-, and long-term challenges.*

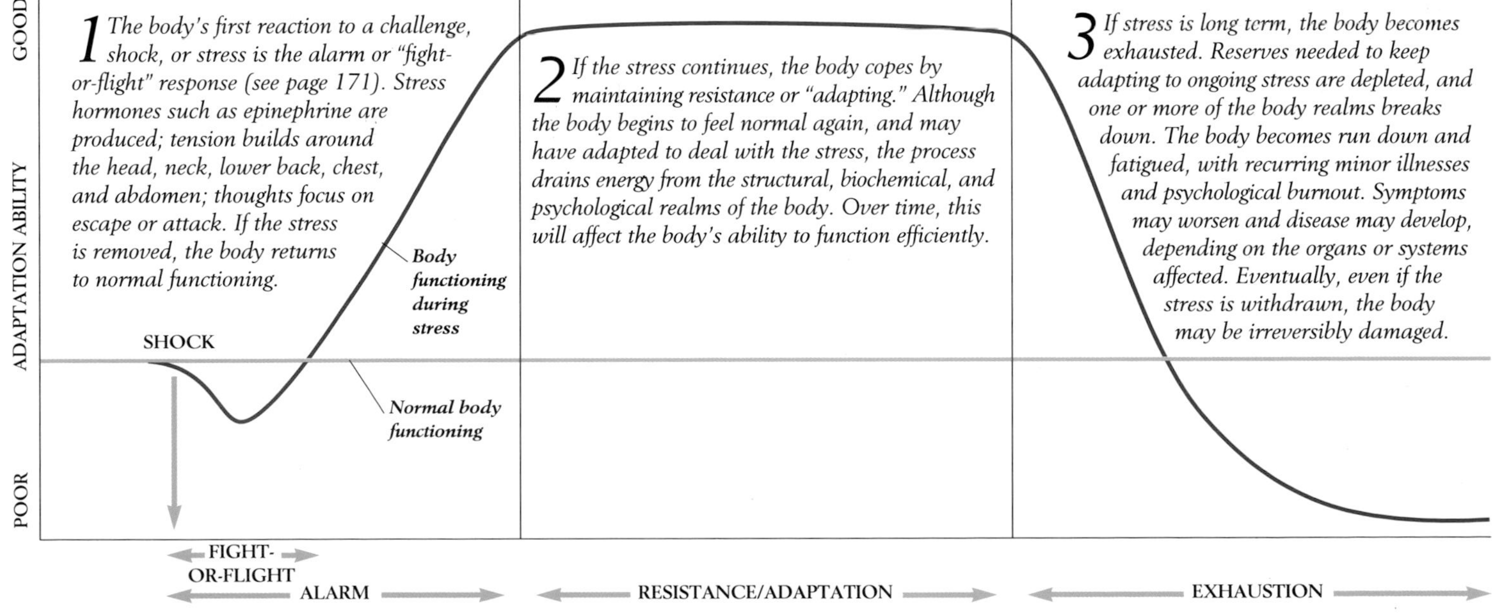

WELL-BEING QUESTIONNAIRE

DIFFERENT ASPECTS OF LIFE can undermine health or support and enhance it. Certain physical factors or psychological strains like an unhappy relationship increase susceptibility to illness. You can increase your resilience by identifying these traits and making the necessary changes in your life. These may be in the realm of "Body," such as diet or exercise, or "Mind," for example finding ways to handle stress or difficult emotions. This questionnaire is designed to enable you to find out more about the different aspects of well-being. The color wheel (see page 33) provides a more general assessment of your overall health.

HOW TO FILL IN THE QUESTIONNAIRE

Go through the entire questionnaire that appears on pages 28–32, checking the colored boxes that apply to you the most. Once you have answered all the questions, return to the beginning and add up your scores for each section of questions. Write your score in the boxes that are provided at the bottom of each column. For each section read General Guidance to find out about the significance of the questions you have answered. Then read Your Score to evaluate the individual aspects of your well-being.

BODY

PHYSICAL WELL-BEING A = *usually* B = *sometimes* C = *never*

	A	B	C
1 *Do you feel well and energetic?*	☐	☐	☐
2 *Are you physically fit enough to do the things you want to?*	☐	☐	☐
3 *Are you free of unexplained physical symptoms?*	☐	☐	☐
4 *Do you get all the sleep you need?*	☐	☐	☐
5 *Do you exercise for at least 20–30 minutes three times a week?*	☐	☐	☐
6 *Do you give yourself time to warm up and cool down before and after exercising?*	☐	☐	☐
7 *Are you comfortable about your weight, shape, and physical condition?*	☐	☐	☐
8 *Given a choice do you walk or use the stairs?*	☐	☐	☐
TOTAL	☐	☐	☐

GENERAL GUIDANCE

Physical fitness helps all the body systems function at their best and is important for the prevention of major diseases. It also boosts energy, helps reduce stress, and benefits emotional well-being. Obesity results from lack of exercise as well as over-eating, and places you at risk of developing diabetes, stroke, arthritis, and other diseases.

YOUR SCORE

- Plenty of As show you are doing your best.
- If you have mostly Bs, find more ways to build exercise into your life (see pages 40–43).
- A high C score indicates that you seldom feel energetic. Before you start an exercise program, get a medical checkup.

RISK-TAKING A = *never* B = *sometimes* C = *frequently*

	A	B	C
1 *Do you smoke?*	☐	☐	☐
2 *Do you use potentially dangerous recreational drugs?*	☐	☐	☐
3 *Do you have more than three alcoholic drinks a day if a man, or two if a woman?*	☐	☐	☐
4 *Do you take risks when driving (such as drinking alcohol, speeding, not wearing a seatbelt)?*	☐	☐	☐
5 *Do you smoke in bed?*	☐	☐	☐
6 *Do you carry a weapon?*	☐	☐	☐
7 *Do you take part in dangerous sports?*	☐	☐	☐
8 *Are you careless when working with toxic or flammable substances?*	☐	☐	☐
TOTAL	☐	☐	☐

GENERAL GUIDANCE

Taking unnecessary risks can endanger not just your life but those of others and it increases stress and emotional problems.

YOUR SCORE

- A majority of A scores indicates a well-adjusted approach to life.
- If you scored mostly Bs, think about re-evaluating your lifestyle in those areas.
- Mostly Cs could mean you are unaware of potential dangers, emotionally disturbed (if so, see a doctor), or have a risk-taking personality (see Psychotherapy & Counseling, pages 160–65). If you answered C to questions 1–3, you may have a problem with substance addiction (see page 296).

BODY

NUTRITION A = *usually* B = *sometimes* C = *never*

	A	B	C
1 *Do you eat a well-balanced, low-fat diet with high-fiber foods and plenty of fresh fruits and vegetables?*			
2 *Do you keep your daily fat intake below 30% of calorie intake (see page 35)?*			
3 *Do you keep your salt and sugar intake down?*			
4 *Do you eat poultry and fish rather than red meat?*			
5 *Do you drink enough fluids to keep your urine pale yellow?*			
6 *Do you rarely skip meals?*			
7 *Do you resist eating when not hungry?*			
8 *Do you avoid junk food and processed food?*			
9 *Do you refrain from following diet fads?*			
10 *Do you minimize your caffeine intake (coffee, tea, cola)?*			
TOTAL			

GENERAL GUIDANCE
What you eat and drink provides energy for cell growth, maintenance, and repair, and for physical and mental activity. A diet low in fats and high in fiber, fruits, and vegetables can protect against disease. Junk and processed foods are low in fiber and high in fats, added sugars, and chemical additives. Fad diets may take weight off, but are difficult to maintain and pounds lost are quickly regained.

YOUR SCORE
- If you scored As, you are doing all you can through diet to ensure well-being.
- If you scored mainly Bs, you should pay more attention to what you eat and drink.
- If your scores are mostly Cs, your diet is unhealthy and you need to learn more about nutrition (see pages 34–37).

FAMILY HEALTH A = *no* B = *yes*

DO YOU HAVE A CLOSE RELATIVE (PARENT, SIBLING, OFFSPRING) WHO HAS HAD ANY OF THE FOLLOWING:

	A	B
1 *Treatment for high blood pressure?*		
2 *A heart attack before the age of 40?*		
3 *Very high cholesterol?*		
4 *Diabetes?*		
5 *Gout?*		
6 *Glaucoma?*		
7 *Breast cancer?*		
8 *Bowel cancer?*		
TOTAL		

GENERAL GUIDANCE
Inheritance predisposes you to some diseases, and certain conditions are passed on in the genes. Even if close relatives lived to an old age, remember that genetic advantages can be undone by an unhealthy lifestyle.

YOUR SCORE
- If you scored As, you may be less at risk of inherited disease, but be aware of the Red Light Symptoms on page 25 and ensure that you have regular checkups.
- If you scored any Bs, talk to your doctor to arrange appropriate checkups, and to be advised of symptoms to watch out for.

BODY MAINTENANCE A = *yes* B = *no*

	A	B
1 *Do you floss your teeth daily?*		
2 *Do you have an annual dental checkup?*		
3 *Do you avoid over-exposure to the sun and use sunscreens when appropriate?*		
4 *If you're ill or injured do you know what to do?*		
WOMEN		
5 *Do you have a cervical smear at least every three years?*		
6 *Do you check your breasts for lumps and changes every month?*		
MEN		
7 *Do you check your testicles for lumps and changes at least every three months?*		
OVER 40		
8 *Do you get a glaucoma test at least every four years?*		
9 *Do you get your blood pressure checked annually?*		
OVER 50		
10 *Have you discussed an occult blood stool test (page 325) with your doctor?*		
11 *Do you get a regular mammogram?*		
TOTAL		

GENERAL GUIDANCE
Regular health checkups are important, particularly as you get older, to identify potential problems while a cure is still possible. While this is especially true if any close relatives have been treated for inherited diseases (see Family Health above), environment and lifestyle contribute to many serious illnesses and can exacerbate any genetic predispositions.

YOUR SCORE
- If you scored high in As, you are monitoring your health well.
- If you scored mainly Bs, you need to learn more about risk factors and how to examine yourself for symptoms. Discuss health screenings with your doctor.

BODY

WORK & ENVIRONMENT A = *usually* B = *sometimes* C = *never*

WORK ENCOMPASSES ANY REGULAR DAILY ACTIVITIES, INCLUDING WORK IN THE HOME

	A	B	C
1 *Are you well enough to work every day?*			
2 *Do you feel secure and satisfied in what you do?*			
3 *Do you feel valued and recognized?*			
4 *Do you feel you have the resources you need?*			
5 *Do get along well with the people you deal with?*			
6 *Do you feel you are learning and developing?*			
7 *Do you look forward to your work day?*			
8 *Is your environment free from pollution (air, noise, chemicals)?*			
9 *Do you feel in control of your workload?*			
10 *Do you sit, stand, or move at work in ways that minimize strain on your back, joints, muscles, and eyes?*			
11 *Do you take enough breaks during the day to keep your mind alert and reduce body tension?*			
12 *Are you happy with your commute between home and work?*			
13 *Do you feel that those closest to you at home are supportive of your work?*			
TOTAL			

GENERAL GUIDANCE

Feeling stimulated and fulfilled in your daily work is an important part of emotional well-being. As well as the nature of the activity itself, the conditions in which you operate are important for both physical and mental health. Although global or national environmental factors may be beyond your control, there is often a lot you can do to minimize risks in the home or workplace.

YOUR SCORE

- If you scored high in As, you should feel on top of your work and find it enjoyable and satisfying.
- A high B score indicates that you would be well advised to examine your job and workplace to find areas for improvement.
- If you scored high in Cs and are unable to control your working conditions, perhaps you should consider the possibility of changing your job because it could be affecting your health. The information on stress (see page 39) and emotions (see pages 44–47) may be helpful.

MIND

LIFE EVENTS A = *no* B = *sometimes* C = *frequently*

IN THE LAST YEAR HAS YOUR LIFE BEEN AFFECTED BY

	A	B	C
1 *The death of an important friend or relative?*			
2 *Changes in close relationships (including marriage and the birth of a baby)?*			
3 *Moving to a new home?*			
4 *A change of job?*			
5 *A lay-off or retirement?*			
6 *Major financial changes?*			
7 *Legal problems?*			
8 *Serious health problems (yours or those of someone close)?*			
9 *Marital or family problems?*			
10 *Problems with friends or neighbors?*			
11 *Ongoing daily hassles that wear you out?*			
12 *Do you think these events have affected you?* A = *hardly at all* B = *moderately* C = *severely*			
TOTAL			

GENERAL GUIDANCE

Remember that the degree to which pressure affects you depends on how you perceive stress, how much you feel in control, and how effective your coping strategies are – whether you exercise, follow a healthy diet, and allow time for relaxation.

YOUR SCORE

- A high A score indicates that you are fortunate to be free of major life stressors. You might consider whether your present strategies for dealing with stress could sustain you through unexpected challenges.
- If you have a majority of Bs, you may be more affected by life events than you realized and should be alert to any possible symptoms of stress (see pages 290–91).
- A high C score shows you need to use stress management techniques and pay attention to other aspects of well-being, such as nutrition, fitness, and emotional support. The following may be useful: stress (see page 39), emotions (see pages 44–47), Relaxation & Breathing (see pages 170–73), Psychotherapy & Counseling (see pages 160–65), Autogenic Training (see page 168), Visualization (see pages 178–79).

MIND

VALUES & CREATIVITY A = *yes* B = *sometimes* C = *never*

	A	B	C
1 *Do you stay aware of political and social issues?*	☐	☐	☐
2 *Is your work consistent with your values?*	☐	☐	☐
3 *Are your leisure activities consistent with your values?*	☐	☐	☐
4 *Are you able to accept people with different values and lifestyles?*	☐	☐	☐
5 *Does your spiritual life sustain you?*	☐	☐	☐
6 *Do you feel your life has a sense of purpose?*	☐	☐	☐
7 *Do you feel you have a place in the scheme of things?*	☐	☐	☐
8 *Do you feel there is enough creativity and stimulation in your life?*	☐	☐	☐
9 *Do you welcome new possibilities?*	☐	☐	☐
10 *Do you feel you can handle uncertainties?*	☐	☐	☐
11 *Do you feel you can handle boredom or lack of stimulation?*	☐	☐	☐
TOTAL	☐	☐	☐

GENERAL GUIDANCE

A contradiction between our beliefs and our way of life creates uneasiness and dissatisfaction that can affect our emotional and ultimately physical well-being. Similarly, everyone has the capacity to be creative, whether growing flowers, cooking supper, or writing music, and the inability to fulfill our creative urges causes frustration and low self-esteem. If you feel comfortable with yourself and where you are going in life, you are less likely to be threatened by unexpected challenges and will have a flexible attitude that enables you to adapt to circumstances.

YOUR SCORE

◆ If you scored high in As, you should feel a sense of commitment, coherence, and control that will enhance your ability to cope with stress.

◆ High B and C scores may indicate a sense of self-doubt and unhappiness and a low resistance to stress and even infection. Make a list of the things you value and enjoy and examine how they fit in with the way you are living. Also look at areas of conflict, and what changes you could make.

COPING WITH STRESS A = *never* B = *sometimes* C = *usually*

	A	B	C
1 *Do you compulsively work, eat, smoke, or drink?*	☐	☐	☐
2 *Do you feel that your life is really out of control?*	☐	☐	☐
3 *Do you experience physical symptoms when stressed (for example, pain, palpitations, exhaustion, breathlessness, indigestion)?*	☐	☐	☐
4 *When you are under pressure, is your mental or emotional life affected, for example, by lost interest in life, fear of disease, sleep disturbance, poor concentration, indecisiveness?*	☐	☐	☐
5 *Do people who know you think of you as being "stressed"?*	☐	☐	☐
6 *Do you find it difficult to relax and enjoy moments of pleasure?*	☐	☐	☐
7 *Is it hard to maintain good relationships with others, even (or especially) those closest to you?*	☐	☐	☐
WHEN YOU ARE UNDER PRESSURE, DO YOU BEHAVE IN A "HOT" WAY ...			
8 *Do you blame other people or feel angry?*	☐	☐	☐
9 *Do you become aggressive?*	☐	☐	☐
10 *Do you fume inwardly?*	☐	☐	☐
... OR IN A "COLD" WAY?			
11 *Do you become withdrawn or deny that there is a problem?*	☐	☐	☐
12 *Do you become panicky?*	☐	☐	☐
13 *Do you blame yourself or feel guilty?*	☐	☐	☐
TOTAL	☐	☐	☐

GENERAL GUIDANCE

How you react to pressure may be influenced by your personality. Some people behave in a "hot" or hostile way, fuming and blaming others, making themselves prone to coronary heart disease. "Cold" reactors may use up energy in trying to ignore the problem or in blaming themselves, and thus deplete their immune system and become vulnerable to infection. Other indications that you are not coping include compulsive or obsessive behavior (see page 290), emotional problems such as insomnia (see page 291), or physical conditions such as indigestion (see page 232).

YOUR SCORE

◆ If you scored a majority of As, you are one of those hardy characters who respond well to challenge.

◆ A majority of B answers indicates that you may deal well in some situations but not others, and would be well advised to learn some coping strategies (see page 38).

◆ If you scored high in Cs, you have a coping style that is particularly vulnerable to stress. The good news is that you can learn to cope but you need to monitor yourself and make a real effort to practice stress management techniques (see page 39).

MIND

EMOTIONS A = *usually* B = *sometimes* C = *rarely*

	A	B	C
1 *Are you unaffected by worry and guilt?*			
2 *Do you find it easy to laugh?*			
3 *Do you express your feelings rather than bottle them up?*			
4 *Can you recall childhood memories without feeling bad?*			
5 *Can you openly share intimate thoughts and feelings?*			
6 *Can you be sensitive to other people's feelings?*			
7 *Are you unaffected by feeling rushed or irritable?*			
8 *Do you avoid undermining yourself with self-criticism?*			
TOTAL			

GENERAL GUIDANCE

A sense of humor, the ability to express yourself and share your feelings, empathy with others, and tolerance of their opinions indicate a strong sense of self-worth and high self-esteem.

YOUR SCORE

◆ Many As mean you have a clear idea of your strengths and weaknesses, are at ease with yourself, and are able to take criticism.
◆ If your score is mostly Bs, use your answers to pinpoint areas that you need to develop.
◆ If you scored highly in Cs, examine your difficulties in communication and your negative opinion of yourself: they could be jeopardizing your well-being.

RELATIONSHIPS A = *usually* B = *sometimes* C = *never*

	A	B	C
1 *Do you have someone with whom you can discuss personal worries or problems?*			
2 *Do you listen to people without interrupting them?*			
3 *Can you accept and deal with conflict in your relations with others?*			
4 *Do you feel no compulsion to seek approval from others?*			
5 *Can you express what you feel or believe without feeling anxious?*			
6 *Are you satisfied with your level of sexual activity?*			
7 *Are you happy with your level of sexual intimacy?*			
8 *Are you satisfied with your use (nonuse) of contraception and/or practice of safer sex?*			
TOTAL			

GENERAL GUIDANCE

Those who have partners with whom to share problems are less likely to get sick and recover faster than those without. If you feel good about yourself it's easier to have close relationships. Sexual activity concerns satisfaction in a purely physical sense, while sexual intimacy concerns the mental aspect of an emotional involvement. Thus it is possible to score A in one and C in the other.

YOUR SCORE

◆ Congratulations if you scored mostly As!
◆ If you scored many Bs, examine the aspects of your relationships that may need attention.
◆ With mostly Cs you could explore ways to improve your self-esteem, ability to relax, and communication skills. See the information on emotions (pages 44–47) and stress (page 39).

LIFE MANAGEMENT A = *yes* B = *sometimes* C = *never*

	A	B	C
1 *Do you include some relaxation time in your daily routine?*			
2 *Do you set yourself realistic goals?*			
3 *Do you organize your time to do things that are important to you?*			
4 *Do you plan ahead for events that may be potentially stressful?*			
5 *Do you feel you can rise to realistic challenges?*			
6 *Do you accept your and others' limitations?*			
7 *Can you make decisions without undue anxiety?*			
8 *Do you decide what you want or feel and say so – specifically and directly?*			
9 *Do you allow others to share tasks and responsibilities?*			
10 *Do you get the balance between work and recreation about right?*			
TOTAL			

GENERAL GUIDANCE

Managing your life to achieve balance and control involves self-confidence, self-esteem, a sense of priorities, assertiveness, the ability to say "no," and planning ahead. It also means making time for things that maintain inner harmony and help you cope with challenge.

YOUR SCORE

◆ A majority of As shows your attitude toward life is positive.
◆ High in Bs; use these questions to examine which areas you could manage better.
◆ A high C score means you may feel that life is out of control, others take advantage, and you cannot cope with everyday problems. The following may help: stress (see page 39), Relaxation & Breathing (see pages 170–73), and Psychotherapy & Counseling (see pages 160–65).

YOUR OVERALL WELL-BEING

THE COLOR WHEEL IS DESIGNED to help you identify at a glance which areas of your life might need improvement. Use dots to mark the total number of As, Bs, and Cs you scored in each section of the questionnaire (on pages 28–32) on the relevant segments of the color wheel. The inner, middle, and outer zones of the wheel are color-coded to match your scores for A, B, and C respectively.

INTERPRETING YOUR RESULT

Together the two halves of the wheel – Body and Mind – make up an overall picture of your health. By looking at the number of dots in each circle you can quickly assess your overall well-being, and see whether there is an imbalance in the health of your body and mind.

THE COLOR WHEEL

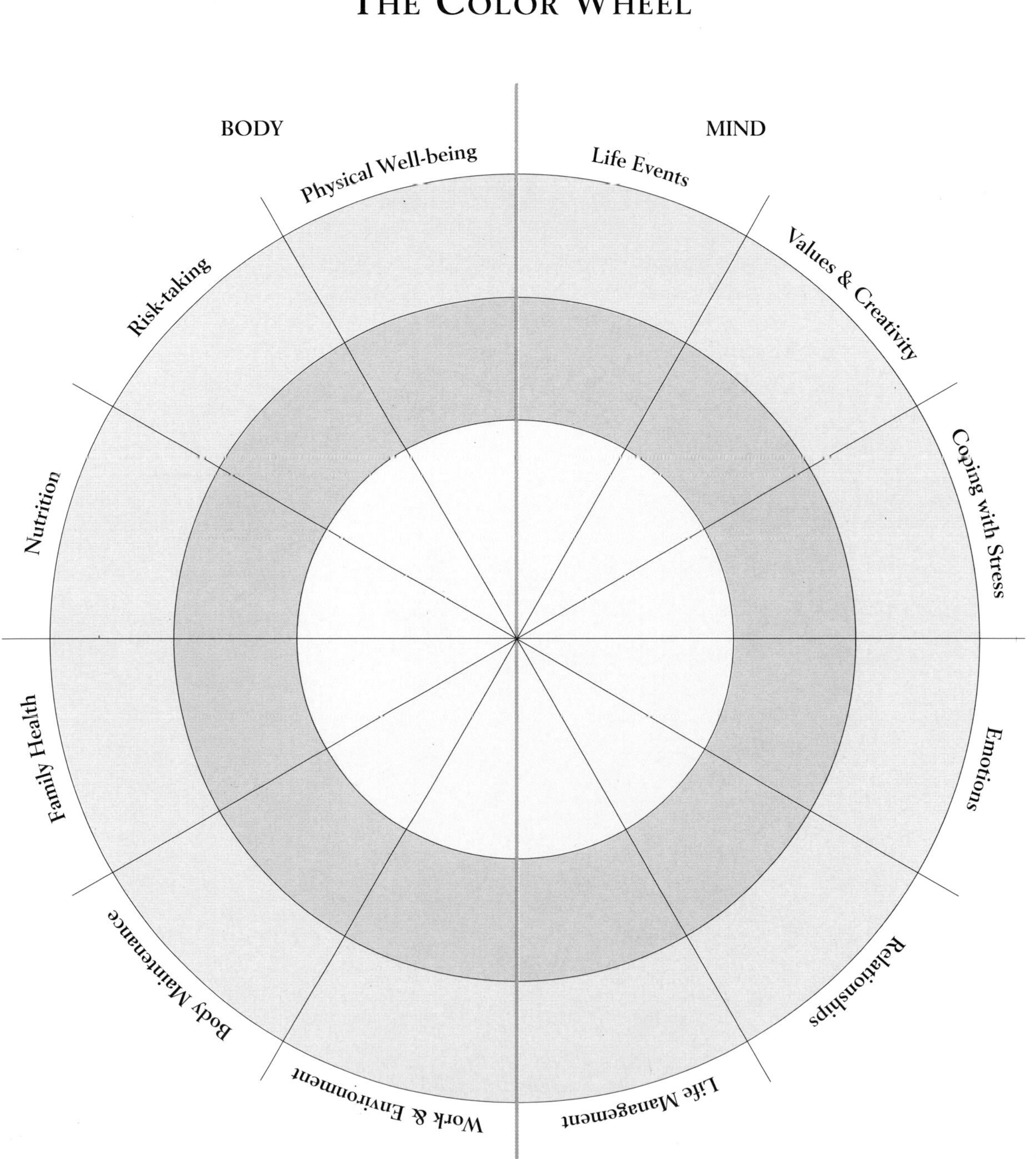

INNER CIRCLE A

The inner circle (A) represents optimum well-being. The more scores you have in this area, the stronger and better equipped you are to deal with stress and illness.

MIDDLE CIRCLE B

Scores in the middle zone (B) mean that while things could be worse, they could also be better. Examine these areas in your life for ways of making improvements.

OUTER CIRCLE C

Any score in the outer zone (C) is cause for concern. A high number of dots in a particular outer zone (C) indicates an area of your life that requires specific attention.

A BALANCED DIET

ALTHOUGH EVERYBODY'S NEEDS VARY, eating the right balance of foods can make a big difference to your health. A healthy diet should consist of about 15% protein, 50% carbohydrates, and 30% fats, and it is also important to get plenty of fiber, vitamins, minerals, and water.

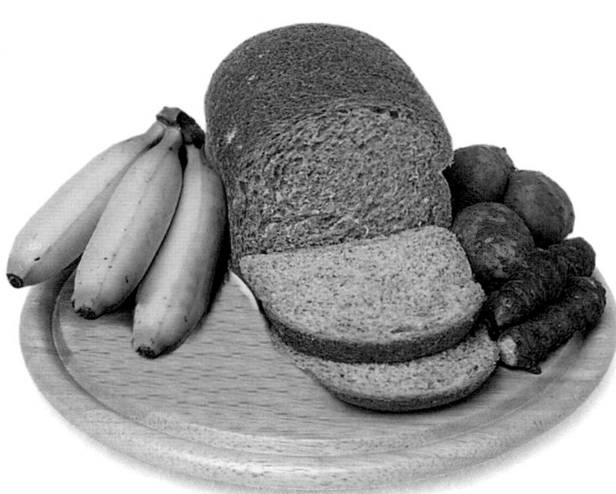

***A healthy diet** should consist of up to 50% carbohydrates, the body's main source of energy. Choose complex carbohydrates, such as bananas and bread, that have the additional benefits of vitamins and fiber.*

CARBOHYDRATES

Carbohydrates are our largest and most immediate source of energy. The body transforms them into glucose, the body's basic fuel, and glycogen, which is stored in the liver and muscles and can be converted to glucose when necessary. There are two main types of carbohydrate: simple and complex.

Simple carbohydrates are basic sugars. They are rapidly absorbed to provide instant energy and have no nutritional value in themselves. Sources include cane or beet sugar as well as sugars found in fruit, honey, vegetables, and milk.

Complex carbohydrates are broken down more slowly than simple sugars. They are compounds of several sugars and tend to be stored as glycogen. Found in starchy foods such as bread, pasta, rice, potatoes, legumes, and cereal grains, and in root vegetables such as sweet potatoes, complex carbohydrates tend to have a nutritional bonus of fiber (see page 36), vitamins, and minerals.

VITAMINS

Only vitamin D can be produced efficiently by the body. All other vitamins must be obtained from our diet. Although only tiny amounts of each are needed, they are essential to life.

Vitamin A

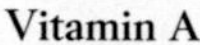

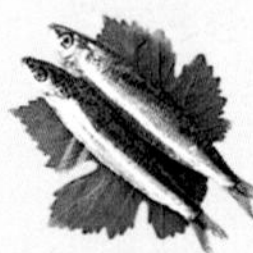

Action: *Promotes good vision, maintains skin and mucous membranes and, as an antioxidant, may protect against some cancers*
Sources: *Oily fish, liver, butter, cheese, margarine, eggs, carrots, tomatoes, apricots, spinach, broccoli*

Vitamin B_1 (thiamine)

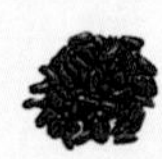

Action: *Needed to turn food into energy*
Sources: *Dried beans, whole grains, brown rice, nuts, bulgur wheat, whole-wheat pasta and bread, lean meat, fish, yeast extract*

Vitamin B_2 (riboflavin)

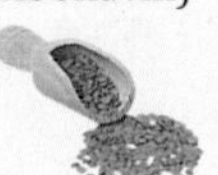

Action: *Helps turn food into energy*
Sources: *Lentils, nuts, dairy products, eggs, liver, lean meat, yeast extract, green leafy vegetables*

Niacin

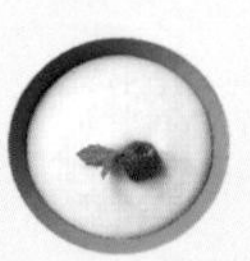

Action: *Involved in the synthesis of DNA; important for the nervous and digestive systems, and the release of energy from food*
Sources: *Dairy products, liver, chicken, turkey, oily fish, whole-wheat bread, brown rice, yeast extract, brewer's yeast, nuts*

Vitamin B_6 (pyridoxine)

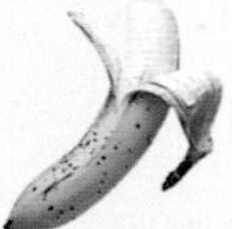

Action: *Involved in brain function, production of antibodies, formation of red blood cells, and helps release energy from protein*
Sources: *Bananas, whole grains, dried beans, eggs, nuts, oats, fish, liver, brown rice, whole-wheat bread, green leafy vegetables, yeast extract*

Vitamin B_{12}

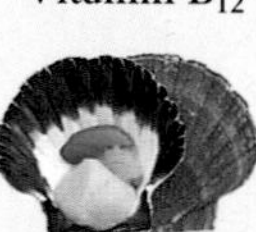

Action: *Helps protect nerves and is necessary for cell division and formation of red blood cells*
Sources: *Shellfish, white and oily fish, liver, kidney, red meat, eggs, milk, cheese, yogurt*

Biotin

Action: *Helps produce energy and maintains skin, hair, bone marrow, and glands producing sex hormones*
Sources: *Whole-wheat bread, brewer's yeast, yeast extract, brown rice, dairy products*

Folic acid (folate)

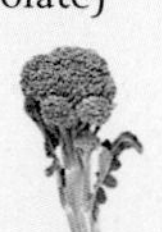

Action: *Helps form new cells, especially red and white blood cells; helps prevent birth defects such as spina bifida*
Sources: *Broccoli, green cabbage, wheat germ, legumes, nuts, yeast extract, liver*

Pantothenic acid

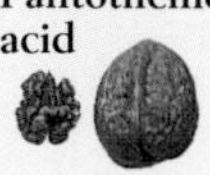

Action: *Helps release energy from food, form antibodies, and maintain nervous system and skin*
Sources: *Nuts, brewer's yeast, yeast extract, kidney, liver, wheat germ, soy flour*

Vitamin C

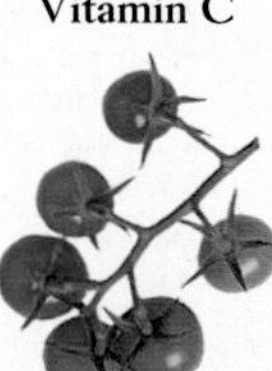

Action: *Needed for healthy gums, teeth, bones, and skin. Makes neuro-transmitters, aids iron absorption and wound healing, is antioxidant, and helps protect against infection*
Sources: *Tomatoes, citrus fruits, black currants, strawberries, kiwi fruit, mango, papaya, spinach, other dark green vegetables, potatoes*

Vitamin D

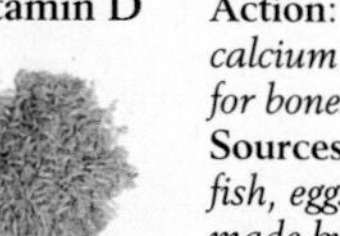

Action: *Essential for absorption of calcium and phosphorus, necessary for bones and teeth*
Sources: *Brown rice, milk, oily fish, eggs, butter, margarine; also made by the skin in response to sunlight*

Vitamin E

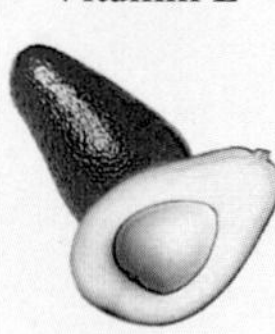

Action: *Protects body tissues by preventing polyunsaturates from forming free radicals; a powerful protector against heart disease*
Sources: *Avocados, nuts, seeds, vegetable oils, eggs, whole grains, olives, asparagus, spinach, blackberries, whole-wheat bread, brown rice, salmon, tuna*

Vitamin K

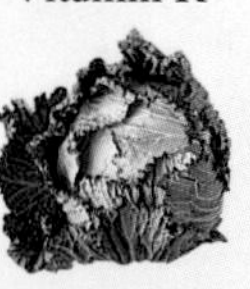

Action: *Helps form proteins and prevent blood clotting*
Sources: *Green leafy vegetables, especially green cabbage, broccoli, brussels sprouts*

PROTEIN

Every cell and organ of the body needs protein, in the form of amino acids, for growth, maintenance, and repair. Protein is also used to make enzymes that help digestion and produce antibodies and hormones. It is not stored directly in the body (any excess is burned as energy or converted to fat), so a fresh supply is needed every day; however, most Westerners, especially meat-eaters, get more than they need. Protein-rich foods include meat, poultry, fish, eggs, soybeans, cheese, cereal grains, legumes, and nuts.

***Sources of protein** include meat, fish, cheese, and eggs. As protein is not stored in the body, it must be obtained daily from food.*

FATS

Fats, which are composed of fatty acids, are the most concentrated source of food energy, providing twice as many calories as carbohydrates or protein. A certain amount of fat is necessary for healthy functioning, but too much can cause serious health problems. There are three types of fat: saturated, unsaturated (including mono- and polyunsaturated), and trans. Saturated and monounsaturated fat can be made by the body, so are not strictly needed in the diet. Too much saturated fat (found in fatty meat, hard cheese, and butter) can raise blood-cholesterol levels and lead to obesity and heart disease. Monounsaturated fat, found in olives, avocados, nuts, and seeds, is healthier than saturated fat. Polyunsaturated fat contains essential fatty acids, which are vital for health and can only be supplied by food. Sources include most vegetable oils and oily fish. Trans fats, which are associated with heart disease, are manufactured by converting unsaturated vegetable oils into saturated fats.

***Fats are vital** for health in small amounts. They are the only source of essential and other fatty acids. Oily fish, vegetable oils, and nuts are good sources of essential fatty acids.*

MINERALS

Although most minerals take up only about 3–4% of our weight, we cannot survive without them. Exactly how minerals work, or how much of each is needed, is still a subject of controversy. Some, such as potassium, are needed in fairly large amounts, while others, such as iodine, are needed in such tiny doses that they are known as "trace elements."

Calcium
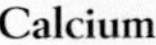
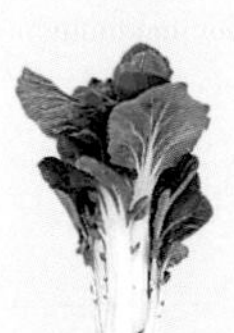
Action: *Helps blood clotting and muscle function, regulates heartbeat, and is needed for growth and maintenance of strong bones and teeth; it is especially important in women to prevent osteoporosis after menopause*
Sources: *Cabbage and other green leafy vegetables, milk, and dairy products (including low-fat), eggs, canned sardines, and other bony fish*

Chloride
Action: *Regulates fluid and circulation of ions in the bloodstream, and helps formation of stomach acid*
Sources: *Salt*

Chromium
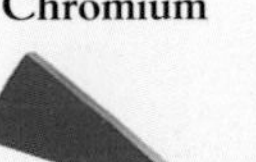
Action: *Regulates blood sugar and cholesterol*
Sources: *Cheese, egg yolks, red meat, liver, whole-grain cereals, seafood*

Copper
Action: *Builds bones and connective tissue and helps iron absorption*
Sources: *Mushrooms, organ meats, shellfish, nuts, seeds*

Fluoride
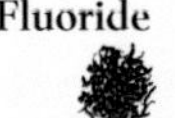
Action: *Protects against tooth decay*
Sources: *Tea, tap water, toothpaste*

Iodine
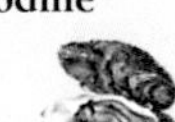
Action: *Vital for hormone secretion by thyroid gland*
Sources: *Seafood, iodized table salt, seaweed*

Iron
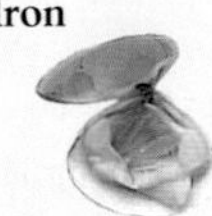
Action: *Carries oxygen to blood cells*
Sources: *Shellfish, liver, red meat, dried fruits, legumes, whole-wheat bread, fortified cereals, dark green leafy vegetables*

Magnesium
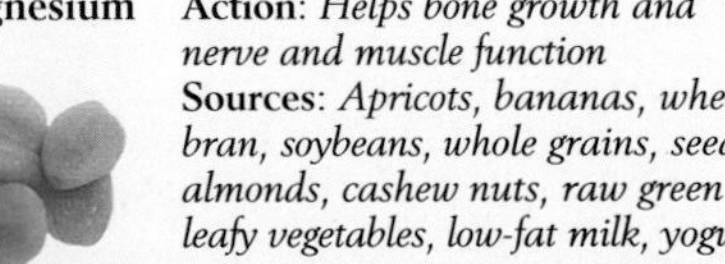
Action: *Helps bone growth and nerve and muscle function*
Sources: *Apricots, bananas, wheat bran, soybeans, whole grains, seeds, almonds, cashew nuts, raw green leafy vegetables, low-fat milk, yogurt*

Manganese
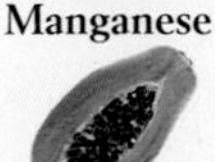
Action: *Used for bone growth and cell function; works as an antioxidant*
Sources: *Fruits, nuts, whole grains, legumes, vegetables, tea, egg yolks*

Molybdenum
Action: *Needed for DNA production*
Sources: *Legumes, whole grains, organ meats, yeast, green leafy vegetables*

Phosphorus
Action: *Used for energy metabolism, nutrient absorption, and healthy bones and teeth*
Sources: *Seafood, white fish, meat, poultry, egg yolks, milk, beans, nuts, dried peas*

Potassium
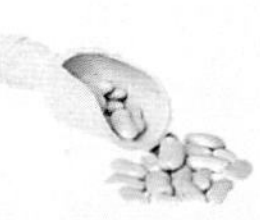
Action: *Regulates heartbeat, fluid, and circulation of ions in the bloodstream, helps muscle contraction, transfers nutrients to cells, and aids nerve function*
Sources: *Dried peas and beans, dried fruits, citrus fruits, bananas, avocados, peanut butter, potatoes*

Selenium
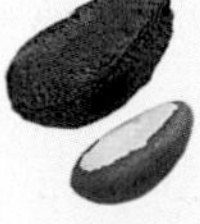
Action: *Works with vitamin E as an antioxidant and helps sexual development*
Sources: *Brazil nuts, whole-grain cereals, whole-wheat bread, muesli, organ meats, red meat, poultry, white fish, tuna, shellfish, dairy foods, egg yolks, lentils, avocados, garlic, tomatoes*

Sodium
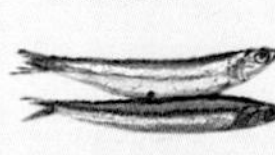
Action: *Helps regulate fluid balance (with potassium), and aids nerve and muscle function*
Sources: *Anchovies, salt, yeast extract, ham, bacon*

Sulfur
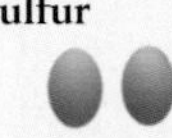
Action: *Helps produce protein*
Sources: *Animal and vegetable protein*

Zinc
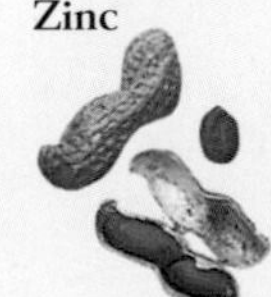
Action: *Vital for normal growth and sexual development, used for immune function and enzyme action, and works as an antioxidant*
Sources: *Peanuts, sunflower seeds, liver, red meat, poultry, eggs, cheese, seafood, oysters*

HEALTHY EATING

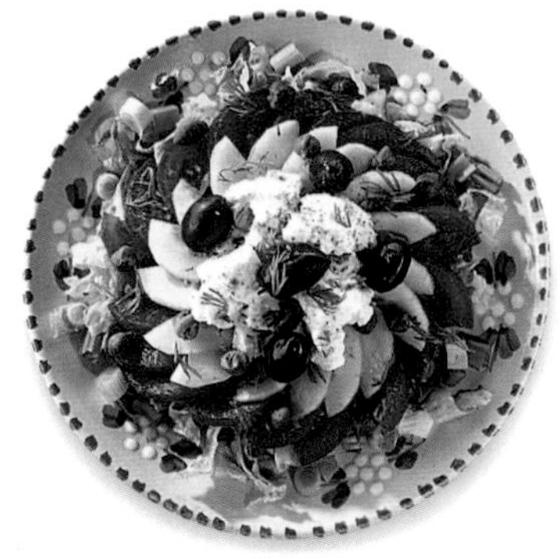

***A nutritious salad** does not have to be dull – remember that eating should be a pleasure.*

JUST AS FILLING A CAR WITH GOOD FUEL makes it run smoothly and efficiently, fueling our bodies with the kind of food that provides optimum nutrition is one of the best ways to achieve good health. In fact, scientists are discovering that certain foods actually protect against disease. Carrots and broccoli, for example, contain beta-carotene, which appears to be able to help the immune system destroy cancer cells. Healthy eating, however, also means eating less of the foods that are bad for us and avoiding foods that might contain harmful additives and pesticides.

Fad diets, based on extreme quantities or combinations of food, should be treated with caution and followed only under expert advice. It is surprisingly easy to miss out on essential nutrients and damage your health through malnutrition.

WHO NEEDS SUPPLEMENTS?

Ideally, eating a sensible well-balanced diet would mean we had no need for nutritional supplements, but there is growing evidence that the mass-processing of food may destroy some vitamins and minerals. Supplements can sometimes be beneficial; for example, additional folic acid for pregnant women can dramatically reduce the occurrence of spina bifida and other birth defects. Extra selenium, a mineral that helps prevent cancer and which may be at dangerously low levels in the Western diet, could also be worthwhile. However, care should be taken with vitamins and mineral supplements. Excess vitamin A, B_6, and iron, for example, can cause health problems, and increasingly it appears that benefits lie in the way food components work together, rather than in individual vitamins and minerals.

THE IMPORTANCE OF FIBER

Dietary fiber is made up of a complex group of substances, and although largely composed of carbohydrates (see page 34), it is not broken down by the body for energy. Fiber is found only in plant foods and, because it is resistant to digestive enzymes, passes through the gut without being absorbed, helping to soften and increase the bulk of the stool. Insoluble fiber (found in rice, nuts, wheat bran, whole grains, and dried fruits) speeds the passage of food through the intestines and may help prevent the buildup of carcinogens that could cause cancer of the colon. Water-soluble fiber (found in oat bran, legumes, fruits, and vegetables) lowers blood-cholesterol levels and inhibits the absorption of glucose into the bloodstream, preventing a sudden rise in blood sugar, which is particularly important for diabetics.

ADDITIVES & PESTICIDES

Not all additives are bad: some are necessary to keep food safe from fungi and bacteria and to prevent it from spoiling. Ascorbic acid (vitamin C),

GUIDELINES FOR OPTIMUM NUTRITION

Most dietitians and nutritionists agree on certain guidelines for optimum nutrition. Many of these are based on traditional eating habits of people in southern Italy and Greece, areas with a history of low rates of long-term disease and high life expectancy.

- Make a third of your daily diet starchy complex carbohydrates such as bread, pasta, rice, potatoes, and whole grains.
- Eat at least seven portions a day of fruits and vegetables, preferably organic.
- Obtain protein from poultry, fish, legumes, cereal, and low-fat dairy products, rather than red meat.
- Use skim milk and low-fat dairy products instead of full-fat foods.
- Eat oily fish for essential fatty acids.
- Use olive oil or other mono-unsaturated oils for salads and cooking.
- Eat plenty of foods high in fiber (see right).
- Steam vegetables rather than frying or boiling.
- Drink fruit juices and enough water to keep your urine pale.

***Foods high in fiber**, such as rice, nuts, legumes, and whole grains, prevent constipation, help lower blood cholesterol, and protect against bowel disease.*

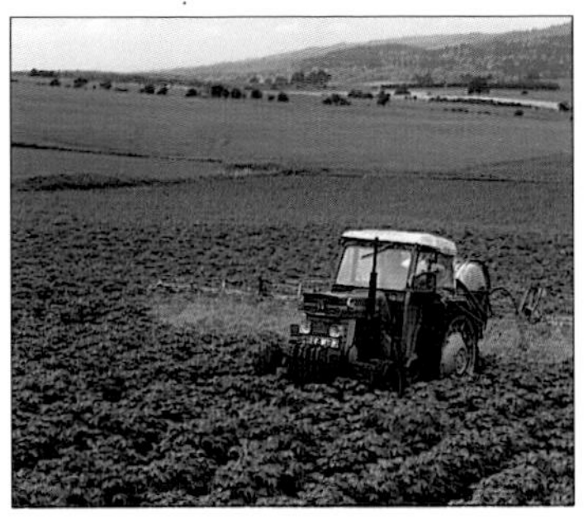

Pesticides are used to prevent damage to crops, especially when large quantities of attractive produce bring huge profits.

for example, is used to prevent fruit juices from turning brown and to prevent fatty foods from going rancid. Other natural and synthetic additives are used to color and flavor food. However, some additives do have potential side effects, which can vary from vomiting to asthma or behavioral problems. Nitrites and nitrates used to preserve processed meats and smoked fish may convert to potentially carcinogenic nitrosamines, and their intake should be limited. Pickled foods are also said to contribute to cancer.

There is also concern that toxins can enter the body via food, damaging cells and causing illness. Fruits and vegetables may harbor traces of pesticides; antibiotics and growth hormones are given to livestock and farmed fish to protect and fatten them; and fish and shellfish from polluted waters may contain unacceptable concentrations of heavy metals, such as mercury, cadmium, and lead.

Try to reduce the threat to your health by choosing organically grown fruits and vegetables that have not been sprayed with pesticides, and organically farmed meat and eggs. Remember that large fish from the top of the food chain, such as swordfish and pike, are most likely to accumulate excessive toxic metals.

ANTIOXIDANTS

Exciting research since the late 1980s has highlighted the role of antioxidants in protecting against cancer, heart disease, premature aging, and other health problems. Antioxidants work by seeking out and deactivating free radicals, which are molecules produced by the body as part of its defense against bacteria. In the few seconds that free radicals exist, they can damage DNA (see glossary) and affect cholesterol so that it "furs up" arteries. Chemicals, cigarette smoke, and industrial pollution can also increase free-radical levels. The body produces some antioxidants but we need to obtain more from our diet.

The main antioxidant nutrients are vitamins A (as beta-carotene), C, and E, and the minerals selenium, zinc, manganese, and copper. Bioflavonoids, found in some fruits and vegetables, including blackberries, black currants, lemons, plums, and cherries, also have antioxidant properties. Carotenoids, which are substances similar to beta-carotene, can help protect against damage by environmental toxins. They are found in tomatoes, spinach, broccoli, turnips, brussels sprouts, red peppers, garlic, onions, yogurt, and wheat germ.

MOOD FOODS

The stimulating effects of caffeine are well known, but other foods can also affect mood. Chocolate contains chemicals and stimulants that can lift the spirits. High-protein foods, such as meat, milk, and eggs, can produce feelings of calm because they contain an amino acid, tryptophan, that produces serotonin, a mood-enhancing neurotransmitter (see glossary). Starchy and sugary carbohydrate-rich foods also increase blood sugar and are thought to raise serotonin levels. Low levels of serotonin may be linked to depression and hostility, and low blood sugar to irritability, depression, and mood swings.

FOODS TO LIMIT OR REPLACE

There is a general consensus among experts that certain types of foods should be limited or replaced.

- Keep the number of calories obtained from fat at or below 30% of your daily total intake of calories.
- Limit intake of red meat and cheeses, which are high in saturated fat.
- Limit saturated-fat intake to less than 10% of total fat calories.
- Replace butter with a low-fat spread or soft margarine, high in polyunsaturated fats and low in trans fats, and spread it thinly.
- Avoid junk and processed foods loaded with preservatives, colorings, and flavorings.
- Limit sugar intake so that blood sugar levels remain even.
- Limit salt intake – avoid adding salt to meals and eating salty foods, such as potato chips and processed meats.
- Reduce caffeine intake by limiting tea, coffee, cola drinks, and chocolate. Drink herbal teas and water instead.
- Limit alcohol intake, although drinking one glass of red wine a day may lower the risk of heart disease.

Plums and blackberries *are good sources of antioxidants, which can help protect against heart disease and cancer.*

A midday meal of complex carbohydrates and protein, such as fish with whole-wheat pasta or whole-wheat bread, can help avert the after-lunch energy slump. A heavy meal containing saturated fats may cause sleepiness.

THE BENEFITS OF EXERCISE

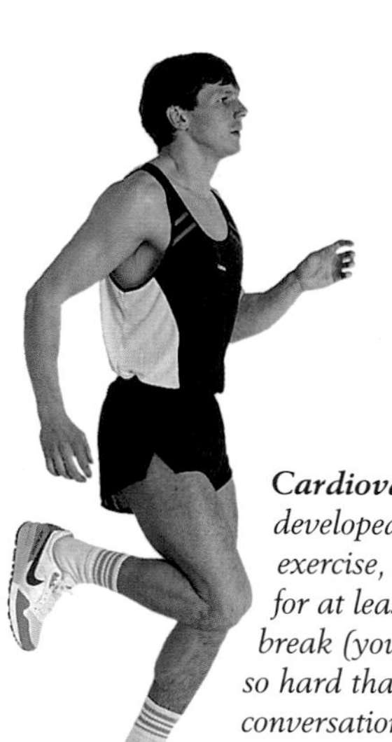

FIT FOR LIFE
Physical fitness requires cardiovascular endurance, muscular endurance and strength, and flexibility. Getting 20–30 minutes' aerobic exercise 3–5 times a week brings definite health benefits.

Cardiovascular endurance *is developed by vigorous aerobic exercise, such as jogging, sustained for at least 12 minutes without a break (you should be puffing but not so hard that you can't carry on a conversation). Aerobic exercise oxygenates the muscles and enables the heart to pump more efficiently.*

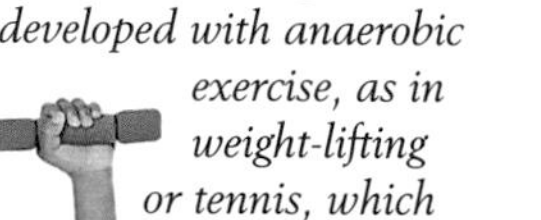

Muscular endurance *is built up with repeated exercising of large muscle groups, as in circuit training or swimming.*

Muscular strength *is developed with anaerobic exercise, as in weight-lifting or tennis, which consists of brief bursts of intense activity.*

Flexibility *is achieved by stretching muscles and is maintained by activities such as golf or yoga. It keeps connective tissue from shortening and tightening, prevents muscle pulls and tears, relieves pain, boosts muscle strength and tone, and helps prevent injury. Flexibility can enhance body awareness and appearance, increase energy, and improve circulation.*

THE BENEFITS OF EXERCISE have been researched, and evidence in its favor is overwhelming. Regular exercise improves the function of the heart and lungs and strengthens muscles to give more stamina. It keeps joints mobile, increases circulation so that the skin looks healthier, helps prevent heart disease and prostate, colon, and breast cancer, lowers high blood pressure and cholesterol levels, reduces the risk of diabetes, and helps weight loss. Exercise may help alleviate premenstrual tension and menstrual pain, and strengthens bones by increasing their mineral content, which reduces the risk of osteoporosis.

EXERCISE FOR ENERGY & WELL-BEING

Research has revealed that exercise can improve mood, lift depression, boost self-esteem, lessen anxiety, and enable us to cope better with stress. It encourages sound sleep, improves immune function and helps us live longer. All human activity – physical or mental – is powered by energy converted from food that has been eaten and oxygen that has been breathed into the lungs. Sedentary people often feel less energetic than those who exercise regularly. Exercise actually increases the body's ability to produce energy effectively. A flexible body with good muscle tone, and with an efficient heart and lungs well synchronized with the circulation, can help create a sense of physical wholeness. This makes us feel energized and ready to deal with life's demands.

PHYSICAL FITNESS

Being physically fit is not just a matter of running up the stairs without panting. Physical fitness depends on good circulation, physical strength and stamina, and a supple body (see left). Cardiovascular endurance is the ability of the heart, blood vessels, and blood to carry oxygen to the cells and to carry waste products away from them. Muscular endurance is the capability of muscles to maintain repeated exercise, and muscular strength is a capacity to carry, lift, push, or pull a heavy load. Flexibility is the ability of joints to move through their full range of motion – they will not move easily

OPTIMUM HEART RATE

Your optimum heart rate during exercise should ideally be kept at 60–80% of your maximum heart rate, which you can establish by subtracting your age from 220. People who exercise regularly learn what their optimum heart rate feels like. As you become fitter, you will need to step up the intensity of exercise to maintain your optimum heart rate.

To calculate heart rate, place two fingers on the pulse at the side of your neck or on your wrist. Count the beats for 15 seconds, then multiply the number by four.

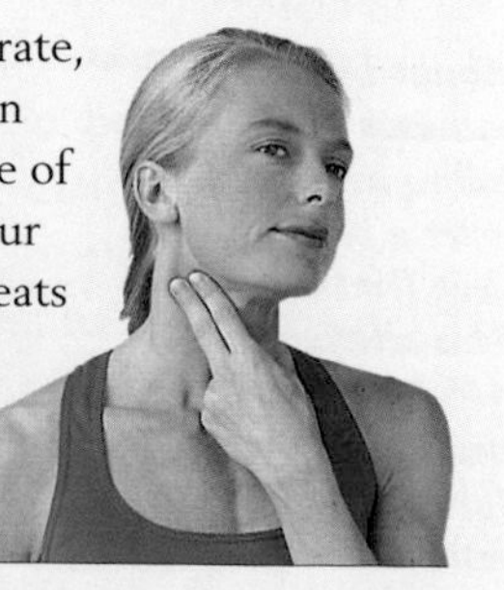

if muscle fibers are too taut. Aerobic exercise is vigorous activity requiring a sustained supply of oxygen, which is pumped to the muscles via the blood. Anaerobic exercise consists of brief bursts of activity during which there is no time for blood to pump oxygen to the muscles, so they draw on chemical processes that produce lactic acid, a waste product that can cause muscle fatigue and cramps.

If you stop exercising, the benefits gained can be lost within a matter of weeks. Therefore if you are very busy, or restricted by an injury, it's better to maintain a reduced exercise routine rather than give up altogether.

In 1995, a study of 10,000 men at the Cooper Institute for Aerobics Research in Dallas found a 44% drop in the risk of death for those who improved from being unfit to fit through aerobic exercise. There was also a reduction of risk between men of moderate- and high-level fitness.

MOTHERHOOD & EXERCISE
Some form of moderate exercise can be beneficial during pregnancy when practiced with care. Avoid contact and high-risk sports such as riding or skiing.

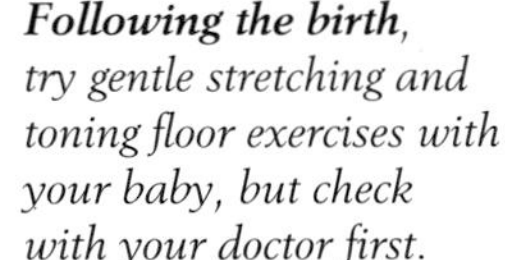

***During pregnancy**, yoga and gentle stretching can be beneficial. Walking and swimming are especially good for flexibility and circulation.*

***Following the birth**, try gentle stretching and toning floor exercises with your baby, but check with your doctor first.*

EXERCISE FOR CHILDREN

Schools can no longer be counted on to provide the optimum amount of exercise for children and, because of safety concerns, many children no longer walk to school. They lack opportunities to climb and run around and can risk setting a precedent for an inactive adult lifestyle. Sports and exercise help bone and muscle development, physical coordination, and social interaction with other children. If sending your child to out-of-school classes such as gymnastics or dancing, make sure that teachers or clubs do not make excessive demands on a child's time and energy, and check that instructors have appropriate qualifications and are registered with relevant organizations. There are also plenty of activities that families can do together, such as swimming, skating, and cycling.

BOOSTING BRAINPOWER

Exercise can boost brainpower. As we grow older, keeping fit helps feed the brain with oxygen and maintains mental alertness. In one study, sedentary older people showed improvement in various mental tasks after four months of moderate exercise. To function, the brain depends on glucose and oxygen carried in the cardiovascular system. If there are insufficient amounts of these, brain cells die, giving weight to the old adage that if you don't use it, you lose it. Some researchers believe that exercise requiring coordination and mental agility, such as tennis, may generate more connections between nerve cells.

EXERCISE & MOOD

Exercise is nature's antidepressant. Physiological changes in the body and brain can induce elation when we exercise, and depression and anxiety when we do not. During exercise, body temperature rises by two or three degrees, giving a sense of warm relaxation. Endorphins, the body's natural opiates, are released, and the alpha brain waves associated with relaxation (see page 175) become more dominant. Sustained exercise burns the stress chemicals accumulated during an inactive day and, after exercise, the body's natural relaxation response returns body and mind to a regenerative state. It might take 6–8 weeks for exercise to change the body and improve body image, but it can change your mood at once. Vigorous activity is usually followed by 1–1½ hours of calm and euphoria, and higher self-esteem may be reported after only one session.

Aerobic exercise, such as brisk walking, jogging, cycling, or swimming, is best for mood enhancement. Coordinating your movements with your breathing helps to stop you from overexercising and may even help to induce a state of "relaxed awareness" (see page 174).

EXERCISE TIPS

- Warm up for 5–10 minutes before exercising to increase heart rate and blood flow, stretch the muscles, and reduce the risk of injury.
- Cool down afterward with slower movements and stretching exercises to prevent muscle cramps and stiffness.
- Set sensible goals, especially if you haven't exercised for a while. Build up gradually so you are less likely to become fatigued and dispirited.
- Drink plenty of fluids to replace what is lost in sweat, during and after exercise, even if you don't feel thirsty.
- Stop if you feel any pain. At first muscles may feel sore after exercising.
- Wear suitable training shoes.

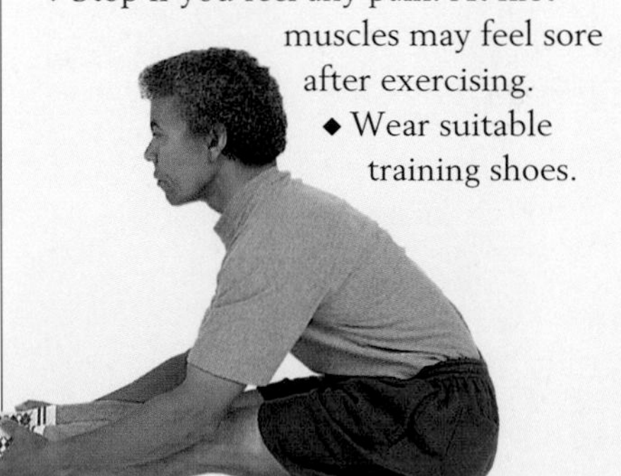

CHOOSING AN ACTIVITY

FINDING AN ACTIVITY THAT SUITS YOUR PERSONALITY will greatly add to your motivation and enjoyment of exercise. People who relish competition or company, for example, may see solo lap-swimming more as a punishment than a pleasure, while daydreamers may find it tedious to keep track of tennis scores. Ask yourself what are your reasons for exercising (see box, opposite), weigh any practical considerations that need to be taken into account, then choose activities that suit you.

WHICH ACTIVITY?

It is a fact that if you enjoy a form of exercise, you are more likely to stick with it. Prevent boredom by varying exercise; for example, try skipping sometimes instead of running.

***Walking**, which has a host of health benefits, can easily be incorporated into a daily routine.*

***Tennis** is good for agility and coordination, and helps build up muscular strength.*

***Running or jogging** is the aerobic exercise par excellence, but don't attempt it until you can walk briskly for 2 miles (3 km) without difficulty. Always wear well-cushioned shoes that bend at the ball of the foot.*

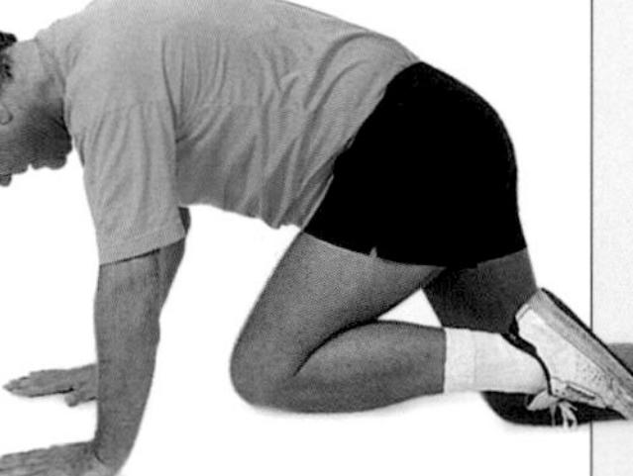

***Exercise classes** vary from stretching and weight training to step aerobics, jazz dance, and dynamic yoga.*

PRACTICAL CONSIDERATIONS

Try to make exercise as much a part of your routine as possible, and consider costs and availability: for example, a health club may strain your budget, while walking requires only the price of a pair of good shoes. Swimming is one of the best aerobic exercises, working the heart and lungs as well as two-thirds of the body's muscles. Muscle strength, endurance, posture, and flexibility all benefit from swimming, and no undue strain is placed on the joints.

HOW FIT ARE YOU?

1 *Do you get some form of aerobic exercise:*

A *Only rarely?*

B *Two or three times a week?*

C *At least four times a week?*

2 *If asked to climb three flights of stairs would you:*

A *Look for an elevator instead?*

B *Struggle to the top with difficulty?*

C *Reach the top without stopping or undue puffing?*

3 *Every day do you walk on average:*

A *As little as possible?*

B *About 1 mile (1.5 km)?*

C *About 2–3 miles (3–5 km)?*

4 *If going out to work or on errands, do you:*

A *Travel by car or by public transportation?*

B *Walk part of the way?*

C *Sprint if necessary to catch a bus or train?*

5 *After work or on weekends do you mostly:*

A *Slump in front of television or read?*

B *Carry out active tasks in the house or garden?*

C *Engage in sports or exercise?*

YOUR SCORE

- **Mostly As**: You would be wise to start an exercise program as soon as possible, but consult your doctor first.
- **Mostly Bs**: The spirit may be willing, but the flesh is a little weak. You should try to make more effort.
- **A mix of Bs and Cs**: You are probably in reasonable shape but should keep an eye on yourself.
- **Mostly Cs**: Congratulations – you are very fit. Keep it up.

If you are 45 or over, or are pregnant, consult a doctor before starting a vigorous exercise program, especially if your lifestyle has previously been sedentary. If you have a history of heart or lung disease, high blood pressure, high cholesterol levels, recurrent chest pain, or obesity, or if you are a heavy smoker, you should also check first with your doctor.

***Downhill skiing** helps develop balance, agility, and coordination, while cross-country skiing provides a more complete aerobic workout and exercises more muscle groups than any other sport.*

GETTING MOTIVATED

Starting a new exercise regime can be difficult, since the less energetic you feel, the less you want to embark on a daunting program of activity. If you have been inactive, you are bound to feel some muscle soreness and fatigue at first and it can take several weeks to stop feeling lethargic at the prospect of exercise.

Remember that if you enjoy an activity, you will stick with it longer. Half of those who begin an exercise regime are said to abandon it after six months. The key is to think of exercise as a form of joy, pleasure, and relaxation rather than as a duty or chore. Find an activity that brings quick benefits, such as feeling better, having fun, learning new skills, or keeping weight down – these can help to keep up motivation. Activities of moderate intensity such as walking, particularly with a companion, may be more enjoyable than vigorous activities. If you can stay with a regular program for six months, the chances are you will continue – you will have begun to see yourself as an active person.

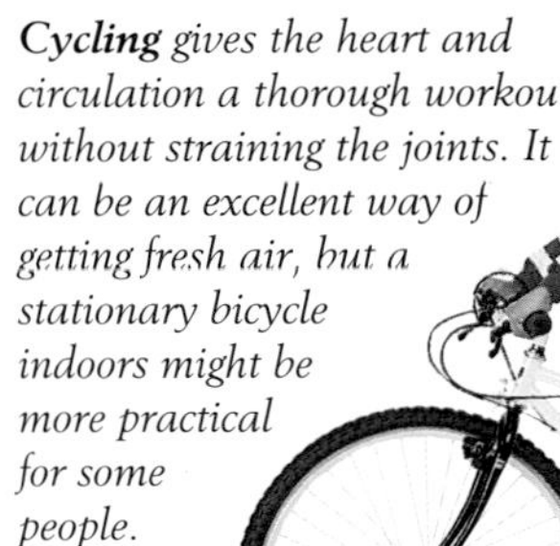

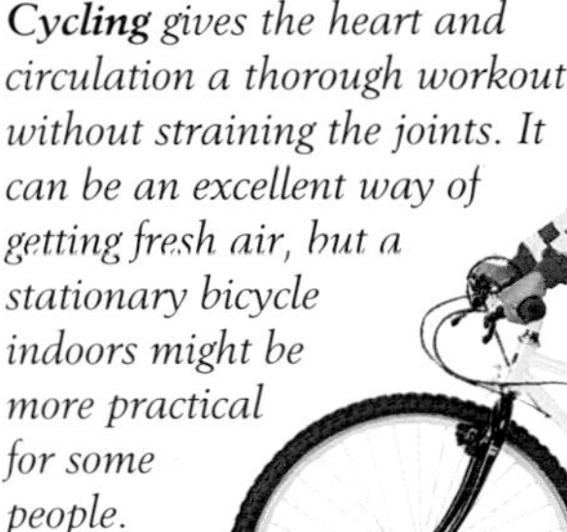

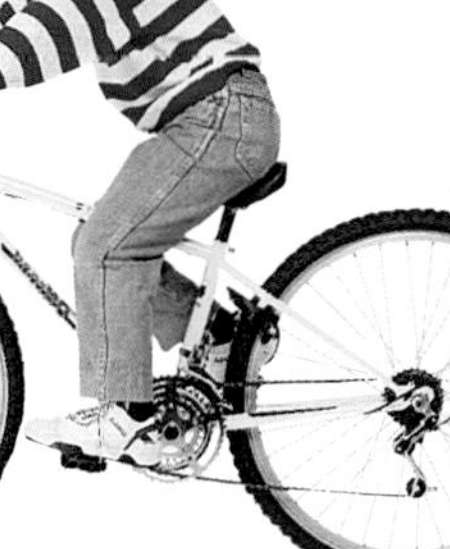

***Cycling** gives the heart and circulation a thorough workout without straining the joints. It can be an excellent way of getting fresh air, but a stationary bicycle indoors might be more practical for some people.*

WHAT TYPE OF EXERCISE?

1 *When exercising, do you like to:*

A *Push yourself as hard as you can?*

B *Keep pace with a companion?*

C *Set your own speed and limits?*

2 *Do you see exercise as an opportunity to:*

A *Let off steam?*

B *Socialize?*

C *Be reflective?*

3 *When exercising, is the presence of other people:*

A *An inducement to perform as well as you can?*

B *What you look forward to most?*

C *Daunting, disconcerting, or distracting?*

4 *The most pleasure when exercising comes from:*

A *Pitting yourself against others?*

B *Improving on your last performance?*

C *The delight of physical activity?*

5 *Your incentive to exercise is:*

A *Overall physical zest?*

B *To feel and look good?*

C *To enhance your sense of control?*

YOUR SCORE

◆ **Mostly As:** You thrive on competition and like to test your limits. Consider tennis, basketball, marathon running, and triathlons.

◆ **Mostly Bs:** You like the benefits of exercise but also enjoy being with other people. Consider joining a gym, a health club, or a walking or cycling group, and playing regular tennis or badminton for competition.

◆ **Mostly Cs:** For you, exercise is an opportunity for mental relaxation, meditation, and quiet satisfaction in physical activity. Consider a regular routine of repetitive exercise that you can practice alone, such as walking, running, or swimming.

***Dancing** exercises the heart, lungs, and muscles, and the social aspect is an added bonus. Choose from tango, salsa, jazz, ballet, or any other form of energetic dance.*

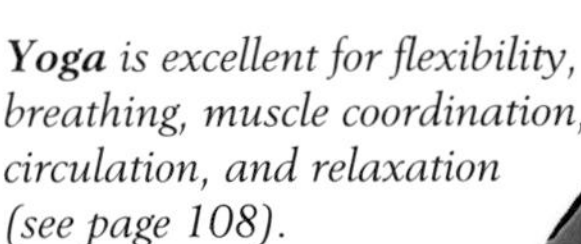

***Yoga** is excellent for flexibility, breathing, muscle coordination, circulation, and relaxation (see page 108).*

COPING WITH DIFFICULT EMOTIONS

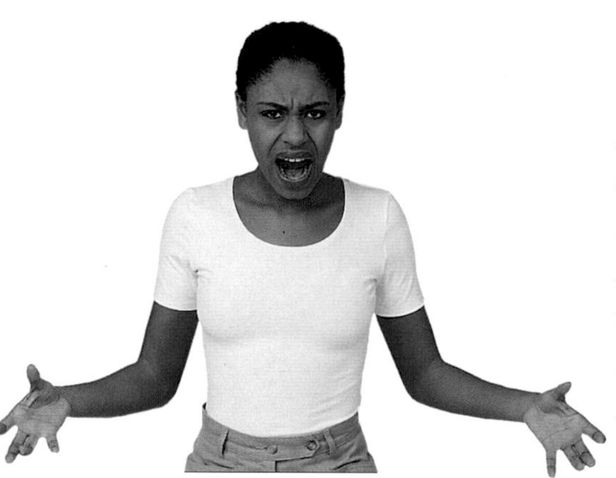

***The way people handle** difficult emotions, such as anger or frustration, can have a profound effect on physical health.*

WE LAUGH WHEN WE ARE HAPPY and cry when we are sad; we talk of being "racked with grief," "gnawed by guilt," and "burning with rage." Our feelings and emotions are not just an inescapable part of being human, but, it seems, a demonstrable expression of the link between the mind and body. Scientists have found evidence of this "interconnectedness" in the waves of hormonal substances known as endorphins that are triggered by pleasure, and in the racing heart and surge of stress hormones associated with anger and fear. Our thoughts prompt moods that are reflected in physiological reactions and can have an impact, for better or worse, on well-being.

EXPRESSING EMOTION

We have different ways of feeling and dealing with emotions, depending on the makeup of the body and nervous system, as well as on upbringing and experiences, and the culture in which we live. In Mediterranean countries, for example, grief at the loss of a loved one can be expressed openly without censure, while in northern European societies, the bereaved may be expected, at least in public, to be "strong" and to "bottle up" their tears to spare others discomfort. Our physical constitution is also said to play a role in our way of coping with feelings. The ability to manage stressful situations and "internal stressors," for example, might be influenced by individual differences in body or brain structure.

At Harvard University, a long-term study of male graduates, published in 1988, found those who were generally optimistic as students to be healthier in later life than pessimists, who were prone to more health problems.

PROBLEMS WITH EMOTIONS

Negative as well as positive emotions have their place in life. It is natural to fear danger, to feel anxiety about the unknown, anger at powerlessness, or sadness in the face of loss. Learning to express emotion in a healthy and appropriate way should be part of growing up.

Sometimes, however, emotions can be so strong and confusing that it can help to talk them through with someone – perhaps a good friend or counselor (see page 160). Otherwise, feelings that threaten to overwhelm us or that seem socially unacceptable, such as anguish or rage, may be held in check, even becoming unconscious. They may then surface in other ways – in unreasonable anger with family members, for example, or in excessive intake of alcohol. Letting yourself cry in an environment in which you feel secure acts as a physical and emotional safety valve: cortisol, a stress hormone, is shed in tears.

Problems can also arise when one kind of emotion predominates, since we need a palette of emotional colors to deal with life's many predicaments. According to British psychologist Hans Eysenck, and in line with traditional theories, if one style of emotional reaction predominates, it can disturb our inner balance so that we eventually become sick.

HOW HOSTILE ARE YOU?

Constant feelings of hostility have been linked with an increased incidence of heart disease. Consider the following to assess your tendency to hostility:

- Is your immediate reaction to everyday frustrations, such as a slow line in the supermarket, or being stuck behind a slow truck, to blame somebody else? Do you then feel anger toward them? Do you express it with some kind of aggressive action?
- Listen to the way you talk. Hostile people are deeply self-involved and litter their conversation with "I, me, my, mine." Their constantly irritated manner becomes habitual.

If someone gets trapped in a particular mood or feeling, all experiences are interpreted in the light of that mood, thus reinforcing it. For example, if you feel "down" and depressed, you tend to view everything pessimistically: you expect the worst and blame yourself.

So our view of the world has implications for well-being. Pessimists tend to lack self-esteem, something that reinforces many other difficult emotions – jealousy, hostility, guilt, and anxiety, to name a few – and that is a significant internal stressor. But overcoming poor self-esteem (see box, page 46) provides the "hardiness" to deal effectively with stressful events. Even quite small shifts in self-perception can bring about profound changes in life.

There is some research suggesting that "cold responders," people who persistently respond to stress by withdrawing and blaming themselves, and who seldom get angry, cry, or express other feelings, may be more prone to immune-related diseases. "Hot responders," those who persistently blame others when under pressure, may place a different kind of strain on the body.

THOUGHT-STOPPING

This method, adapted from cognitive behavioral techniques (see page 164), helps to avoid dwelling on negative and stress-inducing thoughts and memories.

- When you become aware that your thoughts are taking a negative turn, shout "Stop!" in your head.
- Then switch your mind to a pleasant subject that you enjoy thinking about, such as a favorite beautiful scene. The theory is that the mind cannot deal with two opposing feelings at once, and so the first, negative emotion is defused.

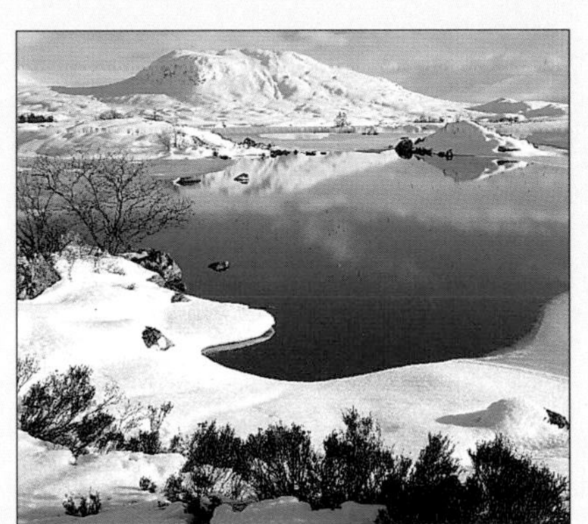

ANGER & HOSTILITY

Anger can be a perfectly appropriate emotion. However, "type A" behavior (driven, tense, competitive, aggressive, and quick to anger) is linked with an increased risk of heart disease. Research, in particular by psychiatrist Dr. Redford Williams, Director of Behavioral Research at Duke University Medical Center, North Carolina, shows that the relevant trait is hostility. This is not a flash of hot temper, nor the surge of anger that can precipitate the will to live, but rather a constant corrosive feeling of annoyance and irritation toward people and surroundings. Dr. Williams compares it to a small dose of poison every day.

When angry, hostile people experience greater physiological responses, such as increased blood pressure and the release of stress hormones, which place more strain on the body. These people are also more likely to smoke, drink alcohol, and overeat, all of which are habits detrimental to health. Their behavior provokes hostility in others so that conflict escalates, and can socially isolate them. While some experts believe that a deficiency of serotonin, the neurotransmitter linked with mood enhancement, may be involved, others point out that it is possible for people to change the way they feel and behave.

Constant feelings of cynical mistrust, anger, and aggression are not only risky for the heart, but are even suspected of contributing to cancer.

CHANGING YOUR EMOTIONAL HABITS

Hostility, pessimism, and anxiety clearly erode quality of life, and they may also undermine health. Changing these habits of mind may be a key to well-being, so researchers are investigating ways to help people who get stuck in a negative frame of mind to experience more positive feelings.

Habitual cold responders may have to learn how to become "hotter"; hot responders to "cool down." Psychoanalytic therapists see these habits as rooted in childhood experiences; cognitive and behavioral therapists would teach techniques for handling thoughts, feelings, and behavior (see box, above); and humanistic therapists would encourage experimentation with a greater range of expression (see pages 160–65).

Try to improve your relationships with others by listening to what people say. In return, they will respond more positively to you. Learn self-assertion and communication skills, practice tolerance, trust, and forgiveness, confide in a friend or partner, and get involved in your community.

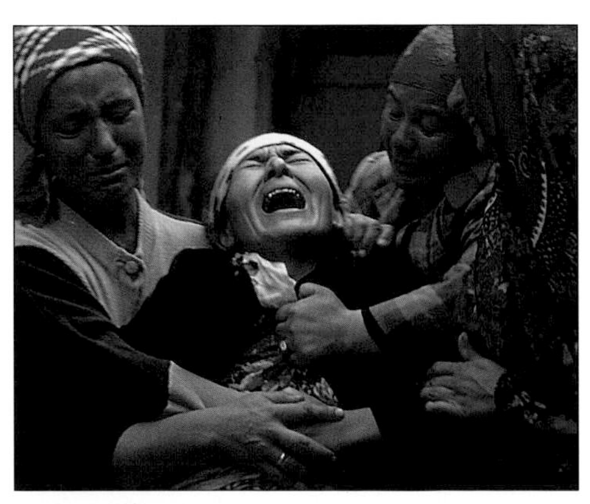

***Strong emotions**, such as grief or despair, can overwhelm, both physically and mentally, if they are "bottled up." In Mediterranean countries it is accepted for people to grieve openly.*

THE POWER OF POSITIVE EMOTIONS

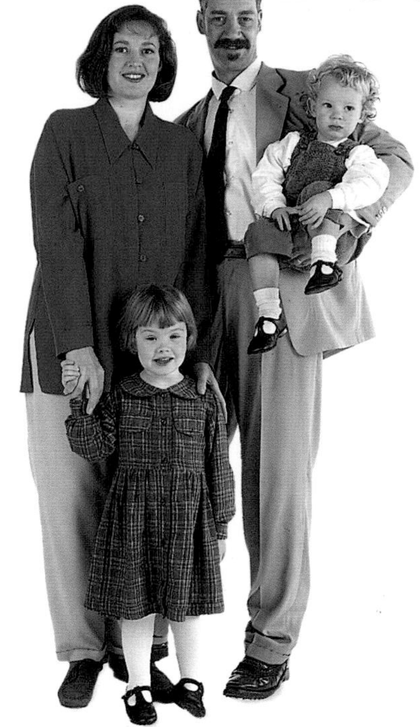

***Close and supportive** family and friends can be as beneficial to your physical health as they are to your emotional well-being.*

RESEARCH SHOWS A STRONG LINK between happiness, optimism, and good health and between increased well-being, and the body's potential to heal itself. Exercises in positive thinking may be beneficial (see opposite), but more powerful still are positive emotions, such as hope and joy. Not surprisingly, close and supportive relationships with friends and family, and a sense of humor, can help engender positive feelings. Being able to express emotions that lie beneath the surface, through art or music, for example, also contributes to a full emotional life and a resilient outlook.

FRIENDS & FAMILY

A network of friends and family may be more important than we realize: a readiness to find emotional sustenance through others is a strong element in the pattern of healing and well-being. The more isolated we are, the less healthy we are likely to be, since it can be difficult to have a rich emotional life alone. Although religious affiliation has been linked to better mental and physical health (see page 13), the feeling of loving and being loved, and of being part of a supportive community, may have much to do with this, rather than faith alone. Several studies in the US have shown that the support of family and friends improves the quality of survival time for patients with heart disease or breast cancer (see page 19), even though some of these patients were not physically healed and eventually died. The expression of deep emotions such as anger and love was important in "healing the soul," and enabled terminally ill people to find a grace in dying.

HOPE & HUMOR

Hope is a component of optimism. It need not be unrealistic – in fact, hope can mean facing up to a problem and then looking for ways forward. Dr. Stephen Greer, a specialist in cancer psychology, links hope to a quality he calls "fighting spirit." His research, undertaken while at King's College Hospital, London, showed that women with breast cancer who could harness their anger and fear in this way lived longer than those who did not (see page 19).

The ability to laugh, and opportunities to do so, make for a brighter emotional landscape. People with a sense of humor tend to suffer less fatigue, tension, anger, and depression in response to stress than those without. Laughter eases muscle tension, deepens breathing, improves circulation, and releases endorphins, the body's natural pain-relieving opiates. It also raises levels of immunoglobulin A, an antibody in the mucous lining of the nasal cavity, and helps release hormonal substances called cytokines that promote the activity of "natural

***Laughter makes you feel good**, but it also has a host of physical benefits. Laughing relaxes tense muscles, eases fatigue, and improves circulation.*

BEATING LOW SELF-ESTEEM

Professor Herbert Benson and Eileen Stuart of the Mind/Body Medical Institute of New England Deaconess Hospital and Harvard Medical School suggest you try to become aware of the origins of poor self-esteem.

Think of your life as a bus with every significant person from your past on board. When they start to criticize you with questions such as "Why are you so clumsy?" ask yourself:

- Who is the driver of the bus?
- Who is in control?
- Who do I want as passengers?

Taking over the driver's seat yourself could mean asking some of the passengers to get off the bus – permanently.

killer" white blood cells. These cells specialize in fighting off invading bacteria and viruses, and in destroying potential tumor cells.

Some hospitals encourage mirth as therapy, by providing organized entertainment, but humor is also a generally optimistic way of looking at the world – a wry smile in a moment of tension, the refusal to take oneself too seriously. As a coping mechanism, it is an affirmation of life, an expression of joy, compassion, hope, love, and playfulness.

Research in the 1970s and 1980s on women with breast cancer found that 80% who had a "fighting spirit" were still alive after 10 years, and 45% after 15 years, while of those who accepted diagnosis stoically or who felt helpless, only 17% were still alive.

ENCOURAGING POSITIVE EMOTIONS

If you find your mind continually focusing on negative, pessimistic, and anxious thoughts, you may be depressed. Discuss this with your doctor. Positive emotions may be lying beneath the surface, and you should work each day to encourage them. If you lack confidence and feel anxious, you may find it useful to practice a form of visualization in which you recall happy occasions in your life and try to reexperience the feelings associated with them. Visualization can also help to improve self-esteem, activate the body's self-healing powers and even reduce pain (see page 178).

A US study in *Social Science in Medicine* in 1988 found that people who had never expressed how they felt about unpleasant or unspeakable events were more prone to feeling sick than others. Reporting the events tended to improve their health, but expressing their emotions verbally or in writing led, in the longer term, to a radical increase in their sense of well being.

Art and music help express emotions that may be difficult to articulate, by penetrating to the intuitive and unconscious part of the mind. Playing or listening to music, chanting, and drumming all have a profound power to stir the emotions and change mood.

POSITIVE THINKING

When you feel good about yourself you can accept your own imperfections. Being under stress and unable to cope, however, can undermine self-esteem and make you interpret every unfortunate event as the end of the world. Try to change the perspective by "reframing the image" – you are not a failure if you do not succeed, but rather a success for trying. If you feel overwhelmed by a stressful situation, stop and relax, and control your breathing (see page 170), then reflect on how best to deal with it. Sometimes it helps to put aside a problem until it can be dealt with more effectively, but beware of procrastination. Taking action – making a difficult telephone call, for example – may be the best way to tackle a situation. If you feel unable to face a decision, making a list of pros and cons might suggest solutions and compromises.

***Learn meditation**, yoga, or qigong to help calm your mind and focus your thoughts (see pages 174, 108, and 99).*

BE MORE POSITIVE

These are simple ways to help develop more positive feelings about yourself and your circumstances.

***Doing something to help** other people, whether voluntary work or visiting a sick neighbor, can help you feel good.*

***Keeping a diary** is a discipline that can help build a sense of inner stability.*

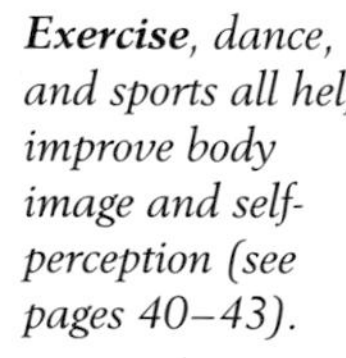

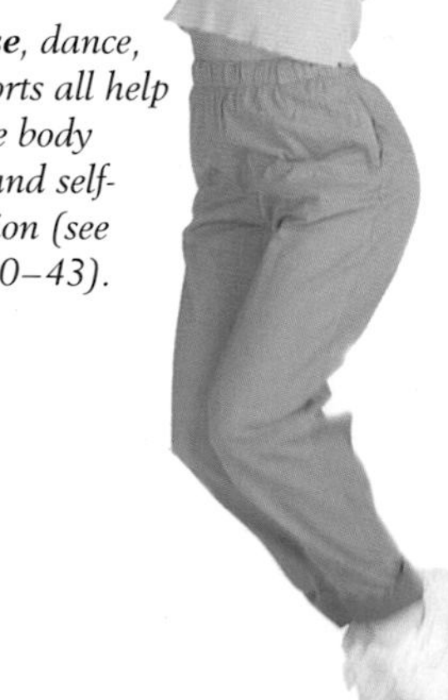

***Exercise**, dance, and sports all help improve body image and self-perception (see pages 40–43).*

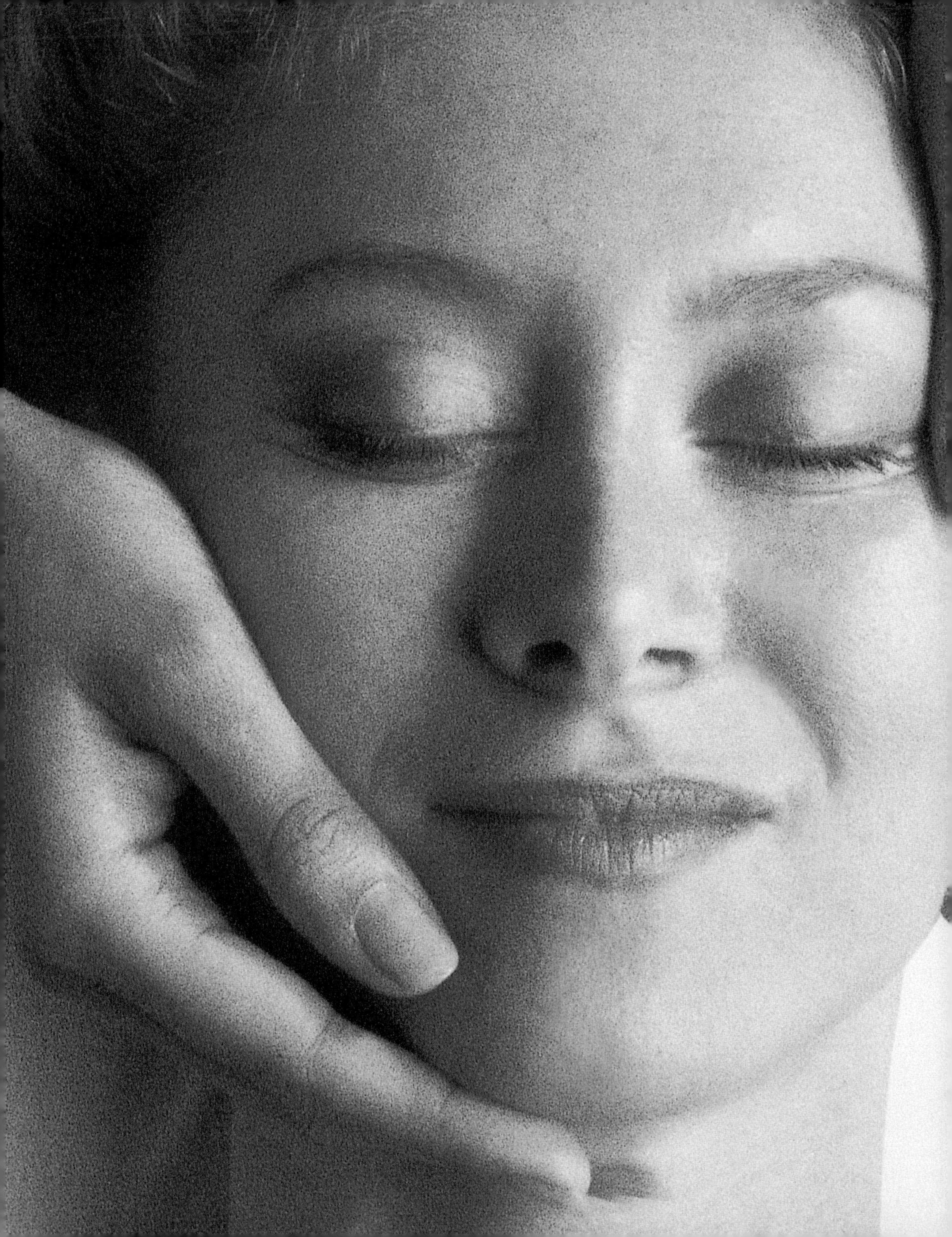

KEY HEALING THERAPIES

3

There are many complementary approaches to health, often with a confusing overlap of influences and theories, and an immense variety of methods for diagnosis and treatment. With the increasing popularity of complementary medicine, the number of therapies available has grown enormously. But how do they work? What does treatment involve? How safe are they, and which therapy is best for you?

The detailed and practical information in this section will enable you to understand therapies ranging from ancient Eastern practices, such as acupuncture, to treatments that focus on the mind, like counseling. It will help you make a more informed decision about which therapy could be the best option to improve your health and well-being.

Over 90 of the most widely used therapies are featured. Quick-reference information boxes summarize their main uses and rate them according to factors such as evidence of efficacy and the opinion of the medical establishment. Practitioners demonstrate exactly what happens in consultation and treatment sessions, there is information on self-help techniques, and the principles behind the therapies are explained. The latest research into therapies is evaluated, guidance is given on how to choose a practitioner, and a question-and-answer flowchart helps determine the most suitable type of therapy for you as an individual.

HOW TO CHOOSE A THERAPY

YOU ARE LIKELY to respond better to a therapy if its principles fit with your ideas on well-being and if you are comfortable with its approach. This questionnaire helps assess your ideas and attitudes about health. There are no right or wrong answers, but these questions should give you an idea of the approaches that might suit you best. Use the well-being questionnaire (see page 28) to help explore the various factors in your life that can influence your health, then fill in this questionnaire to help guide you toward those therapies that most suit your personality and philosophy.

QUESTIONNAIRE

Circle the boxes according to whether you agree with the statements, then see whether most of your circles fall in the A, B, or C columns. Assess the results with the conclusions and flowchart opposite. Use this in conjunction with the therapies section and the guidelines on finding a practitioner (see page 318).

1 *If you had to choose seven of the following, which would you consider most essential to your health?*

	A	B
Well-balanced diet and healthy eating habits.	yes	no
Plenty of exercise and fresh air.	yes	no
The ability to deal with stress.	no	yes
Relaxation techniques and time for myself.	no	yes
Material security.	yes	no
Spiritual development.	no	yes
Family and friends.	no	yes
The flow of healing energy through me.	no	yes
Elimination of toxins and waste products.	yes	no
A body structure that functions precisely and efficiently.	yes	no

CONCLUSION

◆ **Mostly As**: Your beliefs about health tend to be physically oriented, and the condition of your body and your environment are very important to you.

◆ **Mostly Bs**: You are psychologically oriented, so intangible factors, such as emotions, spiritual harmony, or a "vital force," play a fundamental role in your concept of health.

2 *How responsible are you for your health?*

	A	B
If I become ill, I have the power to make myself well again.	yes	no
Often I feel that no matter what I do, if I am going to get sick, I will get sick.	no	yes
If I see an excellent practitioner regularly, I am less likely to have health problems.	yes	no
It seems that my health is greatly influenced by accidental happenings or events.	no	yes
I am directly responsible for my own health.	yes	no
I can only maintain health by consulting a health professional.	no	yes
My physical well-being depends on how well I take care of myself.	yes	no
Other people play a big part in whether I stay healthy or become sick.	no	yes
When I feel ill, I know it is because I have not been taking care of myself properly.	yes	no
I can pretty much stay healthy by taking good care of myself.	yes	no
Even when I take care of myself, it's easy to get sick.	no	yes
When I'm sick, I have to let nature and time heal my body.	no	yes

CONCLUSION

◆ **Mostly As**: Well-being is something you personally encourage in yourself, and you like to be actively involved in any treatment.

◆ **Mostly Bs**: Good health is largely a matter of luck and you are content to put yourself in the hands of practitioners and let them take control.

3 *How do your personal likes and dislikes affect the type of therapy you choose? (For "no," circle both boxes.)*

	A	B	C
I am happy to be touched or massaged.	yes	no	no
I don't mind swallowing pills and can usually remember to take medicine regularly.	no	yes	no
I am comfortable exploring my feelings with another person.	no	no	yes
I like the idea that I can use my mind to influence my health.	no	no	yes
I would be prepared to change my diet radically if required.	no	yes	no
I can tolerate the idea of having needles stuck in me.	yes	no	no
Taking remedies helps me feel I'm getting better.	no	yes	no
I am comfortable talking things through in a group or sharing experiences.	no	no	yes
I don't mind getting undressed in front of a practitioner.	yes	no	no
I want to be able to talk freely and privately about the things that bother me.	no	no	yes
I am comfortable with a practitioner manipulating my body.	yes	no	no
I like to feel that my body is clean inside and functioning well.	no	yes	no

CONCLUSION

◆ **Mostly As**: You are likely to be at ease with touch & movement therapies that involve physical manipulation (see pages 54–115).

◆ **Mostly Bs**: You might consider medicinal therapies using diet, medicines, or remedies (see pages 116–57).

◆ **Mostly Cs**: You may find that mind & emotion therapies help, since you are open to exploring emotional factors (see pages 158–90).

Analyzing Your Results

Use the results of the three sections to determine which approach is most likely to suit you. You may find that more than one approach appeals.

Section 1

Mostly As: You are most likely to prefer a body-oriented therapy.

- **Section 2**
  - **Mostly As:** You are most likely to prefer a patient-led therapy.
    - **Section 3**
      - **Mostly As:** You might consider a touch & movement therapy (see pages 54–115) which, once learned, you can follow on your own, for example, aromatherapy, Alexander technique, do-in, yoga.
      - **Mostly Bs:** You may prefer a medicinal therapy (see pages 116–57) in which you can take some responsibility, for example, naturopathy, hydrotherapy, nutritional therapies.
      - **Mostly Cs:** You might consider a mind & emotion therapy (see pages 158–90) which you can practice alone on your own time, for example, relaxation & breathing, flotation therapy, light therapy.
  - **Mostly Bs:** You are most likely to prefer a practitioner-led therapy.
    - **Section 3**
      - **Mostly As:** You may prefer a touch & movement therapy (see pages 54–115) with strong practitioner involvement, for example, massage, chiropractic, osteopathy, shiatsu.
      - **Mostly Bs:** You might consider a medicinal therapy (see pages 116–57) with firm practitioner guidance, for example, Western herbalism, orthomolecular therapy, clinical ecology.
      - **Mostly Cs:** You may prefer a mind & emotion therapy (see pages 158–90) with strong practitioner support, for example, hypnotherapy, Autogenic Training, biofeedback, art therapy.

Mostly Bs: You are most likely to prefer a spiritually oriented therapy.

- **Section 2**
  - **Mostly As:** You are most likely to prefer a patient-led therapy.
    - **Section 3**
      - **Mostly As:** You might consider a touch & movement therapy (see pages 54–115) which, once learned, you can follow on your own, for example, Aston-Patterning, acupressure, qigong, t'ai chi ch'uan, polarity therapy.
      - **Mostly Bs:** You may prefer a medicinal therapy (see pages 116–57) in which you can take responsibility, for example, biochemic tissue salts, Bach Flower Remedies, crystal therapy, magnetic therapy.
      - **Mostly Cs:** You might consider a mind & emotion therapy (see pages 158–90) which you can follow alone in your own time, for example, self-hypnosis, meditation, visualization, the Silva method.
  - **Mostly Bs:** You are most likely to prefer a practitioner-led therapy.
    - **Section 3**
      - **Mostly As:** You may prefer a touch & movement therapy (see pages 54–115) with strong practitioner involvement, for example, reflexology, Rolfing, bioenergetics, acupuncture.
      - **Mostly Bs:** You might consider a medicinal therapy (see pages 116–57) with firm practitioner guidance, for example, anthroposophical medicine, homeopathy, Chinese herbalism.
      - **Mostly Cs:** You may prefer a mind & emotion therapy (see pages 158–90) with strong practitioner support, for example, psychotherapy & counseling, sound therapy, music therapy, color therapy.

Other Important Factors

We should expect to be able to make informed choices about therapies, but the amount of objective information available is still small. Be an informed "consumer," aware that stories in the media can make vague statements about unspecified conditions, and that claims for fantastic results and superhuman well-being may not be founded on accurate studies.

Nor is it true that all complementary therapies are safe and harmless.

The instincts you have about a therapy or a practitioner are important, as belief and trust play a significant role in healing (see page 17). Make sure that your practitioner is reputable and well trained, using the guidelines on finding a practitioner on page 318.

Also consider the following points:

- Is scientific evidence of a therapy's efficacy important to you?
- Are you influenced by the personal recommendation of a friend?
- Is your doctor's opinion of a therapy's efficacy important?
- Is a particular therapy suitable for any specific health problem you have?

HOW TO USE THIS SECTION

THE FOLLOWING PAGES offer information on over 90 therapies, in three broad groups (outlined below). These categories are necessarily vague, however, since therapies cannot easily be pigeonholed and they often overlap in approach. Diagnostic techniques are explained in a later section (see page 191). You will find advice on choosing a therapy on page 50, with guidelines on finding a practitioner and useful addresses starting on page 318.

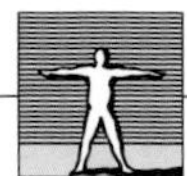

TOUCH & MOVEMENT THERAPIES

This section covers those therapies that treat the body primarily as a structure. Practitioners work on muscles, bones, and joints to promote relaxation and stimulate the circulation. Some touch & movement therapies are thought to have an influence on emotional as well as physical tension.

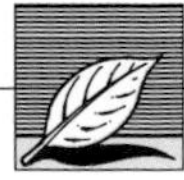

MEDICINAL THERAPIES

The medicinal section focuses on therapies, such as homeopathy and herbalism, that work on a biochemical level, or even a subtle "vibrational" level, claiming to affect the body's cells. Treatment is often taken internally, usually by mouth, or applied directly to the body as creams or lotions.

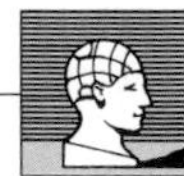

MIND & EMOTION THERAPIES

In the mind & emotion category, the emphasis is on the emotional, spiritual, and psychological aspects of health. Within this section are included therapies, such as meditation and biofeedback, that may directly affect body functions such as heart rate, brain waves, and breathing.

SAFETY ISSUES

We strongly advise you to consult a doctor before embarking on any nonconventional methods. For some health problems, drugs, surgery, or psychiatric treatment are unavoidable, and conventional medication should never be abandoned on the advice of a complementary practitioner. It is essential that you read the precautions below and the red light symptoms on page 25, as well as the guidelines for choosing a practitioner (see page 318).

PRECAUTIONS

- Consult a doctor before embarking on any nonconventional form of treatment if you have any medical condition or symptoms of illness.
- Do not stop taking any prescribed medication without first consulting your doctor.
- Tell your complementary practitioner about any prescribed medication you are taking, and any other complementary treatments you are receiving.
- Tell your doctor about any complementary treatments or remedies you are taking.
- Do not embark on vigorous exercise without first consulting a doctor if you have any serious medical condition, such as back pain, high blood pressure, or heart disease, or if you are pregnant.
- Advise your practitioner if you have any sexually transmitted disease.
- Do not begin a course of complementary therapy without first consulting your doctor if you are pregnant, or if you are trying to conceive.
- Consult your doctor before allowing babies or infants to receive complementary treatments, since some treatments, such as enemas and certain herbal remedies, are unsuitable for small children.
- See your doctor if symptoms persist or worsen.

THERAPY RATINGS

Therapies are assessed according to five categories using the following ratings symbols:

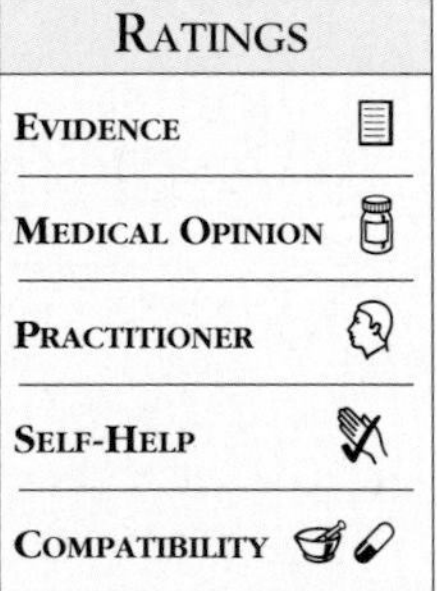

RATINGS
EVIDENCE
MEDICAL OPINION
PRACTITIONER
SELF-HELP
COMPATIBILITY

EVIDENCE

***Good scientific trials with positive results**: There is a credible base of research evidence for the efficacy of this therapy.*

***Some research studies**: There are some published studies, but no well-designed clinical trials and little conclusive evidence.*

***Anecdotal**: Evidence of efficacy is purely via oral tradition or word of mouth; any research has been inconclusive or in some cases negative.*

MEDICAL OPINION

***Positive**: Doctors are generally well disposed toward this therapy and happy for their patients to receive it.*

***Open-minded**: Doctors might not be totally convinced of the efficacy of this therapy, but they concede that it may help some people.*

***Negative**: Doctors would not be happy for patients to receive this therapy, as they do not think it works, and may even consider it harmful.*

***Divided**: Some doctors may be well disposed, but others are skeptical.*

PRACTITIONER

***Essential**: This therapy should not, or cannot, be attempted without guidance from a qualified practitioner.*

***Recommended**: While supervision may not be essential, it is definitely to be recommended initially or if you have a serious condition.*

***Not essential**: It is perfectly possible to learn about this therapy from books, videos, or tapes; while supervision may help, it is not necessary.*

SELF-HELP

***Self-Help possibilities**: It is possible to practice this therapy on yourself, either self-taught or on the advice of a practitioner.*

***No self-help**: Do not try any treatment without the supervision of a practitioner.*

COMPATIBILITY

With conventional medicine

***No precautions**: This therapy may be combined with conventional treatment.*

***Caution**: Consult a practitioner, since in certain circumstances treatment may be incompatible with conventional medicine (see also precautions).*

With complementary medicine

***No precautions**: This therapy may be used with other complementary techniques.*

***Caution**: Consult a practitioner, since in certain circumstances the therapy may be incompatible with other complementary approaches (see also precautions).*

Typical Therapy Pages

Below are sample pages that show the typical coverage of a therapy. Annotations explain how the pages are organized and how information is presented.

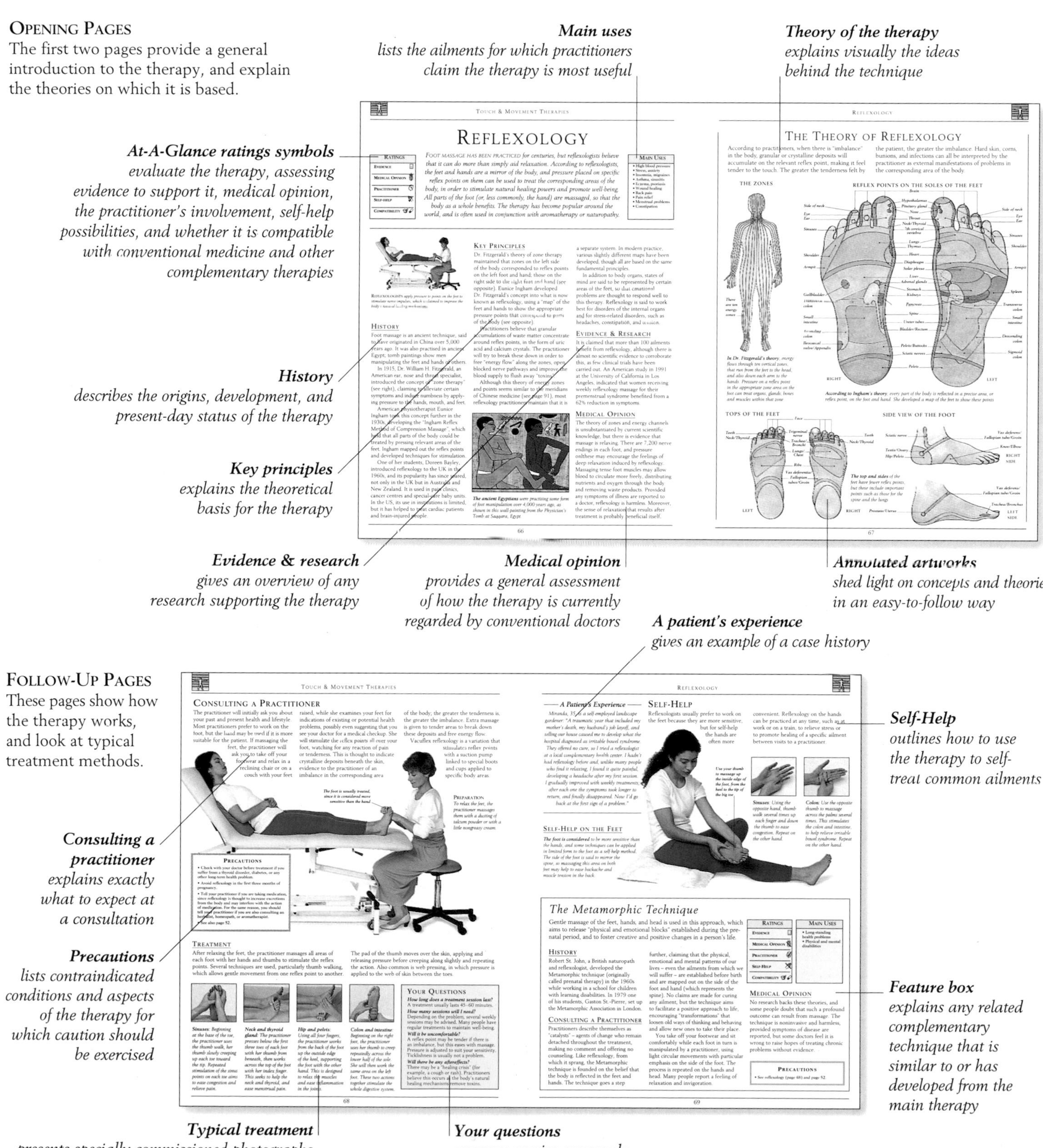

Touch & Movement Therapies

The skin and touch. Muscle and movement. Nerves that sense and coordinate. Our earliest awareness of being alive is deeply connected to all these. Learning what it was like to touch and be touched, to reach out and hold things, to take our first steps: these fundamental experiences shaped how each of us feels and behaves today.

When a practitioner uses touch, the body and mind respond at many levels: in addition to a purely sensory response, pressure and stretching on skin and muscles affect tension in the body, changes occur in breathing and circulation, and certain nerve chemicals may be released. These reactions may be relaxing or stimulating, and can be triggered by the treatments grouped as touch therapies.

Movement – the actions we make with our bodies – is an equally powerful force. We may not realize it, but the way in which we stand, sit, walk, or gesture with our hands expresses a sense of who we are and how we feel about ourselves. Language, too, is important, and movement is bound up so instinctively with our sense of purpose in life that we

Qigong exercise

describe life as a "journey" and speak of "running into trouble" or "walking on the straight and narrow." When we talk of "tension" or wanting more "freedom," we are connecting at some intuitive level to feelings of stretching and bending, of having room to move and maneuver. The power of therapies in which movement plays a key part lies in their ability to tap into this vital link.

Acupressure self-help

THE THERAPIES

MASSAGE *page 56* ♦ BIODYNAMIC MASSAGE *page 61* ♦ AROMATHERAPY *page 62*

MEDICAL AROMATHERAPY *page 65* ♦ REFLEXOLOGY *page 66*

THE METAMORPHIC TECHNIQUE *page 69* ♦ CHIROPRACTIC *page 70*

NETWORK CHIROPRACTIC *page 75* ♦ OSTEOPATHY *page 76*

CRANIOSACRAL THERAPY *page 81* ♦ ROLFING *page 82* ♦ ASTON-PATTERNING *page 83*

HELLERWORK *page 84* ♦ THE FELDENKRAIS METHOD *page 85*

THE ALEXANDER TECHNIQUE *page 86* ♦ TRAGERWORK *page 88*

BIOENERGETICS *page 89* ♦ ACUPUNCTURE *page 90*

AURICULAR ACUPUNCTURE *page 94* ♦ ACUPRESSURE *page 95* ♦ SHIATSU *page 96*

DO-IN *page 98* ♦ THAI MASSAGE *page 98* ♦ QIGONG *page 99* ♦ T'AI CHI CH'UAN *page 100*

POLARITY THERAPY *page 102* ♦ HEALING *page 104* ♦ THERAPEUTIC TOUCH *page 106*

REIKI *page 107* ♦ YOGA *page 108* ♦ DANCE MOVEMENT THERAPY *page 112*

THE BATES METHOD *page 114* ♦ OTHER THERAPIES *page 115*

Rolfing treatment

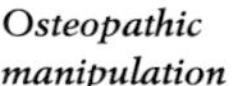

Osteopathic manipulation

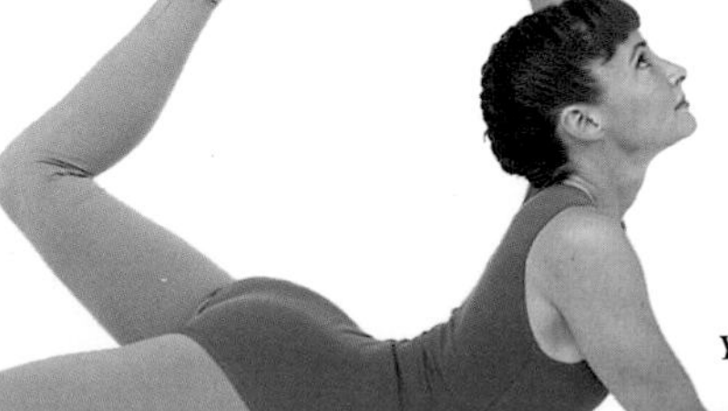

Yoga posture

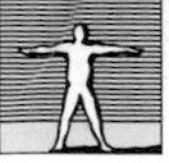

MASSAGE

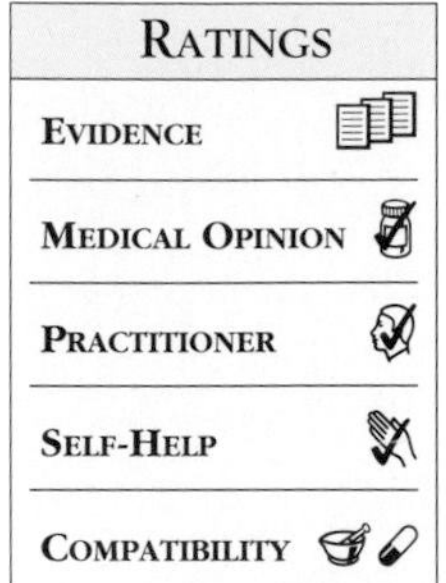

RATINGS

- EVIDENCE
- MEDICAL OPINION
- PRACTITIONER
- SELF-HELP
- COMPATIBILITY

MASSAGE HAS BEEN USED for thousands of years as a simple and effective method of attaining and maintaining good health, and its benefits have long been recognized in many cultures throughout the world. Therapeutic massage can be used to promote general well-being and enhance self-esteem, while boosting the circulatory and immune systems to benefit blood pressure, circulation, muscle tone, digestion, and skin tone. It has been incorporated into many health systems, and different massage techniques have been developed and integrated into various complementary therapies.

MAIN USES

- Stress-related conditions, such as insomnia & headaches
- Muscle & joint disorders, such as arthritis & back pain
- Pain relief
- High blood pressure
- Depression & anxiety
- Digestive disorders, such as constipation

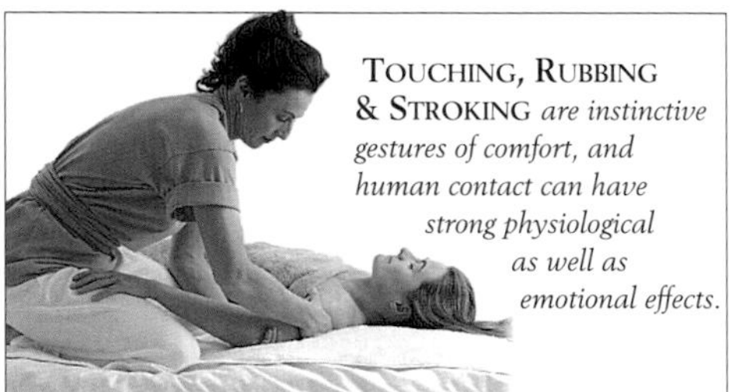

TOUCHING, RUBBING & STROKING *are instinctive gestures of comfort, and human contact can have strong physiological as well as emotional effects.*

HISTORY

Massage may be the oldest and simplest form of medical care. Egyptian tomb paintings show people being massaged, and ancient Chinese and Indian manuscripts refer to its use in treating diseases and injuries. Greek and Roman physicians valued it as a principal method of relieving pain: Julius Caesar was given a daily massage to treat neuralgia. Hippocrates, the "father of medicine," wrote in the 5th century B.C., "The physician must be experienced in many things, but assuredly in rubbing … for rubbing can bind a joint that is too loose, and loosen a joint that is too rigid."

Ayurveda, the traditional Indian system of medicine, places great emphasis on the therapeutic benefits of massage with aromatic oils and spices, but in the West religious ambivalence about potential links between sin and the stimulation of the senses gave massage a dubious image.

Doctors such as Ambroise Paré, a 16th-century physician to the French court, praised massage as a treatment for various ailments, but it was a Swedish gymnast, Per Henrik Ling, who restored therapeutic massage to general favor throughout Europe at the end of the 19th century. Physiotherapy, originally based on Ling's methods, was established with the foundation in 1894 of the Society of Trained Masseurs.

During World War I patients suffering from nerve injury or shell shock were treated with massage. St. Thomas's Hospital, London, had a department of massage until 1934. However, later breakthroughs in medical technology and pharmacology eclipsed massage as physiotherapists began increasingly to favor electrical instruments over manual methods of stimulating the tissues.

At the same time, some brothels were masquerading as "massage parlors," and through this, massage acquired unsavory connotations of prostitution.

This image is fading as awareness of the value and therapeutic properties of massage grows. In both the US and UK nurses are bringing massage therapy into conventional health care, and massage theory and practice are being included in nursing degree programs. Increasingly, massage is used in intensive care units, for children, elderly people, babies in incubators, and patients with cancer, AIDS, heart attacks, or strokes. Most American hospices have some kind of bodywork therapy available, and it is frequently offered in health centers, drug treatment clinics, and pain clinics.

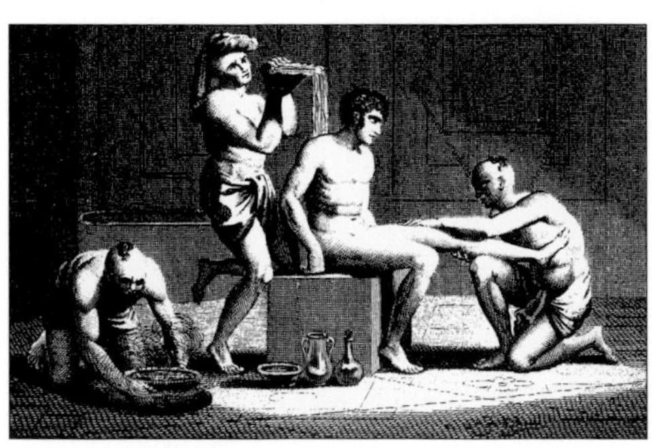

In ancient civilizations *massage was considered highly beneficial: Hippocrates advocated a daily scented bath and massage with oil for good health.*

A variety of massage techniques have also been incorporated into several other complementary therapies, such as aromatherapy, reflexology, Rolfing, Hellerwork, and osteopathy.

KEY PRINCIPLES

All forms of touch are perceived through the skin, which is the body's largest sensory organ. In the embryo, the sense of touch is the earliest to develop, and human babies, in common with primates and other mammals, thrive when in close contact with their mothers.

Thousands of specialized receptors in the dermis (the second layer of skin) react to external stimuli, such as heat, cold, and pressure, by sending messages through the nervous system to the brain. Gentle massage or stroking can trigger the release of endorphins, the body's natural pain-killers, and induce a feeling of comfort and well-being. Stronger, more vigorous massage may help to stretch tense and uncomfortable muscles and ease stiff joints, improving mobility and flexibility.

Massage can aid relaxation, directly affecting the body systems that govern heart rate, blood pressure, respiration, and digestion. While not a cure for specific complaints, the resulting sense of well-being from massage can lower the amount of circulating stress hormones, such as cortisol and norepinephrine, that can weaken the immune system.

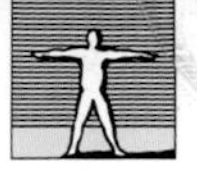

THE THEORY OF MASSAGE

Per Henrik Ling's "Swedish movement treatment," grounded in anatomy, forms the basis for the techniques used in the West today, which are often still referred to as Swedish massage. Ling laid great emphasis on therapeutic massage, or "medical gymnastics," to stimulate the functioning of the body.

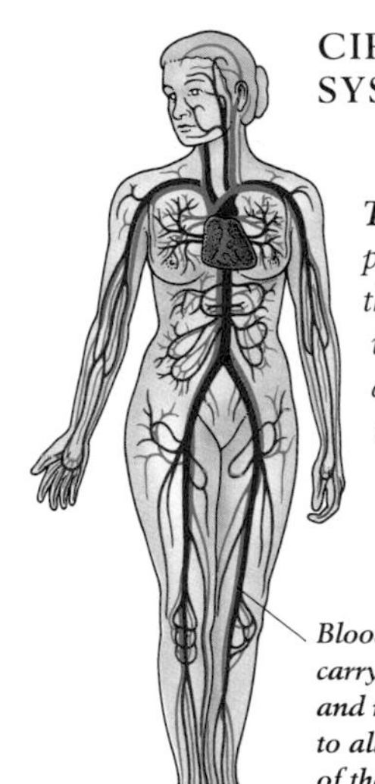

***The circulatory system** (see page 242): Stimulation of the circulation by massage improves the supply of oxygen and nutrients to body tissues and enhances skin tone.*

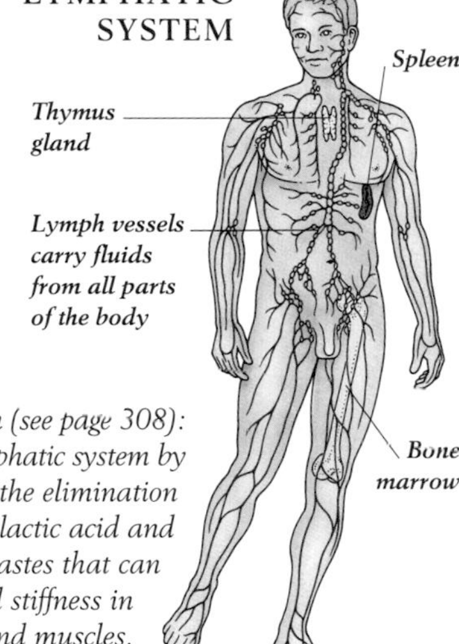

***The lymphatic system** (see page 308): Stimulation of the lymphatic system by massage improves the elimination from the body of lactic acid and other chemical wastes that can lead to pain and stiffness in the joints and muscles.*

THE BASIC TECHNIQUES

Stroking, or *effleurage*, is a gentle action for all parts of the body to aid circulation and relax tense muscles. Kneading, or *petrissage*, stretches and relaxes muscles, and is particularly useful for fleshy areas such as thighs. Friction, or *frottage*, is deep, direct pressure to release tension in the muscles around the spine and shoulders. Hacking, or *tapotement*, uses a brisk percussive action on fleshy, muscular areas.

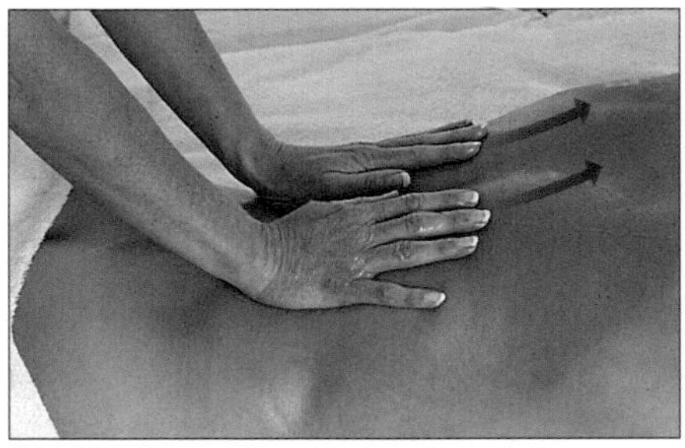

***Stroking**: The hands glide smoothly and rhythmically over the skin, either alternately or in a slow fanning or circular motion.*

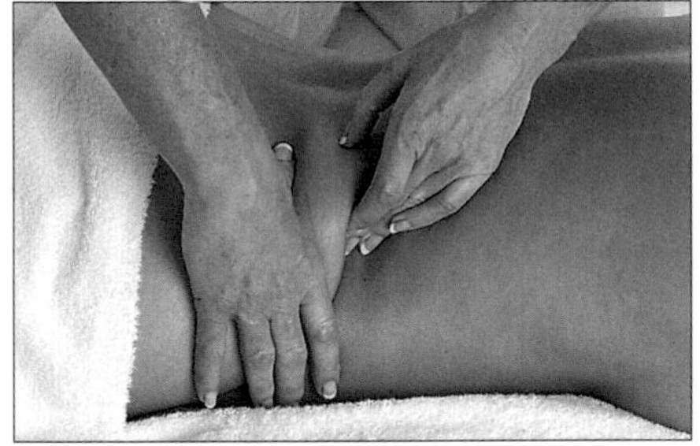

***Kneading**: This action is like kneading dough, using alternate hands to squeeze and release flesh rhythmically between fingers and thumbs.*

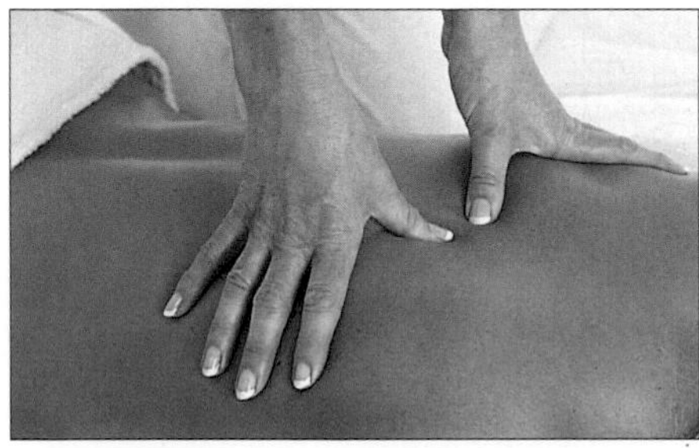

***Friction**: For deep penetration, steady pressure from the thumbs is applied to a static point next to the spine, or in small circles on the skin.*

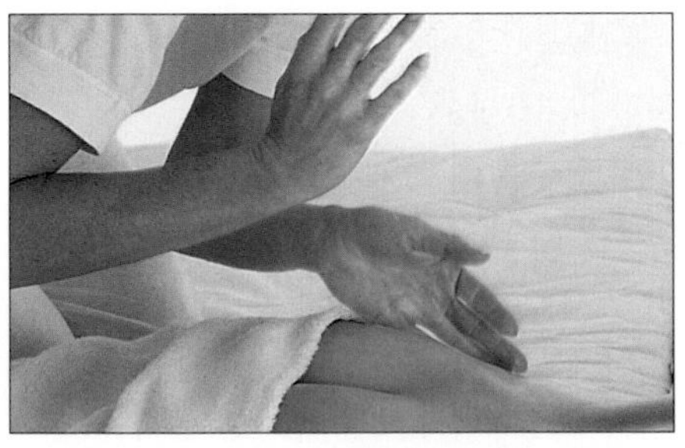

***Hacking**: With hands relaxed and working quickly over the skin, the sides of the hands deliver alternate short, sharp taps on the body.*

Psychologically, massage releases tension and reduces anxiety so that people feel more serene and better equipped to cope with the stresses of life. Awareness of the way in which the mind and body interact can be heightened, thereby enabling people to take greater responsibility for their personal well-being.

EVIDENCE & RESEARCH

An extensive body of research now exists to support the therapeutic claims of massage, much of it performed in the US at the Touch Research Institute (TRI), University of Miami School of Medicine, Florida. A study at the TRI in 1986 revealed that premature babies who were stroked daily gained 47% more weight, were more active, and left the hospital on average six days earlier than nonstroked babies. In 1992 the Institute reported that teenagers hospitalized with anorexia and bulimia expressed a better body image and less anxiety and depression after massage. In 1993 TRI researchers found that when HIV-positive men were massaged daily they produced more of the natural killer cells that destroy invading bacteria and viruses, that asthmatic children breathed more easily and suffered fewer attacks when massaged by their parents, that in diabetic children, glucose levels fell to normal after four weeks of massage, and that office workers who received a 15-minute midday back and shoulder massage reported heightened alertness and showed lower stress hormone levels.

In trials at the Royal Marsden Hospital, London, in 1995, massage was shown to reduce anxiety and improve quality of life in cancer patients.

Massage has also been shown to benefit the giver. At the Touch Research Institute in 1993, foster grandparents who gave shoulder massages to young abused children reported improved self-esteem and less depression.

MEDICAL OPINION

Evidence of the therapeutic advantages of massage, both in clinical studies and from patient's reports, is so overwhelming that most doctors would endorse it. While it may be seen as an adjunct to the usual medical methods, many doctors do not think to recommend it routinely or to refer patients to a massage therapist.

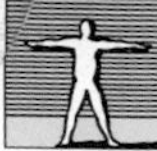

Consulting a Practitioner

At your initial treatment, you will be asked briefly about your medical history, lifestyle, and general state of health, including any current medication.

Western massage is usually given on a special table, but a futon mattress or thick blanket on the floor can be used. For a whole body massage it is usual to undress, though you may prefer to keep on your underwear. A towel is placed over you, as much for warmth as for dignity, exposing only the relevant part of the body to be massaged. At the end, you are covered up warmly and left to savor the experience for a few minutes.

According to the technique used and the degree and rhythm of the pressure, massage can make you more alert or calm you down. It may even put you to sleep. Sometimes massage can arouse temporary feelings of sadness or lightheadedness that may be signs of emotional release.

Western massage, shown here, is based on Ling's techniques, but over the years variations have been developed. Remedial massage, for instance, focuses on specific conditions such as muscle strains, while manual lymph drainage, a gentle, pumping massage, aims to speed the removal of waste products by stimulating the lymphatic system. Biodynamic massage (see page 61) concentrates on releasing emotions or "bioenergy" believed to be trapped within the body.

Eastern massage includes acupressure techniques such as shiatsu, *tuina*, and do-in (see pages 95–98) that emphasize pressure rather than stroking, and aim to balance energy forces in the body according to Eastern philosophy.

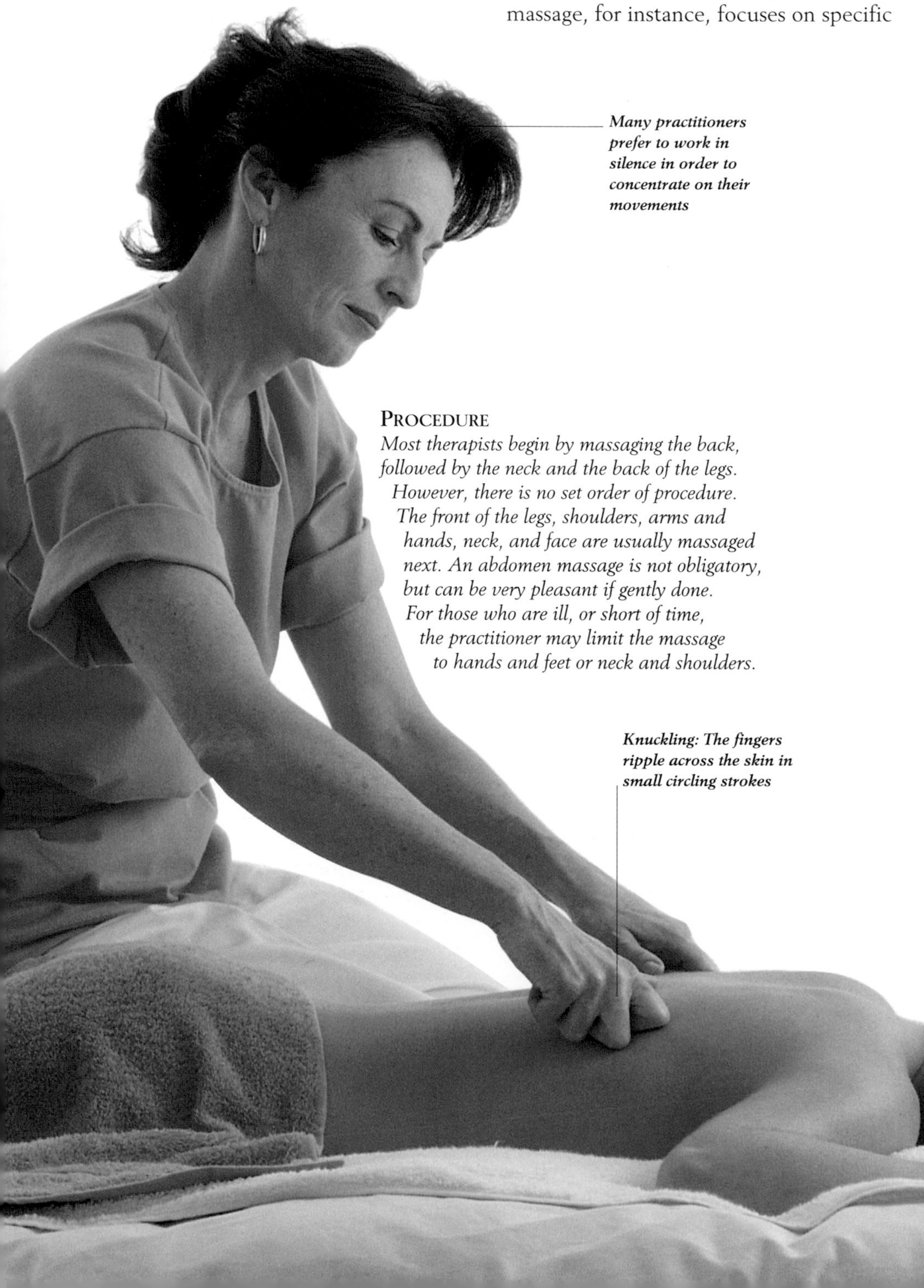

Many practitioners prefer to work in silence in order to concentrate on their movements

Procedure

Most therapists begin by massaging the back, followed by the neck and the back of the legs. However, there is no set order of procedure. The front of the legs, shoulders, arms and hands, neck, and face are usually massaged next. An abdomen massage is not obligatory, but can be very pleasant if gently done. For those who are ill, or short of time, the practitioner may limit the massage to hands and feet or neck and shoulders.

Knuckling: The fingers ripple across the skin in small circling strokes

Using Oil

Practitioners usually work with a light vegetable oil or cream so that their hands glide over the skin. Aromatic essential oils may be added (see pages 62–65).

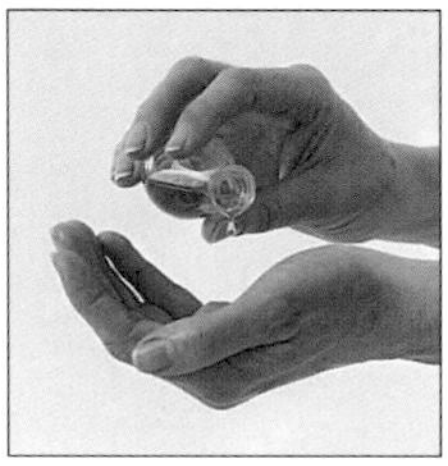

1 About a teaspoon of the chosen oil is poured into the palm of the hand.

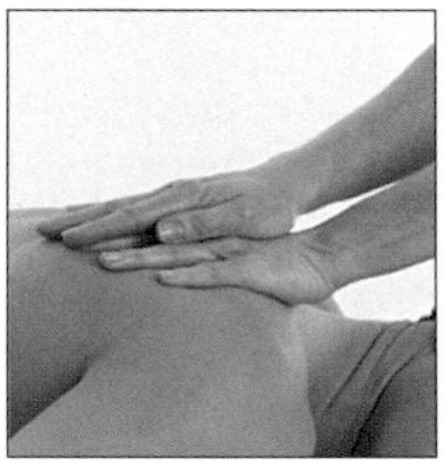

2 The oil is warmed between the hands, then stroked gently onto the body.

Precautions

- Seek medical advice before having a massage if you suffer from phlebitis, thrombosis, varicose veins, severe acute back pain, or fever.
- Swellings, fractures, skin infections, or bruises should not be massaged. Lumps and swellings should be checked by your doctor.
- Massage of the abdomen, legs, and feet should not be given during the first three months of pregnancy.
- Cancer patients are best treated by specially trained practitioners who know which areas to avoid and which kind of massage is appropriate.
- See also page 52.

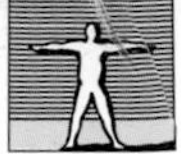

BACK MASSAGE

To begin a back massage, the practitioner may relax the body with gentle strokes. She might then use other soothing techniques, such as circular or fanlike strokes on the back and neck, followed by crisscrossing over the body with her hands to create figure eights up and down the back, pulling up at the sides of the body, and never pressing directly on the spine.

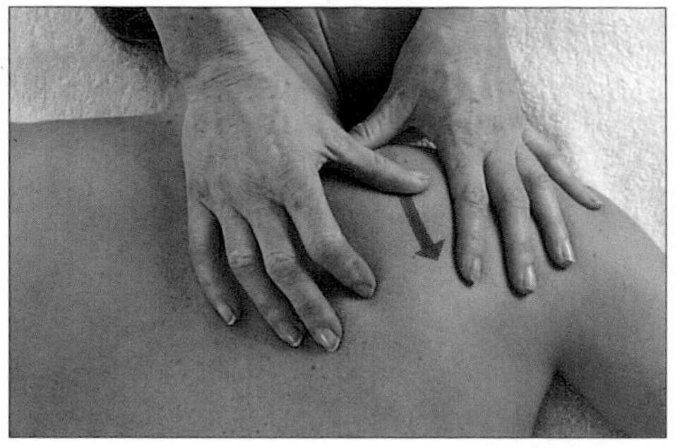

1 The practitioner works to release taut muscles down each side of the neck and out to the top of the shoulder, stroking with firm movements, one thumb following the other.

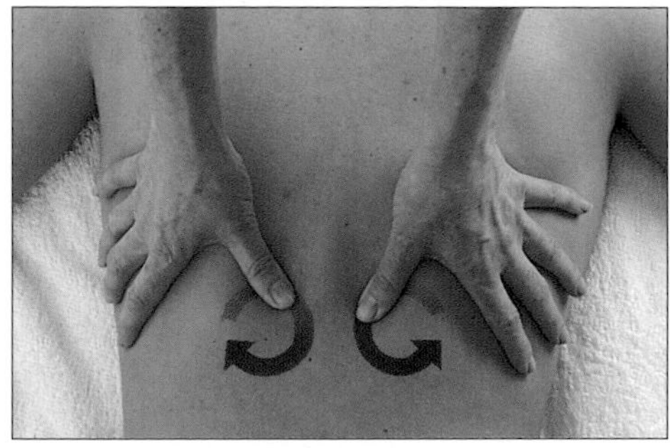

2 Using the thumbs to make large, flat circles, the practitioner massages next to the spine from the shoulders to the small of the back. Making the circles smaller and increasing the pressure can produce a more penetrating effect on tense areas.

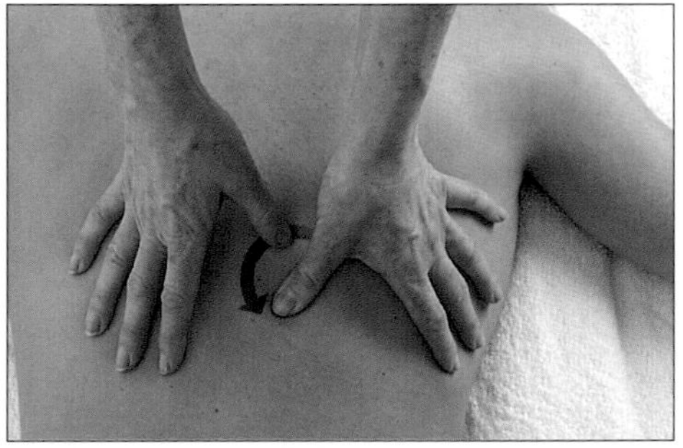

3 Now working down each side of the spine alternately, the practitioner makes a full circle with one thumb and a half circle with the other. The hands work alternately, stroking away from the spine and creating a continuous flowing effect.

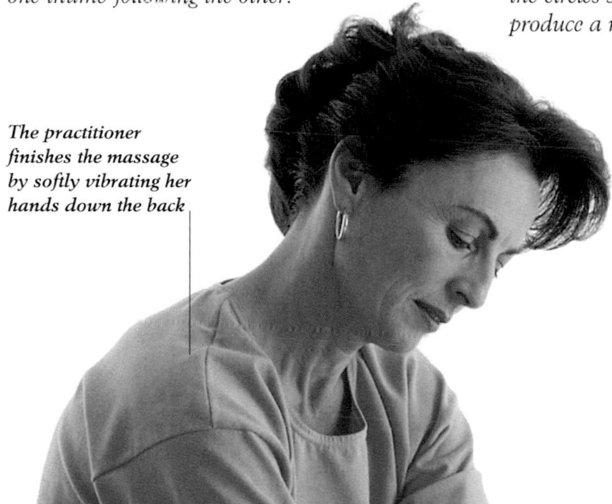

The practitioner finishes the massage by softly vibrating her hands down the back

4 Static pressure on either side of the spine follows, working from the base of the neck to the pelvis, along the tops of the shoulders and into the scalp. The practitioner slowly leans on her thumbs, holds for 5–9 seconds, then releases. Less pressure is used on the neck, base of the skull, and the scalp.

5 The practitioner may finish with gentle movements, such as slow strokes with alternate hands down the back. Then, using one hand on top of the other, she softly vibrates her hands down the back, taking care not to exert direct pressure on the spine.

YOUR QUESTIONS

How long does a treatment session last?
A full body massage takes roughly 60 minutes, or 90 minutes if the face is included in the massage.

How many sessions will I need?
As many as you like and can afford.

Will it be uncomfortable?
Massage therapy should be a pleasant and soothing experience. Tell the practitioner if you feel any discomfort and he or she will ease the pressure.

Will there be any aftereffects?
Right after treatment you may feel very sleepy. Drinking a glass of water is a good idea. You may ache a little the next day but this will soon wear off.

A Patient's Experience

Vicky, a newspaper reporter, used to spend hours on the telephone, cradling the receiver on her shoulder while she took notes: "I was getting headaches and generally feeling very stressed, with constant aches in my neck and shoulders. A friend suggested massage, though it seemed a little self-indulgent to me. The therapist said that years of strain were locked in my shoulders, and at first the massage was a little uncomfortable, particularly if she kneaded me strongly. After sessions every two weeks, the tension gradually left my muscles and the headaches lessened. I learned what real physical and mental relaxation felt like, and my company gave me a phone headset that leaves my hands and shoulders free."

Leg Massage

Keeping the rest of the body covered, the practitioner works on the legs and feet, massaging first one leg, then the other. Many of the movements can be applied to both the front and the back of the legs.

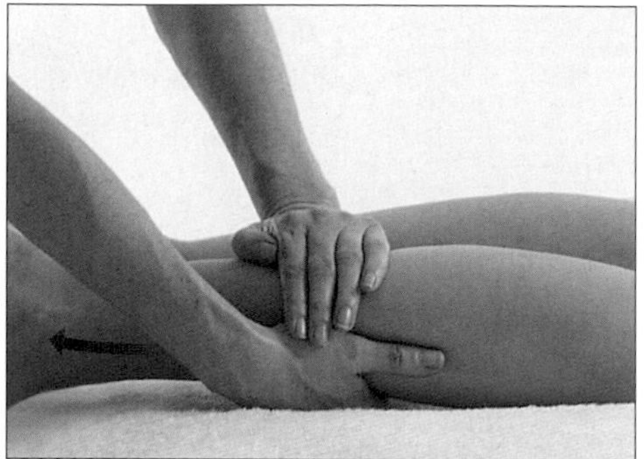

1 With one hand on each side of the calf, fingers facing forward, the practitioner strokes firmly up the length of the leg. She then gently glides her hands back down the leg, sliding her outer hand under the leg and the other hand over the top.

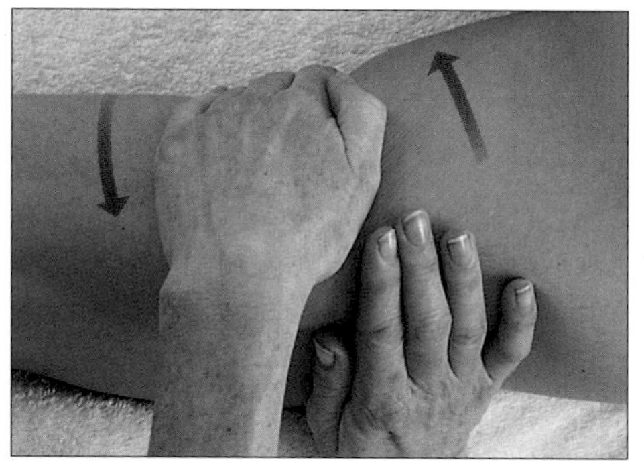

2 Placing one hand on either side of the thigh, the practitioner brings her hands together, easing the flesh up toward the top of the leg. She then releases the pressure, crisscrosses her hands to the other side of the leg, and repeats the stroke.

3 Moving down to the lower leg, the practitioner repeatedly strokes firmly up the calf to the knee and glides back to the ankle, using her palms and then her forearms. The calf may be kneaded with alternate hands, and a soothing foot massage may follow. The entire sequence is then repeated on the other leg before the practitioner begins to work on the front of the legs.

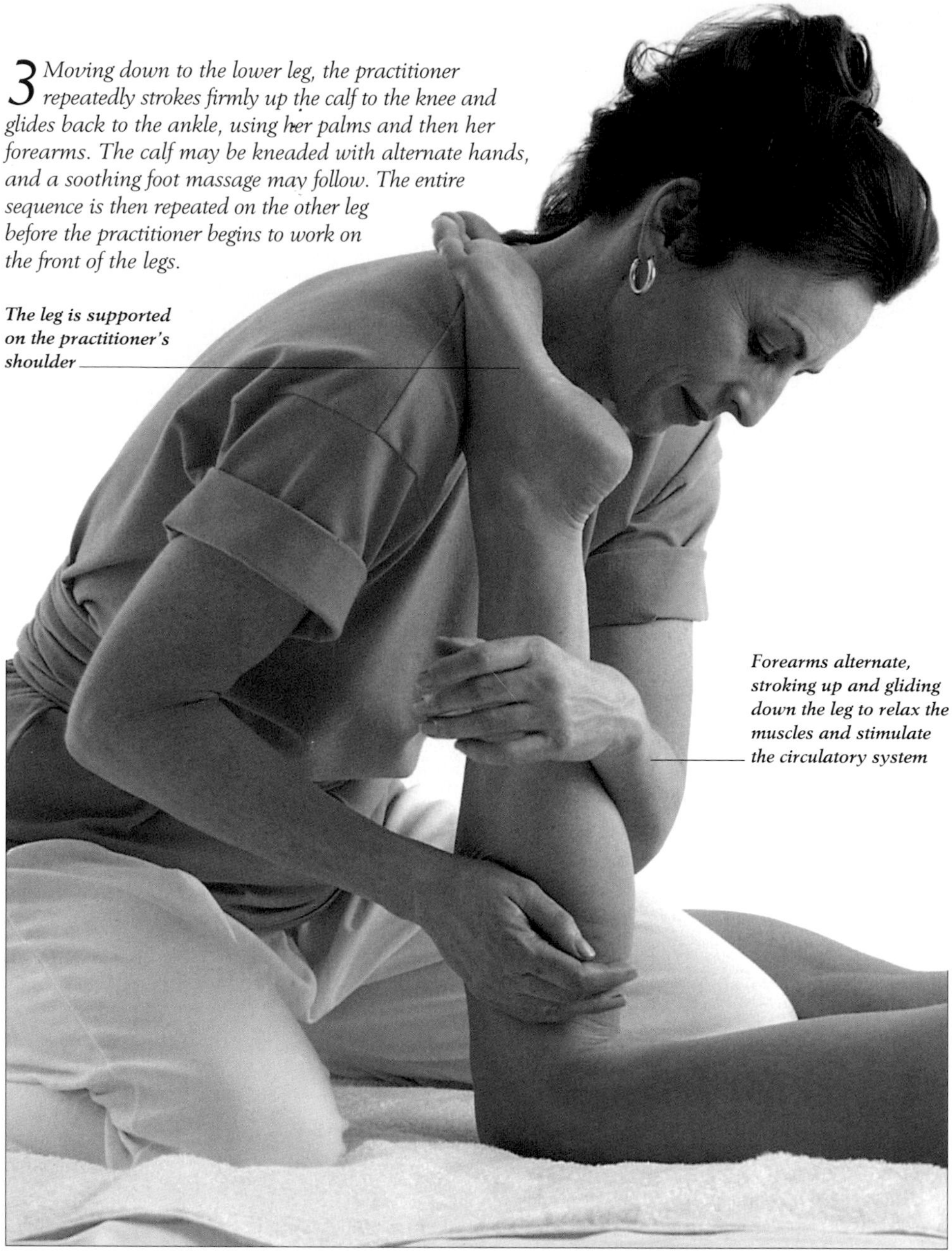

The leg is supported on the practitioner's shoulder

Forearms alternate, stroking up and gliding down the leg to relax the muscles and stimulate the circulatory system

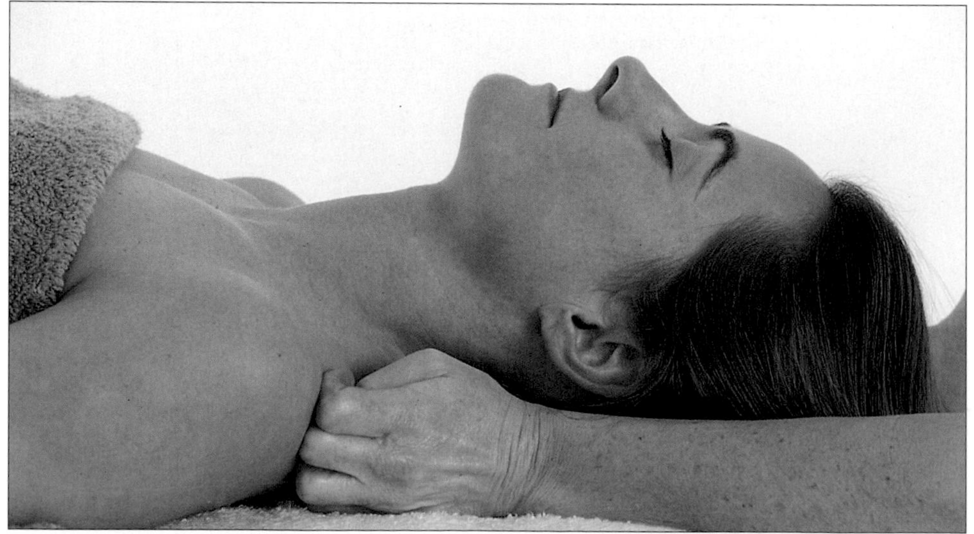

Shoulder Massage

To ease tension in the shoulders, the practitioner may begin with fanning strokes over the collarbone and shoulders, then use slow strokes with the hands moving up the back of the neck. Circular pressure may be applied all over the back of the neck and at the base of the skull, followed by circular pressure and knuckling down the chest from the collarbone out over the pectorals and shoulders.

***The practitioner** uses her knuckles to loosen taut neck muscles. Resting her forearms on the floor, she gently massages the area by rotating her fingers against the base of the neck.*

SELF-HELP

You can easily massage yourself, though it is not quite as relaxing as being massaged by someone else. If you work slowly and rhythmically, however, you should be able to release tension in your body and soothe away aches and pains.

THIGH MASSAGE

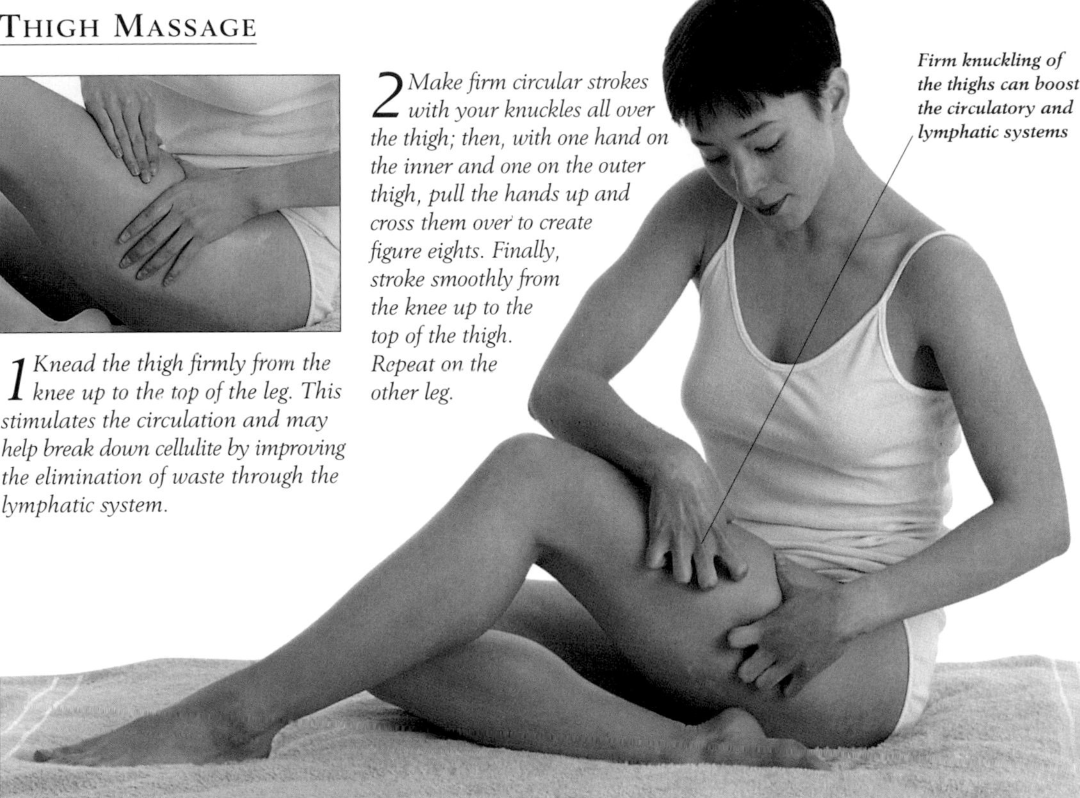

1 Knead the thigh firmly from the knee up to the top of the leg. This stimulates the circulation and may help break down cellulite by improving the elimination of waste through the lymphatic system.

2 Make firm circular strokes with your knuckles all over the thigh; then, with one hand on the inner and one on the outer thigh, pull the hands up and cross them over to create figure eights. Finally, stroke smoothly from the knee up to the top of the thigh. Repeat on the other leg.

Firm knuckling of the thighs can boost the circulatory and lymphatic systems

HAND MASSAGE

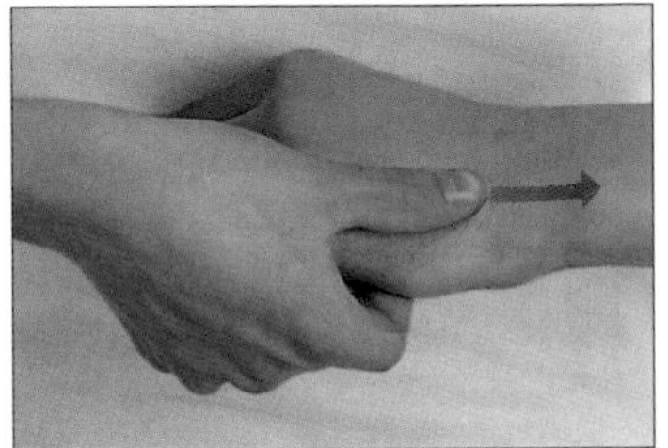

1 After gently stroking the whole hand to relax and warm it, use your thumb to stroke from the knuckle of your little finger down the tendon toward the wrist. Repeat for each finger.

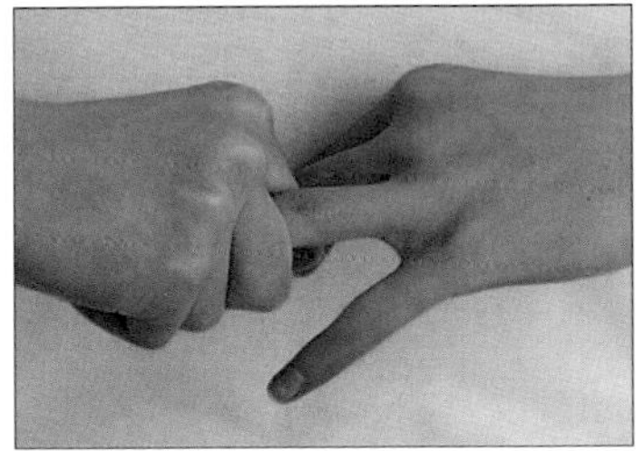

2 Gently grip a finger between the joints of the first two fingers of the other hand. Slowly slide the finger down, pulling with a corkscrewlike motion. Repeat twice on each finger and thumb. Apply knuckle pressure to the palm, then gently stroke it. Repeat on the other hand.

Biodynamic Massage

This form of massage aims to release energy bound up in the muscles and gut, causing physical and emotional pain. Discussion is encouraged, and techniques can be soothing and soporific, or more vigorous.

HISTORY

This approach was developed in the 1960s by Gerda Boyesen, a Norwegian-born psychologist and physiotherapist. She subsequently discovered that her ideas were similar to those of Wilhelm Reich (see page 89). According to his theory of "armoring," suppressed emotions can cause muscular tensions, trapping energy. This may be released by working simultaneously on the body and mind. In 1975 Boyesen founded an institute in London to train practitioners and treat patients; centers later opened in Europe and in Australia. However, this therapy is not well known in the US.

CONSULTING A PRACTITIONER

Practitioners believe that the intestine digests not only food, but stress and trauma, a process known as "psychoperistalsis," which, they claim, can be improved with massage. You lie undressed on a massage table, covered by a blanket. Swedish massage is combined with techniques such as "lifting" the limbs to detect and free trapped "bioenergy," which is released through the abdomen. A stethoscope is applied to the abdomen to monitor progress – the more gurgles the better. Talking is encouraged if the practitioner feels the massage is raising any issues.

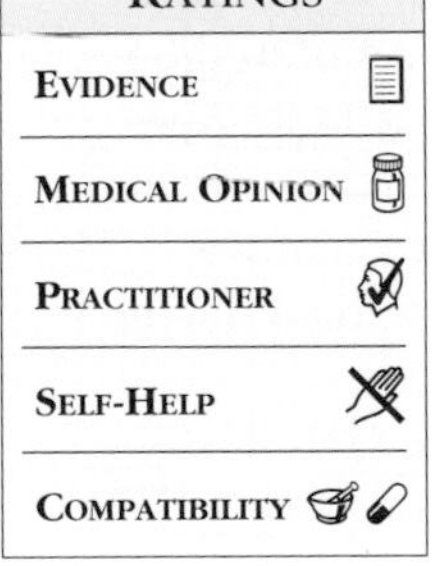

RATINGS
EVIDENCE
MEDICAL OPINION
PRACTITIONER
SELF-HELP
COMPATIBILITY

MAIN USES

- A range of physical ailments, including stress-related conditions, such as backache, headaches & depression
- Digestive disorders

MEDICAL OPINION

The idea that the gut reacts to emotions is familiar, but most psychotherapists and doctors find the use of bowel noises to monitor psychological changes unusual.

PRECAUTIONS

- See massage (page 58) and page 52.

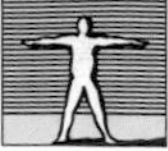

CONSULTING A PRACTITIONER

At your first session, the practitioner will need to know about your medical history and your lifestyle, including the condition of your skin, your diet, and sleeping patterns, and any exercise you do. She will ask whether you want the treatment to alleviate particular health problems, to be a general tonic, or to be an aid to emotional well-being. The aromatherapist will either select those oils she considers most appropriate, or invite you to choose your preferred aromas from a range of bottles. A trained practitioner will use only high-quality oils, free from synthetic additives that may adversely affect the properties of an oil. The oils are diluted in a vegetable-based carrier oil such as almond or grapeseed for massage, or blended in a lotion or cream for external application.

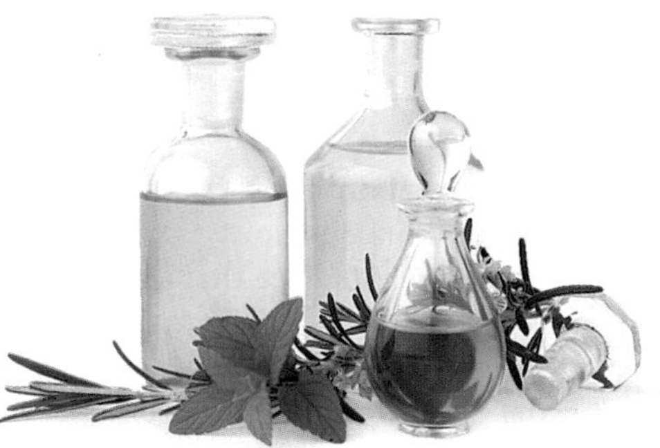

***Essential oils** are combined with vegetable-based carrier oils for use in massage and skin care. Once the essential oils have been diluted in this way, they must be used within a few months or their therapeutic properties will deteriorate.*

Although acupressure techniques are also sometimes used, an aromatherapy massage is usually based on Swedish massage techniques (see page 57), which aim to relieve tension in the body and improve circulation. This, practitioners believe, allows oil molecules absorbed into the bloodstream during massage to pass efficiently through the body to the nervous system. The massage will also stimulate the lymphatic system, which helps to remove metabolic wastes from the body.

If inhalations are recommended, your practitioner will give you specific oils or blends to use at home.

PRECAUTIONS

- Use inhalations with care if you have asthma or are prone to nosebleeds.
- Be sure the practitioner is qualified if you are pregnant, epileptic, or have high blood pressure.
- Never swallow any oils, except under the supervision of a medically trained practitioner.
- Never use undiluted essential oils on the skin (apart from lavender oil on burns and tea tree oil on insect stings). Do not apply near the eyes.
- Keep essential oils away from open flames and from children.
- See also massage (page 58) and page 52.

YOUR QUESTIONS

How long does a treatment session last?
A full body massage lasts about 60 minutes; a face massage lasts 30 minutes.

How many sessions will I need?
As many as you like, or are felt necessary.

Will it be uncomfortable?
The massage should not be painful; tell your practitioner if it causes discomfort.

Will there be any aftereffects?
You may feel sleepy and your muscles may ache for a short time after a massage.

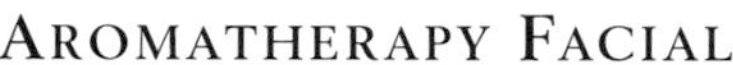

AROMATHERAPY FACIAL

Many people first experience aromatherapy as part of a facial treatment. Before beginning to massage, the practitioner cleanses the skin and may apply hot washcloths to open the pores in preparation for the massage with scented oils or creams.

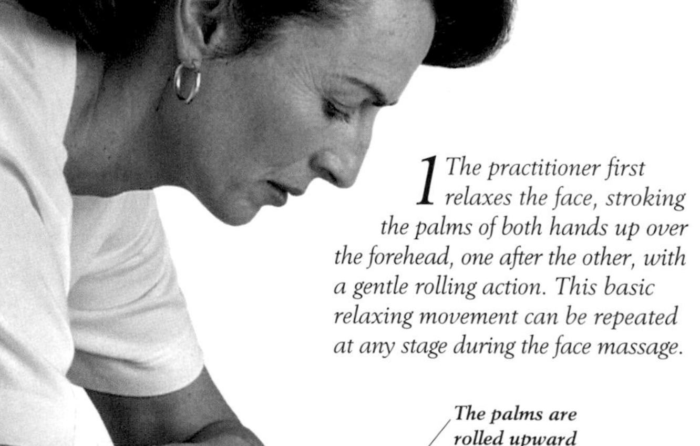

The palms are rolled upward over the forehead

1 The practitioner first relaxes the face, stroking the palms of both hands up over the forehead, one after the other, with a gentle rolling action. This basic relaxing movement can be repeated at any stage during the face massage.

2 To release tension, the practitioner makes circular strokes around the face from the center of the forehead to the chin and back again, crossing the hands on the upward strokes. The movement is repeated several times.

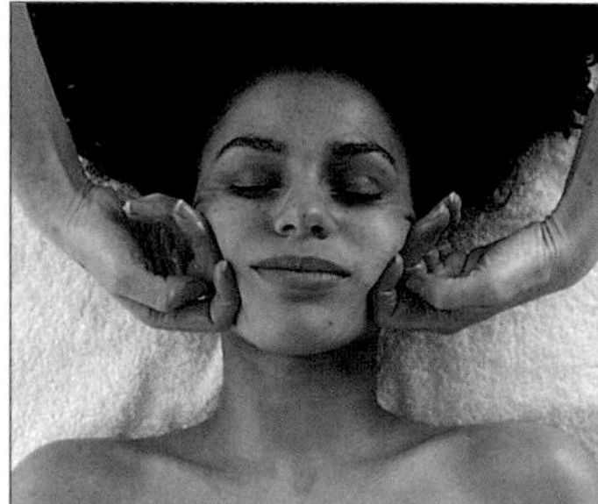

3 The jaw muscles are often tense and can be relaxed by massaging with the knuckles. Working with a rhythmic circular motion, the practitioner massages outward from the cheeks to the joints of the jaw.

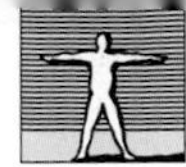

SELF-HELP

Use only pure essential oils free from additives, and pay attention to instructions for dilution. In addition to their use in massage, oils can be inhaled, vaporized, or added to baths. Inhalations are thought to be highly effective, since the olfactory receptors have direct links with the brain. They can be used for respiratory conditions, such as phlegm, sore throats, colds, and coughs, or as part of a skin care routine. Use with caution if you are asthmatic. Vaporizers and scented baths can be relaxing or invigorating, depending on the oil chosen.

Vaporizers: To scent a room, place 2–3 drops of oil in the bowl with a little water and place over the lighted candle.

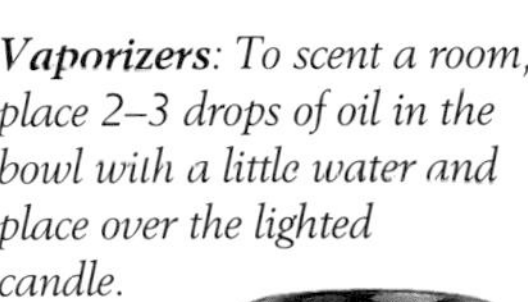

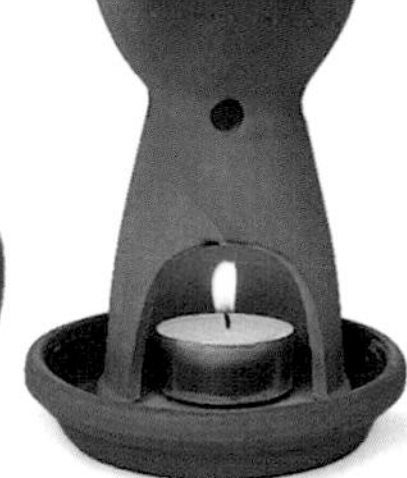

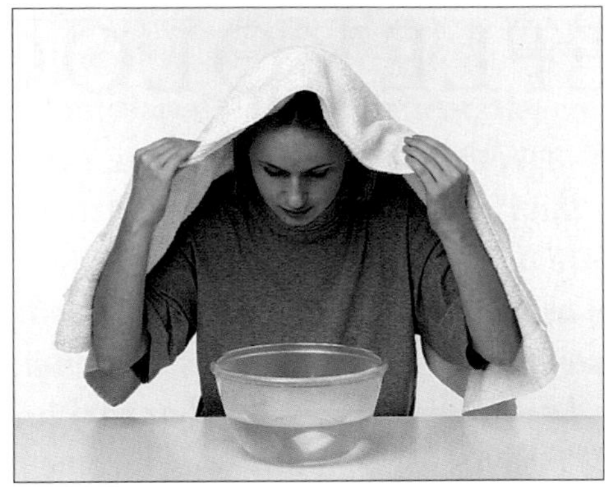

***Inhalations**: Add 4 drops of essential oil (2–3 for peppermint or eucalyptus) to a bowl of steaming hot water and lean over the bowl with head covered by a towel and eyes closed. Inhale for up to 10 minutes. Alternatively, place 4–5 drops of oil on a tissue, hold it to your nose and take deep breaths. Do not inhale directly from the bottle.*

***Aromatherapy baths**: Add 6 drops of essential oil to a warm bath, and relax in it for at least 10 minutes. Geranium, lavender, sandalwood, and neroli are all excellent bath oils, and fresh rose petals may also be added.*

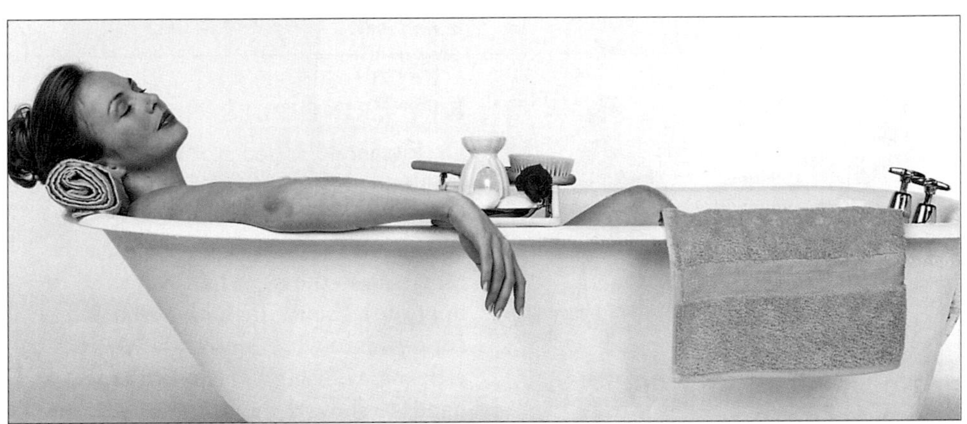

Aromatherapy: Medical Applications

Medical aromatherapists, unlike aromatherapists, prescribe oils for internal use. They have an approach similar to herbalists, but consider their oils to be more effective than herbs, since the oils are concentrated by distillation.

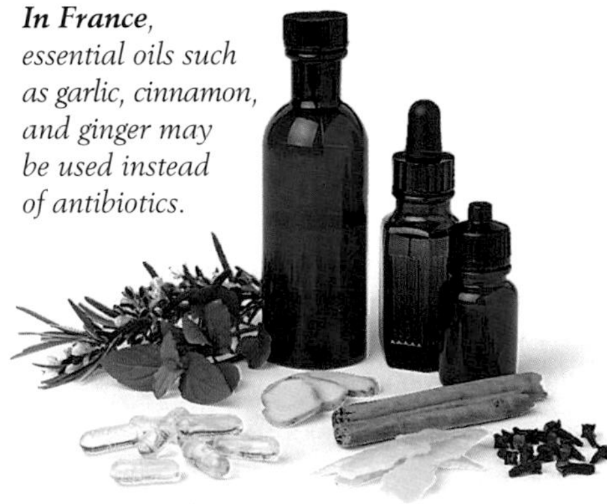

***In France**, essential oils such as garlic, cinnamon, and ginger may be used instead of antibiotics.*

HISTORY

The study of the pharmacology and chemistry of essential oils is a relatively recent branch of medical research. It is known as medical aromatherapy (or, increasingly in the UK, as aromatology). Although essential oils were used during World War I to treat wounded soldiers, it was not until the 1960s that doctors in France, such as Dr. Jean Valnet, began to study their medicinal use in treating burns, cancer, diabetes, and tuberculosis. Some French doctors and hospitals now regularly administer oils, and there is growing interest in the UK and in Australia and New Zealand.

CONSULTING A PRACTITIONER

Diagnosis is based on a thorough knowledge of the patient's medical history and a full medical examination. The practitioner will prescribe essential oils, derived from plants, to be taken by the patient either orally, rectally, vaginally, or by inhalation or massage. Some practitioners in French hospitals employ an aromatogram, a laboratory technique used to determine which oil is deemed best for treating particular conditions in patients.

RATINGS

EVIDENCE	
MEDICAL OPINION	
PRACTITIONER	
SELF-HELP	
COMPATIBILITY	

MAIN USES

- Genitourinary infections, cystitis & candidiasis
- Constipation
- Skin conditions, especially psoriasis
- Anxiety & stress (particularly following major surgery)
- Insomnia
- Depression

MEDICAL OPINION

Outside France, this therapy is not widely practiced and doctors are more cautious about the internal use of plant extracts. In the US, although the therapy is neither licensed nor illegal, its use is uncommon. As of 1996, one practitioner is working in the British National Health Service, treating a range of disorders.

PRECAUTIONS

- Essential oils should be taken internally only under medical supervision.
- See also aromatherapy (page 64) and page 52.

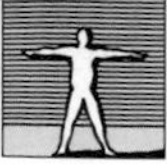

Consulting a Practitioner

The practitioner will initially ask you about your past and present health and lifestyle. Most practitioners prefer to work on the foot, but the hand may be used if it is more suitable for the patient. If massaging the feet, the practitioner will ask you to take off your footwear and relax in a reclining chair or on a couch with your feet raised, while she examines your feet for indications of existing or potential health problems, possibly even suggesting that you see your doctor for a medical checkup. She will stimulate the reflex points all over your foot, watching for any reaction of pain or tenderness. This is thought to indicate crystalline deposits beneath the skin, evidence to the practitioner of an imbalance in the corresponding area of the body; the greater the tenderness is, the greater the imbalance. Extra massage is given to tender areas to break down these deposits and free energy flow.

Vacuflex reflexology is a variation that stimulates reflex points with a suction pump linked to special boots and cups applied to specific body areas.

The foot is usually treated, since it is considered more sensitive than the hand

Preparation
To relax the feet, the practitioner massages them with a dusting of talcum powder or with a little nongreasy cream.

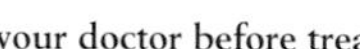

Precautions

- Check with your doctor before treatment if you suffer from a thyroid disorder, diabetes, or any other long-term health problem.
- Avoid reflexology in the first three months of pregnancy.
- Tell your practitioner if you are taking medication, since reflexology is thought to increase excretions from the body and may interfere with the action of medication. For the same reason, you should tell your practitioner if you are also consulting an herbalist, homeopath, or aromatherapist.
- See also page 52.

Treatment

After relaxing the feet, the practitioner massages all areas of each foot with her hands and thumbs to stimulate the reflex points. Several techniques are used, particularly thumb walking, which allows gentle movement from one reflex point to another. The pad of the thumb moves over the skin, applying and releasing pressure before creeping along slightly and repeating the action. Also common is web pressing, in which pressure is applied to the web of skin between the toes.

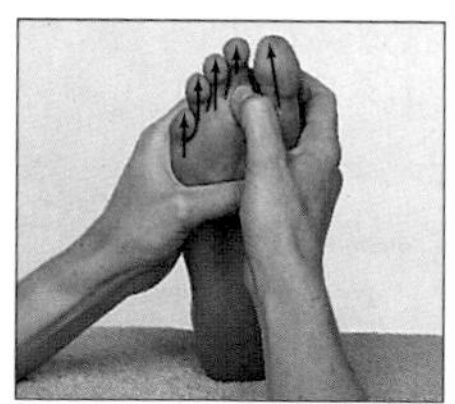

***Sinuses**: Beginning at the base of the toe, the practitioner uses the thumb walk, her thumb slowly creeping up each toe toward the tip. Repeated stimulation of the sinus points on each toe aims to ease congestion and relieve pain.*

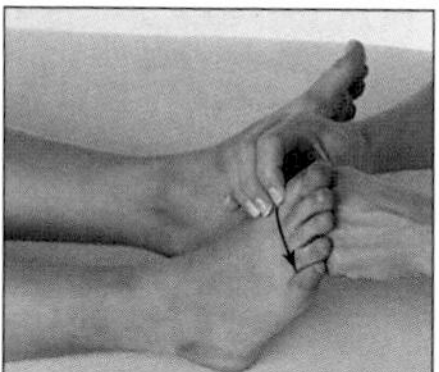

***Neck and thyroid gland**: The practitioner presses below the first three toes of each foot with her thumb from beneath, then works across the top of the foot with her index finger. This seeks to help the neck and thyroid, and ease menstrual pain.*

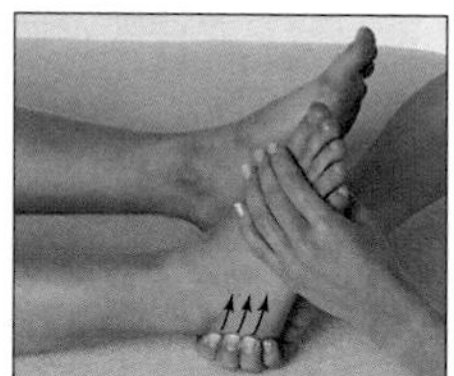

***Hip and pelvis**: Using all four fingers, the practitioner works from the back of the foot up the outside edge of the heel, supporting the foot with the other hand. This is designed to relax the muscles and ease inflammation in the joints.*

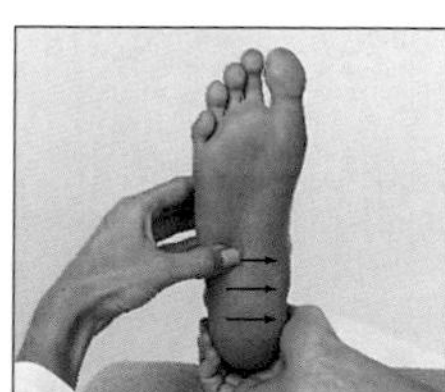

***Colon and intestine**: Beginning on the right foot, the practitioner uses her thumb to creep repeatedly across the lower half of the sole. She will then work the same area on the left foot. These two actions together stimulate the whole digestive system.*

Your Questions

How long does a treatment session last?
A treatment usually lasts 45–60 minutes.

How many sessions will I need?
Depending on the problem, several weekly sessions may be advised. Many people have regular treatments to maintain well-being.

Will it be uncomfortable?
A reflex point may be tender if there is an imbalance, but this eases with massage. Pressure is adjusted to suit your sensitivity. Ticklishness is usually not a problem.

Will there be any aftereffects?
There may be a "healing crisis" (for example, a cough or rash). Practitioners believe this occurs as the body's natural healing mechanisms remove toxins.

A Patient's Experience

Miranda, 35, is a self-employed landscape gardener: "A traumatic year that included my mother's death, my husband's job layoff, and selling our house caused me to develop what the hospital diagnosed as irritable bowel syndrome. They offered no cure, so I tried a reflexologist at a local complementary health center. I hadn't had reflexology before and, unlike many people who find it relaxing, I found it quite painful, developing a headache after my first session. I gradually improved with weekly treatments; after each one the symptoms took longer to return, and finally disappeared. Now I'd go back at the first sign of a problem."

SELF-HELP ON THE FEET

***The foot is considered** to be more sensitive than the hands, and some techniques can be applied in limited form to the foot as a self-help method. The side of the foot is said to mirror the spine, so massaging this area on both feet may help to ease backache and muscle tension in the back.*

SELF-HELP

Reflexologists usually prefer to work on the feet because they are more sensitive, but for self-help the hands are often more convenient. Reflexology on the hands can be practiced at any time, such as at work or on a train, to relieve stress or to promote healing of a specific ailment between visits to a practitioner.

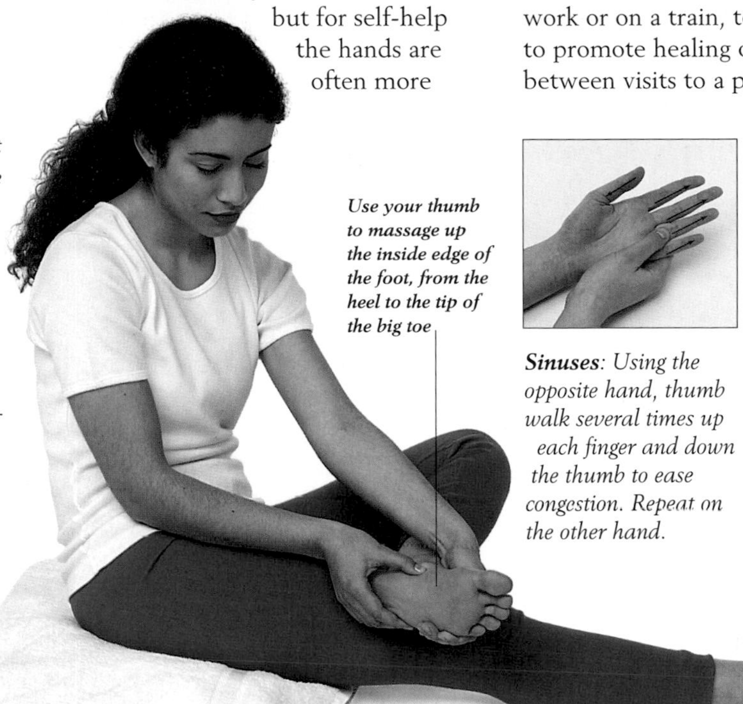

Use your thumb to massage up the inside edge of the foot, from the heel to the tip of the big toe

***Sinuses**: Using the opposite hand, thumb walk several times up each finger and down the thumb to ease congestion. Repeat on the other hand.*

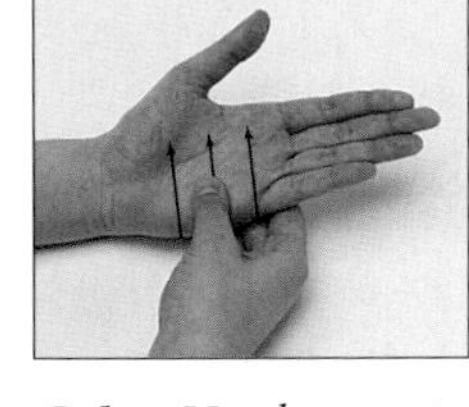

***Colon**: Use the opposite thumb to massage across the palms several times. This stimulates the colon and intestine, to help relieve irritable bowel syndrome. Repeat on the other hand.*

The Metamorphic Technique

Gentle massage of the feet, hands, and head is used in this approach, which aims to release "physical and emotional blocks" established during the prenatal period, and to foster creative and positive changes in a person's life.

RATINGS
EVIDENCE
MEDICAL OPINION
PRACTITIONER
SELF-HELP
COMPATIBILITY

MAIN USES

- Long-standing health problems
- Physical and mental disabilities

HISTORY

Robert St. John, a British naturopath and reflexologist, developed the Metamorphic technique (originally called prenatal therapy) in the 1960s while working in a school for children with learning disabilities. In 1979 one of his students, Gaston St.-Pierre, set up the Metamorphic Association in London.

CONSULTING A PRACTITIONER

Practitioners describe themselves as "catalysts" – agents of change who remain detached throughout the treatment, making no comment and offering no counseling. Like reflexology, from which it sprang, the Metamorphic technique is founded on the belief that the body is reflected in the feet and hands. The technique goes a step further, claiming that the physical, emotional and mental patterns of our lives – even the ailments from which we will suffer – are established before birth and are mapped out on the side of the foot and hand (which represents the spine). No claims are made for curing any ailment, but the technique aims to facilitate a positive approach to life, encouraging "transformations" that loosen old ways of thinking and behaving and allow new ones to take their place.

You take off your footwear and sit comfortably while each foot in turn is manipulated by a practitioner, using light circular movements with particular emphasis on the side of the foot. The process is repeated on the hands and head. Many people report a feeling of relaxation and invigoration.

MEDICAL OPINION

No research backs these theories, and some people doubt that such a profound outcome can result from massage. The technique is noninvasive and harmless, provided symptoms of disease are reported, but some doctors feel it is wrong to raise hopes of treating chronic problems without evidence.

PRECAUTIONS

- See reflexology (page 68) and page 52.

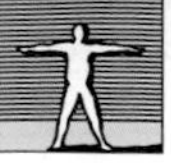

CHIROPRACTIC

RATINGS
EVIDENCE
MEDICAL OPINION
PRACTITIONER
SELF-HELP
COMPATIBILITY

DEVELOPED IN THE LATE 19TH CENTURY by Daniel D. Palmer, chiropractic seeks to diagnose and treat disorders of the spine, joints, and muscles with techniques of manipulation, and to maintain the health of the central nervous system and organs. Practitioners believe that when body systems are in harmony, the body has the ability to heal itself from within. As a result of its success in treating back problems, headaches, and sports and other injuries, chiropractic is the most widely practiced branch of complementary medicine in the West, with around 60,000 practitioners worldwide.

MAIN USES

- **Spine & neck disorders**
- **Muscle, joint & postural problems**
- **Sciatica**
- **Headaches, migraine**
- **Gastrointestinal disorders**
- **Tinnitus, vertigo**
- **Menstrual pain**
- **Asthma**

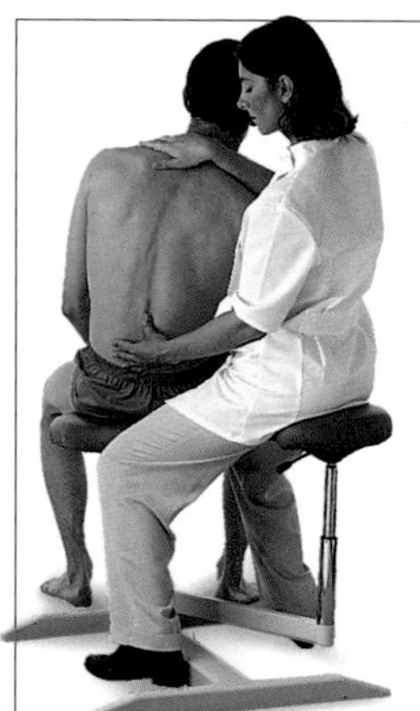

CHIROPRACTORS *carefully examine the spine and vertebrae, since the spine is the "communication highway" between the brain and the body.*

HISTORY

The term chiropractic comes from the ancient Greek *cheiro*, meaning hand, and *praktikos*, doing; literally, "done by hand" or "manipulation." Spinal manipulation has been practiced since at least the 5th century B.C., and variations, such as Native American "back-walking," are found all over the world.

Chiropractic was developed in 1895 by a Canadian, Daniel D. Palmer, who tested his theories by manipulating the spine of his janitor, deaf for 17 years after a back injury. This reportedly caused a shift and the janitor's hearing returned.

In 1906 Palmer was jailed for practicing medicine without a license, but his son, B. J., continued his methods. The therapy was popular during the early 20th century, spreading to Australia, New Zealand, and Europe, but doctors were skeptical, and in the 1960s the American Medical Association (AMA) condemned it as an "unscientific cult." A 12-year legal battle ensued, which the AMA lost in 1987. Now recognized in American health care, chiropractors work in hospitals and sports clinics. British chiropractors built up research evidence to support their case; in 1994 the Chiropractors' Act allowed them to be state-registered as health professionals. In Australia, official recognition of chiropractic in 1978 led to the world's first government-funded course.

KEY PRINCIPLES

Chiropractic sees the body as a naturally healthy system. Along with its mechanical structure of bones, joints, and muscles, it has a power source, lubrication, and wiring. The key to the system is the spine, which links the brain to the body, affecting how the body functions. Any distortion to the spine affects other parts of the body.

Chiropractors regard individuals as more than a set of bones, nerves, and muscles. They claim that treatment can ease muscle tension resulting from stress or problems in internal organs, such as the intestine or uterus. When the skeletal structure functions smoothly, the body's natural healing processes are free to keep the entire system working in harmony.

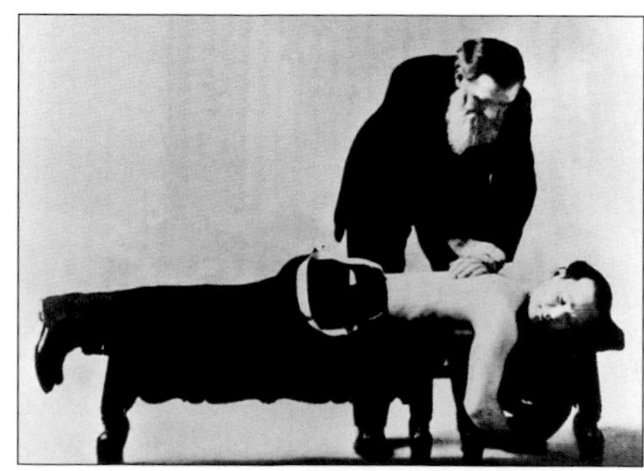

***Palmer, above**, founded a chiropractic school in the US in 1897, but the first license to practice was not issued until Kansas passed a state law in 1913.*

EVIDENCE & RESEARCH

A substantial body of scientific research now exists to support the efficacy of chiropractic for acute lower back pain. Recent studies have found it not only clinically convincing but also cost-effective.

Studies at the College of William and Mary in Williamsburg, Virginia (1992), showed that chiropractic compared favorably with traditional medical treatments in terms of effectiveness and cost. A study by the Rand Corporation in Los Angeles (1992) marked the first time that representatives of the medical community went on record stating that chiropractic is an appropriate treatment for certain causes of lower back pain.

In 1990 and 1995 the *British Medical Journal* published results of multicenter trials that showed that patients receiving chiropractic treatment for lower back pain improved more than those receiving standard hospital outpatient care.

Studies undertaken by the Australian Centre for Chiropractic Research in 1991 showed chiropractic to be twice as effective as standard medical health care for back injuries, with major savings in compensation for injury at work.

MEDICAL OPINION

Thanks to positive studies in reputable journals, medical opinion is generally well disposed. Yet most doctors know little about chiropractic and are unsure how to incorporate it into their practice. Outside the US, it is still unusual for a chiropractor to work in a conventional medical setting, but as research accumulates and the profession establishes legal codes of practice, the situation is likely to improve.

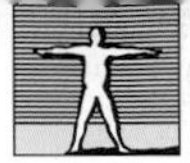

THE THEORY OF CHIROPRACTIC

The spine is the most important support in the body structure, and it protects the nervous system – the communication highway between the brain and the body. Any spinal misalignments, known to chiropractors as "subluxations" or "fixations," not only cause back pain, but may affect the functioning of the whole body. Treatment focuses on joint manipulation; some methods resemble those used in osteopathy (see page 77).

THE SPINE & NERVOUS SYSTEM

***The spinal cord** is the link that carries the nerves to the rest of the body. Any disruption to this link affects not only the muscles, nerves, and ligaments of the back, but also of the neck, shoulders, arms, and legs.*

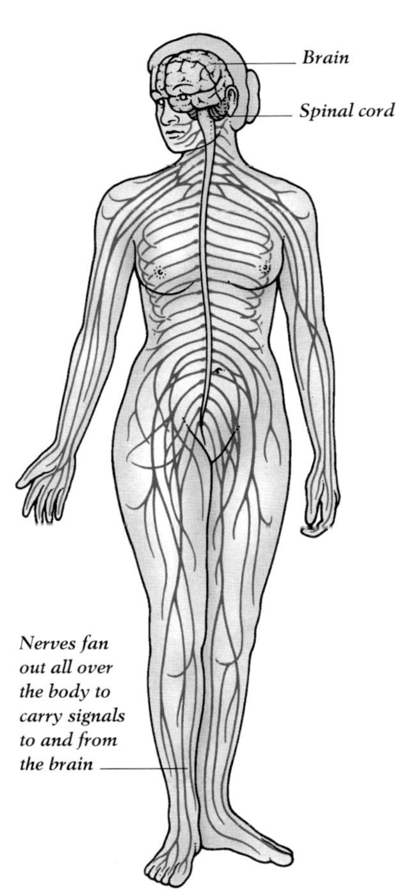

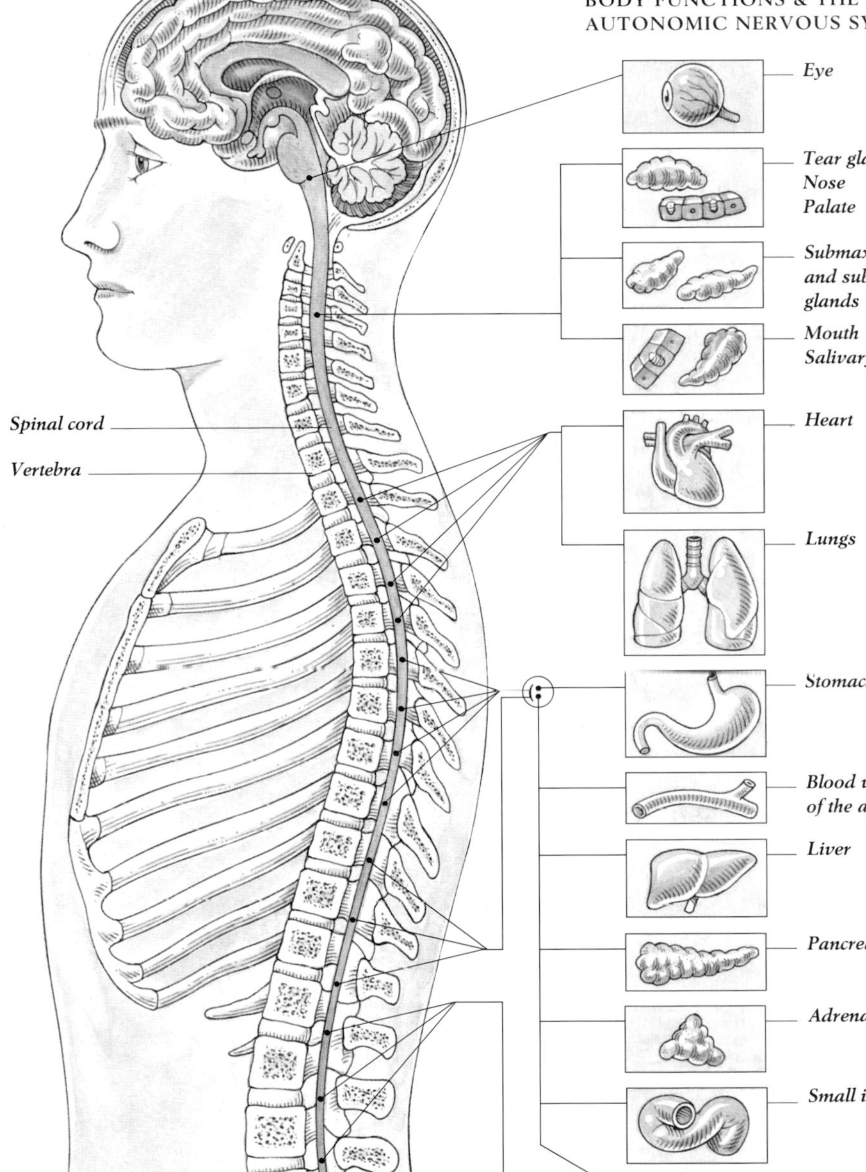

AUTONOMIC NERVOUS SYSTEM

***Protected within the spine**, this system regulates seemingly automatic internal body functions such as sweating, digestion, and heart rate. The nerves to each of these body systems emerge from the spine at particular vertebrae. Any strain, damage, or distortion of the spine can interfere with these nerves, causing disruption to the smooth working of the internal organs, glands, blood vessels, and the heart, and preventing homeostasis – the body's self-regulating and healing processes (see page 26).*

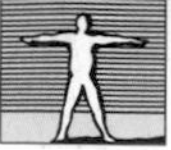

Consulting a Practitioner

The practitioner begins by taking a detailed medical history, both of current and past problems, including any past injuries or surgery that may have contributed to your condition. She will ask about your lifestyle and work, and observe your posture and gait; she may also carry out some diagnostic tests. Your diet and any recreational drugs (including caffeine and tobacco) will be noted, and you will be asked how you sit at your desk, what exercise you get, and even what kind of bed you have.

The practitioner will maneuver you into various positions so that she can examine the functioning of your spinal column, joints, and muscles. You will be asked to stand, sit, or lie on a specially adjustable chiropractic table which enables even sufferers of severe back pain to be lowered from a standing position.

Treatment usually begins with your second consultation, after any diagnostic tests have been returned. The practitioner usually uses precise and well-controlled techniques known as "adjustments," although sometimes other, less forceful techniques might be employed, or gentle touch applied along the spine, skull, and pelvis.

Surgery is never used, and if drugs or treatment other than chiropractic is considered necessary, such as in the case of severe inflammation, you will be referred to your doctor or a suitable specialist.

Precautions

- Tell your chiropractor if you have osteoporosis or inflammation, signs of infection, tumors, circulatory problems (particularly aneurysms), or a recent fracture. While chiropractors may decide not to treat some of these conditions, they are skilled in pain relief methods that can ease discomfort in some of the conditions listed.
- See also page 52.

A physical examination will be necessary, so expect to undress to your underwear; if you feel uncomfortable, a gown will be provided

Checking the Spine

With the patient seated, the practitioner uses her hands to discover which spinal joints are moving freely and which joints are stiff or "locked." This is known as "motion palpation." The practitioner is usually able to locate the exact source of any general pain.

The practitioner applies pressure to the vertebrae and locates the site of the pain

Adjustable seats allow patient and practitioner to sit in a suitable position

Special Equipment

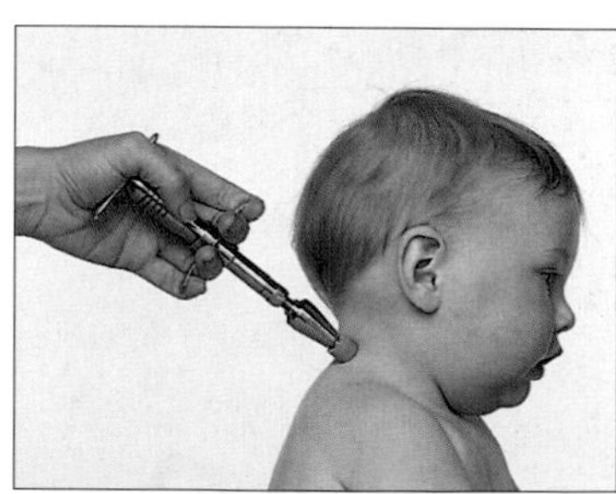

***A rubber-tipped instrument** known as an Activator, rather than the hand, is sometimes used to manipulate the vertebrae. It is used particularly with older patients or babies, since it is designed to deliver a very small, precise, measured thrust. This extra control is important if the patient is frail or delicate, or if the bones are still young.*

Standard Tests

Great care is taken to ensure that diagnosis is precise, so other standard medical, neurological, and orthopedic tests may also be carried out.

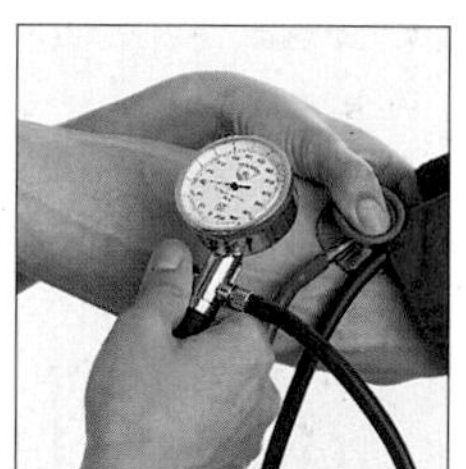

***Blood pressure** is often measured.*

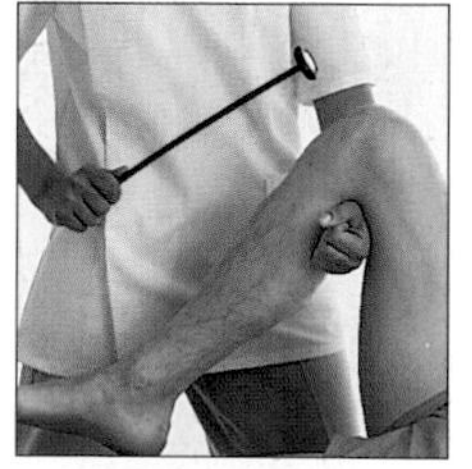

***Reflexes** are tested with a reflex hammer.*

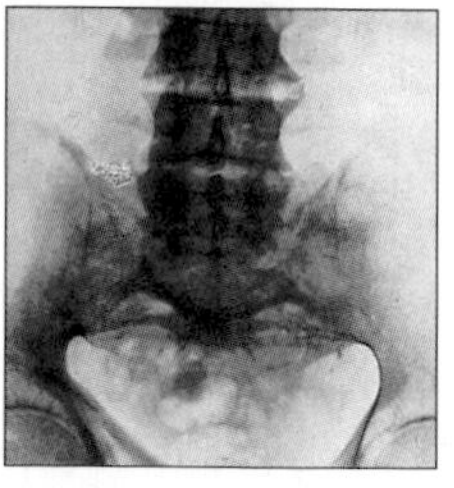

***An X ray** may be taken if considered clinically necessary.*

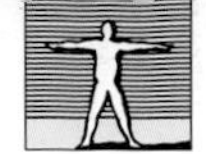

CHECKING THE HIP, PELVIS & LOWER SPINE

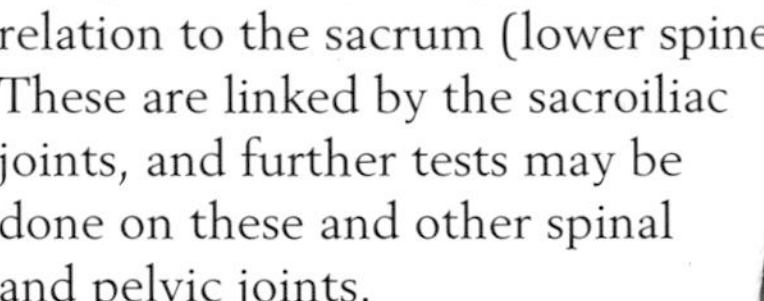

Using her hands, the practitioner tests how the pelvis moves in relation to the sacrum (lower spine). These are linked by the sacroiliac joints, and further tests may be done on these and other spinal and pelvic joints.

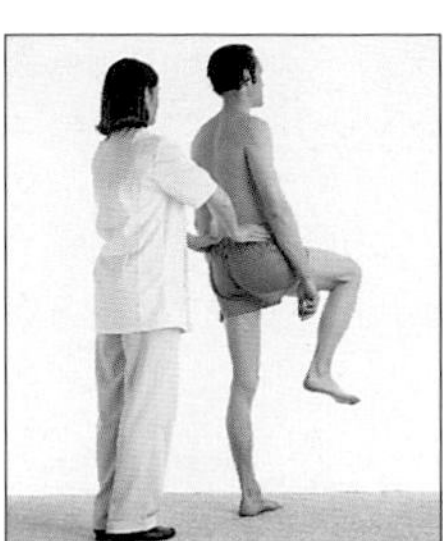

Marching *in place shows the pelvic action.*

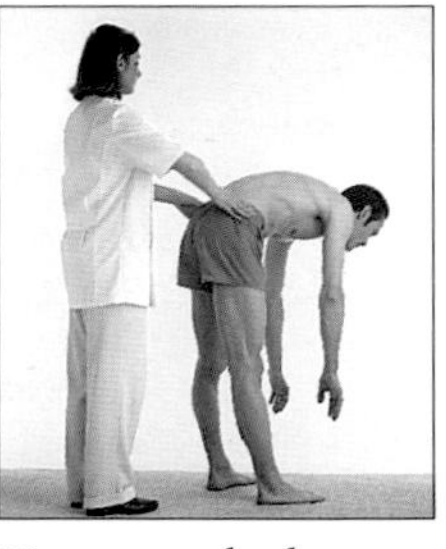

You may *also be asked to bend over.*

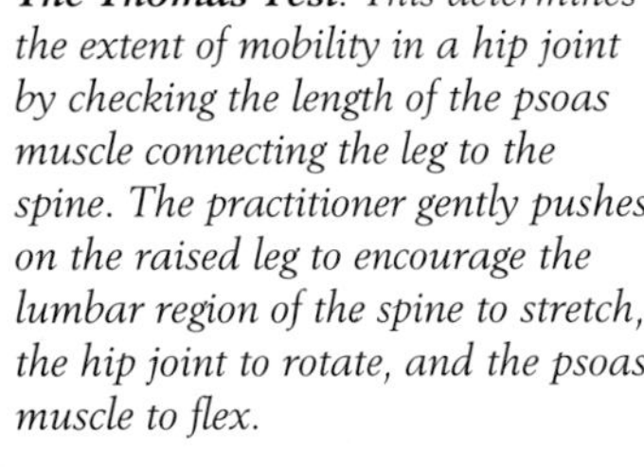

The Thomas Test: *This determines the extent of mobility in a hip joint by checking the length of the psoas muscle connecting the leg to the spine. The practitioner gently pushes on the raised leg to encourage the lumbar region of the spine to stretch, the hip joint to rotate, and the psoas muscle to flex.*

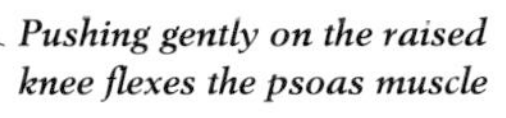

Pushing gently on the raised knee flexes the psoas muscle

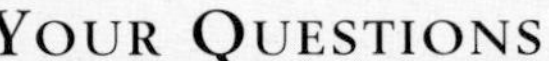

YOUR QUESTIONS

How long does a treatment session last?
The first session is roughly 30–60 minutes; subsequent sessions last 15–20 minutes.

How many sessions will I need?
You may have two or three sessions a week, and weekly sessions later, but this depends on the condition and on how quickly you respond to treatment. Many chiropractors advise maintenance visits to keep potential problems at bay.

Will it be uncomfortable?
Some immediate pain may accompany the adjustment but this eases quickly.

Will there be any aftereffects?
Though athletes frequently compete right after treatment, you may get aches and stiffness for a few days as muscles and joints realign, and feel a little tired for a day as your body recovers.

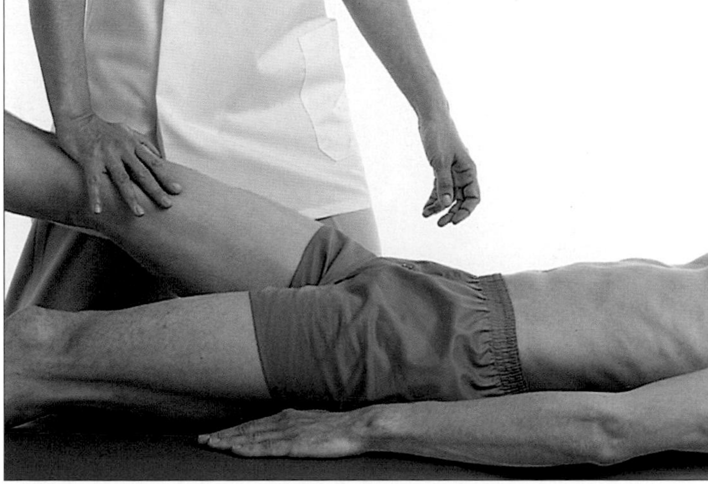

The Psoas Muscle Test: *The practitioner may use this to test the joints between the vertebrae. Asking the patient to raise his leg, she pushes against it, using the groin and upper leg muscles to exert gentle tension on the lower spine. This tests for pain, inflammation, and imbalance.*

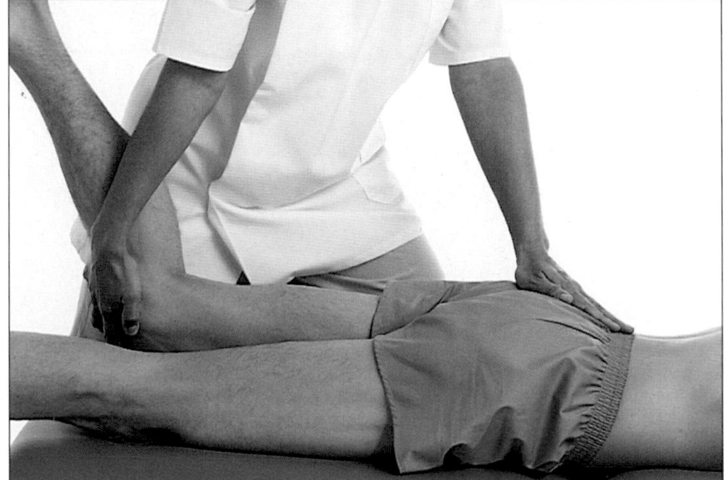

The Yeoman's Test: *If the sacroiliac joints (which link the sacrum to the pelvis) are strained, the patient may experience pain in the lower back and buttocks. The practitioner flexes the patient's leg and extends the thigh to test the joints for any sprain and for mobility.*

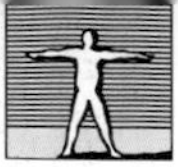

LOWER BACK TREATMENT

Back pain is a commonly encountered health problem, and one with which chiropractic has demonstrated particular success. "Unlocking" a joint by using chiropractic adjustment is usually painless, and can bring immediate relief from pain and an increased range of movement for the patient. With any chiropractic adjustment, there may be an audible, painless "click" in the relevant joint. This is caused by a tiny gas bubble that is created when the pressure in the joint changes, as happens when it is suddenly stretched.

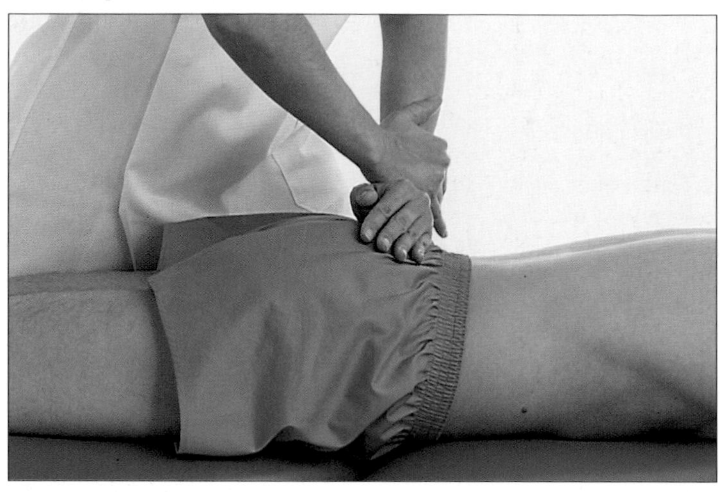

***The Toggle Drop**: This treatment aims to improve mobility in the vertebral joints between the sacrum and pelvis. With hands crossed, the practitioner presses down swiftly to adjust a specific vertebra with a precise thrust.*

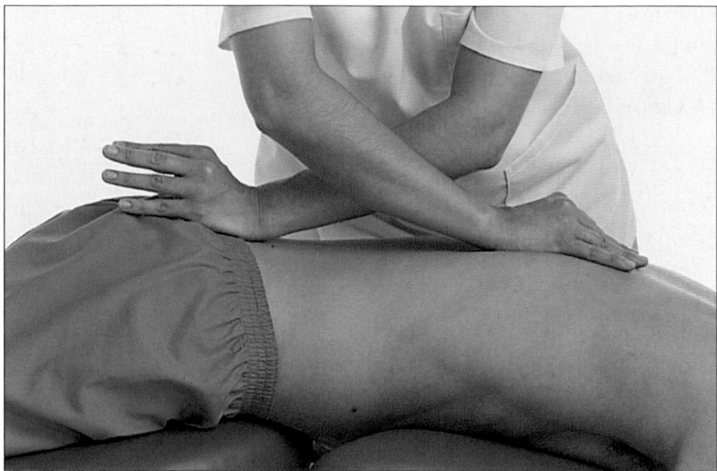

***Spinal traction**: For this maneuver, the table is adjusted to curve the patient's spine slightly. Using precise, gentle pressure, the practitioner pushes with her hands to stretch apart the vertebrae of the lower spine.*

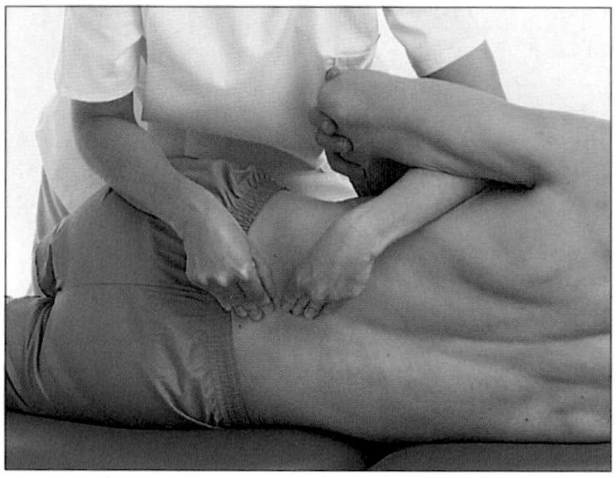

***Release Work**: The chiropractor gently separates the projections of the vertebrae with her fingers to release tension.*

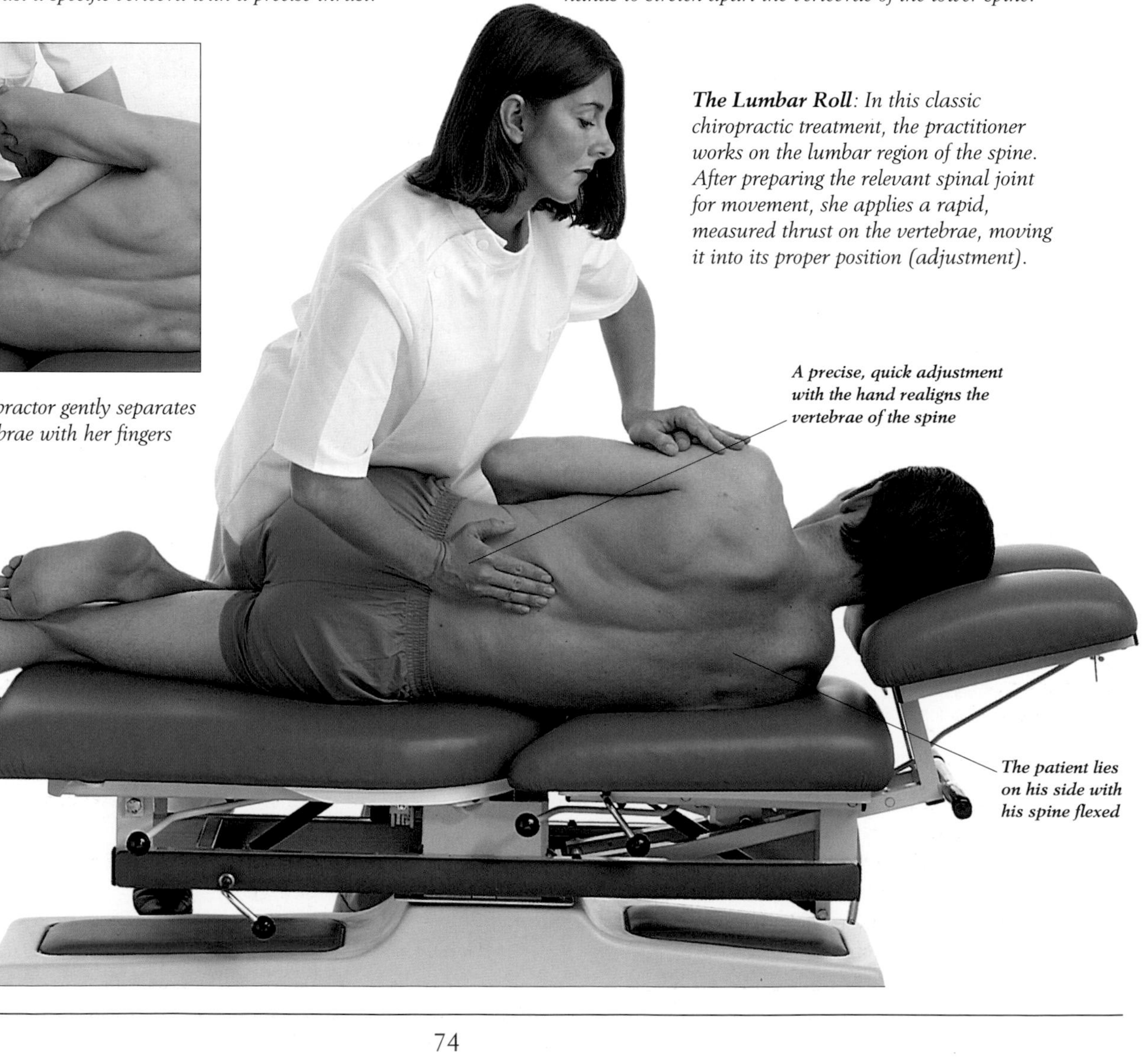

***The Lumbar Roll**: In this classic chiropractic treatment, the practitioner works on the lumbar region of the spine. After preparing the relevant spinal joint for movement, she applies a rapid, measured thrust on the vertebrae, moving it into its proper position (adjustment).*

A precise, quick adjustment with the hand realigns the vertebrae of the spine

The patient lies on his side with his spine flexed

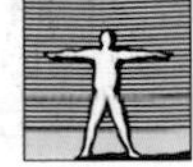

A Patient's Experience

Jenny, aged 45, is a schoolteacher and mother. She had suffered from lower back pain and headaches for some time: "When the chiropractor asked me about past accidents, I remembered being hit by a car when I was ten. On the first visit he made minor adjustments to my lower back and I felt much better, though I was very tired the next day and the pain eventually returned. Further adjustments were made on the next two visits, but it was the fourth visit that provided a turning point. Now I hardly ever have back pain or headaches, and if I get the slightest twinge in my back, I return to my chiropractor for a maintenance session."

MCTIMONEY & MCTIMONEY-CORLEY CHIROPRACTIC

These variations were developed by John McTimoney and Hugh Corley. McTimoney, a British chiropractor practicing in the 1950s, believed that the body constantly compensates for misalignments by making minor structural adjustments, and that the whole body should be reintegrated at each consultation to ensure full alignment. In 1972 he established a school of McTimoney chiropractic in the UK. Corley, also British, trained under McTimoney, but further developed the "whole body" approach with his own techniques, and established a chiropractic college in the UK in 1984 to teach the McTimoney-Corley method. He also designed preventive exercises that allow patients to control problems themselves.

Both methods adjust joints with a rapid thrust followed by immediate release, using the elasticity of ligaments and tendons to encourage misaligned bones to "toggle" back into proper position. McTimoney-Corley chiropractors also practice a gentle technique using only the fingertips. Called the Reflex Recoil Adjustment, it is a light method of vertebral manipulation. These gentle techniques are relatively comfortable to receive, and babies and the elderly may find them particularly acceptable.

Network Chiropractic

This variation was initiated in 1979 by Dr. Donald Epstein, an American chiropractor. Using light, supple movements, practitioners adjust each vertebra in relationship to the rest of the spine, since they believe that the spine protects an essential channel of energy and information to the body.

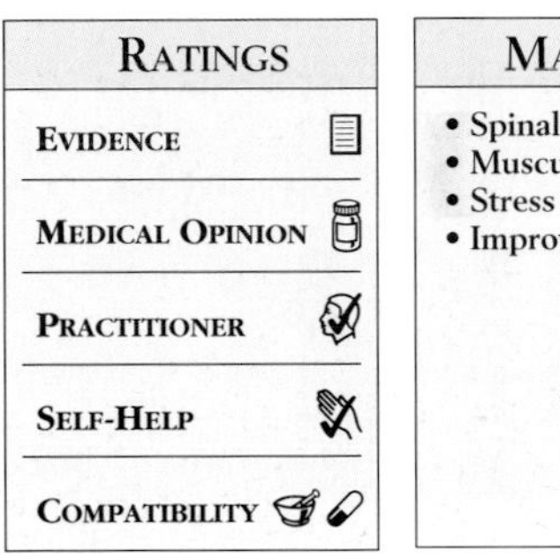

HISTORY

Dr. Epstein's system of Network Spinal Analysis integrates points of agreement from diverse chiropractic approaches. The system diverges in its belief that there are two types of subluxations, structural (arising from physical stresses) and facilitated (arising from emotional stresses). The practitioner addresses them in different ways.

A 1995 survey of 3,000 patients of Network Spinal Analysis conducted by the University of California at Irvine suggests that Network Spinal Analysis is associated with improvements in self-reported health, an important indicator of actual health.

Postgraduate training in Network Spinal Analysis was first offered in the US in 1995. Certification is now granted in the three levels of care that the system provides.

CONSULTING A PRACTITIONER

The practitioner uses a specialized system of evaluating the spine that focuses on the way individual vertebrae interact. She makes adjustments to subluxations, following a unique sequence, or "network." The sequence involves 12 different techniques, which are applied with careful timing.

Facilitated subluxations are generally addressed with the Logan Basic Technique – light steady pressure applied to the spine, mainly in the upper cervical area. Structural subluxations may be addressed with the Toggle-Recoil Technique – a quick thrust with the heel of the hand. The types of adjustments used change according to improvements in spinal function.

At your first consultation the practitioner will take a history of previous chiropractic care and an inventory of physical and mental stresses. She will examine your muscle tone, leg length, and any tension in the ankles and heels, and assess spinal function in respect to breathing. X rays may be taken, but are not standard. Level 1 care then begins.

The goal of Level 1 care, which is usually given three times a week for 1–2 months, is to return as much function to the spine as possible and to increase body awareness. At Level 2, visits twice a week for 2–4 months ease not only the spine, but the whole body. Self-help begins at Level 2, when you have developed sufficient body awareness to be able to focus on specific sites and release any tension.

By this point, the spine is self-correcting. General function and well-being have improved. Some people continue to Level 3, also called Wellness Care. Self-directed, it is determined by each person's needs and goals. Sessions may take place once a week; a quality-of-life inventory is made periodically.

MEDICAL OPINION

Many doctors do not distinguish between the different chiropractic approaches. The effectiveness of the more vigorous manipulations would seem more understandable to a doctor than the gentle maneuvers of Network Chiropractic, which is currently the subject of research studies.

PRECAUTIONS

• See chiropractic (page 72) and page 52.

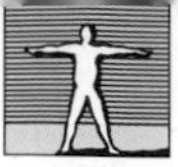

Osteopathy

Ratings	
Evidence	
Medical Opinion	
Practitioner	
Self-Help	
Compatibility	

This holistic approach to diagnosis and treatment originated in the United States in the late 19th century. Practitioners use touch and manipulation of the musculoskeletal system to restore or improve mobility and balance, and thereby enhance well-being. Techniques range from gentle massage to high-velocity mobilization of the joints. Now established alongside conventional medicine in North America, and practiced throughout Europe and Australasia, osteopathy is one of the most respected and widely used complementary therapies, particularly for pain in the back and joints.

Main Uses

- Back & neck pain
- Joint pain, such as arthritis
- Sciatica
- Sports injuries & repetitive strain injuries
- Headaches
- Insomnia, depression
- Menstrual pain
- Digestive disorders
- Asthma

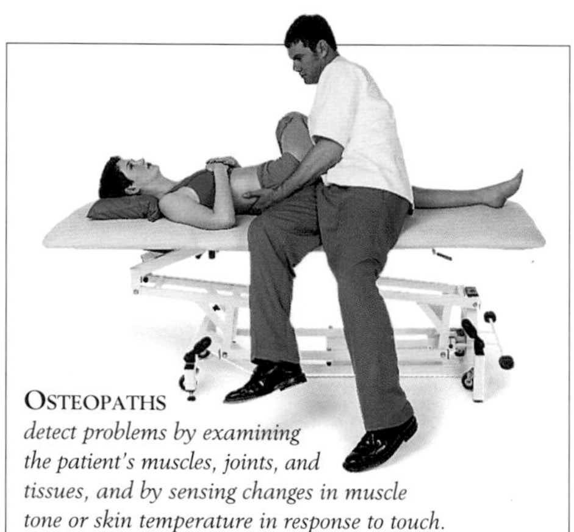

Osteopaths *detect problems by examining the patient's muscles, joints, and tissues, and by sensing changes in muscle tone or skin temperature in response to touch.*

History

Osteopathy, from the Greek *osteon* (bone) and *pathos* (disease), was developed by Dr. Andrew Taylor Still of Virginia, who was an army doctor in the Civil War. Prompted by the tragic deaths of his wife and three of his children from meningitis, in 1872 he devised osteopathy to stimulate the body's self-healing powers.

In 1892 Dr. Still founded the American School of Osteopathy. Despite initial opposition from the conventional medical establishment, the therapy proved popular, receiving a major boost during the flu epidemic of 1919, when the mortality rate for patients in osteopathic hospitals was far below that in conventional hospitals. In 1917 one of Still's pupils, Dr. John Martin Littlejohn, founded the British School of Osteopathy in London.

In the US, osteopaths have been licensed as conventional doctors since 1972. In the UK, osteopathy gained official recognition with the passing of the Osteopathy Act in 1993. Osteopathy is popular in Japan, Australasia, North America, and Europe.

Key Principles

The organs of the body are supported and protected by the musculoskeletal system (see opposite). If this system of joints and muscles is correctly aligned and working well, the tissues of the body, including the brain and nerves, will be healthy, and the circulatory, lymphatic, and digestive systems will function properly. Osteopaths aim to improve the mobility of the joints and soft tissues using various manual techniques.

An osteopath will be as concerned about *why* there is a fault in the musculoskeletal framework as with the physical problem itself, and will look for the reasons behind the problem. For this holistic approach, lifestyle and mental and emotional health are seen as important factors influencing physiological health.

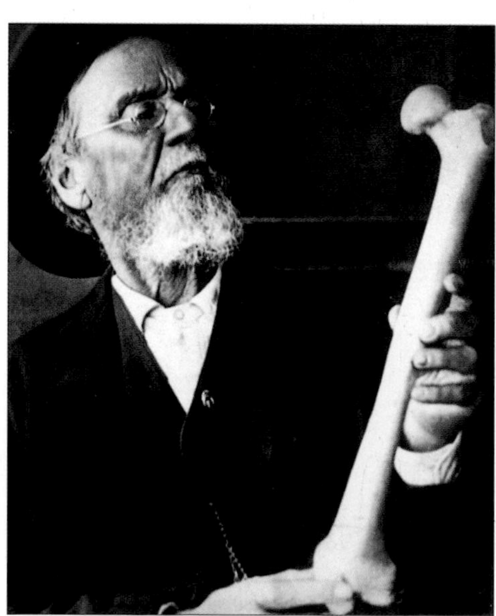

***Dr. Andrew Taylor Still**, who developed osteopathy, considered that all disease was related to the body's musculoskeletal framework.*

Evidence & Research

There has been a considerable amount of research into osteopathy in the US, though not to a consistently high standard. Much evidence is anecdotal and most osteopaths accept that more clinically controlled trials need to be carried out. Research studies are under way in the UK, including Department of Health pilot projects to test the possibility of doctors referring National Health Service (NHS) patients to osteopaths and chiropractors. In 1994, the Clinical Standards Advisory Group recommended that manipulation should be available for NHS patients with acute back pain, and that doctors should work more closely with osteopaths, chiropractors, and physiotherapists.

Two studies, published in the US and UK in 1988 and 1990 respectively, showed that osteopathic manipulation could improve recovery time for lower back pain patients. During the 1940s, an American physiologist used electrical measurements to confirm osteopaths' claims of increased activity in muscles.

Medical Opinion

With official recognition as doctors for over two decades, American osteopaths are part of the medical mainstream, and osteopathy is increasingly being integrated into the practice of medicine worldwide. Although perhaps a third of doctors in the UK refer patients to osteopaths, some are still reluctant to do so, especially when the patient's problem is not musculoskeletal. The establishment of the UK General Council of Osteopaths in 1996 should build a basis for strong cooperation with the medical profession.

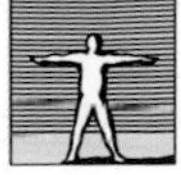

THE THEORY OF OSTEOPATHY

Physical or emotional stress, injury, or poor posture can affect the musculoskeletal system. They can cause pain or impair nerve function locally or elsewhere in the body, and affect the vital organs and respiratory, circulatory, and nervous systems. Osteopathy aims to ease muscle tension and restore bone and joint function to strengthen the body systems and restore the body's ability to heal itself. While chiropractors often concentrate on manipulation of misaligned joints, osteopaths may focus on "soft tissue" treatment to relax muscles and bring back joint mobility.

THE MUSCULO-SKELETAL SYSTEM

Osteopaths believe *that this mechanical system, comprising the bones, joints, muscles, ligaments, and connective tissue, is not merely scaffolding for the rest of the body, but plays a vital part in maintaining health. Any disturbance of this system can cause pain and strain, and affect other body systems (see also page 71).*

Layers of skeletal muscles overlap in intricate patterns
Spine forms a strong, flexible support for the head and body
Musculo-skeletal structure consists of over 600 muscles
An average adult human body contains 206 bones

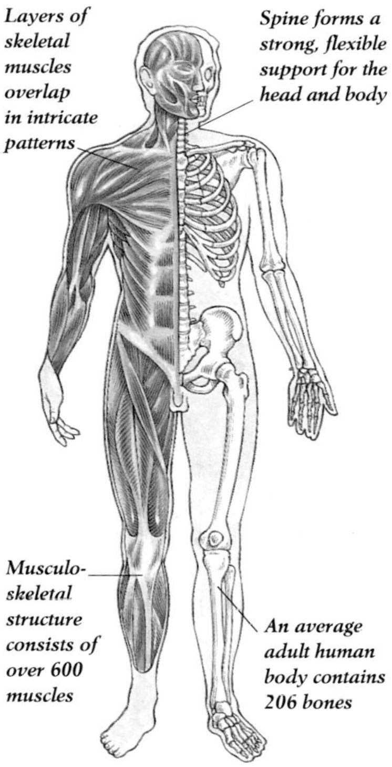

HOW THE BRAIN REGISTERS & RESPONDS TO PAIN

Muscle, bone, and joint pain *registers in the cortex of the brain, but other areas of the brain influence how the mind perceives and adapts to this pain. An osteopath will use soft tissue manipulation and mobilization of the vertebrae around tense areas of the spine to relax the muscles at the local source of the pain. He will also seek to ease tension in other muscles whose nerves pass through the irritated area of the spine, and examine underlying factors, such as poor posture or anxiety, that cause or perpetuate tension either locally or elsewhere in the body.*

Hypothalamus controls automatic body processes, including muscle tension and blood supply to muscles
Thalamus influences the emotions
Hippocampus is involved in memory storage
Frontal lobe of cortex governs ideas and expectations
Cerebellum is linked to posture and muscle tone
Brain stem regulates the release of endorphins
A spinal segment includes all the tissues supplied by the nerves of a particular section of spinal cord
If the spinal joint is affected by injury or strain, it stiffens up and makes the whole segment vulnerable to irritation
The muscle supplied by the spinal joint can be affected by pain and tension spreading out from the joint; if pain and tension persists, it puts strain on other areas as the body tries to adapt
The nerves supplying the muscle can be affected by pain from injury to a muscle; the spinal joints relating to those nerves consequently stiffen

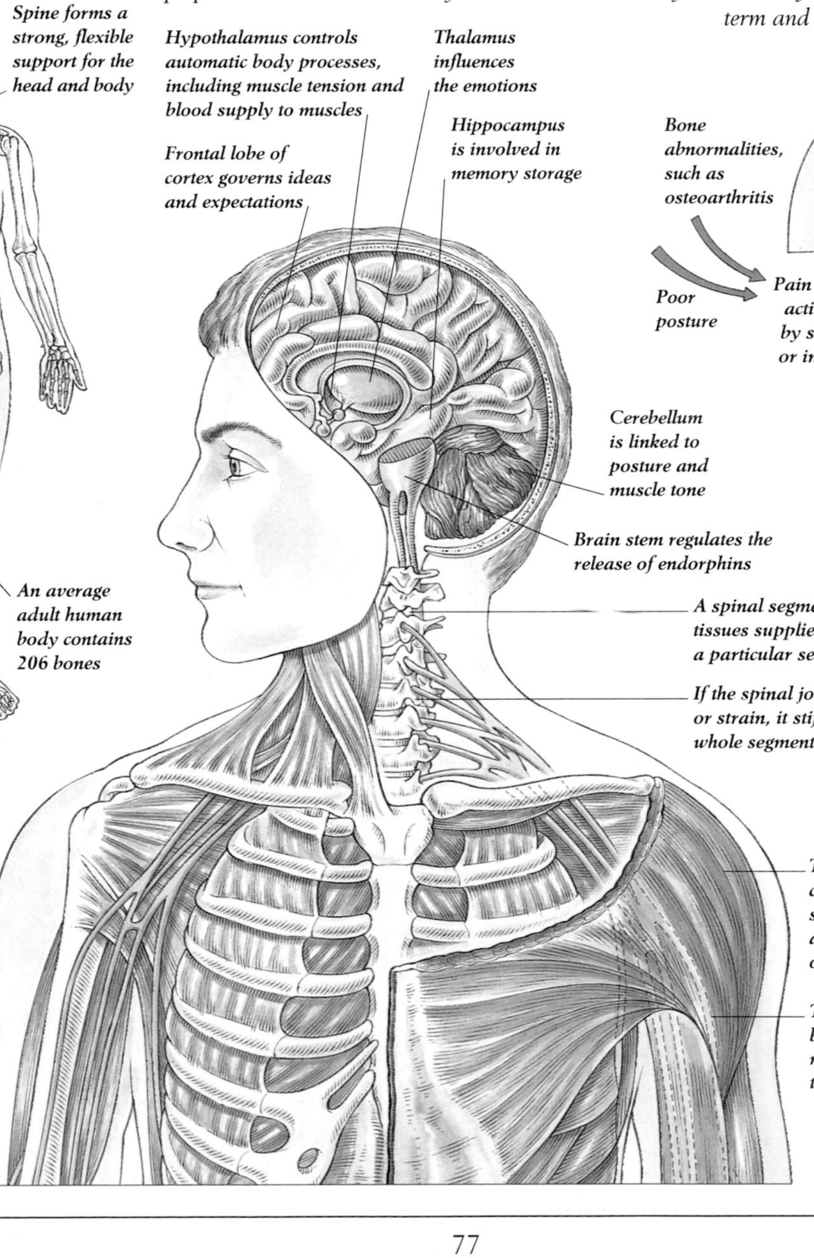

THE PAIN–TENSION CYCLE

The various factors *that contribute to pain can form a vicious cycle. Pain signals (caused by strain or injury or by the buildup of chemical waste products, such as lactic acid) pass from a muscle or joint to the spinal segment that supplies its nerves. This segment then sends back reflex nerve impulses to the muscle that tense the muscle even more. The spinal segment also becomes more open to irritation, and may become more sensitive in the long term and therefore prone to further problems.*

Bone abnormalities, such as osteoarthritis
Poor posture
Pain nerves activated by strains or injuries
Pain nerves activated by chemical waste products in the muscle (cramp)
Spinal reflexes
Muscle tension
Incorrect or excessive moving or lifting
Anxiety or stress

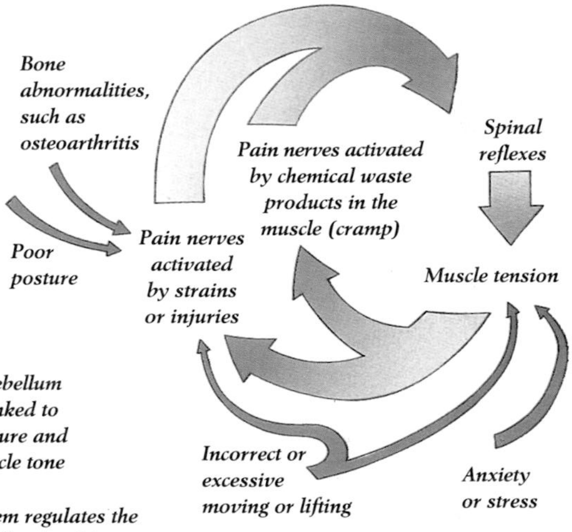

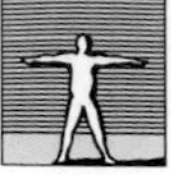

CONSULTING A PRACTITIONER

At the first consultation the practitioner will ask how your symptoms began and what activities make them worse. He will ask about your medical history, especially any past injuries, about any medication you are taking, including homeopathic and herbal remedies, and about your lifestyle, work, and emotional health.

Be prepared to undress to your underwear, so that the practitioner can see as much of your body framework as possible. You may be offered a gown if you feel uncomfortable. In order to assess the way you hold yourself and how the joints are functioning, you may be asked to stand, sit, and lie down on a treatment table. The practitioner will probably examine your muscles for stresses and strains and will ask you to bend in various ways while feeling your spine. Standard medical tests are carried out, and arrangements are made for X rays or blood tests where necessary.

This assessment enables the practitioner to make a diagnosis, and decide whether osteopathy can help or whether you should be referred to another specialist.

Any osteopathic treatment will be tailored to your individual needs and adapted as treatment progresses. It may consist simply of soft tissue treatment, using cradling and light pressure, or it may involve vigorous manipulation of the joints, necessitating some rather unusual positions. Discomfort caused by muscle spasm can disappear after one session, but most patients need a course of treatment.

The main osteopathic procedures range from gentle manipulation of the joints, taking the limbs through their full range of movement, to an abrupt high-velocity thrust that, although painless, can cause the joint to "click" disconcertingly. Other techniques include positioning you so that tension from areas of strain or injury is spontaneously released, "muscle energy techniques," in which you release muscle tension by working against resistance provided by the practitioner, and visceral manipulation, in which the practitioner uses touch and pressure to pinpoint and relieve problems in the internal organs.

The practitioner may recommend exercises and relaxation techniques to follow at home or work.

STANDARD TESTS

Diagnostic procedures include conventional medical tests as well as a full examination of the body's structure.

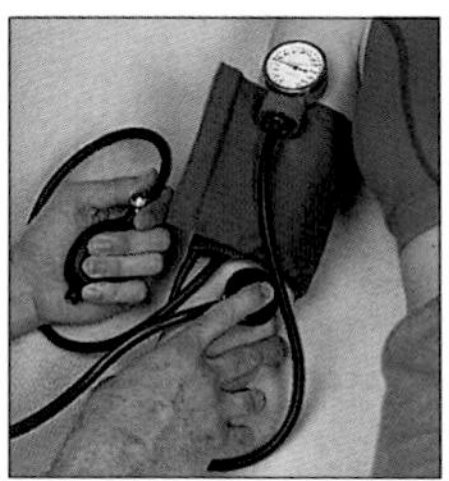

Blood pressure *is measured.*

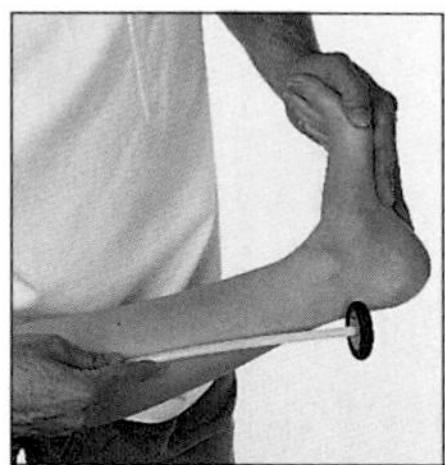

Reflexes *are tested with a reflex hammer.*

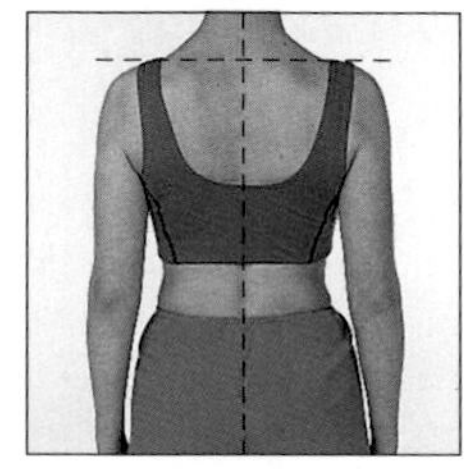

Posture *is examined for asymmetry.*

CHECKING PELVIC ALIGNMENT

The practitioner uses his hands to examine the alignment of the two pelvic bones (the ilia) with the sacrum (the base of the spine) and to check whether one side is higher than the other.

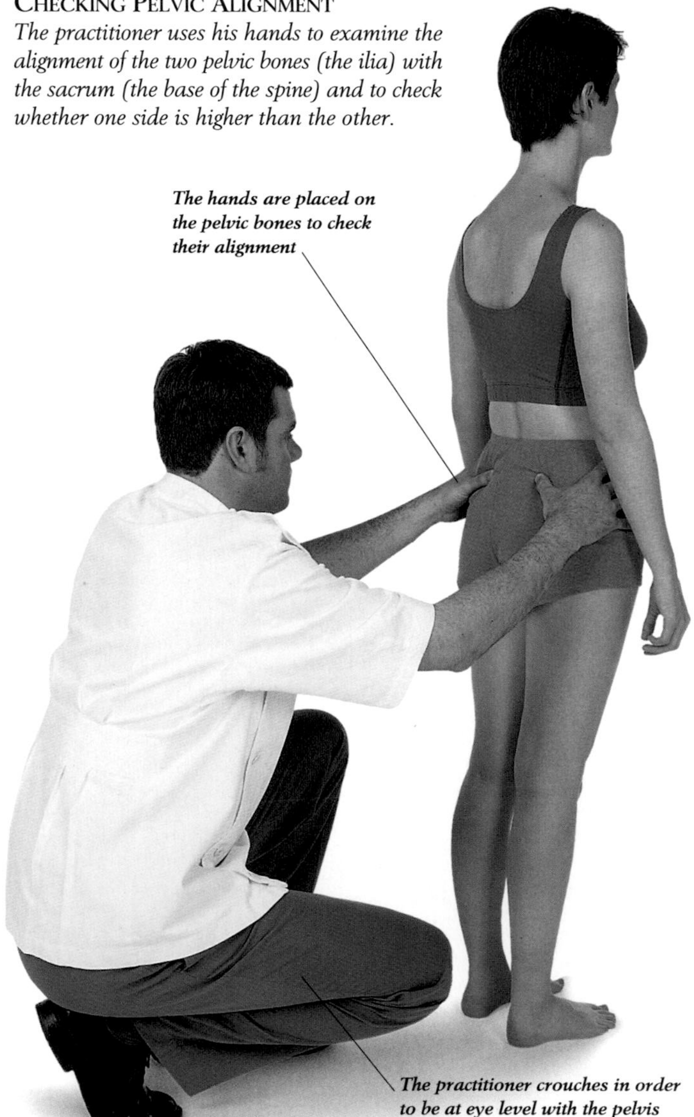

The hands are placed on the pelvic bones to check their alignment

The practitioner crouches in order to be at eye level with the pelvis

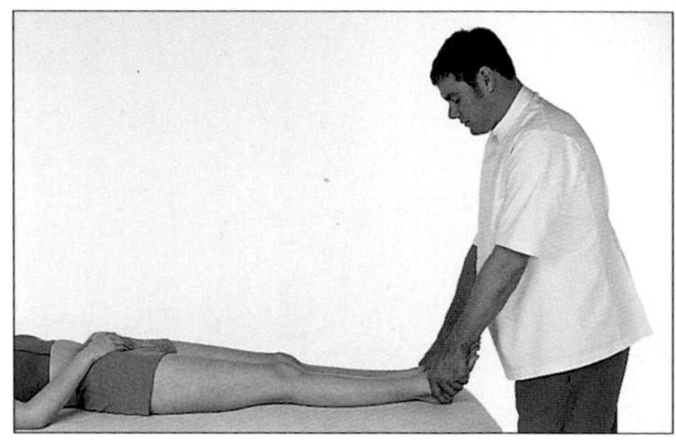

Leg length*: The lengths of the patient's legs are compared. Any discrepancy may indicate a curve in the spine or asymmetry in the pelvis, or show that one leg is structurally shorter than the other.*

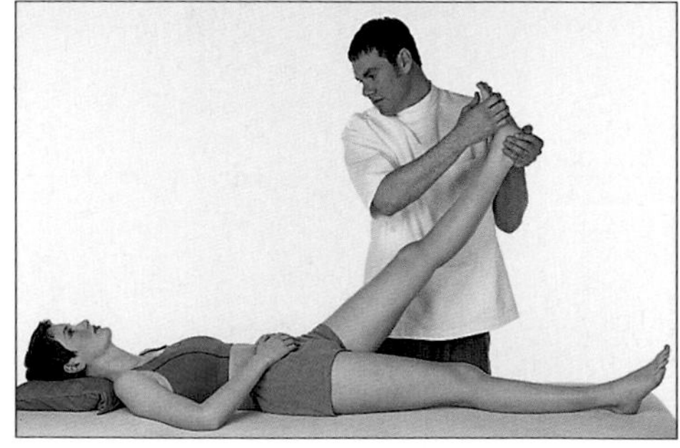

Straight leg raise*: Raising the leg stretches the sciatic nerve and shows the mobility of the lumbar (lower) vertebrae. Pain suggests a disorder in the lumbar spine, usually a disk or joint problem.*

PRECAUTIONS

- Do not have osteopathy if you have bone cancer or any bone or joint infection, such as osteomyelitis.
- Avoid vigorous osteopathic manipulation if you have badly prolapsed disks.
- See also page 52.

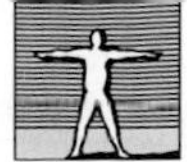

TREATING THE LOWER SPINE

Lower (or lumbar) back pain is a common problem, and one for which osteopathy is often used. Sitting habitually in a slouched position, lifting heavy objects incorrectly, and sports or other injuries all frequently cause lower back pain. The practitioner examines the spine to identify areas of stiffness. He uses soft tissue treatment to relax the area and then may perform precise manipulations, which may be accompanied by a "click" as joints are restored to their full range of movement.

YOUR QUESTIONS

How long does a treatment session last?
The first consultation usually lasts 30–60 minutes; subsequent sessions may last 20–30 minutes.

How many sessions will I need?
One visit may be enough, but three to six sessions are average, depending on your state of health and the problem. More sessions are often needed in old age and for longer-term problems. Some patients have regular sessions as a preventive measure.

Will it be uncomfortable?
Manipulation is not usually painful, but this will depend on the problem.

Will there be any aftereffects?
Some stiffness is common for a day or two following treatment, and strenuous activity should also be avoided during this period.

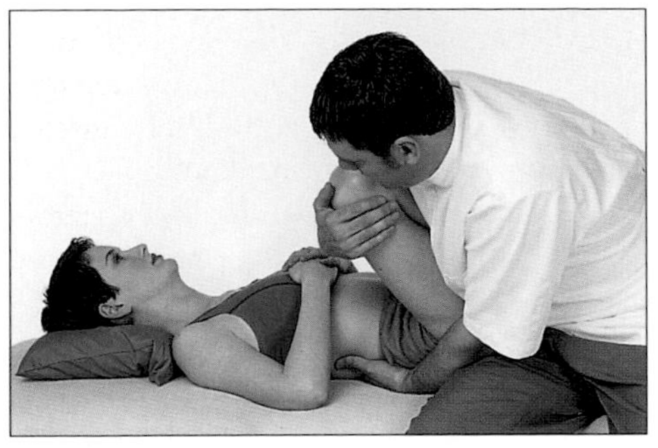

1 With the patient's leg raised and bent to flex and rotate the lumbar vertebrae in the lower back, the practitioner uses his fingers to feel the range of movement of a vertebra and, if necessary, stretch the lumbar spine with a precise movement.

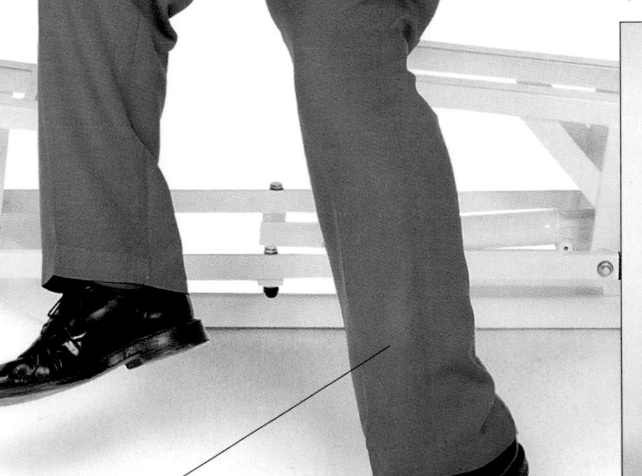

The leg is bent to flex the lumbar vertebrae in the lower spine

The practitioner feels for any restriction of mobility in the spine

Body weight and momentum are used to rotate the patient's vertebrae rhythmically

2 The practitioner repeats this exercise on each lumbar vertebra. As he moves up the spine to examine the next vertebra, he moves the leg to bend and rotate the spine and uses his fingers to monitor the resulting movement of the vertebra.

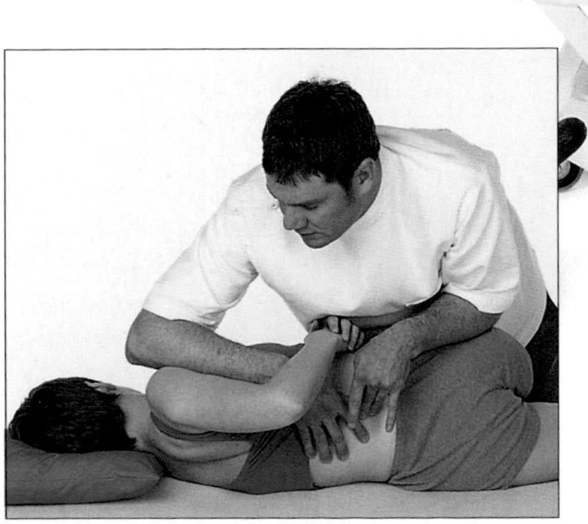

***The Side Roll**: The patient lies on her side with her spine gently rotated to allow the practitioner to target each lumbar vertebra precisely. He examines each vertebra with his fingers to detect and correct any restriction in its range of movement.*

***The Lift**: Pulling the patient's elbows up to "open" her spine, the practitioner uses his body to deliver a high-velocity thrust to a specific area.*

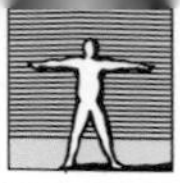

UPPER BACK & NECK TREATMENT

Sprains, stiffness, and injuries such as whiplash or the locking of a vertebra in the neck can be treated with osteopathic manipulation, shown here, or by soft tissue treatment. This uses light massage and rhythmic stretching techniques designed to improve joint mobility by decreasing muscle tension and improving blood supply to the tissue.

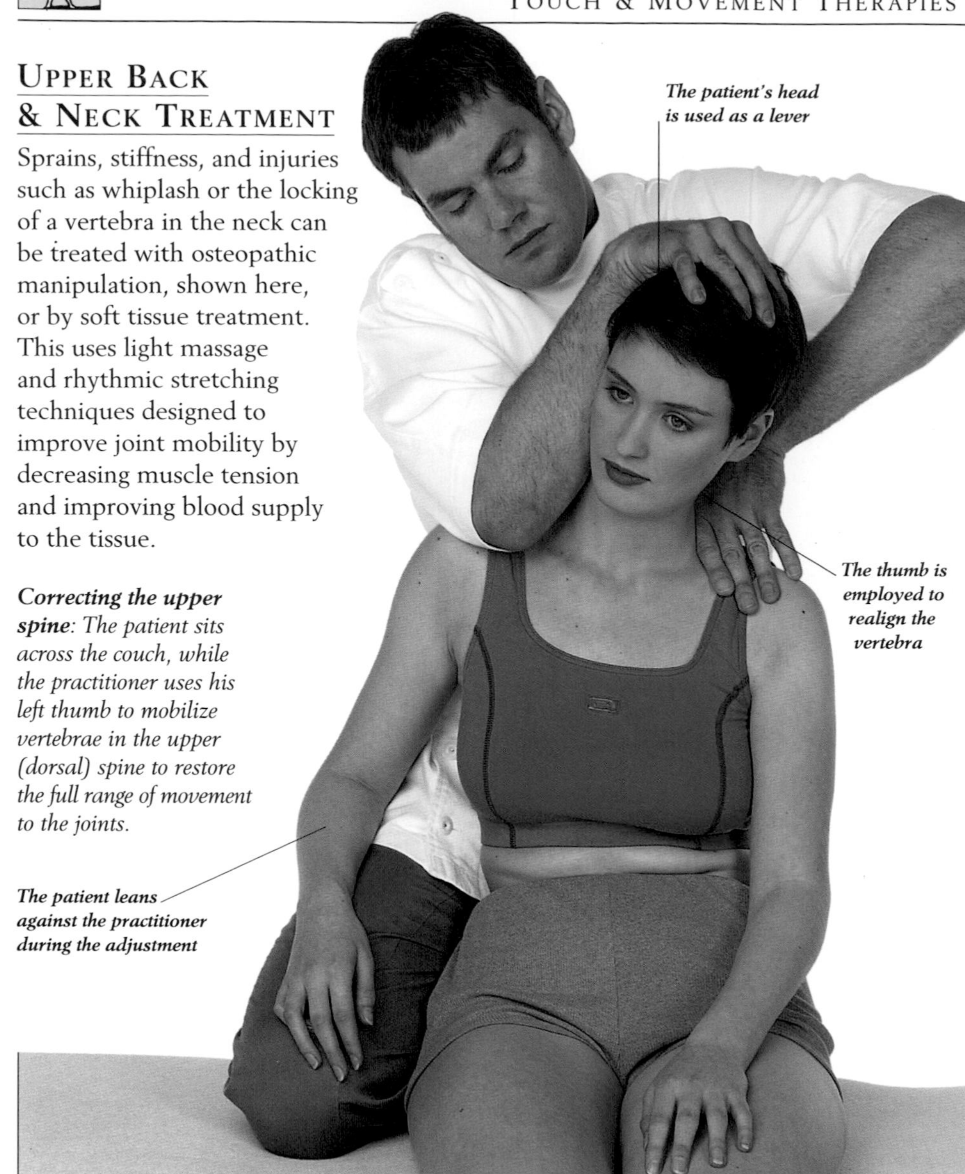

***Correcting the upper spine**: The patient sits across the couch, while the practitioner uses his left thumb to mobilize vertebrae in the upper (dorsal) spine to restore the full range of movement to the joints.*

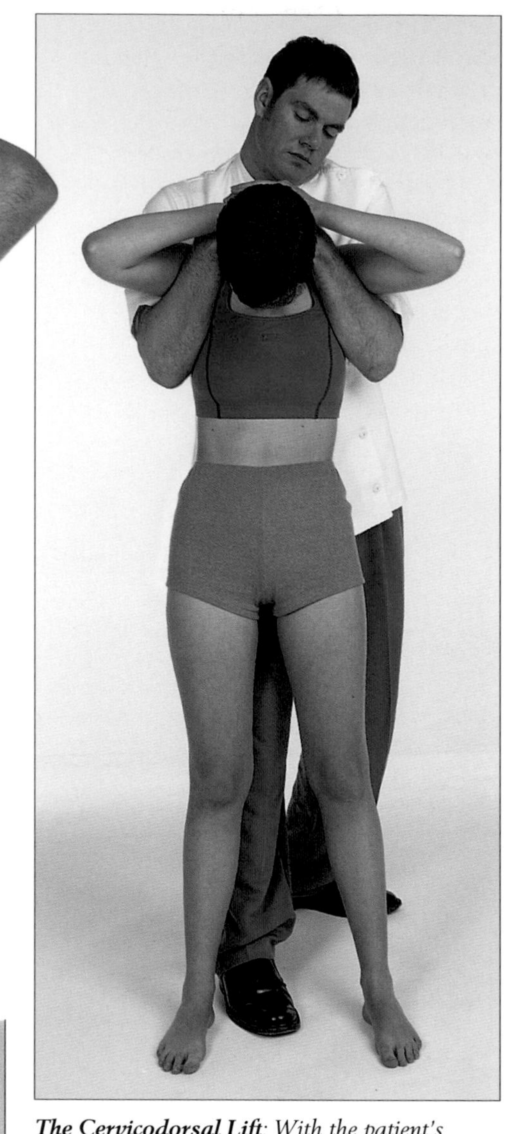

***The Cervicodorsal Lift**: With the patient's hands behind her neck, interlocked with his, the practitioner gently uses his body to stretch and realign her upper spine (cervicodorsal spine).*

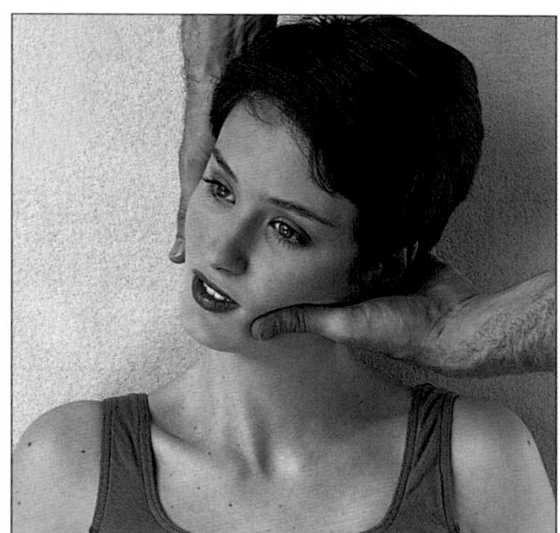

***Correcting the neck (supine)**: For this correction the patient lies face up while the practitioner focuses on the neck (cervical) vertebrae, using the base of his index finger as a lever.*

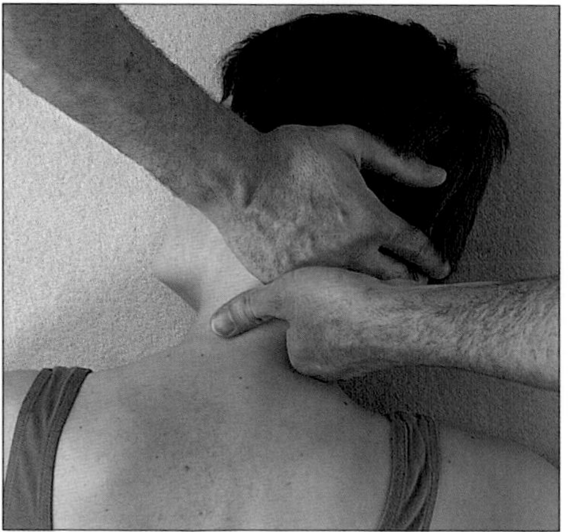

***Correcting the neck (prone)**: Less commonly, the patient may lie on her front as the practitioner corrects the cervical vertebrae in the neck, using the tip or base of his index finger.*

A Patient's Experience

David, 45, works as a chef. He consulted an osteopath while suffering from acute back pain: "I felt a twinge in my back after moving a table and the next day, when I bent over, I collapsed in excruciating agony. I hobbled around to Tom, the osteopath, who was one of our regular customers. He asked me loads of questions, examined me this way and that, and explained that it was a pinched nerve, the culmination of years of minor strains. Tom twisted and turned me to straighten the nerve, and made clicks in my neck, but afterward the pain did ease slightly. He gave me exercises to practice and I went back twice during the following week. Each time my back improved. Now it's fine and I haven't had a problem since."

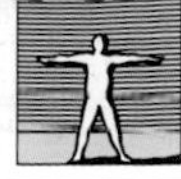

CRANIAL OSTEOPATHY

An American osteopath, Dr. William Garner Sutherland, developed cranial osteopathy in the 1930s. At that time, it was believed that the bones of the cranium (the part of the skull around the brain) fused by adulthood and could not be adjusted. According to Dr. Sutherland, however, these bones, which are separate in babies and young children, do retain flexibility. He also believed that the cerebrospinal fluid, which nourishes and protects the membranes encasing the brain, spinal cord, and sacrum, pulses at a rate of about 6–15 times per minute. This cranial rhythmic impulse (CRI) is difficult to measure with equipment, but practitioners claim to be able to sense it by touch.

Disturbances in the flow of fluid are said to reflect pressures on the cranial bones or injuries and tension in the body, which can be eased by delicate manipulation of the cranial and spinal bones to restore the CRI and boost blood circulation and drainage of lymph and sinus fluids in the head.

Cranial osteopathy may be used for the same conditions as osteopathy, and can be combined with other osteopathic methods. It seems particularly successful on young children with colic, middle ear effusion (glue ear), and recurrent infections, and is often used on babies to correct distortions in the cranial bones caused during birth. If these are not eased back into place, or are knocked slightly out of position later in life, it may lead to physical problems.

Other variations focus less on the bones than on other parts of the cranial system. The reflex approach aims to relieve stress patterns in the body by stimulating nerve endings in the scalp and between the cranial bones. The sacro-occipital technique, preferred by chiropractors, combines elements of cranial osteopathy with craniosacral techniques (see below).

BONES OF THE CRANIUM

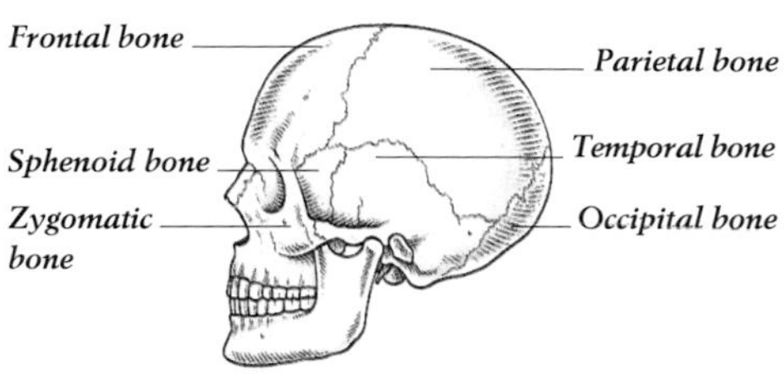

The bones of the cranium *are connected by interlocking joints, or sutures. Cranial osteopathy works to manipulate the bones along these joints.*

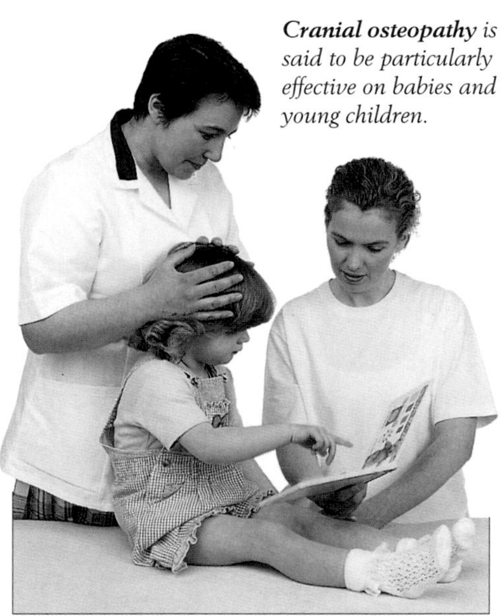

Cranial osteopathy *is said to be particularly effective on babies and young children.*

CranioSacral Therapy

A diagnostic and healing approach based on the application of corrective pressure to the cranium and spine (the craniosacral system), CranioSacral therapy grew out of work with cranial osteopathy in the US during the 1970s. It goes further than cranial osteopathy in claiming that the cranial rhythmic impulse (see above) affects every cell in the body.

RATINGS
EVIDENCE
MEDICAL OPINION
PRACTITIONER
SELF-HELP
COMPATIBILITY

MAIN USES

- Headaches
- Musculoskeletal pain
- Arthritis
- Depression
- Dyslexia & other learning difficulties
- Aftereffects of strokes & meningitis
- Aftereffects of stress or injury

HISTORY

Dr. John Upledger, an osteopath at Michigan State University, developed this approach in the late 1970s. While incorporating some of the techniques practiced in cranial osteopathy, Upledger distinguishes it from osteopathy in being "soft tissue-oriented," "fluid-oriented," and "membrane-oriented" rather than "bone-oriented." The approach is still considered controversial in the UK, though more widely practiced in the US.

CONSULTING A PRACTITIONER

While the bones of the cranium are the focus of cranial osteopathy, CranioSacral therapy focuses on the membranes encasing the brain and spinal cord. Practitioners believe that it is these membranes that generate the cranial rhythmic impulse (CRI) of cerebrospinal fluid, which affects the connective tissues linking all the organs, bones, and muscles of the body. The aim of treatment is to ensure an even, rhythmic flow of CRI.

You will be asked to lie clothed on a treatment table while the practitioner applies subtle pressure with his hands, usually, but not always, on your head or at the base of your spine (the sacrum). Many people report feeling deeply relaxed during treatment, though some experience a spontaneous "unwinding" of tension, believed to result from the release of physical or emotional trauma in the body. One or two treatments of about an hour may be sufficient, but often more sessions are recommended.

MEDICAL OPINION

Doctors skeptical of cranial osteopathy are even more cautious about this. Unlike osteopaths or chiropractors, some CranioSacral practitioners may not have training in anatomy or physiology, and while the therapy is harmless in itself, doctors fear practitioners may fail to recognize serious medical conditions.

PRECAUTIONS

- See osteopathy (page 78) and page 52.

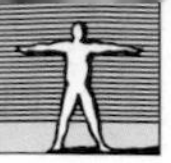

ROLFING

RATINGS
EVIDENCE
MEDICAL OPINION
PRACTITIONER
SELF-HELP
COMPATIBILITY

DR. IDA ROLF, AN AMERICAN BIOCHEMIST, began to develop Rolfing in the 1950s as a system of body education and soft tissue manipulation designed to bring the whole body into vertical alignment. Dr. Rolf believed that the body has a natural symmetry, enabling it to work in harmony with gravity, but that injury, poor posture, or emotional distress could throw it out of alignment. Rolfing has been used by athletes, dancers, and singers to improve breathing patterns and increase suppleness, and many people use it as an aid to physical and emotional well-being.

MAIN USES

- Poor posture
- Sports injuries
- Persistent muscle pain, including neck, shoulder & back pain
- Respiratory problems
- Prevention of postural or stress-related problems
- Promoting health

HISTORY

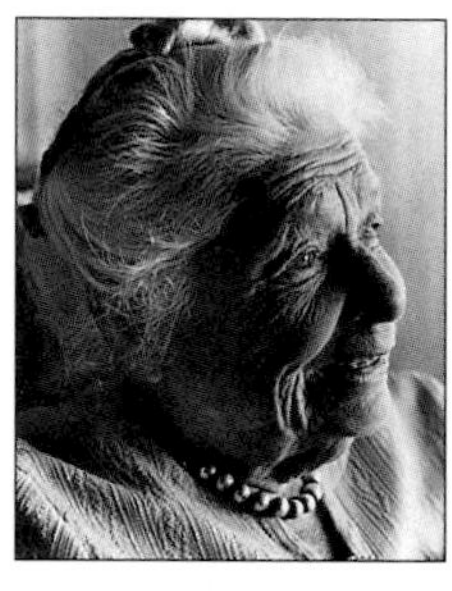

***Dr. Ida Rolf** based her therapy on her knowledge of yoga, physical therapy, and a study of the effects of gravity on the structure of the human body.*

Rolfing, also known as "structural integration," was developed by Dr. Ida Rolf, who became interested in body manipulation after receiving osteopathic treatment for a displaced rib. Dr. Rolf's research led her to conclude that the physical structure of the human body affects its physiological and psychological makeup and is the key to well-being. Her work took many years to gain recognition, but in the 1960s an awakening of interest in the relationship between body and mind, aided by the well-publicized treatment of a number of celebrity clients and the personal growth movement (see page 160), brought Rolfing to the fore as a complementary therapy. In 1971 Dr. Rolf established the Rolf Institute for Structural Integration in Boulder, Colorado. Over 900 practitioners have since been trained by the Institute: most practice in the US, but there are some in Australia, Brazil, and Europe, particularly in Germany and the UK.

KEY PRINCIPLES

Every muscle in the body is enveloped in and separated by a network of thin, elastic connective tissue known as fascia. Rolfers maintain that when the body is subjected to physical or emotional stress, fascia loses pliability and bunches and hardens, so that movement becomes restricted. This process is believed to be gradual, and people subconsciously adapt to cope with the limitations it imposes on the body. They stop breathing easily and moving freely, and as a result they lose their natural vertical alignment. Gradually, the nervous system, circulation, and digestion become impaired, affecting both physical and emotional health and even contributing to premature aging.

Rolfers compare their work to sculpting, realigning the body so that it can work with, rather than against, gravity. In a series of ten sessions they systematically work around the body using firm pressure applied with elbows, fingers, and knuckles to remold the fascia, stretching and opening the soft tissues to correct any misalignment of the head, shoulders, abdomen, pelvis, and legs. Once the body is correctly aligned, aches and pains caused by muscular tension are alleviated.

THE FUNCTION OF FASCIA

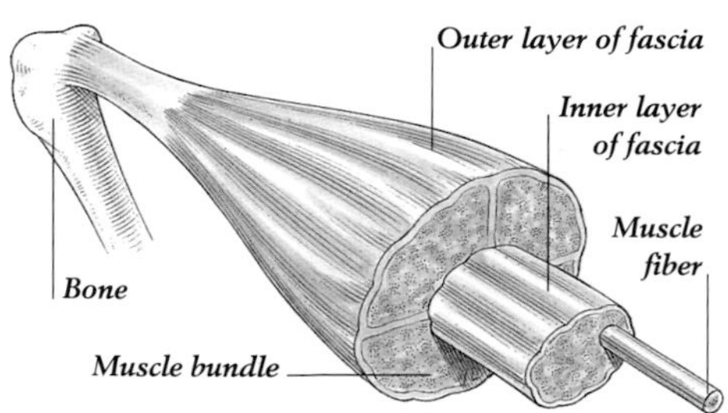

***A kind of connective tissue,** fascia wraps every muscle in the body, forming a sinewy web around and through each layer of muscle. When an area is under strain, fascia shortens and thickens, "storing" tension. Rolfing releases this tension.*

THE BODY'S STRUCTURE

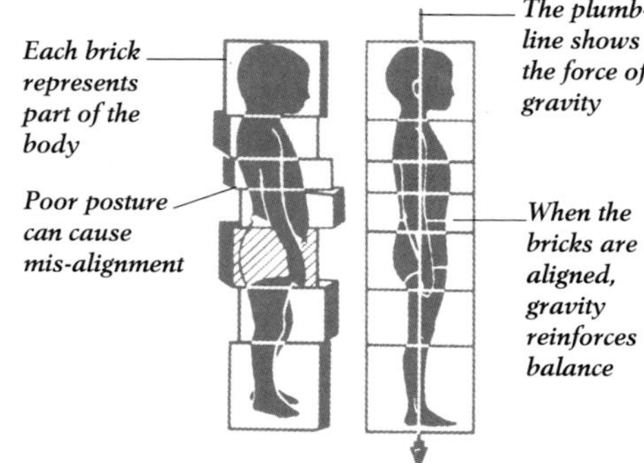

***Dr. Rolf compared the body** to a tower of bricks: any misalignment (above left) puts the structure under stress, but if the bricks are aligned (above right) the structure is stable.*

EVIDENCE & RESEARCH

Clinical studies into Rolfing are limited. However, in 1988, researchers at the University of Maryland found that Rolfing reduced stress, strengthened the body's physical structure, and improved nervous system functioning. In a 1977 study at the University of California at Los Angeles, patients who had received Rolfing exhibited improved posture and body control, and less constrained movements. Rolfing has also been reported to reduce anxiety more efficiently than exercise and to help correct excessive inward curvature of the spine (swayback).

MEDICAL OPINION

Most doctors view Rolfing as a form of massage therapy and see its use as a matter of personal choice, provided the patient is in reasonable mental and physical health, and the practitioner fully trained. Some doctors appreciate its potential value for the treatment of persistent pain.

CONSULTING A PRACTITIONER

Treatment usually consists of ten weekly, one-hour sessions. The practitioner will take a detailed medical and personal history before asking you to undress to your underwear so that she can examine your posture and body structure. Any physical problems revealed are then discussed. Before and after treatment you will be photographed from several angles so that any changes can be recorded. During a session, you lie or sit on a massage table or mat, and the practitioner uses her hands, fingers, knuckles, and elbows in a series of slow movements, often applying considerable pressure that may cause some pain. You will be asked to synchronize your breathing with the manipulation, and sometimes to move your arms and legs in a controlled way. Each session focuses on a particular body area, the final sessions intended to "reset" muscles and fine-tune posture. Treatment can sometimes release memories of emotional anguish. As a follow-up, self-help exercises, known as "movement integration," are often taught.

WORKING ON THE SPINE *In early sessions, the practitioner focuses on areas such as the spine, where the surrounding muscles are close to the surface of the skin.*

The patient breathes in rhythm with the massage

TREATING THE HIPS & PELVIS

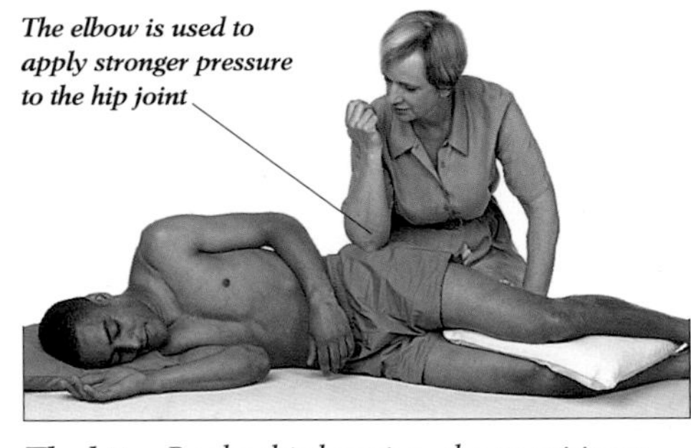
The elbow is used to apply stronger pressure to the hip joint

***The hips**: By the third session, the practitioner starts to apply pressure down the side of the body to lengthen fascia at the hip and increase mobility.*

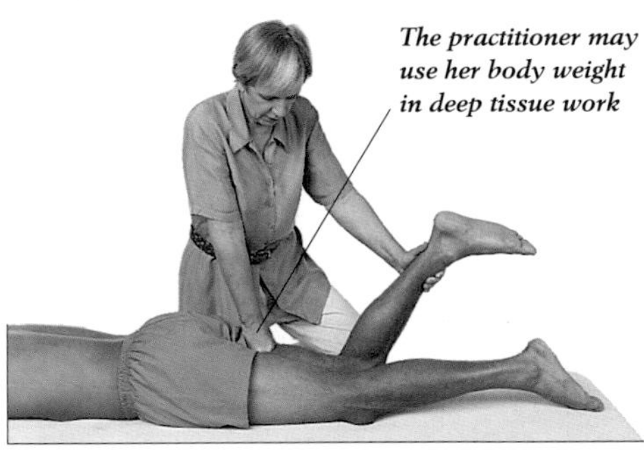
The practitioner may use her body weight in deep tissue work

***The pelvis**: Later sessions focus on deep tissue. The practitioner applies pressure to the back of the legs to aid pelvic mobility and relax the hamstrings.*

PRECAUTIONS

- Avoid Rolfing if you have cancer, rheumatoid arthritis, or any other inflammatory condition.
- See also page 52.

Aston-Patterning

Aston-Patterning, developed in the US, is a system of movement education, bodywork, ergonomics, and fitness training used to facilitate rehabilitation, improve athletic performance, and provide preventive therapy.

HISTORY

Aston-Patterning is named after Judith Aston, a dance and physical education teacher, who was treated by Dr. Ida Rolf after a car accident. Aston-Patterning was originally intended to supplement basic Rolfing techniques. However, while Dr. Rolf worked to align people's bodies to one model, Aston came to see that each person had a unique alignment resulting from body structure, personality, and life experience. Different alignments were viewed as natural adaptations by the body to daily activity.

CONSULTING A PRACTITIONER

After assessing your movement habits, such as walking, sitting, reaching, and lifting, and noting places of tension, the practitioner will design a session specific to your needs. The main components are movement education and bodywork, with ergonomics (such as adjusting your chair or desk to the correct height for your body) and fitness training as needed. The practitioner seeks to help you release tension and achieve your optimal posture by encouraging an even distribution of body weight, and unrestricted movement.

RATINGS

- EVIDENCE
- MEDICAL OPINION
- PRACTITIONER
- SELF-HELP
- COMPATIBILITY

MAIN USES

- Poor posture
- Improving coordination & movement
- Persistent muscle pain, including neck, shoulder & back pain
- Headaches
- Respiratory problems
- Promoting health

MEDICAL OPINION

Most doctors have no basic objection to the method as a form of physical therapy.

PRECAUTIONS

- See Rolfing (above) and page 52.

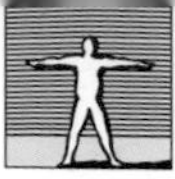

HELLERWORK

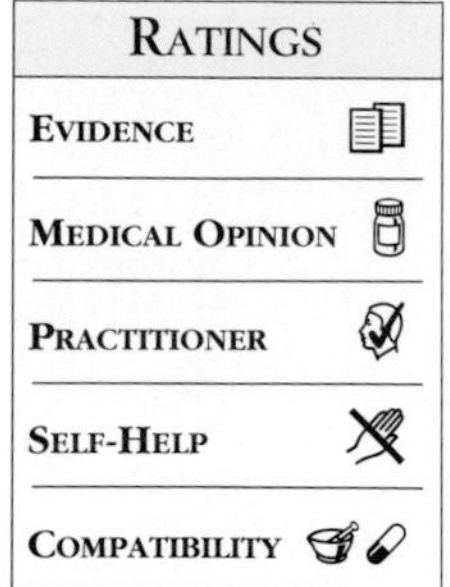

RATINGS
EVIDENCE
MEDICAL OPINION
PRACTITIONER
SELF-HELP
COMPATIBILITY

DEVELOPED IN THE 1970s by an American engineer, Joseph Heller, this therapy combines massage with reeducation in the way the body moves, and an exploration of emotional issues. Heller had worked with Dr. Ida Rolf (see page 82) and shared her ideas about body alignment and releasing muscular tension, but emphasized the therapy's psychoemotional aspects. "The body stores the traumas of our lives in muscular rigidity," he wrote. "When we release the tension in the body and align ourselves with gravity, we take a new stand in life." Hellerwork is worldwide, but mostly practiced in the US.

MAIN USES

- Poor posture
- Persistent muscular pain, including neck, shoulder & back pain
- Respiratory problems
- Prevention of postural or stress-related problems
- Sports injuries
- Promoting health

HISTORY

Joseph Heller trained as an aerospace engineer and studied the effects of gravity and stress on space rockets. His interest in human development and manipulative therapies led him to train as a Rolfer, and in 1975 he became the first president of the Rolf Institute. However, three years later, Heller broke away from the Rolf Institute, arguing that simple restructuring would not produce long-term benefits, and that treatment should be supplemented by exercises and by an exploration of the relationship between body and mind. Since this time, Rolfing has also developed "movement reeducation" exercises. There are over 160 practitioners, mostly in the US, with some in Europe and a few in Australia and New Zealand.

CONSULTING A PRACTITIONER

Comprising 11 sessions of 90 minutes each, a Hellerwork course involves deep tissue manipulation using techniques similar to Rolfing, combined with "movement reeducation," teaching stress-free ways to perform everyday actions. A key feature is "guided verbal dialoguing," in which the practitioner and patient explore emotions triggered by the release of body tension.

An initial interview will be conducted to build up a case history, and photographs taken before and after treatment. Each session concentrates on a particular part of the body and emotions related to it. Firm pressure is applied to release tension in the fascial tissue surrounding the muscles (see artwork, page 82). The first sessions focus on outer "sleeve" muscles, for example in the feet and arms, that control functions learned in childhood, such as standing and reaching. Later sessions concentrate on "core" muscles deeper in the body, for example in the pelvis and spine, and on their relation to repressed emotion; final sessions integrate the work done on the "sleeve" and "core" muscles and explore issues of maturity.

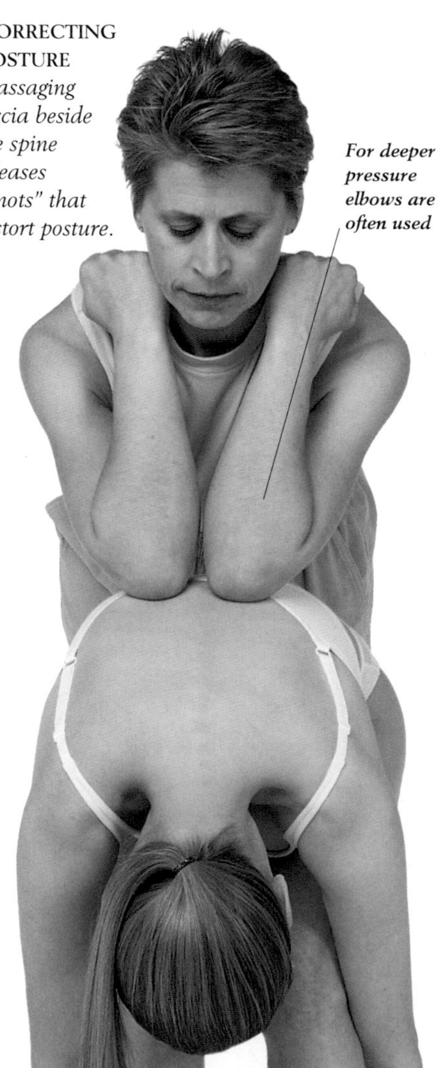

CORRECTING POSTURE *Massaging fascia beside the spine releases "knots" that distort posture.*

For deeper pressure elbows are often used

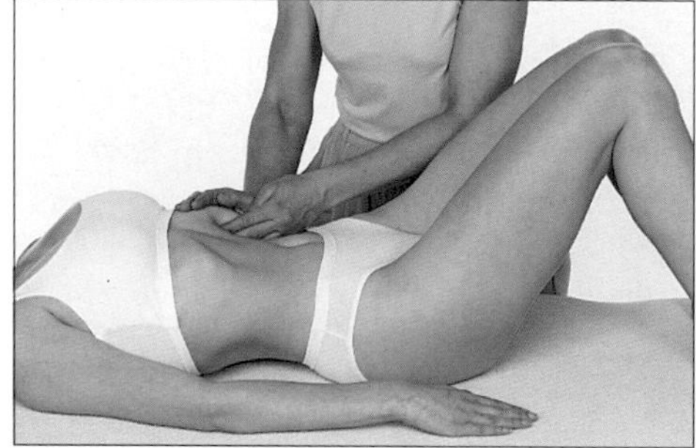

***Breathing** is inhibited by poor posture, which reduces the diaphragm's effectiveness. The practitioner releases diaphragmatic tension and improves flexibility with massage, synchronizing her movements with the breathing of the patient.*

EVIDENCE & RESEARCH

In the 1990s, Hellerwork was practiced on employees at a software company in Portland, Oregon, and found to improve posture and reduce physical stress. Most employees also reported better working relationships and less susceptibility to back pain. The study was, however, uncontrolled and poorly designed.

Any studies on Rolfing techniques also have implications for Hellerwork.

MEDICAL OPINION

So little specific clinical research has been conducted into the practice of Hellerwork that it cannot be said to have any proven effect in cases of disability or rehabilitation after injury. However, it may possibly be of value in preventing muscle strain, promoting health and managing stress.

PRECAUTIONS

- See Rolfing (page 82) and page 52.

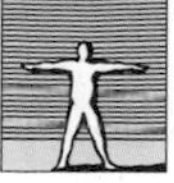

THE FELDENKRAIS METHOD

RATINGS
EVIDENCE
MEDICAL OPINION
PRACTITIONER
SELF-HELP
COMPATIBILITY

THIS SYSTEM OF PHYSICAL REEDUCATION, named after Dr. Moshe Feldenkrais, was developed in the 1940s to explore body awareness, improve flexibility and confidence, and enhance well-being. Practitioners believe that certain habitual postures and movements reflect disruptions in the nervous system, and they teach students to identify and avoid them. Gentle manipulation is used in individual lessons to help those with disorders such as cerebral palsy and multiple sclerosis. Dr. Feldenkrais initially taught in Israel and the United States, but Feldenkrais classes are now held worldwide.

MAIN USES

- Muscle pain
- Back pain
- Learning difficulties
- Neuromuscular conditions, such as cerebral palsy & multiple sclerosis
- Sports injuries
- Strokes & paralysis
- Improved physical & mental well-being

HISTORY

Moshe Feldenkrais was a Russian-born atomic physicist and engineer who worked in France until World War II, when he escaped to England. An enthusiastic soccer player and judo black belt, he began to study human movement when recovering from a serious knee injury. His work was initially based on observation of the spontaneous natural grace of children, which he supplemented with a study of anatomy, physiology, neurology, and psychology. In 1950, he settled in Israel, where he further developed his method and aimed at encouraging ease of movement with "minimum effort and maximum efficiency." He founded the Feldenkrais Institute in Tel Aviv in 1962, and also worked in the US and Europe, using his method to help in many neuromuscular conditions. There are now over 2,500 practitioners worldwide, particularly in Israel, the US, Australia, and Europe.

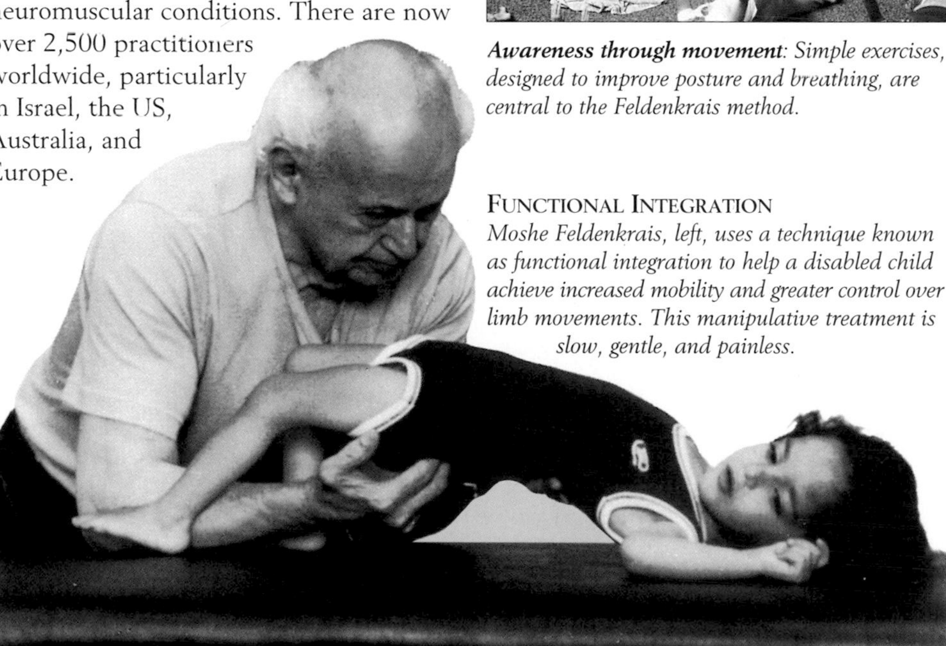

FUNCTIONAL INTEGRATION
Moshe Feldenkrais, left, uses a technique known as functional integration to help a disabled child achieve increased mobility and greater control over limb movements. This manipulative treatment is slow, gentle, and painless.

CONSULTING A PRACTITIONER

Feldenkrais practitioners are essentially teachers of their method, preferring to talk of students or pupils rather than patients. Practitioners believe that our postures and movements reflect the state of our nervous system: for example, somebody suffering from depression often has hunched shoulders. The Feldenkrais method aims to improve physical and mental health by reprogramming movement patterns, and is based on two approaches.

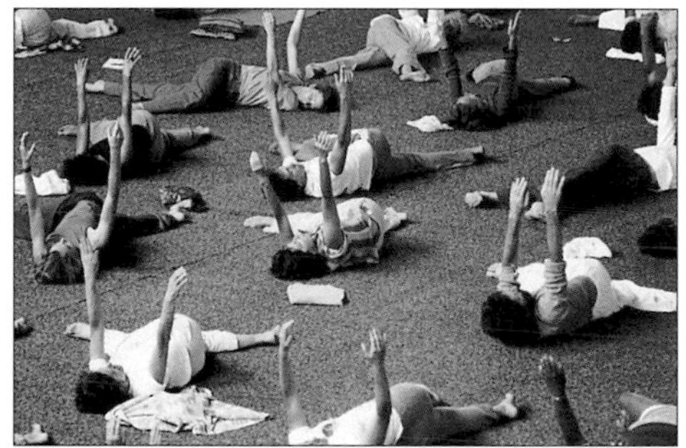

***Awareness through movement**: Simple exercises, designed to improve posture and breathing, are central to the Feldenkrais method.*

The first of these is known as "awareness through movement." It is designed to help you develop body awareness and increased mobility as part of a group by following the practitioner's instructions. This learning experience aims to replace old patterns of movement with new ones, improving breathing and circulation. It is said to benefit both mental and physical performance, and is often used by actors, dancers, and musicians.

The second approach is "functional integration," a one-to-one technique that uses touch and manipulation, and is tailored to your individual needs.

EVIDENCE & RESEARCH

Feldenkrais was noted for his work with severe neuromuscular disturbances, such as cerebral palsy, but the long-term results have not been well studied and there is no direct research on his method. There have been studies in areas such as educational psychology and rehabilitation.

MEDICAL OPINION

Most doctors would find the neurological theory behind the Feldenkrais method plausible and should have no serious medical objection to the use of the therapy alongside conventional physiotherapy. However, without medical research, doctors might hesitate to recommend the method for those with severe disability.

PRECAUTIONS

- See page 52.

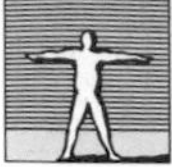

THE ALEXANDER TECHNIQUE

RATINGS
EVIDENCE
MEDICAL OPINION
PRACTITIONER
SELF-HELP
COMPATIBILITY

WITH A FOLLOWING IN MANY COUNTRIES and strong links with the performing arts, the Alexander technique has become one of the most respected and well-established body-oriented therapies. It aims to improve posture so that the body can operate with minimum strain. Young children possess natural poise, but years of hunching and slouching distort the way joints and muscles work. By learning to stand and move correctly, stresses on the body are eased. Alleviating complaints that are exacerbated by poor posture allows all the body systems to function more efficiently.

MAIN USES

- Musculoskeletal problems, back pain
- Stress, anxiety
- Depression
- Headaches
- Gastrointestinal disorders
- Repetitive strain injuries, bursitis
- Postural pain in pregnancy

HISTORY

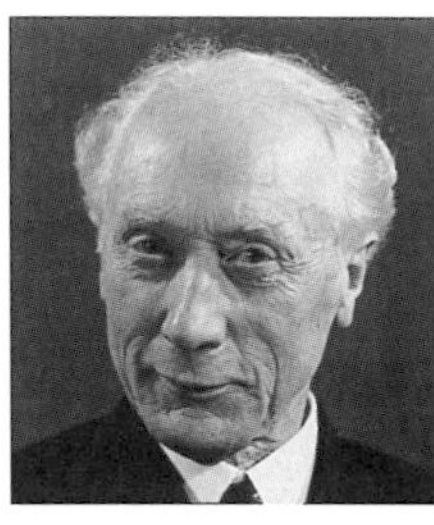

***F. M. Alexander** taught his approach to many prominent people in London during the 1930s. Enthusiastic students included the writers Aldous Huxley and George Bernard Shaw.*

In the late 19th century, Frederick Matthias Alexander, an Australian actor, found that his voice became strained during performances, or disappeared altogether. Studying himself in front of a mirror revealed the cause: before speaking, he pulled his head back and down, arched his back and tensed his arms and legs. The muscles in his throat tightened visibly. Alexander taught himself to release these restrictive reactions and went on to develop the technique that bears his name.

Alexander moved from Australia to London in 1904 and then to the US during World Wars I and II. In 1931 he set up the first training school for teachers of the Alexander technique in London. Praised by numerous educators and scientists, his technique is popular with musicians and actors (it is often studied by drama students). Although the UK has the majority of teachers, the technique has a wide international following, with 1,500 practitioners worldwide.

KEY PRINCIPLES

One only has to compare the grace of a three-year-old child with the slumped back and stooped shoulders of her parents to appreciate the damage done by years of sitting and standing badly, lifting incorrectly, and tensing up with anxiety or self-consciousness. Alexander believed that habitually poor posture influences the way the body and mind function and that, in such cases, it is necessary to relearn basic movements, such as sitting and standing. There are no set exercises; instead Alexander teachers educate students to become aware of "patterns of misuse" in their everyday movements, to pay particular attention to the way they hold their heads, and to align their bodies so that they are balanced and can move in a relaxed, fluid way.

EVIDENCE & RESEARCH

Compared to other complementary therapies, the efficacy of the Alexander technique has been well documented. An ongoing study that began in 1994 at Kingston Hospital, London, indicates that the technique can help relieve persistent back pain. Studies at Columbia University, New York, published in 1984 and 1992, showed that the Alexander technique improved patients' breathing. A series of studies published during the 1960s and 1970s using X rays taken at Tufts University, Boston, revealed that Alexander training increased the length of the subject's neck muscles.

In a UK study published in 1995, music students practicing the Alexander technique performed better and were less anxious. In the 1950s, Dr. Wilfred Barlow, who had trained with Alexander, took photographs of students before and after a course of lessons at the Royal College of Music, London, and found that the students' postures improved significantly.

MEDICAL OPINION

Doctors consider the Alexander technique an approach to poor posture, stress, and persistent back pain. The claims it makes are seen to be reasonable and it focuses on achievable aims. Many doctors recommend lessons to their patients.

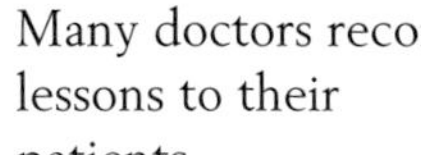

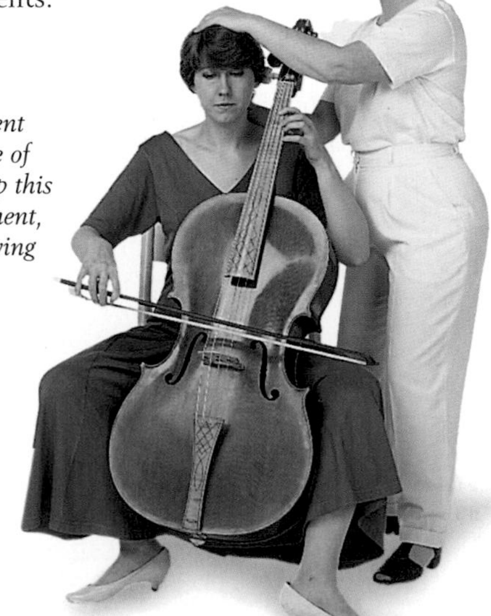

CORRECTING "PATTERNS OF MISUSE"

***Musicians often benefit** from Alexander training to prevent muscle strain, because it teaches students to become aware of and avoid patterns of misuse in their everyday life. To help this musician, the teacher works on the head-neck-spine alignment, and the position of the wrists and elbows. A balanced playing position reduces the risk of repetitive strain injury.*

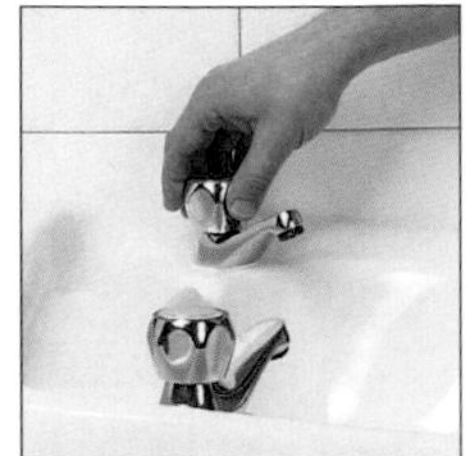

***When turning on a tap**, many people use more force than required, or unnecessarily twist their back. The back and neck should stay relaxed, and the twisting action should come from the arm.*

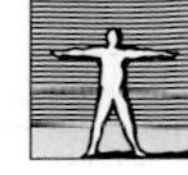

CONSULTING A TEACHER

The Alexander technique, usually taught on a one-to-one basis, can be learned by people of any age. You should wear loose, comfortable clothing. At the introductory lesson you will be asked to stand calmly and move around as the teacher assesses your problem.

The teacher may begin by asking you to lie flat, with your knees bent and your head resting on two or three books. She will make a series of adjustments to your position before helping you to your feet. The aim is to help you become aware of what optimum body posture feels like. The initial process of reeducation takes place while you are lying down because your body is relaxed and the light adjustments of the teacher will have maximum effect.

The rest of the lesson will be spent sitting or standing, while the teacher adjusts your posture and reeducates you to use muscles with minimum effort and maximum efficiency. She will teach you to follow Frederick Alexander's directions: "Free the neck; let the neck go forward and upward; let the back lengthen and widen," and ask you to concentrate on the sensation of sitting or standing without strain. She will also ask you to be aware of how your body is positioned (this is often referred to as "thought in activity").

In later lessons all kinds of movements are examined, such as standing, moving, sitting, lying down, walking, lifting objects – even ironing. You may discover that you use unnecessary force to turn door-knobs and taps, or that if the telephone rings you reach to answer it too abruptly.

One lesson lasts 30–45 minutes and a course consists of 15–30 classes, depending on how quickly you learn, how frequently you can attend (twice a week is ideal), and how much you practice.

PRECAUTIONS

- See page 52.

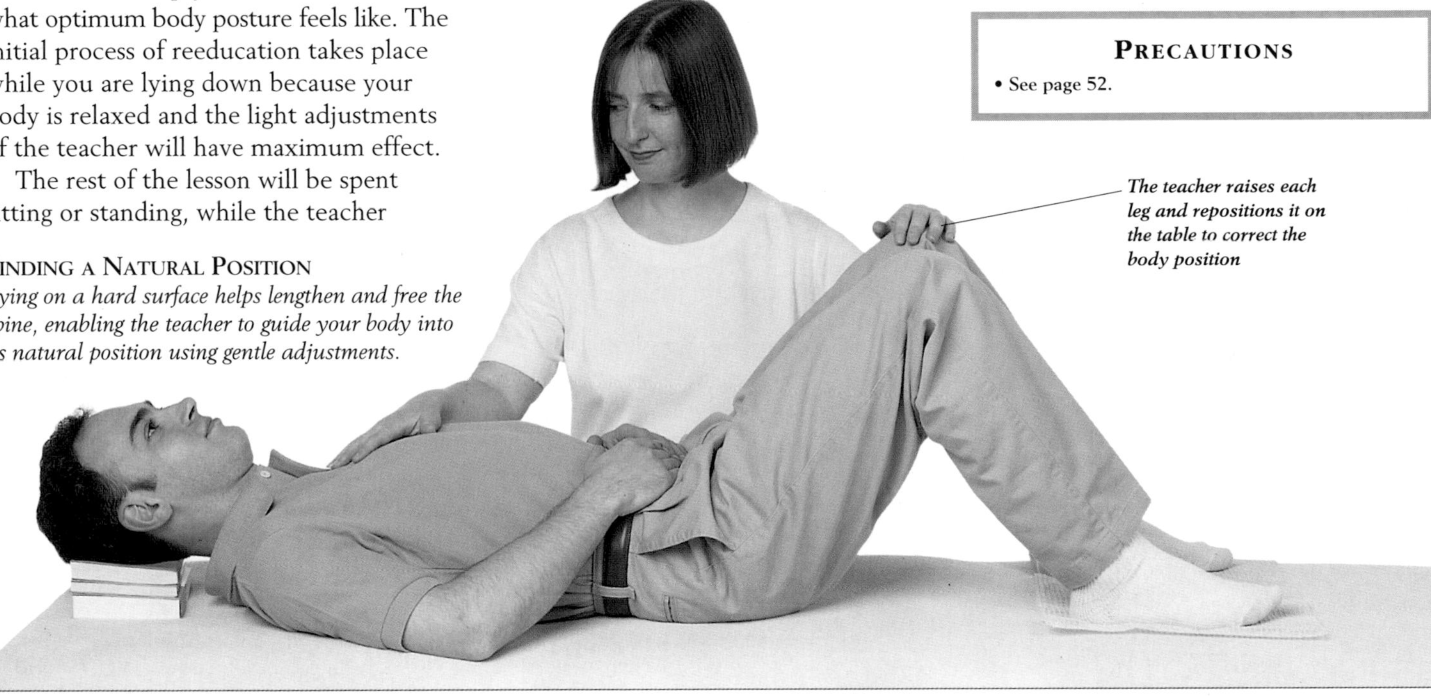

The teacher raises each leg and repositions it on the table to correct the body position

FINDING A NATURAL POSITION
Lying on a hard surface helps lengthen and free the spine, enabling the teacher to guide your body into its natural position using gentle adjustments.

LEARNING TO STAND

An important part of your lesson will involve learning the technique of "thought in activity." You will become aware of how it feels to sit and stand without strain.

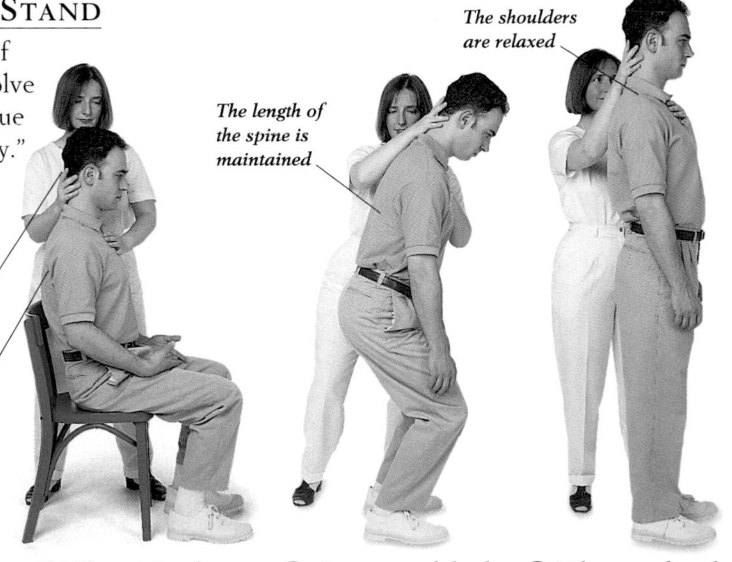

The teacher supports the head and spine to keep them "free" (without strain)

The back is held straight to avoid compressing the spinal joints.

The length of the spine is maintained

The shoulders are relaxed

1 *When sitting, keep the head and spine upright but "free."*

2 *As you stand, lead with the head and try not to jerk it back.*

3 *When standing, let the head remain poised to free the spine.*

SELF-HELP

It is important to learn the principles of the Alexander technique from a teacher, and practice is essential thereafter. Simple exercises can be done lying down for 10–15 minutes twice a day, but don't confine practice to these occasions. Remember to use it at any time and in any situation. If you inadvertently strain a muscle, lie down and follow your "orders."

In the beginning you will have to work hard to retain good posture – poor habits become so entrenched that, initially, slouching and stooping feel natural. With practice, however, maintaining a free neck and spine will become second nature. Many people find that minor nagging ailments such as recurrent backache or headaches gradually improve as they regain a natural posture.

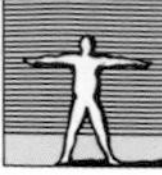

TRAGERWORK

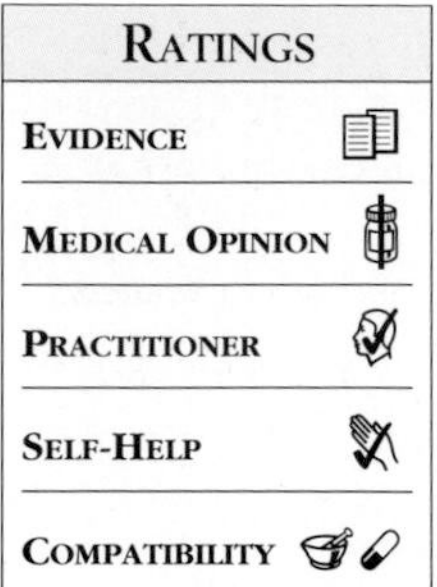

RATINGS	
EVIDENCE	
MEDICAL OPINION	
PRACTITIONER	
SELF-HELP	
COMPATIBILITY	

A GENTLE THERAPY aimed at reintegrating body and mind, Tragerwork, or Trager Psychophysical Integration, was developed by Dr. Milton Trager in the United States. Light, gentle, nonintrusive movements, such as rocking and stretching, help the body to enter a state of profound relaxation. This facilitates the release of deep-seated patterns of physical and mental tension created unconsciously by past traumas and experiences. The approach has gained popularity, particularly in the US, with over 800 practitioners worldwide treating a variety of conditions from poor posture to asthma.

MAIN USES

- Stress-related conditions
- Muscular tension
- Persistent pain
- Poor posture
- Neuromuscular & spinal problems, sciatica
- High blood pressure
- Strokes
- Migraines
- Asthma

HISTORY

Milton Trager, born in Chicago in 1908, was a professional boxer who found that by working on people intuitively with his hands he could ease pain, even helping polio sufferers to walk. He trained as a physical therapist and in 1955 became a doctor, practicing in Hawaii. He also took up Transcendental Meditation (see page 174), which greatly influenced him. In 1975 Trager demonstrated his approach at Esalen, the center of the holistic growth movement in California. It was so successful he set up a practice in California, founding the Trager Institute in 1980.

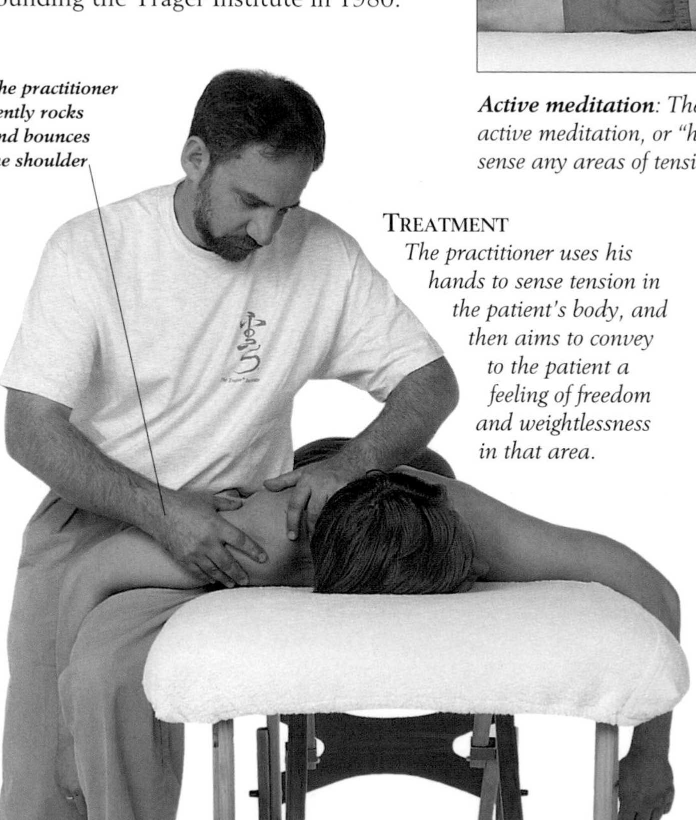

The practitioner gently rocks and bounces the shoulder

TREATMENT

The practitioner uses his hands to sense tension in the patient's body, and then aims to convey to the patient a feeling of freedom and weightlessness in that area.

CONSULTING A PRACTITIONER

A session lasts 60–90 minutes and begins with an assessment. Treatment involves bodywork and may also include instruction in "Mentastics," a self-help movement therapy designed to instill a feeling of freedom and grace in the patient. For bodywork you undress to your underwear. No oil is used, as the skin is not massaged but cradled, stretched, and rocked. The practitioner enters a state of relaxed, active meditation called "hook up," which makes him aware of patterns of tension in the patient's body.

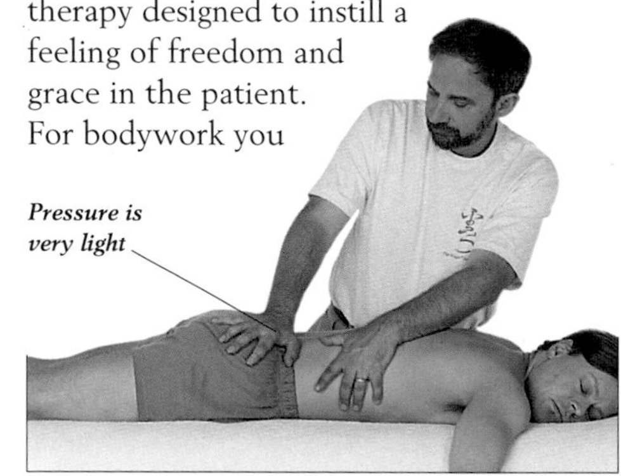

Pressure is very light

Active meditation: *The practitioner's state of active meditation, or "hook up," allows him to sense any areas of tension in the patient's body.*

When areas of tension are located, the practitioner eases the contact pressure (most bodywork increases it) to transmit a sense of freedom and lightness to the patient. The effect is subtle but cumulative; a typical session includes thousands of movements, encouraging the patient to surrender muscular control and "let go." Treatment sets up a ripple effect in tissues, and is said to reach organs inaccessible by conventional massage. One session may be sufficient. Many patients claim to feel lighter and freer from pain after treatment. A Chinese philosopher said he felt like a "dancing cloud" after therapy, and the Chinese ideogram for this often appears on practitioners' T-shirts.

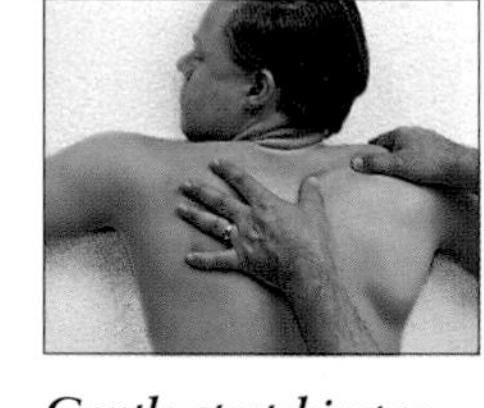

***Gentle stretching** or jiggling of the superficial muscles releases tension in the shoulder.*

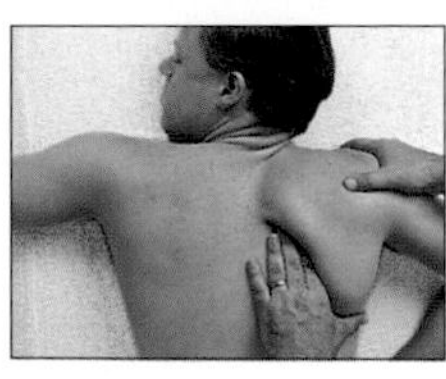

***Cradling** and rocking a joint encourages the patient to give up all conscious control of it.*

EVIDENCE & RESEARCH

In the US, a 1993 study in the journal *Spine* showed that Tragerwork could ease pain, and in a 1986 study, symptoms of lung disease eased after two weeks of therapy.

MEDICAL OPINION

Most doctors remain neutral toward Tragerwork: they feel that it is unlikely to do any harm, and would not object to it as a method of relaxation.

PRECAUTIONS

- Tell your practitioner if you have osteoporosis or thrombosis.
- See also page 52.

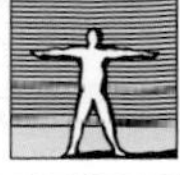

BIOENERGETICS

RATINGS

EVIDENCE	
MEDICAL OPINION	
PRACTITIONER	
SELF-HELP	
COMPATIBILITY	

BIOENERGETICS IS A BODY-ORIENTED form of psychotherapy developed in the US in the 1960s by Dr. Alexander Lowen. An individual's history of dealing with stress or trauma is thought to be "programmed" into the muscles, and practitioners believe that posture and physical tension provide clues to mental attitudes and psychological problems. Bioenergetics exaggerates, then releases, tensions linked with buried memories, enabling past traumas to be explored. Known as Bioenergetic Analysis in North America, where most practitioners are based, bioenergetics is also practiced in Europe and New Zealand.

MAIN USES

- Stress-related conditions, such as irritable bowel syndrome, peptic ulcers, migraines, asthma & fatigue
- Some mental health problems
- Persistent pain
- Personal development

HISTORY

The term "bioenergetics" was first coined by Dr. Alexander Lowen, an American psychotherapist practicing in the 1960s. He was a student of Wilhelm Reich, a follower of Freud who believed that the body, mind, and emotions are closely interrelated. To develop bioenergetics, Dr. Lowen adapted some of Reich's ideas, including his theory of "body-armoring" (adopting defensive postures because of past events). Someone hurt as a child, for example, might hold herself as if warding off blows. Following Freud's practice of encouraging people to relive repressed traumas, Dr. Lowen devised exercises from sources such as t'ai chi ch'uan (see page 100) and Pilates (see glossary).

CONSULTING A PRACTITIONER

After an initial one-to-one assessment, the practitioner may recommend individual therapy sessions, joining a group, or a combination of the two approaches. A session may last roughly 50 minutes, and comfortable clothing should be worn.

Workshops usually contain between 12 and 20 people, and may begin with warm-up movements before a sharing of experiences. Exercises focus on tense areas, such as a "frozen" chest, "locked" pelvis, and tension in the jaw. Attention is paid to "grounding" – the way you stand and balance; practitioners believe that if you are in firm touch with the ground, you will also be in touch with your body and emotions. Key "stress positions," like lying backward over a stool, are often used to build up and unlock emotional energy. Repressed memories may surface, and there may be outpourings of emotion.

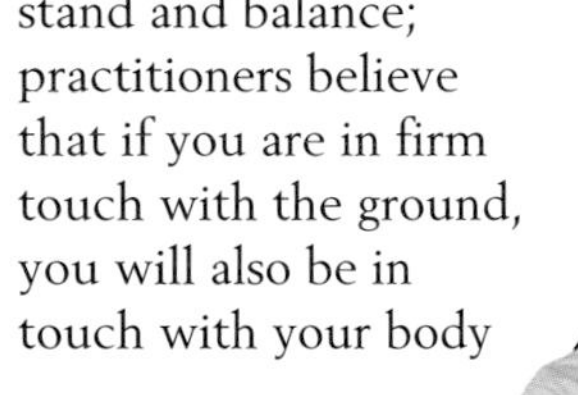

***Grounding**: The patient stands and stretches upward, supported by the practitioner. She focuses on feeling the ground beneath her, and on her body and emotions.*

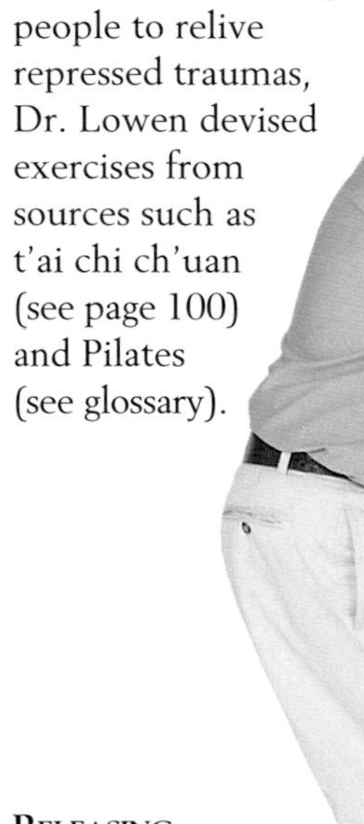

The patient pulls and wrings a rolled towel to release emotion or aggression

The practitioner encourages the patient to express her feelings

RELEASING EMOTIONS

Physical tension is released in exercises like wringing a towel, or hitting a bed with a bat or racquet, which allow the patient to vent her emotions. Such confrontational work can release anger, frustration, or grief.

EVIDENCE & RESEARCH

A number of papers on bioenergetic theories and practice have been published in psychotherapeutic journals, but most evidence is anecdotal: six sessions can be life-changing for some people, while others continue for years.

MEDICAL OPINION

If body and mind are as closely linked as practitioners suggest, then the theory of bioenergetics seems plausible. Any doctor would appreciate that strong feelings may manifest physically – we talk of "tension" headaches, "irritable" bowel, and "nervous" stomachs. But the defenses that lead to feelings being expressed through the body, rather than verbally, are very important, and should be dismantled only at a pace that the patient can handle.

PRECAUTIONS

- See page 52.

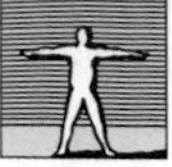

ACUPUNCTURE

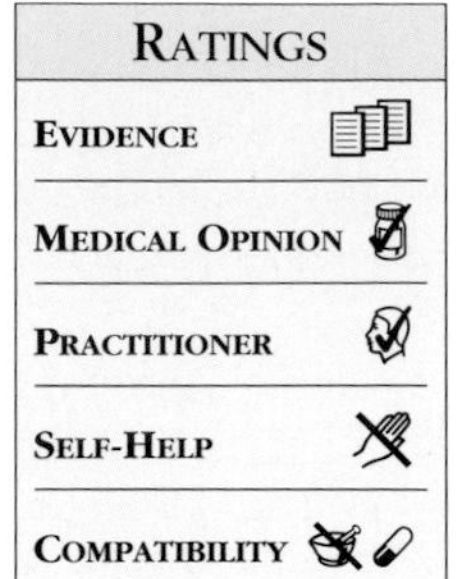

RATINGS
EVIDENCE
MEDICAL OPINION
PRACTITIONER
SELF-HELP
COMPATIBILITY

PART OF TRADITIONAL CHINESE MEDICINE, acupuncture has been practiced in China for thousands of years, but became widely known in the West only in the 1970s, when its use as an anesthetic received sensational press coverage. Practitioners insert fine, sterile needles into specific points on the body as a treatment for disorders ranging from asthma to alcohol addiction, but most often in the West as a means of pain relief. Now one of the most well-known and most widely accepted Eastern therapies, acupuncture is increasingly practiced in a simplified form by medical doctors.

MAIN USES

- Pain relief, anesthesia
- Musculoskeletal problems, arthritis
- Addictions
- Asthma, hay fever
- Depression, anxiety
- Migraines, nausea
- High blood pressure
- Digestive disorders
- Women's health
- Promoting health

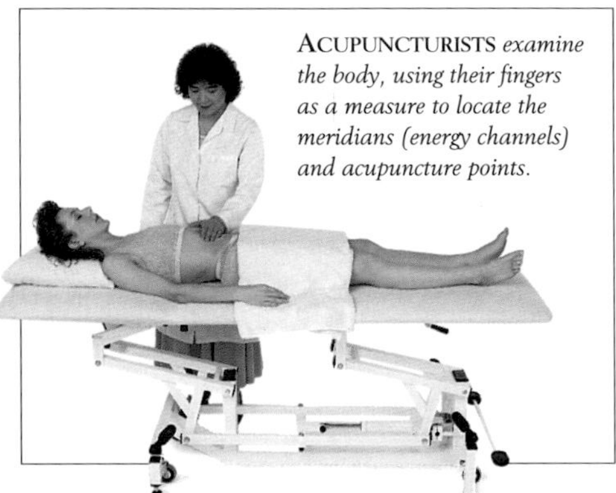

ACUPUNCTURISTS *examine the body, using their fingers as a measure to locate the meridians (energy channels) and acupuncture points.*

HISTORY

Stone acupuncture needles dating back to 3000 B.C. have been found by archaeologists in Inner Mongolia, and acupuncture has been widely practiced in China for around 3,500 years. In the 17th century, doctors and missionaries brought acupuncture to Europe, where it slowly gained a foothold. In 1972, James Reston, a journalist for the *New York Times*, had an emergency appendectomy while in China. He gave acupuncture an enormous boost when he described how it had eased his postoperative pain. Spectacular examples of acupuncture as an alternative to conventional anesthesia during surgery were subsequently reported in the West.

Since the opening of China to the West after the 1970s, many Western doctors have studied acupuncture techniques and use "medical acupuncture," as the practice is known, to supplement conventional treatment in hospitals and pain clinics. In the West, traditionally trained practitioners who are not doctors tend to practice in private clinics. The use of acupuncture in anesthesia is mainly confined to China.

KEY PRINCIPLES

Acupuncture is an element within the Traditional Chinese Medicine (TCM) health system, which also includes herbs (see page 140), acupressure (see page 95), exercise (see page 99), and diet. Fundamental to TCM are the concepts of *yin* and *yang*, opposite but complementary forces whose perfect balance within the body is essential for well-being (see also page 141). *Yin* signifies cold, damp, darkness, stillness, and contraction; *yang* signifies heat, dryness, light, action, and expansion. *Yin* and *yang* are components of *qi* (pronounced "chee"), which is an invisible "life energy" that flows through meridians (channels) around the body (see opposite). There are 12 regular meridians running up and down the body in pairs (six on the left and six on the right). They are mostly named after the main internal organs through which they pass. Six are primarily *yin*, associated with "solid" *yin* organs, such as the liver; six are *yang*, linked to "hollow" *yang* organs, such as the stomach. Two more meridians, the Conception and Governing vessels, provide control of the 12 other meridians.

The even circulation of *qi* around the body is essential for health. Disruption on a meridian can create illness at any point along it; for example, a disorder in the Stomach meridian (passing through the upper gums) could cause a toothache. There are about 365 acupoints along the meridians at which *qi* is concentrated and can enter and leave the body. It is possible to affect the circulation of *qi* at these points, and acupuncturists insert fine needles to stimulate or suppress the flow.

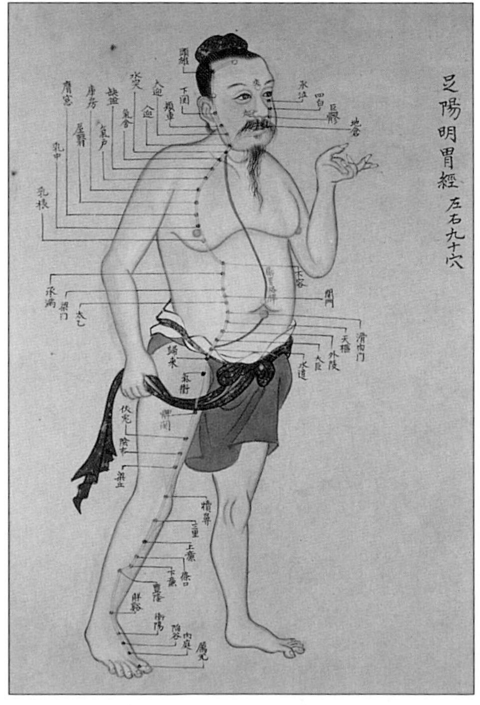

***This medical chart**, typical of those traditionally used by Chinese doctors, illustrates the acupoints along the Stomach meridian.*

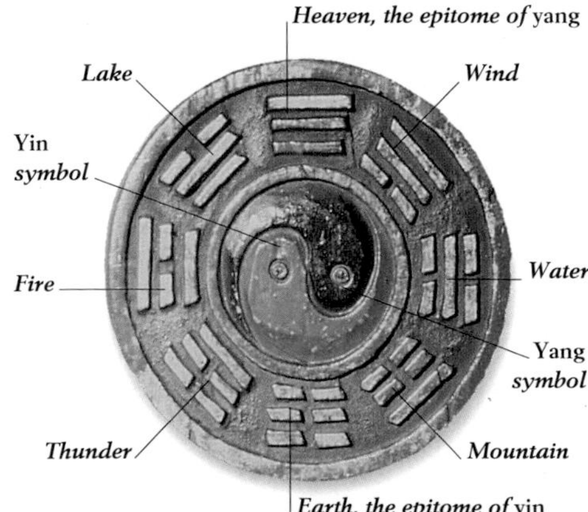

Yin ***and*** yang, *entwined to depict interaction, are also shown as broken and solid lines respectively in eight trigrams representing elements of nature.*

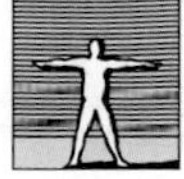

THE THEORY OF MERIDIANS

Qi, an invisible life energy, flows through *yin* and *yang* meridians just below the surface of the skin. Any disruption to the flow disturbs the balance of *yin* and *yang* and leads to illness. Acupuncturists improve the flow of *qi* by inserting needles into specific acupoints on the skin.

MERIDIANS & ACUPOINTS

***Of the 14 major meridians**, 12 take their names from the main body organ through which they pass. The Chinese concept of the organ is broader and less literal than its conventional counterpart. The other two major meridians provide important links for the other meridians.*

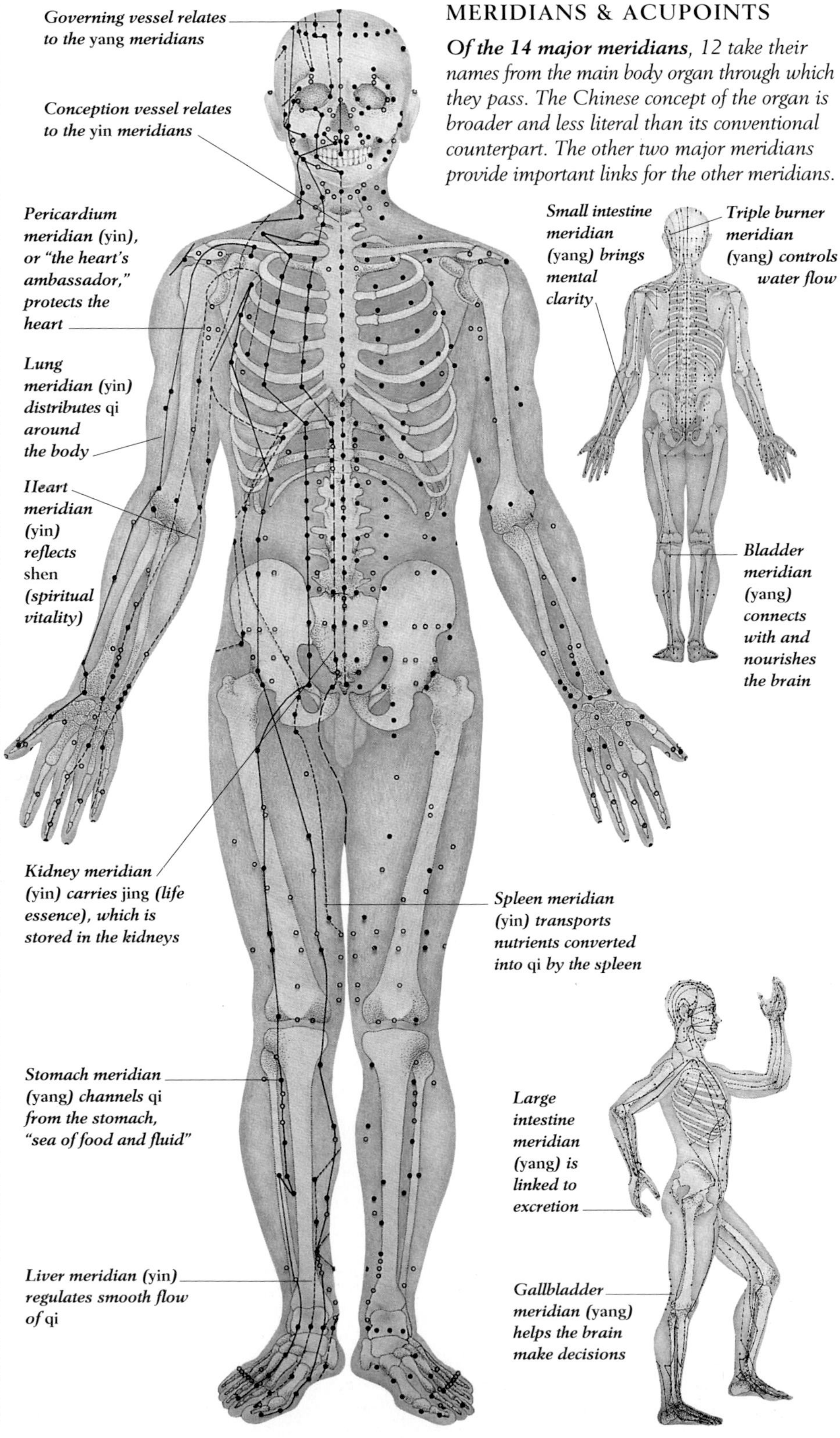

Governing vessel relates to the yang *meridians*

Conception vessel relates to the yin *meridians*

Pericardium meridian (yin), or "the heart's ambassador," protects the heart

Lung meridian (yin) distributes qi *around the body*

Heart meridian (yin) reflects shen *(spiritual vitality)*

Kidney meridian (yin) carries jing *(life essence), which is stored in the kidneys*

Stomach meridian (yang) channels qi *from the stomach, "sea of food and fluid"*

Liver meridian (yin) regulates smooth flow of qi

Small intestine meridian (yang) brings mental clarity

Triple burner meridian (yang) controls water flow

Bladder meridian (yang) connects with and nourishes the brain

Spleen meridian (yin) transports nutrients converted into qi *by the spleen*

Large intestine meridian (yang) is linked to excretion

Gallbladder meridian (yang) helps the brain make decisions

EVIDENCE & RESEARCH

A body of scientific evidence now exists to support the use of acupuncture to treat certain conditions. Some of the most convincing research into the therapeutic effects of acupuncture, published in the *Journal of the Royal Society of Medicine* in 1988, was carried out by Professor John Dundee of Queen's University, Belfast. His research confirmed that stimulating an acupoint approximately 2 in (5 cm) above the crease of the wrist closest to the hand relieved and even eliminated nausea and vomiting in early pregnancy. According to a 1989 study in the *British Journal of Anaesthesia*, the same point could also be used to treat nausea following general anesthesia and chemotherapy.

In 1989, *The Lancet* reported that patients with alcohol addiction responded well to acupuncture. A Swedish study in 1989 found that acupuncture eased post-surgical pain. American studies in 1982 and 1980 showed that it relieved neck pain and lower back pain respectively.

Attempts to relate the meridians' pattern of energy pathways to electrical currents in the body have been unscientific and inconclusive, but some evidence exists for acupoints having lower electrical resistance than nonacupuncture sites. In a Spanish study in 1992, radioactive tracers injected at acupoints seemed to travel along similar pathways to meridians, leading to theories of information transmission linked to neurochemicals rather than to the circulatory or lymphatic system.

MEDICAL OPINION

A growing number of doctors now practice "medical acupuncture," usually for pain relief, although medical opinion on the therapy is still divided. The World Health Organization has identified over 40 conditions treatable with acupuncture, and UK midwives claim to have used it to turn fetuses in the breech position, although no scientifically plausible explanation has been given for this.

Acupuncture may release painkilling endorphins (see glossary). It also may trigger nerve "gate control," in which pressure messages reach the brain faster than do messages of pain. More research is needed: if a communication network of meridians does exist, it has so far eluded definition using modern technology.

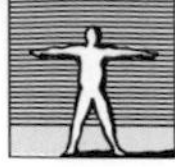

Consulting a Practitioner

On your first visit, the practitioner will take notes on your lifestyle and medical history, and assess your condition using the "Four Examinations" of TCM – *asking, observing, listening* (and smelling), and finally *touching,* in which the most important test is taking the pulse. This is a skilled method of checking the rhythm and strength of all 12 meridian pulses (six on each wrist). There are 28 descriptions, such as "wiry" or "choppy," to categorize the state of each pulse (see page 192). To aid diagnosis, the practitioner may examine other parts of the body. She will then discuss treatment options, which, as well as acupuncture, often include advice on diet and lifestyle, and may involve herbs (see page 140) or acupressure (see page 95). You will then be asked to lie on a treatment table, after removing any clothes covering needle sites (acupoints). The site depends on the disorder and whether the flow of *qi* is to be "warmed," reduced, or increased. Several acupoints may be used: those on the hands and feet are often treated, but sites on the back, abdomen, shoulders, and face are also widely used.

Standard Tests

The tongue and pulse are checked as part of the Four Examinations.

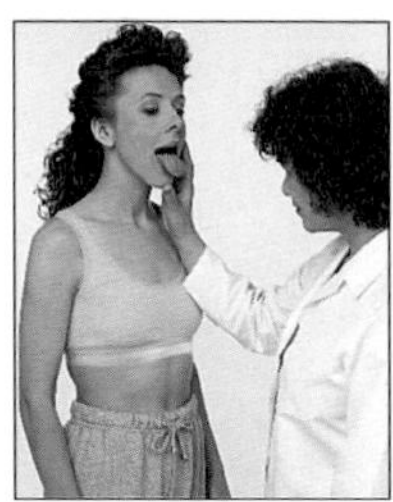

The tongue *reveals imbalances of* yin *and* yang *(see page 193).*

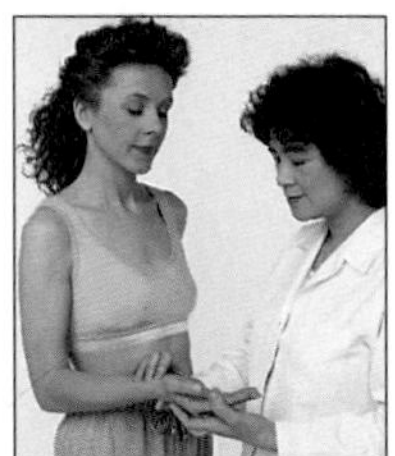

The pulse *is checked for strength and rhythm (see page 192).*

Equipment

Acupuncture needles *vary in length, and are made from stainless steel tipped with steel or copper. Cones of the herb moxa, or moxa-filled burners placed on needles, are used to generate heat on the skin.*

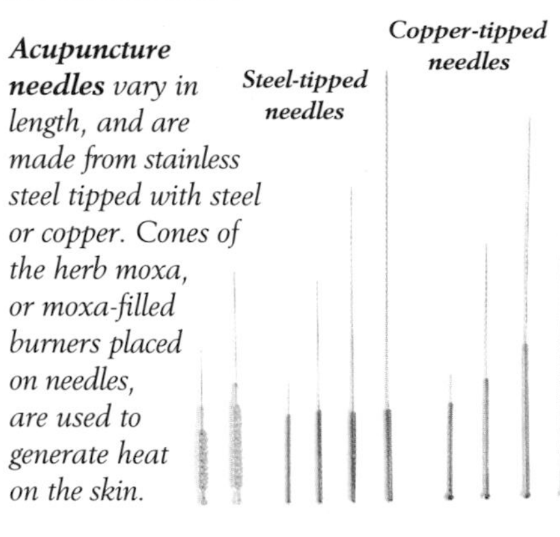

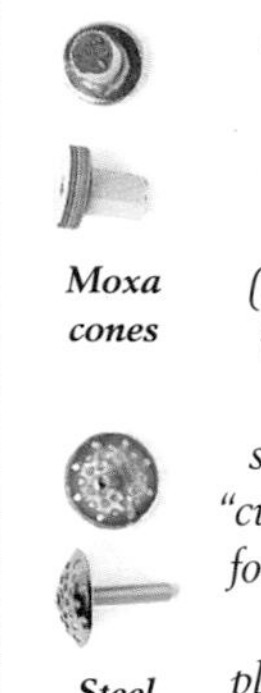

The herb moxa *is burned at an acupoint to generate heat (moxibustion). It is dried and can be rolled into a stick or cone. For "cupping," another form of treatment, glass cups are placed on the skin at an acupoint.*

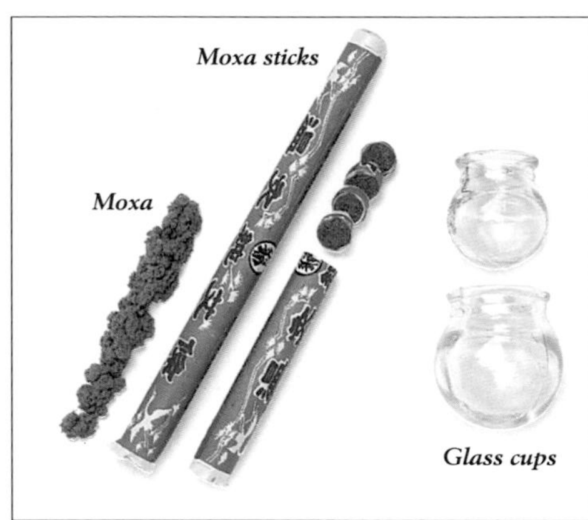

Precautions

- See a qualified practitioner; acupuncture is an invasive therapy and therefore not without risk.
- Ensure that your practitioner sterilizes needles in an autoclave or, preferably, uses disposable needles.
- Tell your practitioner if you are pregnant. Certain acupoints should not be stimulated in pregnancy, except during labor.
- Tell your practitioner if you have a sexually transmitted disease, hepatitis, or AIDS.
- Avoid alcohol, large meals, hot baths or showers, and strenuous exercise (including sex) immediately before or after treatment, since they may counteract its effect.
- See also page 52.

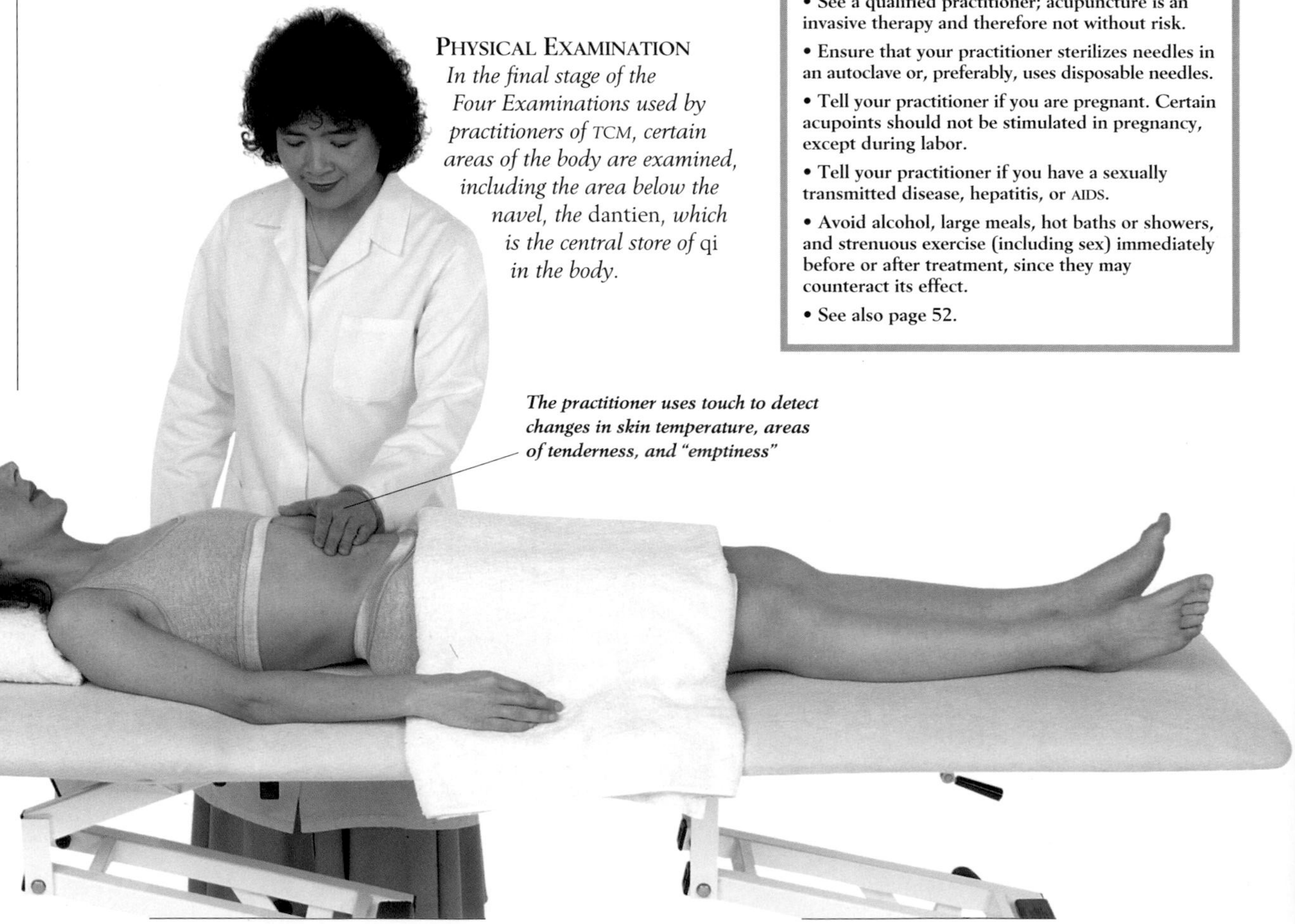

Physical Examination

In the final stage of the Four Examinations used by practitioners of TCM, *certain areas of the body are examined, including the area below the navel, the* dantien, *which is the central store of* qi *in the body.*

The practitioner uses touch to detect changes in skin temperature, areas of tenderness, and "emptiness"

INSERTING THE NEEDLES

The practitioner generally inserts the acupuncture needles to a depth of ⅛–1 in (4–25 mm) depending on the position of the acupoint being treated, although in some cases, practitioners may insert needles to a deeper level. Treatment often involves a combination of acupoints; usually 6–12 needles are used, varying according to the type of acupuncture and the condition of the individual patient. Acupuncture needles may be left in position for a few minutes, as little as a few seconds (especially along the back), or as long as an hour. At the end of the session they are withdrawn swiftly and gently, usually painlessly, without bleeding, and leaving no trace on the skin.

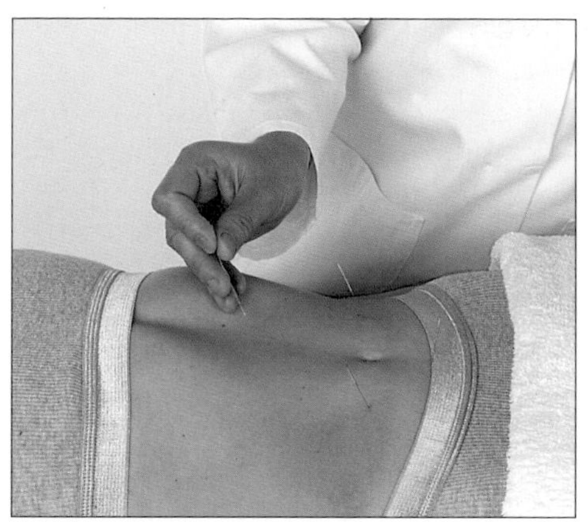

***Insertion is quick**, and usually bloodless and painless, although there is often a pinprick as the skin is pierced. The period for which the needle is left in place depends on its site – here on the Kidney meridian – and the condition being treated.*

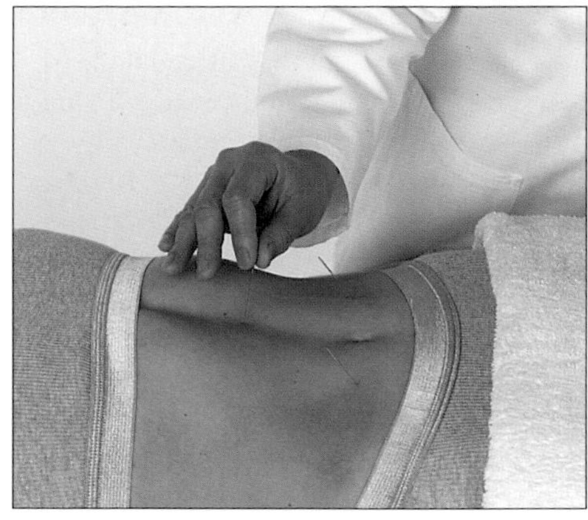

***Twisting the needle** gently between thumb and forefinger, once it is in position, allows the practitioner to regulate the flow of* qi. *This procedure should not hurt, although it may cause a slight numbness or tugging feeling.*

MOXIBUSTION

For some conditions, especially those due to *qi* or *yang* deficiency, such as low back pain, the practitioner burns the herb moxa, generating heat to stimulate acupoints.

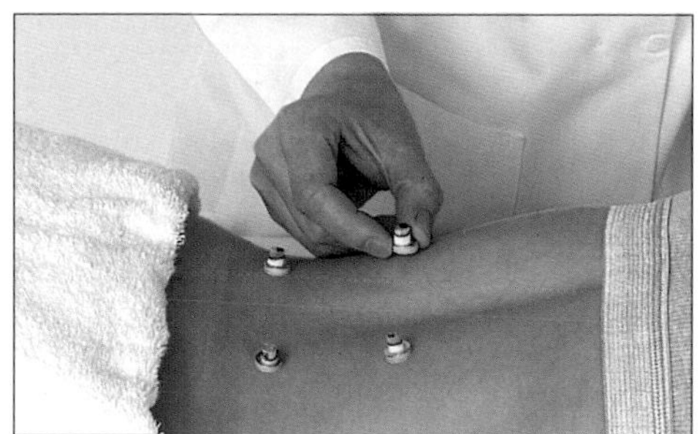

***Moxa cones**, placed here on Kidney and Spleen acupoints, smolder gently on the patient until the heat becomes uncomfortable. Moxa may also be used in a steel burner placed on a needle head.*

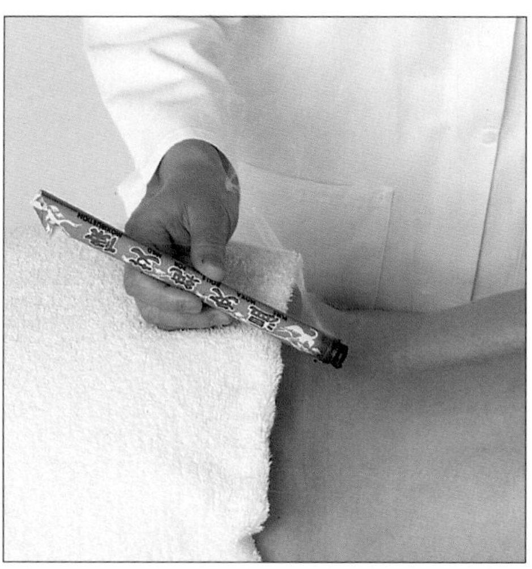

***A moxa stick**, lit like a cigar and held over the acupoint, is an alternative method of treatment. The stick does not touch the skin and is removed when the heat becomes uncomfortable.*

YOUR QUESTIONS

How long does a treatment session last?
Treatment times vary greatly, from 30 to 90 minutes, depending on how long the needles are left in position. The initial consultation will probably be the longest.

How many sessions will I need?
You will usually require between 10 and 20 sessions, depending on your age and on how long you have suffered from the condition. You should expect some improvement after five sessions.

Will it be uncomfortable?
An ache or tingle, known as the "needle sensation," is often felt.

Will there be any aftereffects?
Some people feel tired after treatment and need to rest, or find that their pain worsens for a few hours before getting better. Others may feel rejuvenated.

CUPPING

Glass cups may be placed over the acupoints in order to draw *qi* and blood toward them. As with the use of needles and moxibustion, the aim is to harmonize the body by influencing *qi* at the appropriate point on a meridian. The practitioner can also gain information about the patient's condition by looking at the appearance of the skin during and after treatment: in a healthy person, the skin color quickly returns to normal.

***Glass cups** are placed on Kidney acupoints. The practitioner creates a vacuum in the cup by burning an alcohol-soaked cotton ball in it and placing it on the skin. When the cotton has burned the oxygen, the skin lifts into the vacuum.*

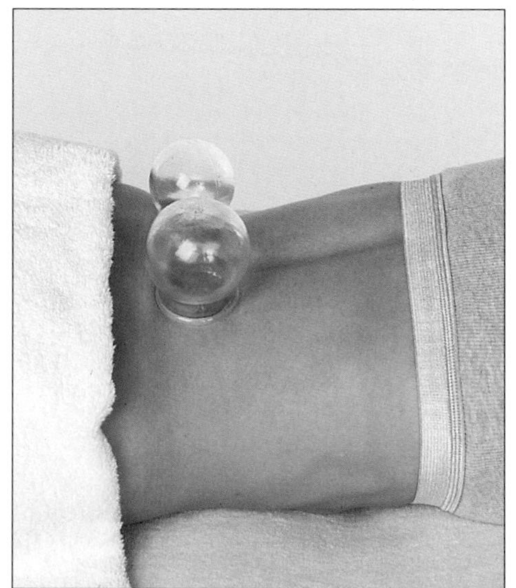

A Patient's Experience

Tim, 35, a computer consultant, had suffered from asthma and bronchitis since childhood: "I was often sick, and fed up with always taking antibiotics, when someone suggested I see an acupuncturist. I can't say I felt great about having needles stuck in me, but after a while I got used to it. The acupuncturist asked me what I ate and how I felt in a way that put my life in context. At first I saw her once or twice a week. She put needles in the top of my head and even in the corners of my eyes, which was pretty weird. There wasn't an overnight change, but now I feel like a different person. I play squash twice a week and I've hardly taken a sick day in the last 12 months."

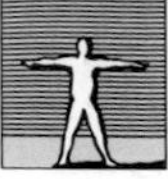

ELECTRO-ACUPUNCTURE

A variation on traditional acupuncture, electro-acupuncture was developed in China in the 1950s. Practitioners apply a low-intensity pulsing electric current to the needles, which is then conducted through to the acupoint to stimulate it. Electro-acupuncture reaches a large number of acupoints simultaneously, and is especially useful as an anesthetic during surgery, avoiding the need for many acupuncturists to work on the patient at the same time.

Laser acupuncture, another variation, directs a fine, low-energy laser beam onto the acupoint. It is particularly useful for patients who have an aversion to needles.

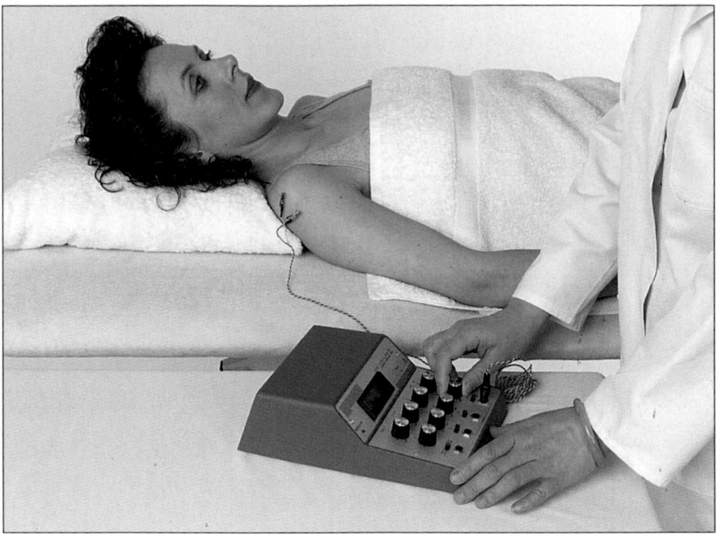

***The practitioner** uses electro-acupuncture to ease the pain of a frozen shoulder. She attaches electrodes, connected to an electro-acupuncture machine, to needles inserted at selected acupoints along a meridian – in this case, the Large Intestine meridian, which runs down the arm. When the machine is switched on, a light electric current is transmitted into the acupoints for a few minutes.*

Auricular Acupuncture

According to Chinese medical theory, there are over 120 acupoints on each ear relating to specific parts of the body. The traditional therapy of auricular, or ear, acupuncture has been adapted by modern practitioners, who now stimulate ear acupoints using needles, laser treatment, and electrical currents.

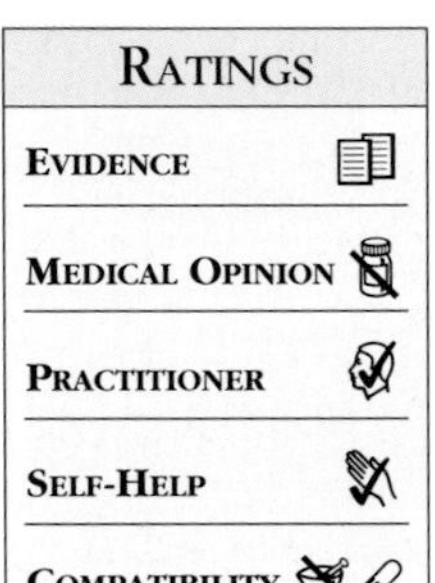

MAIN USES
• Pain relief, anesthesia • Addictions • Sports injuries • Acute pain, including sciatica • Headaches • Digestive disorders, indigestion, nausea • Kidney disorders

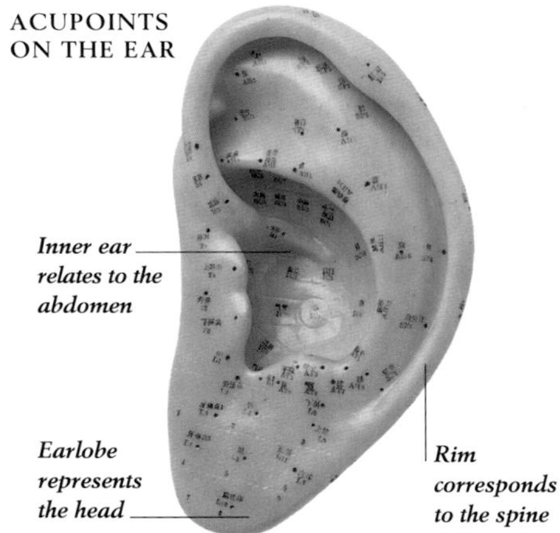

***In auricular acupuncture**, the ear represents an inverted fetus and stimulation of points affects corresponding parts of the body.*

HISTORY

The ear has traditionally been considered an area of great significance in TCM, since it is thought to be crossed by all the major meridians. Practitioners study the ears in detail, observing their color as well as the condition of the skin.

A French doctor, Dr. Paul Nogier, made a study of auricular acupuncture in the late 1950s, based on his observation of the work of a local healer in the town of Lyons. Dr. Nogier developed a theory that the ear corresponded to an inverted fetus, and identified 30 basic points that appeared to have a reflex response in an associated area of the body. He later carried out research in China, where acupuncturists adopted his theories, and he developed a method of pulse diagnosis (see page 192). Dr. Nogier is now regarded as the father of modern ear acupuncture.

CONSULTING A PRACTITIONER

In auricular acupuncture (sometimes known as auriculotherapy or ear acupuncture), diagnosis is based not only on the traditional Four Examinations of Traditional Chinese Medicine (see page 92), but also on a detailed examination of the ear itself. The practitioner will note any signs on the ears, such as flaking skin or blisters, that may point to disharmony in your system as a whole (dry skin, for example, is said to be a common feature of kidney disorders). Treatment is designed to stimulate the acupoints on the ear, over 120 of which have now been suggested. The practitioner may apply gentle pressure to the acupoints with her hands, or use tiny acupuncture needles, a mild electrical current, or laser or infrared light, to stimulate the relevant points. In some cases, needles resembling thumbtacks, with tips about $\frac{1}{16}$ in (1.5 mm) long, are left in place for several days, in order to transmit *qi* to the relevant organ or body part.

MEDICAL OPINION

Although acupuncture is increasingly used in conventional medicine, many Western doctors remain skeptical of the meridian theory and "mapping" of the body in this way. They are likely to find the idea of an ear map of acupoints even more fanciful.

PRECAUTIONS

- Certain acupoints should not be stimulated in pregnancy, except during labor.
- Consult a practitioner if needles left in position for some time become painful or infected.
- See also acupuncture (page 92) and page 52.

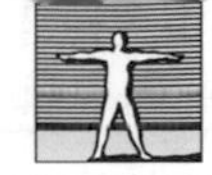

ACUPRESSURE

RATINGS

- EVIDENCE
- MEDICAL OPINION
- PRACTITIONER
- SELF-HELP
- COMPATIBILITY

DESCRIBED AS "ACUPUNCTURE WITHOUT NEEDLES," acupressure probably predates its better-known sister therapy. Part of Traditional Chinese Medicine (see pages 90 and 140), it is based on the theory of qi *("life energy") flowing through channels in the body known as meridians. Finger and thumb pressure is applied to acupoints to relieve specific conditions and to promote harmony and good health. Widely practiced in China, acupressure is less common in the West but gaining popularity. Many acupuncturists use acupressure as part of treatment, and claim it is suitable for self-treating minor ailments.*

MAIN USES

- Musculoskeletal problems, arthritis
- Stress, fatigue, insomnia
- Headaches, migraines
- Depression, anxiety
- High blood pressure
- Nausea
- Digestive disorders
- Women's health
- Promoting health

HISTORY

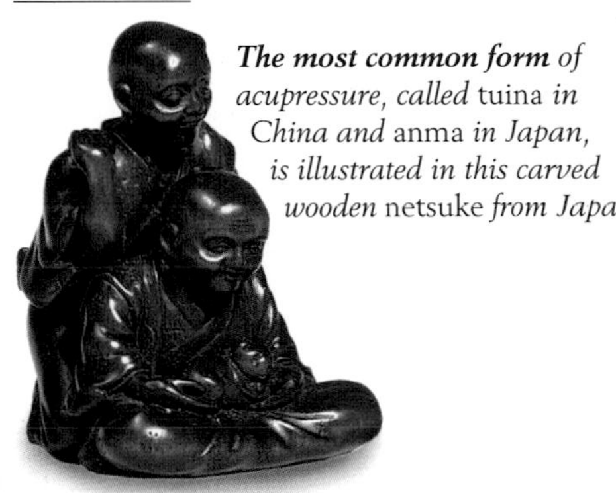

The most common form *of acupressure, called* tuina *in China and* anma *in Japan, is illustrated in this carved wooden* netsuke *from Japan.*

An ancient system of massage aimed at encouraging *qi* ("life energy") to circulate through the body, acupressure probably predates acupuncture (see page 90). However, the theory of stimulating points on the meridians that circulate *qi* (see page 91) remains the same whether it is needles or fingers that are used. While acupuncture developed a high profile in the West during the 1970s, acupressure was imported later. It is regularly practiced by many Chinese people, particularly for self-treating common ailments and boosting the body's immune system.

Tuina is the most common type of acupressure practiced in China. Other forms include *shen tao*, possibly the oldest system and sometimes referred to as the "mother of acupuncture," in which very light pressure is applied with only the fingertips. In *jin shin do*, relatively few acupoints are used and the patient is encouraged to enter a meditative state. The Japanese version of acupressure, *anma*, has developed into what is now called *shiatsu* (see page 96).

CONSULTING A PRACTITIONER

The practitioner will question you about your medical history, and assess you according to the Four Examinations (see page 92). You lie down on a treatment table or on a floor mat. No oils are used and although it is not necessary to undress, you should wear loose-fitting clothes. Sessions usually last 30–60 minutes and you may need up to 20 weekly sessions. Many people have regular treatment to promote health and a sense of well-being.

The practitioner stimulates acupoints using her fingers, thumbs, and even feet and knees. *Tuina*, which translates as "push and grasp," involves vigorous body massage using many different techniques, including one-finger manipulation, as well as rubbing, kneading, and a unique rolling action claimed to recharge the body's energy levels.

SELF-HELP
Points shown here and above may help common ailments. To aid digestion, press the Leg Three Miles point on the Stomach meridian for five seconds to aid digestion.

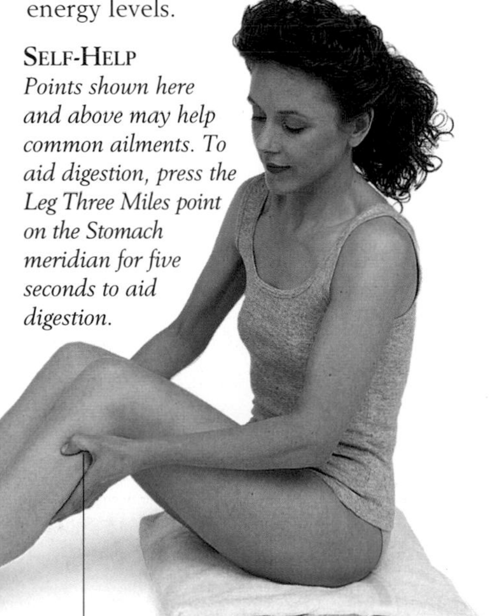

Leg Three Miles acupoint

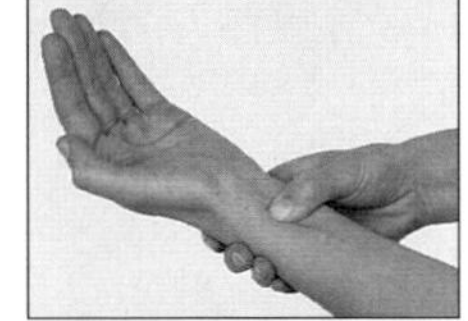

Press the Inner Gate *acupoint below the wrist crease in line with the ring finger to ease nausea or treat motion sickness.*

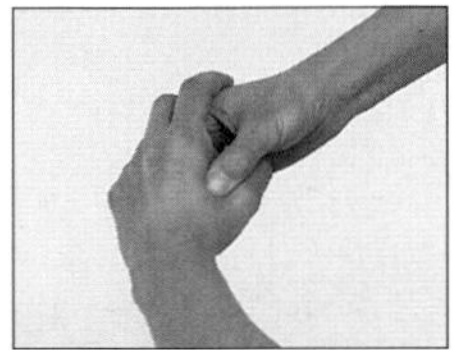

Press the Meeting of the Valleys *acupoint between thumb and forefinger to aid the digestion and to relieve head and face aches.*

Pressure is applied directly down on the skin or angled in the direction of the meridian's flow, and acupoints on both sides of the body are massaged to balance *qi* flow. You should feel a slight discomfort when the acupoint is pressed. Self-help treatment is possible for many ailments and can be practiced at home or work.

EVIDENCE & RESEARCH

Some of the benefits associated with certain acupoints have been confirmed by research (see page 91), but attempts to explain the meridian system of energy channels in terms of Western physiology have proved unsuccessful.

MEDICAL OPINION

Western doctors presume acupressure to be less effective than needles, and find it hard to believe that what is basically a form of massage may be able to influence the internal organs in such a precise way.

PRECAUTIONS

- Certain acupoints should not be stimulated in pregnancy, except during labor.
- See also acupuncture (page 92) and page 52.

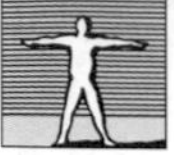

SHIATSU

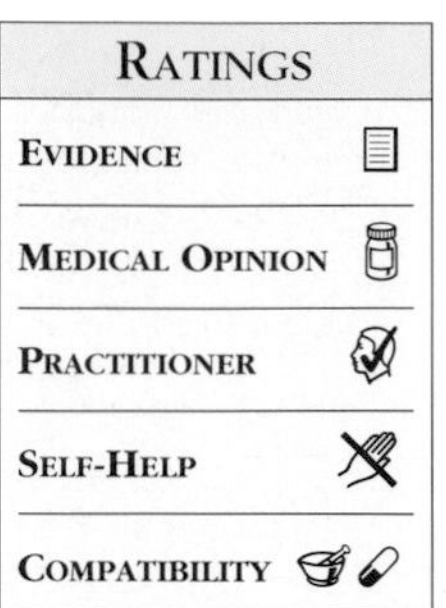

SHIATSU MASSAGE WAS DEVELOPED IN JAPAN early in the 20th century. Although influenced by Western medicine, it has its basis in Traditional Chinese Medicine and follows the same principles of energy and meridians as acupressure (see page 95). The practitioner uses fingers, thumbs, elbows, knees, and even feet in a combination of massage techniques, applying pressure to key points to influence and stimulate energy flow in the body. Shiatsu has become very popular in the West, where it is both practiced by trained practitioners and used as a self-treatment for minor ailments.

MAIN USES

- Musculoskeletal problems, arthritis
- Stress, fatigue
- Insomnia
- Headaches, migraines
- Digestive disorders
- Menstrual pain
- Asthma
- Circulatory problems
- Promoting health

HISTORY

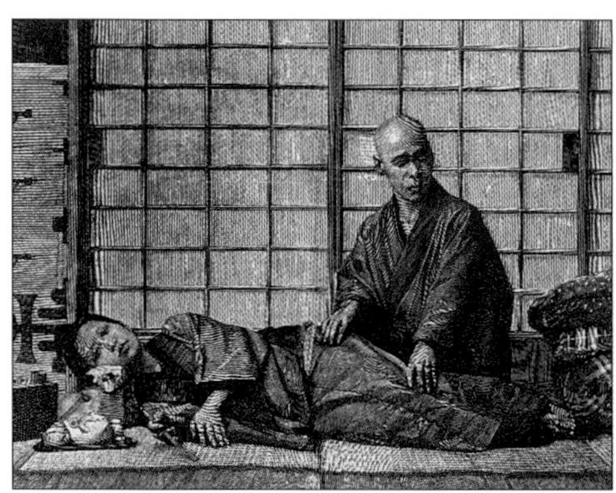

***This engraving** from the late 19th century shows the practice of* anma, *a traditional form of massage in Japan and the forerunner of shiatsu.*

Shiatsu (which translates literally as "finger pressure") has its origins in Traditional Chinese Medicine, introduced into Japan around 1,500 years ago. The most common form of Japanese massage was *anma* (*tuina* in China), which was used for hundreds of years simply as a means of relaxation. The therapeutic potential of this type of massage was rediscovered in Japan early in the 20th century, and a Japanese practitioner called Tamai Tempaku developed what is now known simply as shiatsu by combining the traditional Eastern techniques with a knowledge of physiology and anatomy derived from Western medicine. Schools were founded to promote the new therapy, which received official recognition by the Japanese government in 1964.

Shiatsu is used in Japan by professional therapists to diagnose and treat ailments, and a related version of shiatsu, called do-in (see page 98), is practiced as a form of self-help. There are approximately 1,200 practitioners in the US.

KEY PRINCIPLES

Shiatsu is based on the principles of Traditional Chinese Medicine, according to which "life energy" (*ki* in Japanese and *qi* in Chinese) circulates throughout the body along meridians, or channels, which can be influenced at specific points (*tsubos*, or acupoints) on the body. Stimulating the *tsubos* externally, either by acupuncture (see page 90) or by finger pressure and massage, is said to reduce excess *ki* where its flow is blocked or it is overactive (*jitsu*), and to restore it where it is depleted (*kyo*). Practitioners aim to identify and harmonize the body's *jitsu* and *kyo* patterns.

Practitioners may use a specialized technique called *hara* diagnosis to monitor the flow of *ki* through the internal organs and their meridians (see below and page 194). Treatment techniques vary, with some practitioners working on specific *tsubos*, as in Chinese acupressure, and others using a general massage to stimulate the meridians.

Western practitioners use physiological terms to describe the effects of shiatsu, claiming it regulates the hormonal system and the circulation of blood and lymphatic fluid, aids the elimination of waste products, releases muscle tension, and promotes deep relaxation. They claim that shiatsu works effectively as a general tonic and also enhances the body's self-healing abilities.

EVIDENCE & RESEARCH

There is little evidence specifically relating to shiatsu. Any studies on acupuncture, acupressure, or massage would have implications for this technique.

MEDICAL OPINION

The theory of acupoints and meridians underlying all Traditional Chinese Medicine is unfathomable to doctors and scientists in the West. Some patients report strong sensations after shiatsu, yet for many doctors, the therapy appears to be no more than a highly developed approach to massage. Practitioners' claims for the power of touch and pressure to treat diseases need more research before Western science can accept that shiatsu triggers healing processes.

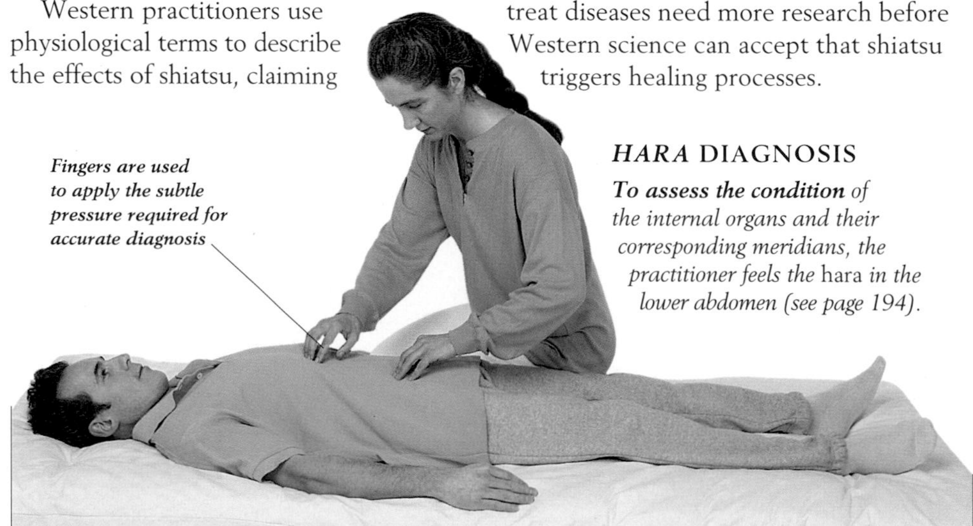

HARA DIAGNOSIS

***To assess the condition** of the internal organs and their corresponding meridians, the practitioner feels the* hara *in the lower abdomen (see page 194).*

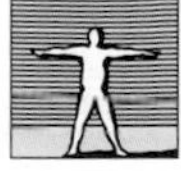

Consulting a Practitioner

The practitioner will be trained in the "Four Examinations" of Traditional Chinese Medicine: she will *ask* detailed questions about your medical history, emotions, lifestyle, and your responses to foods; *observe* your appearance, movements, and posture; *listen* to your voice (wheezing is a sign of poor lung energy, for example, and an angry voice indicates liver energy problems); and use *touch* to take your pulse, using a complex technique characteristic of Eastern medicine (see page 192).

The practitioner may also use *hara* diagnosis; the *hara* consists of "energy centers" in the abdomen, which are said to relate to parts of the body. The practitioner may gently feel the *hara* to detect problems elsewhere in the body (see opposite).

You remain clothed for treatment, but loose, preferably cotton, clothing is advised. So that the practitioner can use her body weight to apply pressure, you lie on the floor, on a mat or a futon. Sessions last about an hour, and several may be needed, depending on your condition. The practitioner may also advise changes in your lifestyle and diet.

Each session covers the whole body and treatment often begins at the point on the *hara* called the *tanden*, three fingers' width below the navel, which is the center of balance and gravity, and is said to be where *ki* is stored. A wide range of techniques may be used, including pressing with the knee or elbow to stimulate blood and *ki* flow, stretching and squeezing to disperse blocked *ki*, rocking to counteract agitated *ki*, and gentle holding on the meridians and *tsubos* to enhance the flow of *ki*. The practitioner may even walk on the soles of your feet (believed to stimulate the kidneys). At the end of the session you will be left alone for a few minutes to relax and absorb the benefits of the treatment.

Although firm and sometimes robust, treatment should leave you feeling relaxed but invigorated. However, after-effects, such as flulike symptoms, may occur; this is the "healing crisis," a sign that the body is trying to expel "toxins," said to be released as *ki* is unblocked.

Treating a Headache

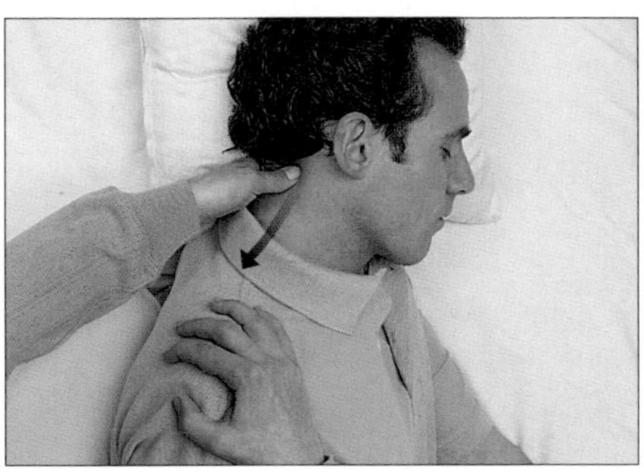

1 *Working on the Gallbladder meridian, the practitioner gently stretches the shoulder away from the head with her right hand and uses her left thumb to massage down the neck.*

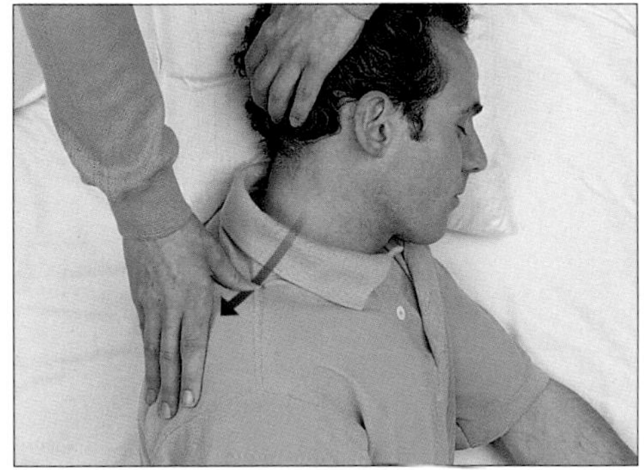

2 *Turning around, she then massages along the top of the shoulder with her thumb. The sequence is then repeated on the other side of the neck. It may also ease sinus pain or earache.*

Precautions

- Tell your practitioner if you are pregnant. Certain *tsubos* should not be stimulated in pregnancy, except during labor.
- Tell your practitioner if you have any long-term condition, such as cancer, AIDS, or CFS; some shiatsu techniques may be unsuitable. This also applies if you have high blood pressure, epilepsy, osteoporosis, thrombosis, or varicose veins.
- Avoid alcohol, large meals, hot baths or showers, and strenuous exercise (including sex) immediately after treatment, as they may counteract its effect.
- See also page 52.

TREATING THE LIVER MERIDIAN

This meridian, which runs along the side of the body, ensures the smooth flow of ki *around the body. Pressure applied along the Liver meridian can address many conditions, from headaches to menstrual pain.*

Supporting herself with this hand, the practitioner ensures pressure is evenly balanced

The thumb applies direct pressure to specific points on the Liver meridian

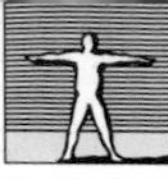

DO-IN

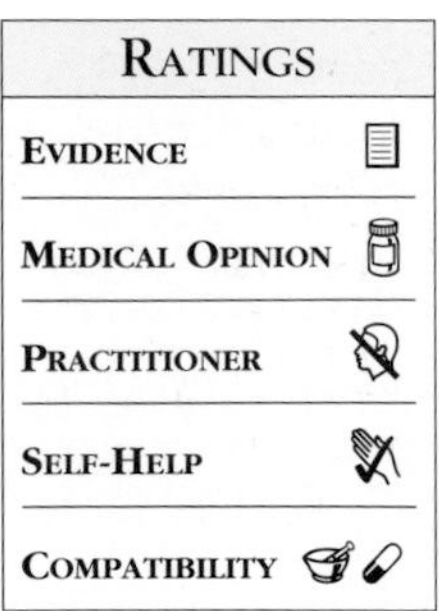

CLOSELY RELATED TO SHIATSU AND ACUPRESSURE, do-in is a form of Japanese self-massage designed to stimulate the flow of ki, *or "life energy," throughout the body (see page 91). Do-in (pronounced "dough-in" and sometimes also spelled* daoyin*) originated as a way of maintaining good health, similar to qigong or yoga, but is now usually practiced as a form of self-help shiatsu. Daily practice aims to tone skin and muscles, improve circulation and flexibility, ease aches and pains, and encourage mental clarity and emotional stability. Do-in is not very well known in its own right in the West.*

MAIN USES

- Musculoskeletal problems, arthritis
- Stress-related conditions, such as insomnia
- Depression, anxiety
- High blood pressure
- Migraines, nausea
- Digestive problems
- Women's health
- Promoting health

CONSULTING A PRACTITIONER

Patients receiving shiatsu (see page 96) often learn do-in without realizing it, through the self-help exercises that their shiatsu practitioner may teach. Do-in developed in Japan and China as a self-help health maintenance program. The practitioner will teach you exercises to encourage the flow of *ki*, including controlled breathing, meditation, stretching, percussion (tapping), and applying pressure to acupoints, or *tsubos*. A typical exercise is encircling your arm with your hand, then "pushing" *ki* to the fingertips and out of the body. Focusing your mind and breathing is important to renew *ki* in the body. Do-in is best practiced upon awakening or just before going to bed.

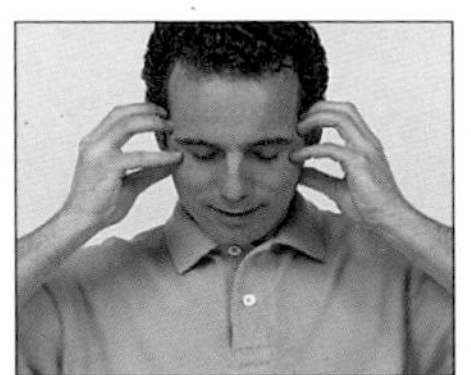

***Eyestrain**: Use your fingertips to massage* tsubos *on the temples.*

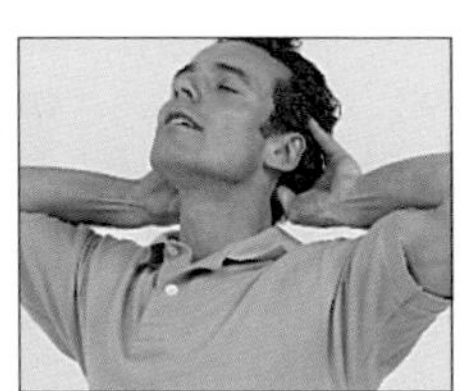

***Headache**: Stimulate the base of the skull with your thumbs.*

MEDICAL OPINION

While the theory of meridians and *ki* can arouse skepticism in doctors, few would doubt the benefits of massage and regular relaxation and breathing exercises.

PRECAUTIONS

- See shiatsu (page 97) and page 52.

THAI MASSAGE

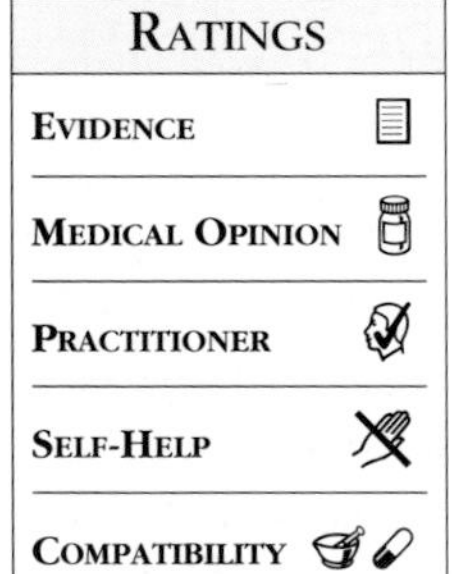

JIVAKA KUMAR BHACCHA, physician to the Buddha, is said to have developed Thai massage over 2,500 years ago in India. The original Ayurvedic techniques were reputedly brought to Thailand by Buddhist sages from India in the 3rd century B.C. *Some are depicted in stone at Phra Chetuphon Temple, Bangkok. Acupressure techniques were later added by Chinese settlers, creating a unique blend of Indian and Chinese health systems. Modern Western visitors to Thailand brought the techniques to Europe and the US, and some have incorporated Western massage strokes into the treatment.*

MAIN USES

- Pain relief
- Musculoskeletal problems, such as backache & arthritis
- Stress-related conditions, such as headaches & insomnia
- Poor posture
- Circulatory problems
- Promoting health

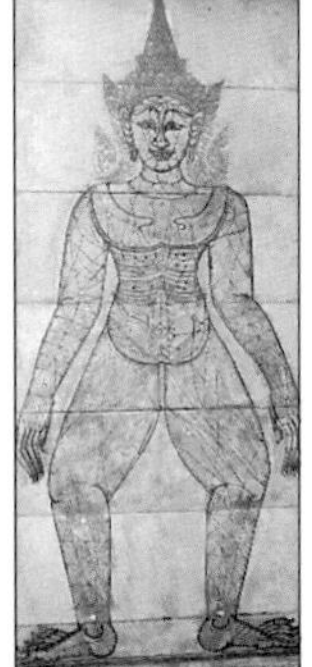

***This 19th-century** Thai manuscript depicts some of the 72,000 "vital force" channels and acupoints on the body.*

CONSULTING A PRACTITIONER

Thai massage is a hybrid of the Chinese and Ayurvedic healing systems. The practitioner will use hands, feet, and elbows to massage channels and points on the body through which *prana*, or "vital force," is said to flow (see pages 144–45). This concept is similar to Traditional Chinese Medicine's theory of meridians (see page 91). Treatment involves a great deal of gentle stretching, bending, and pulling, intended to restore or improve the flow of *prana*. It is also designed to induce a trancelike state that is believed to be psychologically beneficial.

MEDICAL OPINION

Doctors are dubious about theories that encompass meridians and *prana*, since they cannot be medically explained, but massage itself is recognized as therapeutic.

PRECAUTIONS

- See massage (page 58), acupuncture (page 92), and page 52.

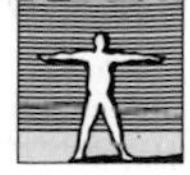

QIGONG

RATINGS
EVIDENCE
MEDICAL OPINION
PRACTITIONER
SELF-HELP
COMPATIBILITY

QIGONG (PRONOUNCED "CHEE GONG") translates literally as "energy work." A component element of Traditional Chinese Medicine, it is an ancient system of movement, breathing techniques, and meditation, which is designed to develop and improve the circulation of qi, or "life energy," around the body. Qigong is believed to help both body and mind to function at an optimum level, increasing vitality and encouraging self-healing mechanisms. Suitable for all ages and levels of ability, it is practiced daily by more than 60 million people in China and is fast growing in popularity in the West.

MAIN USES

- Fatigue
- Stress-related conditions
- High blood pressure, heart disease
- Conditions of old age
- Musculoskeletal pain & stiffness
- Promoting health

HISTORY

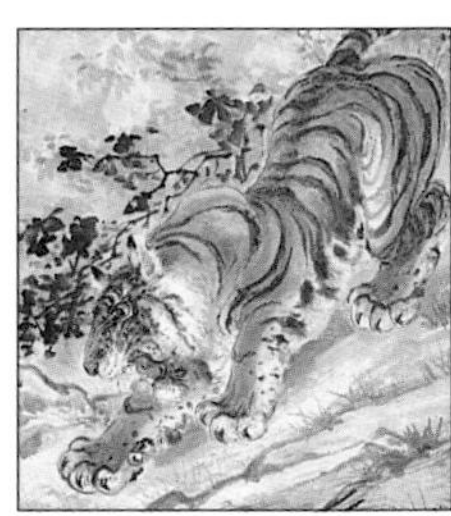

***The movements** of wild animals helped inspire qigong. A 3rd-century B.C. doctor devised "Five Animal Play." This included stretching out the arms in front, like a tiger, to ease tension in the lungs.*

The Chinese have always used breathing and movement as methods of healing, and people living near the Yellow River 4,000 years ago used dance to ward off arthritis.

These ancient practices are said to have been based on the instinctive movements of animals and they were used to promote balance, strength, and healthy organs. Over the centuries the exercises developed into qigong. In 1955, the first qigong clinic was founded in Heibei province, but during the Cultural Revolution (1966–69) qigong was suppressed. The system is now reestablished throughout China.

QIGONG EXERCISES

***Child Worships the Buddha** strengthens the legs and "lightens" the body, promoting a calm state.*

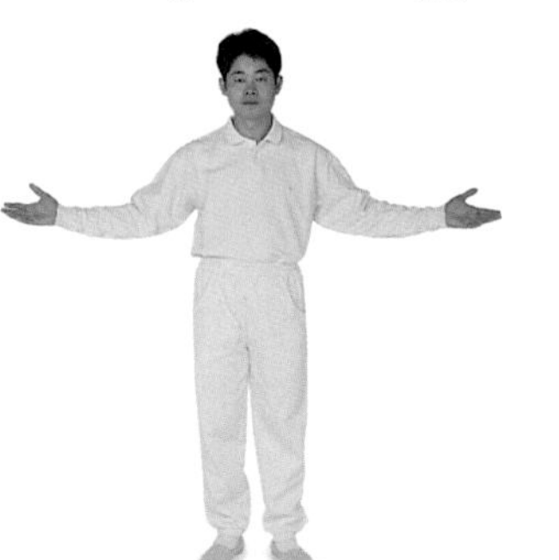

1 Stand balanced. Open your arms, breathing in deeply.

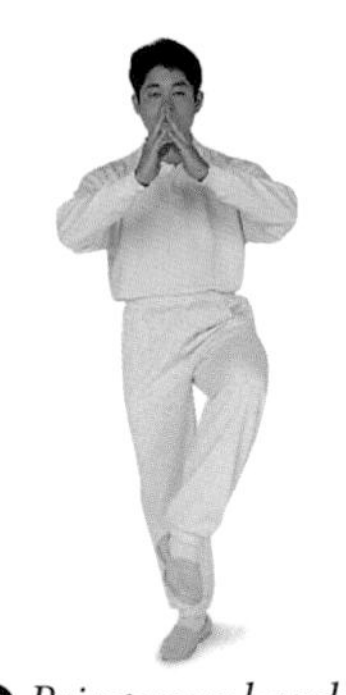

2 Bring your hands together in front of you. Raise your left leg.

Qi is directed down the body into the legs

Holding this position is good for leg strength

Body "sinks" into position as the right knee bends

3 Rest your left leg on your right knee. As you breathe out, gently bend your right leg.

CONSULTING A PRACTITIONER

The practitioner will teach you exercises and meditation techniques to stimulate *qi* in the meridians and acupoints (see page 91). You will learn to recognize sensations of *qi*, and use your mind, or "intention," to guide it in ways that calm your mind and enhance the functioning of your body. Qigong exercises can be performed in any order: you repeat each one six times to start with, building up as you feel ready. The basic postures are easy to learn and suitable for anyone, including the aged and infirm. Many can be performed anywhere, even in a wheel-chair, or in bed. Clothing should be loose and comfortable, and flat, flexible shoes are recommended rather than sneakers. In addition to teaching exercises, master practitioners are said to be able to "emit external *qi*" to heal others.

***Rainbow dance:** Qi is channeled through the arms and directed from the hand down to the acupoint at the top of the head. This exercise may help relieve headaches.*

EVIDENCE & RESEARCH

Chinese research since the 1980s claims that qigong can increase blood flow to the brain and other vital organs and improve the functioning of body systems. Unfortunately, few of these studies exist in translation and some are incomplete.

MEDICAL OPINION

"Qi" and "emitting external *qi*" sound improbable. Doctors will accept these claims only when backed up by scientific theory and research. Nonetheless, many doctors are impressed by their patients' experiences of "healing" encounters.

PRECAUTIONS

- See page 52.

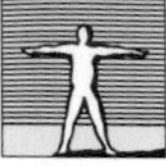

T'AI CHI CH'UAN

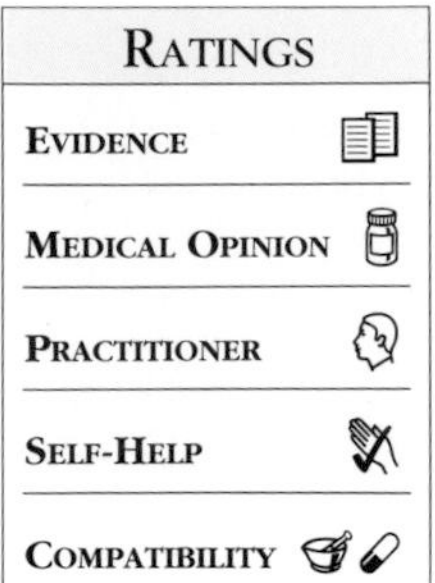

RATINGS
EVIDENCE
MEDICAL OPINION
PRACTITIONER
SELF-HELP
COMPATIBILITY

OFTEN KNOWN SIMPLY AS "T'AI CHI," this Chinese movement therapy was reputedly practiced by Taoist monks in the 13th century, but its exact origins are difficult to trace. A dynamic form of qigong (see page 99), t'ai chi is a noncombative martial art that uses breathing techniques and sequences of slow, graceful movements to improve the flow of qi, *or "life energy," calm the mind, and promote self-healing. T'ai chi is often described as "meditation in motion" and is performed daily by millions of Chinese people all over the world. In the West its popularity is rapidly increasing.*

MAIN USES

- Stress-related conditions, such as anxiety & tension
- Conditions of old age
- Enhancing mental & physical control
- Improving vitality
- Calming the mind
- Promoting health

HISTORY

Derived from the words for "great," "ultimate," and "fist," t'ai chi ch'uan can be loosely translated as "supreme ultimate power." One legend says that Chang San Feng, a 13th-century Taoist monk, devised the movements after dreaming about a snake and a crane engaged in a dancelike fight: the bird is said to have represented universal consciousness, the snake to have embodied nature's powers of regeneration. Chang San Feng reputedly combined these dancelike movements with traditional Taoist breathing exercises to create t'ai chi. Another ancient legend holds that t'ai chi was developed as a martial art by monks forbidden to carry weapons. A more modern belief is that it was created about 400 years ago by a retired Chinese general, Chen Wang Ting, from Henan province.

T'ai chi was suppressed during the Cultural Revolution (1966–69), but it has since been promoted by the Chinese government as a form of preventive health care. In the West it is now one of the most popular movement therapies for all ages.

KEY PRINCIPLES

As an element of Traditional Chinese Medicine, the aim of t'ai chi is to ensure the smooth flow of *qi*, or "life energy," through the body's meridians (see page 91). Practitioners believe illness is caused by an imbalance of *qi*, although t'ai chi is practiced more as a form of preventive health care than as a response to an ailment.

Genuine t'ai chi involves "empty hand forms," "weapons forms" (with sword, spear, and broadsword), "pushing hands," and "standing like a tree" (*zhan zhuang*). As a noncombative martial art, t'ai chi is used for spiritual and mental clarity. It should ideally be practiced outdoors, so that the universal *qi* of the earth can join with the body's internal *qi*.

Today there are five major styles of t'ai chi: *Chen, Yang, Wu, Woo,* and *Sun. Yang* (the most commonly practiced in the West) is a rhythmical style performed as a slow series of postures, linked into one long, flowing exercise. The *short form* version consists of 24 movements and can be performed in 5–10 minutes, while the *long form* version of 108 movements takes 20–40 minutes. The sequences bear symbolic names like "snake creeps down to water" and "stork cools its wings." They are designed to focus body and mind in harmony to encourage an even flow of *qi*.

EVIDENCE & RESEARCH

Research indicates that t'ai chi relaxes the muscles and nervous system and benefits posture and joint flexibility. In 1996, a trial in Atlanta found t'ai chi could help improve the health of elderly people. A study published in the UK *Journal of Psychosomatic Research* in 1992 showed that t'ai chi could reduce symptoms of stress. In a 1989 study, American researchers found that t'ai chi improved breathing without straining the heart.

MEDICAL OPINION

Many doctors might value t'ai chi as a form of exercise and as a relaxation and breathing technique. Most would, however, be wary of the theory of *qi* and meridians.

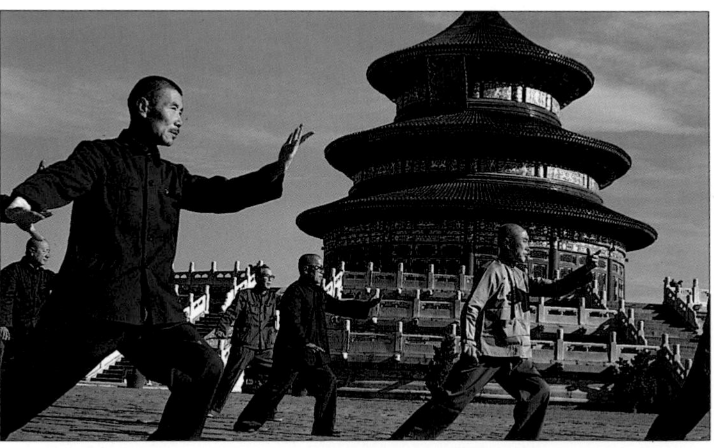

***In China** any piece of open land may be used for daily practice of t'ai chi, and men and women of all ages participate. This group is practicing in front of the Temple of Heaven in China's capital city, Beijing. Styles of t'ai chi vary, but grace, concentration, and control are common to all forms.*

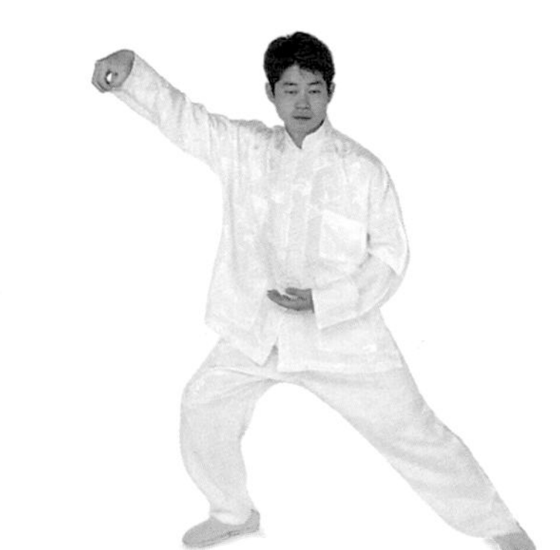

***This posture** from the Single Whip sequence shows the martial aspect of t'ai chi; an imaginary sword is held in the upper hand.*

CONSULTING A TEACHER

Although video courses are available, it is better to attend classes with a teacher, who can explain the philosophy of t'ai chi and ensure that sequences are learned correctly. Classes range from one-to-one to groups of 15–30. The teacher will not take a case history, but you should tell him of any current medical condition. Loose, comfortable clothes are recommended, and flat-soled shoes (not sneakers). The teacher will begin with gentle warm-up exercises, before instructing you in t'ai chi movements. You are advised not to overexert yourself, and t'ai chi should not make you feel sore or stiff. Sessions will be calm and unhurried, focusing on breathing and state of mind to encourage a calm, meditative state. Daily practice is ideal, with weekly sessions considered the minimum for any noticeable benefit. Repetition and refinement of postures are the key to improvement.

PUNCHING

This sequence improves arm and leg strength and generates *yang qi* (see page 141). *Qi* is generated within the *dantien* (in the abdomen) and the postures distribute it around the upper body.

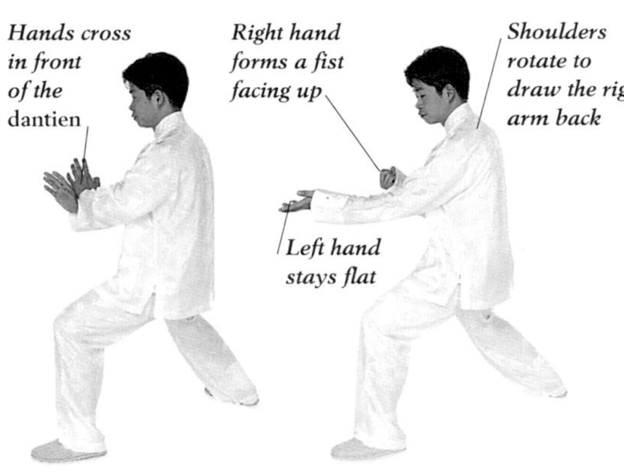

Right fist now faces down

The outstretched arm carries the power through to the fist

The whole upper body is used to generate the power of the punch

Qi is carried up the back and through the shoulder as the upper body swivels

Weight is centered in the lower body

1 *Stand with your feet wide apart and knees slightly bent. Rest your left hand on your right in front of your abdomen, where your* dantien *is located.*

2 *Bend your legs a little more. Swing your hands wide, palms out, then bring them back to the center, left hand in front, right hand in a fist behind.*

3 *Transfer the weight to your right foot and twist your body to the left. To release the punch, pull your left hand back and send your right fist forward. Center your weight, and swing your upper body into the movement. The sequence can be performed as controlled, slow postures or as a powerful, fast action.*

CLOUD HANDS

This gentle series of movements develops *yin qi* (see page 141), and helps to balance *qi* in the body. It also strengthens the arms and legs, and can be performed repeatedly as a flowing sequence.

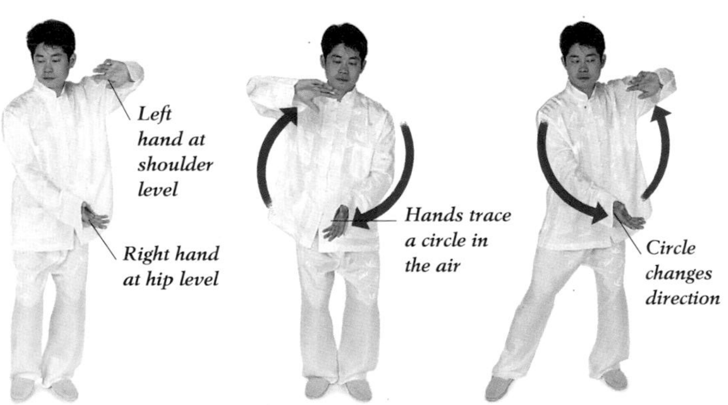

1 *Put your weight on your right leg, slightly raising your left leg. Raise your left hand, palm out, and bring your right hand, palm up, below it.*

2 *Shift the weight onto the other leg; make a large counter-clockwise circle with your hands so that your right hand is in the higher position.*

3 *Step to the right, transfer your weight to the left foot, and make a clockwise circle with your hands. This movement can be repeated many times.*

> **PRECAUTIONS**
>
> • See page 52.

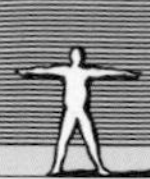

POLARITY THERAPY

RATINGS
EVIDENCE
MEDICAL OPINION
PRACTITIONER
SELF-HELP
COMPATIBILITY

IN THIS BLEND OF WESTERN THERAPIES, Traditional Chinese Medicine and Ayurveda, well-being is said to be the result of an unobstructed flow of "life energy" around the body. This energy corresponds in nature to qi *in Traditional Chinese Medicine (see page 140) and* prana *in Ayurveda (see page 144), and is thought to move in currents around the body between positive and negative poles. Practitioners aim to rebalance or restore energy flow by means of touch, nutritional advice, exercise, and counseling. The therapy is well established in the US and growing in Europe.*

MAIN USES

- Migraines
- Fatigue, lethargy, CFS
- Menopausal problems, PMS
- Stress
- Allergies
- Digestive disorders, such as irritable bowel syndrome
- Back pain
- Arthritis

HISTORY

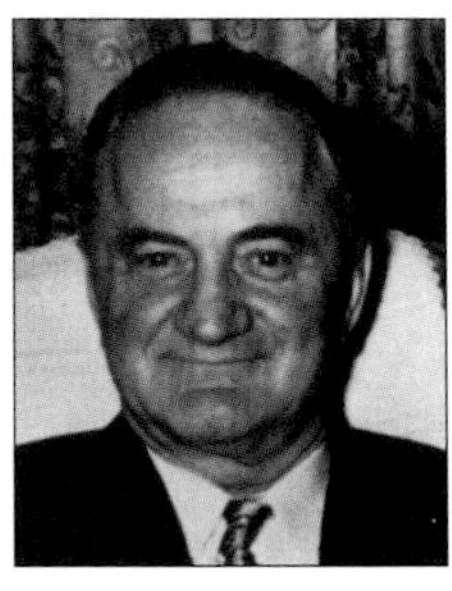

Dr. Randolph Stone, *who drew on elements of Eastern and Western medicine to develop polarity therapy, believed that "the awareness of life as energy currents ... is the key to the natural art of health-building."*

Polarity therapy was developed in the late 19th century by Dr. Randolph Stone, who was born in Austria, but spent his working life in the US as a naturopath, osteopath, and chiropractor. In search of a unifying healing principle, he studied Eastern medical traditions and came to the conclusion that all pain or illness is due to an imbalance of life energy, and that well-being and deeper self-understanding result when life energy is able to flow without interruption or stagnation.

Dr. Stone conducted many teaching seminars on polarity therapy, mostly aimed at the medical profession. In 1984 the American Polarity Therapy Association was set up, and over 150 practitioners have since been certified.

KEY PRINCIPLES

Polarity therapists see the body as a system of energy fields, and believe that life energy is kept in constant motion by the pull of opposing poles, which act like magnets. The head and right side of the body are the positive pole, and the feet and left side are the negative pole. The center of the body, along the line of the spinal cord, is neutral. Energy flows clockwise between the poles, passing along the central channel, where there are five neutral energy centers of ether, air, fire, water, and earth. These correspond in position to Ayurvedic *chakras* (see page 109) and in character to the Five Elements of Traditional Chinese Medicine (see page 141). Each center has a particular function: ether controls the throat and hearing; air regulates respiration, the lungs, circulation, and the heart; fire governs digestion; water controls glands and emotions; and earth governs excretion.

Illness and poor health are considered to be the result of stagnation and depletions in the energy currents, and practitioners may use one or more of a number of therapies to restore balance: therapeutic "bodywork," nutritional advice, "polarity yoga" or stretching exercises, and counseling.

ENERGY FIELDS

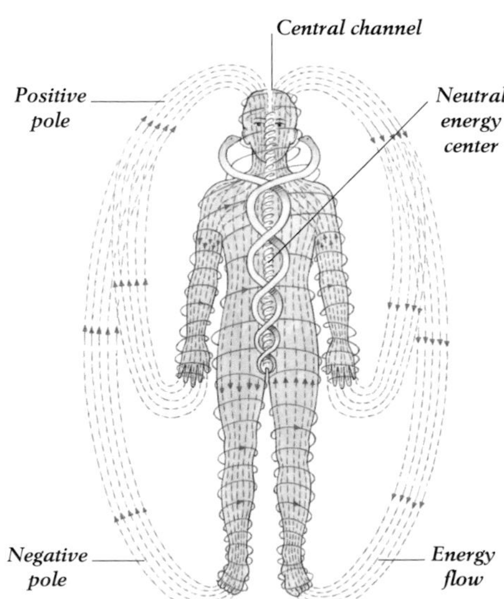

A field of electromagnetic currents *is said to surround the body. At its heart are the five neutral energy centers of ether, air, fire, water, and earth.*

For bodywork, touch and manipulation techniques are used to pinpoint and relieve stagnation and encourage the free flow of energy around the body.

Food is believed to contribute directly to the quantity and quality of this energy. Poor nutrition and digestion may be at the root of many physical problems, and practitioners often prescribe cleansing or detoxifying diets to eliminate harmful products that may have accumulated in the body. A "health-building diet," containing plenty of fresh fruit and vegetables, may then be recommended.

Polarity yoga exercises, based on the body's natural movements, consist of simple postures designed to help maintain muscle tone, release toxins, and strengthen the spine. They are accompanied by gentle rocking, stretching, and vocal expressions, said to open up the flow of energy.

Counseling is used when practitioners feel that negative thoughts are impeding energy flow. They believe that the mind has a direct impact on the way the body works, and that counseling helps to enhance self-awareness and self-esteem and encourage a positive attitude.

EVIDENCE & RESEARCH

No clinical trials have been carried out so far. This is partly due to lack of funding and partly because practitioners have no background in research.

MEDICAL OPINION

To date, there is no scientific evidence for the theory of "life energy" flow. The treatments, however, seem harmless, as long as caution is exercised when embarking on detoxifying diets.

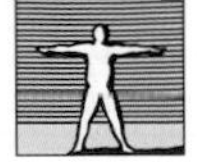

CONSULTING A PRACTITIONER

The practitioner will begin by asking questions about your medical history and lifestyle. In most cases, you then lie on a treatment table while the practitioner assesses your energy flow using polarity bodywork. It is not essential to undress, and you can be examined through clothing if you prefer.

The practitioner usually starts by moving her hands around your head, then down toward your feet, up the body over the five energy centers, finishing back at your head. She will employ different levels of pressure: *neutral*, a light, fingertip touch to restore body awareness and balance; *positive*, which aims to stimulate energy by stroking, molding, and rocking the body; and *negative*, which uses deep, sometimes uncomfortable manipulation of body tissue to stimulate the flow of energy. Most people find bodywork profoundly relaxing, but it is possible that in clearing areas of stagnation, it may induce an emotional outburst of anger, grief, or mirth.

The practitioner may show you exercises to follow at home and recommend a "health-building" cleansing diet with plenty of fruit and vegetables (see below). If she believes negative thoughts are contributing to the problem, she may suggest counseling (see page 163).

BODYWORK TECHNIQUES
The practitioner uses her left or right hand to restore energy flow at the negative and positive poles of the body. The pressure applied will vary but she will ease it if you find it uncomfortable.

The practitioner applies pressure with her fingertips to the abdomen

The right hand is believed to be the positive energy charge

The left hand corresponds to the negative energy pole

> **PRECAUTIONS**
> - Consult your doctor before following a detoxifying diet.
> - See also page 52.

SELF-HELP

Your practitioner may suggest simple polarity yoga exercises to be carried out at home and that require only a few minutes daily to complete, together with a specific diet or detoxifying regime. Dr. Stone believed strongly in the cleansing and healing power of fruit and vegetables. A diet might therefore include steamed or boiled vegetables, soups, fresh juices, and herbal teas, such as the polarity liver flush and tea (right).

POLARITY YOGA

Keep the shoulders back to avoid slouching
Breathe deeply to calm the mind
Bend forward from the hip

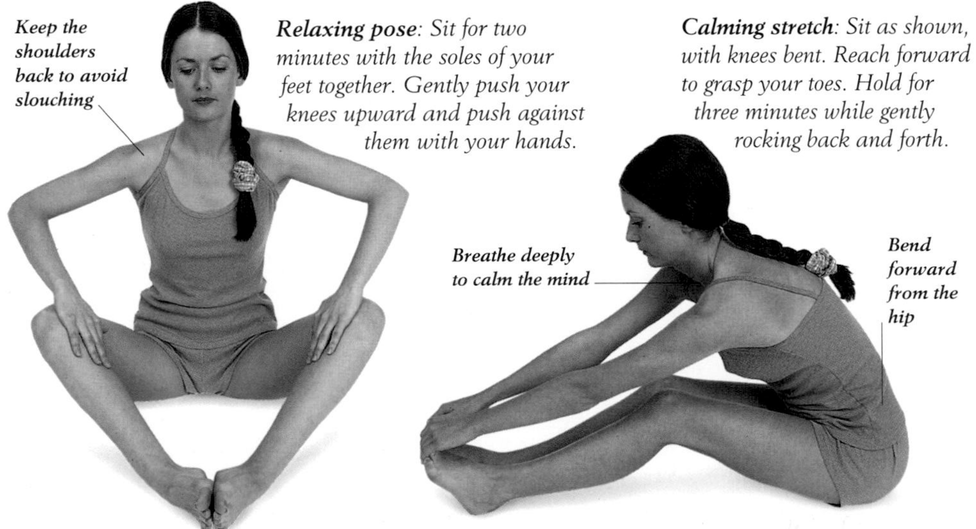

***Relaxing pose**: Sit for two minutes with the soles of your feet together. Gently push your knees upward and push against them with your hands.*

***Calming stretch**: Sit as shown, with knees bent. Reach forward to grasp your toes. Hold for three minutes while gently rocking back and forth.*

POLARITY LIVER FLUSH & TEA

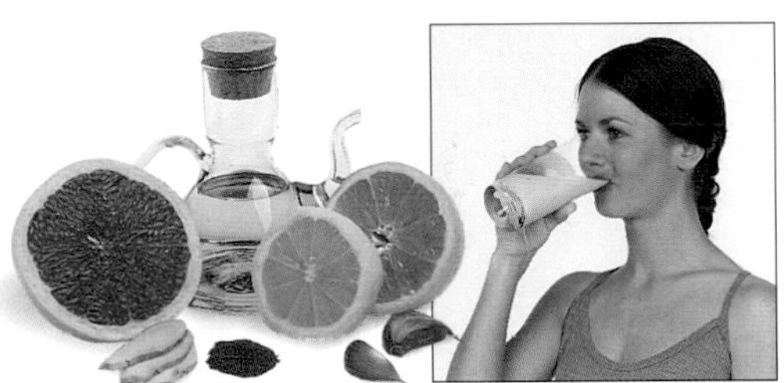

1 The liver flush aims to cleanse the liver, kidneys and bowel. Drink the flush first, which blends lemon, orange, and pink grapefruit juices with olive oil, garlic, ginger, and cayenne pepper.

Tea is left to infuse for ten minutes

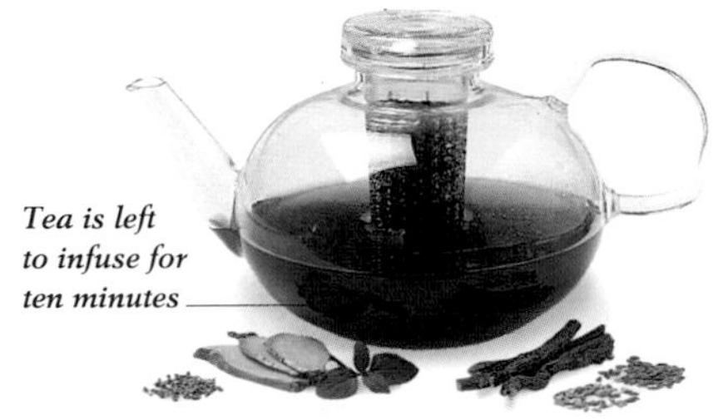

2 Polarity tea should always follow the liver flush. An infusion of linseed, fenugreek, anise, fennel seed, licorice root, peppermint leaves, and slices of ginger, it is an acquired taste.

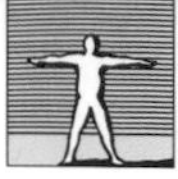

Healing

Ratings	
Evidence	
Medical Opinion	
Practitioner	
Self-Help	
Compatibility	

Healing, sometimes known as the "laying on of hands," is part of the ancient religious and magic practices of many cultures, past and present, encompassing a wide range of belief systems. Healers describe their work as the "restoration to health by nonphysical means." They channel benign healing energy to the patient to activate natural self-healing mechanisms, either through the laying on of hands or at a distance by thought or prayer. In the late 20th century, medical science began to acknowledge the possible benefits of healing, and it is offered in some hospitals, mostly in the UK, to support conventional treatment.

Main Uses

- Chronic pain, post-operative pain
- Healing wounds
- Stress-related conditions, such as depression & anxiety
- Tension headaches, migraines
- High blood pressure
- Menstrual problems

History

Cultures throughout the world have a tradition of healing linked to shamanism, religious ritual, or magic. Priests in ancient Egypt were said to have cured the sick by the laying on of hands, and there are many examples of miraculous cures in the Bible.

By the Middle Ages, the work of spiritual healers was viewed with suspicion by the Christian church, which often attributed their power to witchcraft. One tolerated practice was the visiting of holy shrines by the sick. Usually tombs of saints, or places associated with divine visions, healing shrines such as Lourdes in France and Knock in Ireland still draw thousands of pilgrims every year. In the 20th century some churches have revived early Christian traditions of healing in special services.

Reports of healers using "auras," or psychic energy fields, were common in the 19th century. Reflecting a centuries-old practice, aura healing was part of a wider interest in the "subtle body" that emerged in Europe and the US at this time. It became fashionable to attend seances held by mediums said to communicate with the spirit world and, in some cases, to channel healing powers from the spirits of the dead. One of the most famous spiritualist healers was the British medium Harry Edwards (died 1976), who claimed Louis Pasteur and Joseph Lister among his spirit guides.

In the UK today, around 8,000 people belong to healing organizations, and many more practice as unregistered healers. Since the 1970s, healers have been permitted to work in British hospitals when requested by patients or medical staff, and a few practice regularly in a number of hospitals, pain clinics, and cancer units. Some British doctors refer patients to healers, and several include them in their practice.

In the US, healing is not a separate therapy, but may be offered in offices or innovative hospitals by health professionals including doctors, osteopaths, and acupuncturists. Acceptance varies by state law. Public interest exists in some other countries.

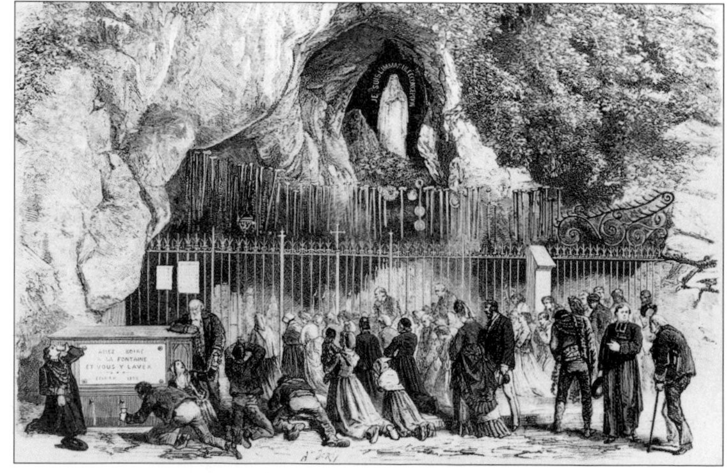

***A 19th-century illustration** showing pilgrims at the shrine of Lourdes in southern France. The waters from a spring in the grotto are believed to have the power to effect miracle cures, and thousands of people visit this shrine every year.*

Key Principles

Most healers believe therapeutic changes take place in the patient's soul during treatment, prompting biological responses. Traditionally, healers worked in the name of a spirit or god, and many healers today believe in a spiritual or divine presence and purpose behind the therapy. Some interpret this power as a form of "energy," a "channel," or a "guide." Others believe extraterrestrial beings are involved, or rationalize their work using theories from quantum physics, Jungian analysis, or New Age philosophy. There is a confusing overlap of ideas, and it can be difficult to distinguish between the forms of healing. Major differences usually lie in the source attributed to the healing energy, and the way it is transferred.

Most practitioners are ordinary people without any particular qualifications, who see themselves as channels for, rather than possessors of, healing energy. The energy's nature varies according to the healer's beliefs. Healing ability is seen by some as a special gift; others consider it to be a natural talent shared by all.

Specific forms of healing include Therapeutic Touch (see page 106), reiki (see page 107), and those listed here:

Aura healing: Healers claim to see "bands" or "fields" of changing colors or radiance, representing a nonphysical "auric" body that reflects the patient's state of health. Aura healers place their hands on or near the patient and visualize "healing" colors, sometimes involving Ayurvedic *chakras* (see page 145) or color therapy (see page 186).

Spiritualist healing: Practitioners claim that an entity from the "spirit world" takes over their body while they are in a trance

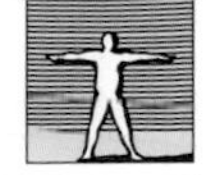

and performs healing through them.

Spiritual healing: Like spiritualists, spiritual healers regard themselves as conductors of supernatural healing forces but they do not associate these with the spirits of the dead.

Faith healing: While most healers regard themselves as channels for an impartial force, faith healers believe that without the patient's faith in their personal powers or those of the deity or cult leader they represent, there can be no cure.

Absent healing: One or more healers visualize a transfer of healing energy from themselves to a distant recipient. This type of healing may include prayer.

Evidence & Research

There is no explanation as to how healing is induced, but trials allegedly demonstrate its beneficial effects. In 1993 Dr. Daniel Benor, an American healer, reviewed 155 studies and claimed 60% had significant results, notably in cases of high blood pressure, anxiety, and wound healing. However, his review was unsystematic, and whether healing triggers specific biological changes remains debatable.

A controversial trial in 1988 on 400 heart patients at San Francisco General Hospital claimed that absent healing by prayer seemed to help patients in recovery.

Studies with animals and plants are sometimes considered more convincing than those on humans because the results cannot be attributed to a placebo effect. In laboratory tests, healers have apparently extended the life of blood cells and accelerated growth of plants. The UK healer Matthew Manning is said to have accomplished this. In another series of experiments in the 1970s, laboratory mice recovered more quickly from anesthesia when treated by healers.

Medical Opinion

"Healing energy" so far defies scientific explanation, although there is a substantial, occasionally convincing, body of research into its effects. A placebo response or autosuggestion (see page 167) may explain some successes, but a collection of 700 American case studies reporting spontaneous, "miraculous" recoveries from a range of problems makes disturbing reading for skeptics. Many doctors reason that healing can at least offer patients comfort in severe cases where medicine has little to offer.

Consulting a Practitioner

Depending on the type of healer, a consultation may take place at a church, the practitioner's home, your home, or a center or clinic. You will usually be asked informal questions about your complaint, medical history, and lifestyle. You will then sit or lie down while the healer sits or stands beside you. The healer will usually spend a few moments "centering" himself, relaxing and focusing his mind, before mentally "attuning" to you.

Healers often regard their hands as amplifiers or conduits of healing power, placing them on or slightly above the site of the problem in order to stimulate your healing processes. The healer may assess your energy field by touching you lightly with his hands, or by making sweeping movements around you, to detect any sensations of heat or cold that might indicate an energy "imbalance." Once attuned, he will consciously try to connect with the source of healing energy, allowing this to flow through himself into your body.

Lighted candles or soft music may be used to encourage a calm and peaceful atmosphere. When healing is part of a Christian church service, prayers for the patient's recovery and hymns will be used. Other rituals, such as incantations, may be used, depending on the belief system.

The healing session may last from a few minutes to over an hour. There are unusual cases of patients who claim to have been cured after one session, but a much longer course of treatment is generally advised. A rapport with the practitioner is not essential, but you must be comfortable with the healer and with the philosophy on which the healing is based. You should also remember that the benefits of healing may be more psychological than physical.

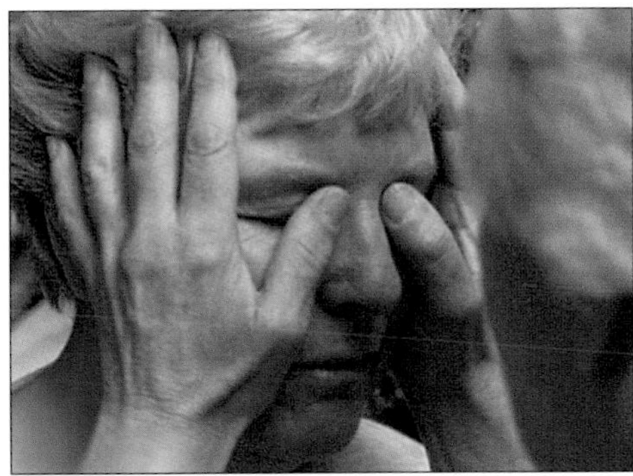

***Healers often say** that their hands feel hot during the healing process and many feel energized by the experience. Patients frequently report sensations of warmth, cold, or tingling, or even dizziness.*

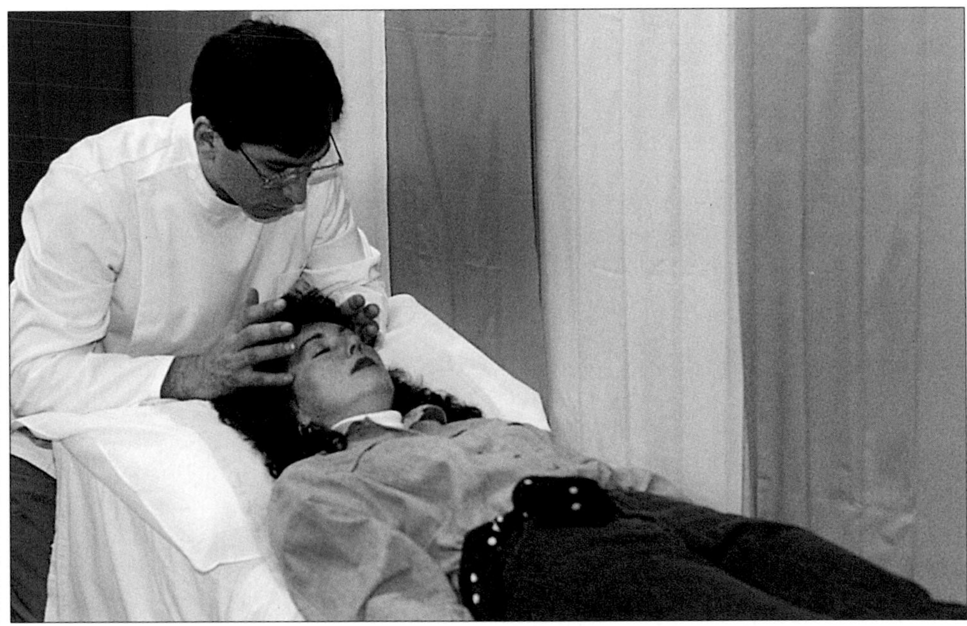

***A healer uses his hands** to connect with the aura or energy field of the patient, mentally attuning to her to awaken her healing processes. Some studies show that during treatment the healer's brain waves often slip into a pattern similar to that reported in people who meditate (see page 175). The same changes in the patient's brain waves may follow.*

Precautions

- Avoid healers who charge excessive fees, who promise a cure, or who imply that any failure to recover reflects your lack of faith.
- See also page 52.

THERAPEUTIC TOUCH

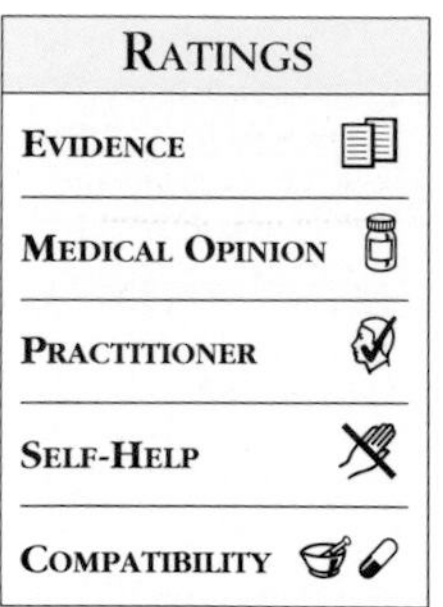

DESCRIBED AS A MODERN FORM of the laying on of hands (see page 104), this method of healing was first used in American teaching hospitals in the early 1970s. Practitioners believe that the body has unique energy fields, defined in terms of quantum physics, and they use their hands to rebalance disruptions in the flow of energy and stimulate the patient's natural powers of self-healing. Therapeutic Touch is taught in over 80 North American colleges, and is widely practiced by nurses in American hospitals to supplement conventional treatment. It is becoming increasingly popular in Britain and Australia.

MAIN USES

- Stress-related conditions, such as fatigue & headaches
- Pain relief, especially from musculoskeletal problems & following surgery
- Wound healing
- Menstrual problems
- Lymphatic & circulatory disorders

HISTORY

In the late 1960s, Dr. Dolores Krieger, Professor of Nursing at New York University, learned the technique of laying on of hands from a healer, Dora Kunz. Concerned about the impersonal nature of the patient–nurse relationship, she sought ways to bring the therapeutic power of this technique into nursing. In 1972 Dr. Krieger began teaching what she called "Therapeutic Touch" (TT) to her students. At least 30,000 nurses use it in American clinics and hospitals. Increasing numbers of nurses in the UK are learning TT and the British Association of Therapeutic Touch was launched in 1994. About 100 nurses practice TT in Australia.

CONSULTING A PRACTITIONER

Therapeutic Touch presupposes that people have individual "energy fields" interacting with one another and with the environment as part of a universal energy force. These fields are thought of in scientific, rather than mystical, terms.

During treatment, the practitioner will try to "attune" her energy field with yours so that disturbances in your "energy flow" are balanced and your body's healing powers can work freely. She will sit beside you and "center" herself, relaxing and focusing on the care that she will give you. When ready, she places her hands 2–6 in (5–15 cm) above your body and gently moves them over it to assess any changes or blockages in your energy field. She may feel these as "warm," "cold," "tingly," or "buzzy" sensations. Using sweeping movements, she will try to treat areas of imbalance, perhaps by visualizing healing energy directed from her body to yours.

A session may last 10–15 minutes. Many people report a sense of relaxation and relief from pain, and increased well-being. Pent-up emotions may be released and breathing can become easier.

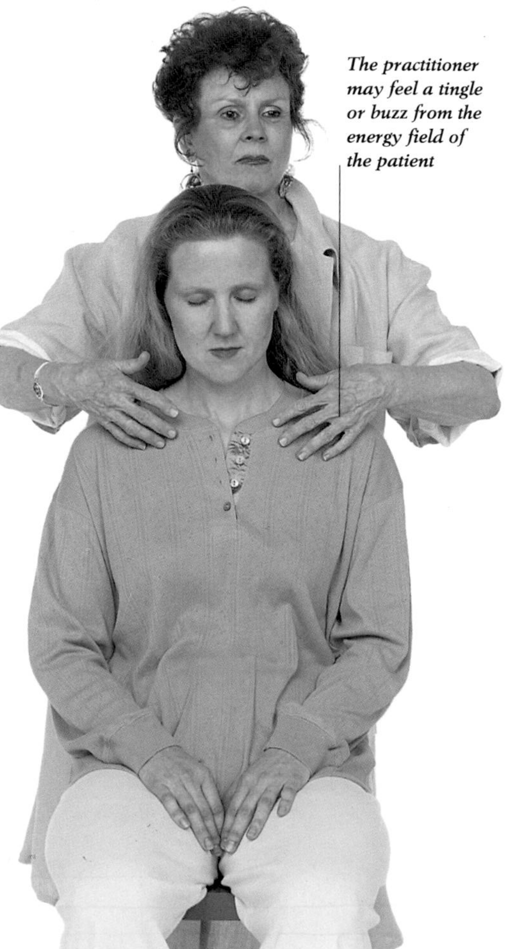

The practitioner may feel a tingle or buzz from the energy field of the patient

ASSESSING THE ENERGY FIELD
The practitioner passes her hands over the body, without making contact, in order to determine the state of the patient's energy field.

This practitioner sweeps her hands over the patient

REPATTERNING THE ENERGY FIELD
Healing energy is directed through the hands to influence the pattern of the patient's energy field. Some practitioners place their hands on the area, some sweep their hands over it.

EVIDENCE & RESEARCH

Studies carried out in the 1960s by Dr. Krieger showed that hemoglobin levels increased in some patients receiving TT. Later studies in the 1980s showed that TT was more effective than simple touch in allaying anxiety and relieving tension headaches. A 1997 US study revealed that TT could reduce the effects of stress on the immune system.

MEDICAL OPINION

A growing number of nurses are taking an interest in TT, and using it in hospitals. Despite this, the medical establishment is still fairly skeptical, although the best research in this area is difficult to deny.

PRECAUTIONS

- Treatment should be given with extra care if you are elderly or pregnant, or if it is your baby that is being treated; if you have a head injury, psychosis, or shock; or if you are emaciated.
- See also page 52.

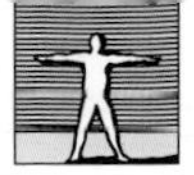

REIKI

RATINGS

EVIDENCE	
MEDICAL OPINION	
PRACTITIONER	
SELF-HELP	
COMPATIBILITY	

A FORM OF JAPANESE SPIRITUAL HEALING, reiki has its foundations in ancient Tibetan Buddhism, and was apparently forgotten until its rediscovery in the late 19th century. Practitioners draw on "reiki energy," channeling it to areas of need in themselves and their patients. They borrow terminology from physics, claiming that reiki acts at an atomic level, causing the body's molecules to vibrate with higher intensity and thus dissolving energy blockages that lead to disharmony and disease. Reiki is becoming popular in the West, with over 200,000 initiates in North America, Europe, and Australasia.

MAIN USES

- Stress-related conditions, including headaches, fatigue, insomnia & anxiety
- Emotional distress
- Pain relief
- Practitioners claim that reiki can be used to treat any physical, mental, or emotional disorder

HISTORY

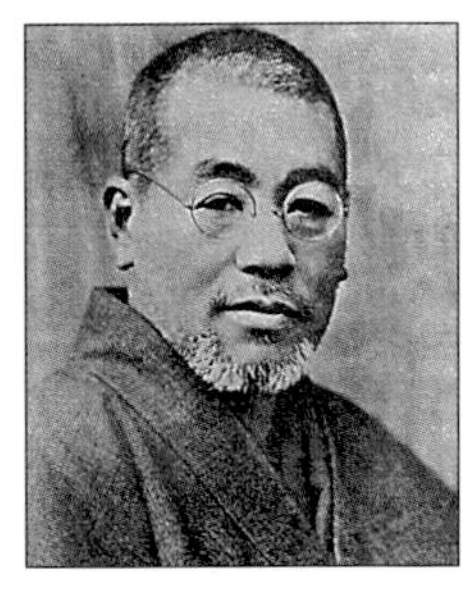

***Dr. Mikao Usui**, the founder of reiki, was a Japanese theologian who studied the secret of Christ's healing power. Usui spent 14 years seeking the secrets of healing, and claimed that the answer came to him in a vision.*

The Japanese word reiki is derived from *rei* ("universal") and *ki* ("life energy"). The ancient reiki healing practices of Tibetan Buddhism were believed to have been lost over the centuries, until Dr. Usui rediscovered and reinterpreted them in the late 19th century. One of his pupils, Dr. Chujiro Hayashi, passed on this knowledge to Hawaio Takata, a Japanese woman living in Hawaii, who introduced reiki in the West in the 1970s. In 1981, her pupils formed the Reiki Alliance, which now has over 800 members worldwide.

CHANNELING ENERGY

Practitioners channel ki, *or "life energy," to the patient to rebalance and replenish areas where it is depleted. Channeling reiki is also said to clear the practitioners' own energy blocks, encouraging inner strength and self-growth.*

The practitioner directs reiki energy through his hands to the patient

CONSULTING A PRACTITIONER

Reiki aims to promote health, maintain well-being, and help people attain a higher consciousness. Practitioners say that before acting as a channel for reiki, their physical and spiritual (or "etheric") bodies need to be "attuned" according to ancient and secret symbols revealed to initiates in three stages over years. Once the healing channel is opened, it is thought to remain active for life and can be used when required.

You are asked to "formulate your intent" (to say what you wish the practitioner to treat), but since it is thought that reiki "works for the highest good," it may not necessarily offer a cure. Each treatment session lasts about an hour. You lie clothed on a treatment table and the practitioner holds his hands on or over your body in 12 basic positions for about five minutes each; four are on the head, four on the front of the body and four on the back. This is said to balance the body's energy centers, or *chakras* (see page 109). Some patients may feel relaxed after treatment; others feel invigorated. Reiki may also be practiced as a form of absent healing (see page 105).

EVIDENCE & RESEARCH

Virtually no controlled studies have been made to support the claims of reiki. However, heat-sensitive photographs of a practitioner's hand, taken before and during treatment, reportedly show an intensification of heat during healing.

MEDICAL OPINION

The principles on which reiki is based lie far beyond the realm of conventional science, and most doctors would regard it as little more than an exotic-sounding healing ritual. While the concepts and terminology may seem far-fetched, some doctors might see reiki as an artistic and imaginative adjunct to health care, provided that the physical disease is being dealt with by conventional treatment.

PRECAUTIONS

- See page 52.

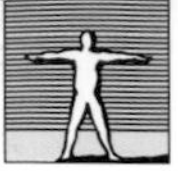

YOGA

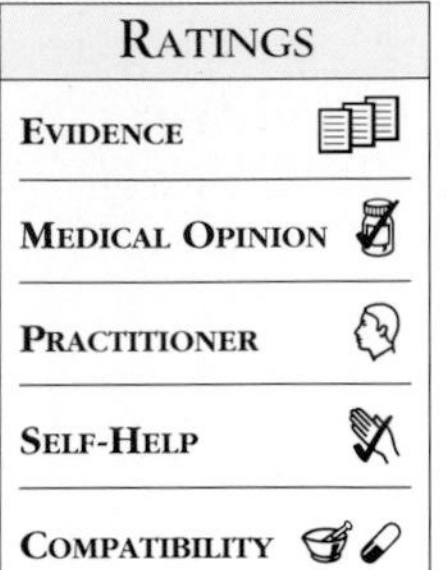

BEST KNOWN IN THE WEST as a form of gentle exercise consisting of body postures and breathing techniques, yoga is in fact a complete system of mental and physical training, originally developed as preparation for spiritual development. It has been practiced for thousands of years in India as part of Ayurveda (see page 144), and has now become popular around the world. In the West it is valued more for its physical than spiritual benefits, such as its ability to increase suppleness and vitality, and to relieve stress. Yoga has now been incorporated into a number of Western health regimes.

MAIN USES

- Stress, fatigue, CFS
- Headaches, migraines
- Depression
- Circulatory disorders
- Asthma, bronchitis
- Rheumatoid arthritis
- Digestive disorders
- Back pain
- Menstrual problems, including PMS
- Improved mobility

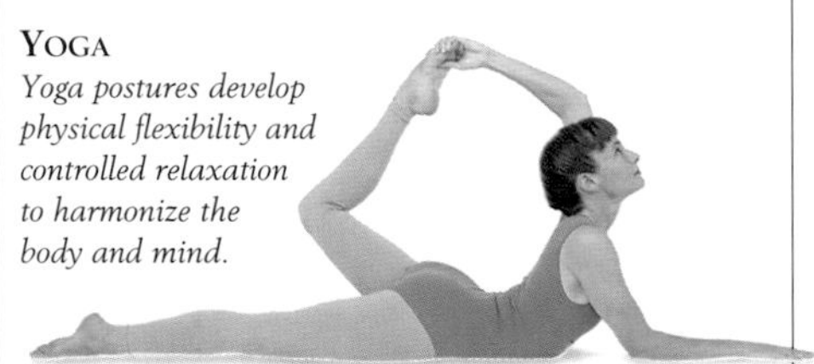

YOGA
Yoga postures develop physical flexibility and controlled relaxation to harmonize the body and mind.

HISTORY

The word yoga (from the same root as the English "yoke") is Sanskrit for "union." The system originated over 4,000 years ago in India, where it was traditionally practiced by Hindu ascetics, or yogis. Patanjali, the father of yoga, defined the path of the yogi in his *Yoga Sutras* (or aphorisms) in the 3rd century B.C. (see right). Yoga was introduced to the West in the 19th century, when scholars translated ancient Hindu religious texts. Initially it attracted few followers, but has grown enormously in popularity since the 1960s, along with many other Eastern disciplines promoting well-being. By 1996, 500,000 people in the UK alone were doing yoga. It is part of some American health care programs, such as Dr. Ornish's regime for reversing heart disease (see page 243).

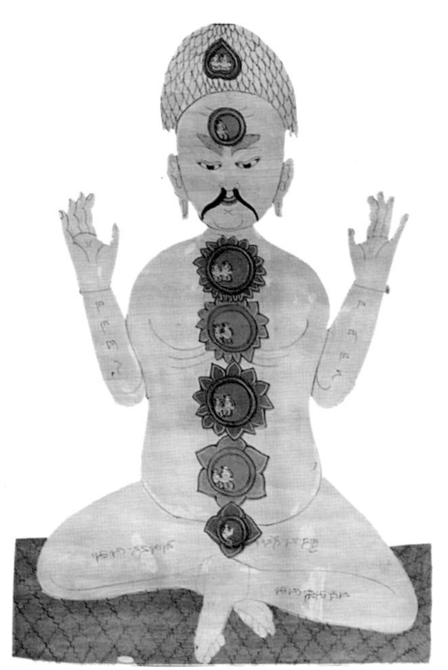

The seven* chakras *(see opposite) are symbolically represented as floral-petaled patterns on this ancient Hindu manuscript from Nepal.

KEY PRINCIPLES

In its purest form, yoga is a fully integrated system controlling all aspects of life. In the "Eight Limbs of Yoga," the yogi Patanjali described a series of increasingly spiritual stages on the path to enlightenment. These begin with ethical guidelines, including healthy eating habits and high levels of personal hygiene, and progress through the practice of *asanas* (physical postures) and *pranayama* (breathing techniques) to meditation and, eventually, withdrawal to the supreme level of pure consciousness.

Today there are many types of yoga, including yoga therapy to maintain health and help specific medical conditions, and ashtanga, or power yoga. While meditation is central to some forms of devotional yoga, the most popular form in the West is hatha yoga, using *asanas* and *pranayama*. Breath is seen as the outward form of *prana* ("life energy"), and controlled breathing regulates *prana* in the body (see opposite).

Hatha means "balance," reflecting the balance of mind and body; a serene mind produces regular breathing and a relaxed body. Conversely, a relaxed body promotes steady breathing and a calm mind. *Asanas* are designed to benefit both mind and body; performed slowly and deliberately, they are coordinated with the breathing. Each *asana* has an individual shape and it is important to maintain these shapes correctly. Regular practice is preferred, since it helps to maximize the benefits of performing the *asanas*.

EVIDENCE & RESEARCH

Most research has been carried out using gentle forms of yoga; so far no medical evidence exists to substantiate claims for more advanced forms. Some reputable studies have, however, confirmed that yoga can benefit a range of conditions. One well-known study from the 1960s was done at the Menninger Foundation in Texas, where researchers developing biofeedback techniques found that yoga meditation clearly affects the heart and circulation.

A 1990 study in *The Lancet* showed that yoga breathing reduced the frequency of asthma attacks, and at Oxford University in 1993, psychologists found yoga breathing more effective for restoring energy than relaxation or visualization. In the *British Journal of Rheumatology*, a 1994 study indicated that yoga therapy could benefit people with rheumatoid arthritis.

MEDICAL OPINION

The medical establishment is skeptical of some of the claims of yoga (for example, that yoga can affect the nervous system and hormone levels), but most doctors would not object to it as an exercise or relaxation technique, and many would acknowledge that it deserves closer examination as a treatment for conditions such as heart disease. The development of yoga therapy, which uses specific *asanas* and *pranayama* to treat medical complaints, is likely to be followed with considerable interest.

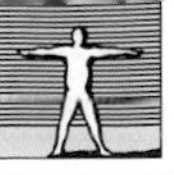

THE THEORY OF YOGA

Yoga *asanas* and relaxation techniques were developed to bring physical and spiritual benefits. *Asanas* are designed to have an impact on the physical body, stimulating nerve centers and organs. Spiritual benefits are derived from using breathing techniques and meditation to influence the flow of *prana*, or life energy, which flows through the "subtle" (nonphysical) body in invisible "energy channels," known as *nadi*. When mind and body are in harmony, the individual can focus on spiritual goals by practicing the higher discipline of meditation.

THE *CHAKRAS*

In more esoteric yoga teachings, the *chakras* are centers of life energy, situated in the subtle body – seat of the senses, emotions, and intellect. Seven *chakras* ascend in order of spiritual refinement along a central channel, the *Sushumna*. *Chakras* are linked to nerve centers along the spinal cord and, like them, are thought to be influenced by *asanas*. Each *chakra* is symbolized by an exact number of lotus petals and, according to some schools of yoga, is associated with a specific mantra or sound, such as "Om" or "Ram." These are used in meditation and breathing exercises to act on the *chakras*.

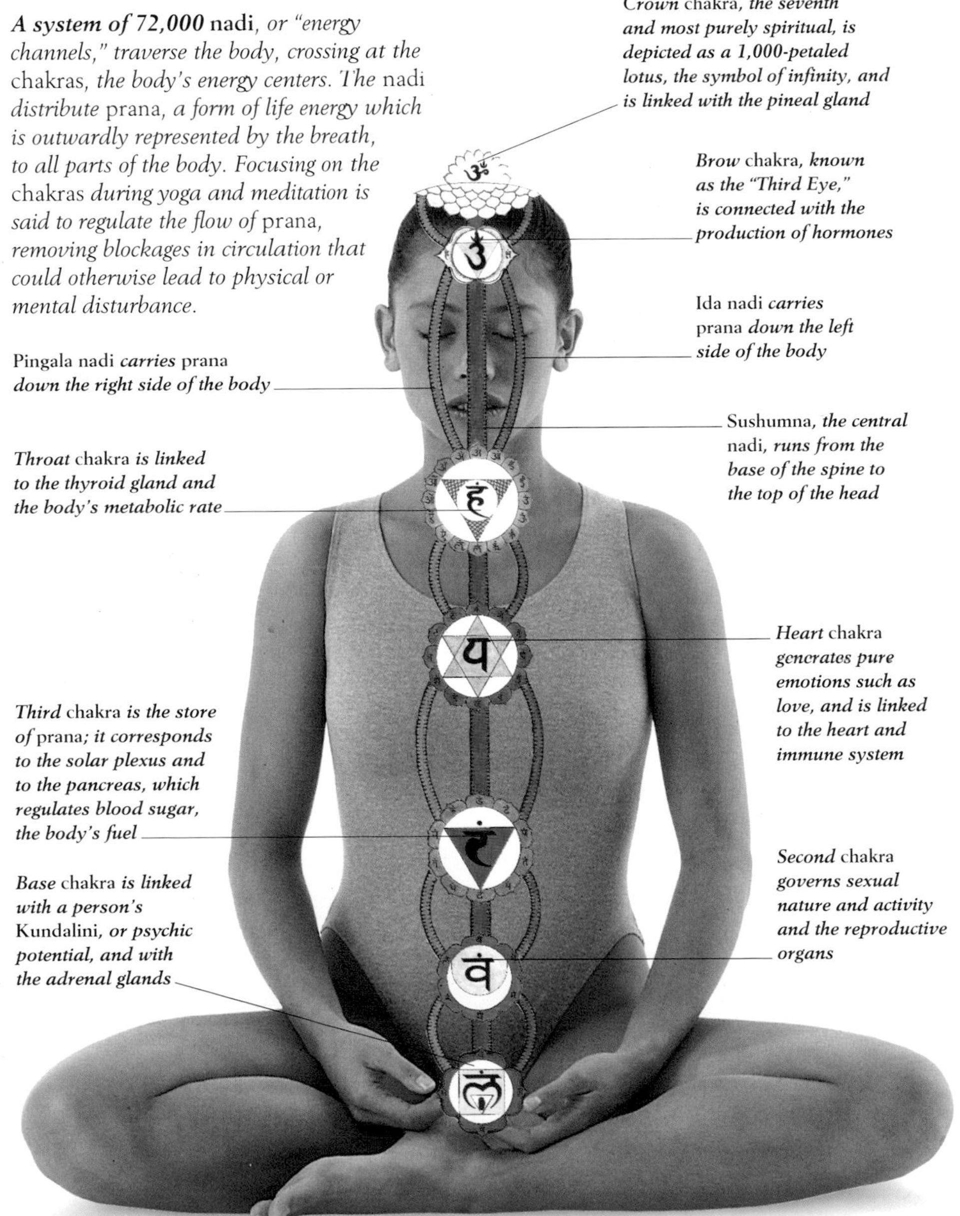

A system of 72,000 **nadi**, *or "energy channels," traverse the body, crossing at the* chakras, *the body's energy centers. The* nadi *distribute* prana, *a form of life energy which is outwardly represented by the breath, to all parts of the body. Focusing on the* chakras *during yoga and meditation is said to regulate the flow of* prana, *removing blockages in circulation that could otherwise lead to physical or mental disturbance.*

PHYSICAL BENEFITS

Hatha yoga has a physiological effect on muscle tone and circulation. Various *asanas* are believed to affect the autonomic nervous system (see page 71) and endocrine glands, which regulate internal functions, including heart rate and hormone production.

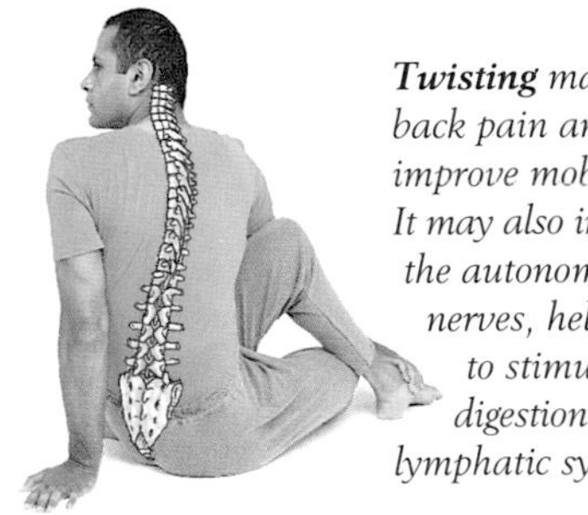

Twisting *may ease back pain and help improve mobility. It may also influence the autonomic nerves, helping to stimulate digestion and the lymphatic system.*

Veins carry blood back to the heart

Arteries carry blood out from the heart

Headstands *relax the heart by allowing blood to flow from the legs to the upper body. Meditative* asanas *such as this are said to improve circulation and stimulate the brain.*

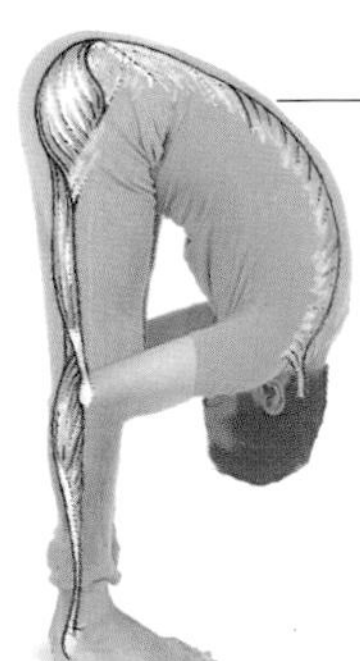

Bending forward *with the head down lengthens the spine, stretches the back muscles, and increases the supply of oxygen to the brain.*

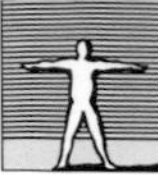

DANCE MOVEMENT THERAPY

RATINGS
EVIDENCE
MEDICAL OPINION
PRACTITIONER
SELF-HELP
COMPATIBILITY

A METHOD OF EXPRESSING THOUGHTS and feelings through movement, dance movement therapy as practiced today was developed in the United States in the 1940s. Participants attend weekly sessions given by trained therapists, in which they are encouraged to move freely, sometimes to music. Dance movement therapy can be used by people of all ages to promote self-esteem and gain insight into emotional problems, but it is also practiced to help those with serious mental and physical disabilities. As such, it is widely used in the United States, and is becoming established around the world.

MAIN USES

- **Work with the blind, deaf & elderly & those who have been abused or traumatized**
- **Physical & mental disability, autism, learning difficulties**
- **Depression, anxiety, psychotic conditions**
- **Behavioral & eating disorders**

HISTORY

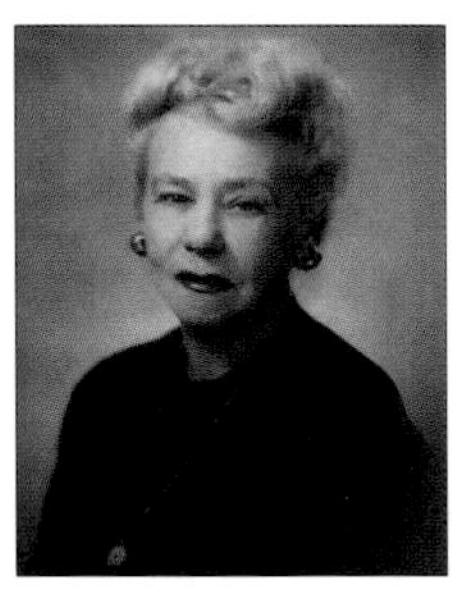

***Marian Chace**, a dance teacher, helped pioneer dance movement therapy in Washington D.C. She found that rigid or repetitive behaviors could be released by encouraging patients to move freely.*

Throughout history, society has exploited the link between body movement and emotion, using movement to let off steam, whip up battle frenzy, arouse passion, and exorcise evil spirits. The use of expressive movement as a tool in psychotherapy was explored at the turn of the 20th century by Carl Jung (see page 160) and by Wilhelm Reich (see page 89), and later by Rudolf Laban. A choreographer and movement analyst born in Bratislava, Laban emigrated to Britain at the outbreak of World War I. He believed that by observing nuances of movement or facial gesture, the analyst could learn much about the patient's emotional state.

In the 1940s, partly in response to the large number of people physically and emotionally damaged after World War II, a small group of professional dancers in the US began to develop a form of therapeutic dance movement. Prominent among them was Marian Chace, who used the therapy in her work with schizophrenics.

Well established in the US, and widely accepted by the American medical profession, dance movement therapy is gaining recognition in Australia and the UK. It is most likely to be encountered in health care centers, schools, and prisons.

KEY PRINCIPLES

Babies and young children express themselves through their bodies before they learn to talk. Their feelings are conveyed through movements, such as kicking or clenching their fists with anger, or jumping and wriggling for joy. Children are quite natural and spontaneous in their actions, but in later life the thoughts, emotions, and physical experiences that shape their personalities are influenced by their social surroundings, and the link between feeling and actions becomes less spontaneous and more conditioned. Adults still reveal themselves through body language; however, many of these feelings are expressed unconsciously.

In dance movement therapy, movement, and particularly the sensual, rhythmic response aroused by dance and music, is used as a way of bypassing the conscious mind and making contact with the inner emotional world. To do this, patients explore a range of movements and learn to overcome physical limitations and cope with disabilities. The aim is to evoke images that raise important emotional issues, which the practitioner will help the patient to explore further through dance in the later stages of therapy. In this way, hidden emotions can be expressed in a nonverbal way, and subsequently accepted by the conscious self.

Dance movement therapy works equally well for highly articulate people and for those less able to express themselves in words, including people with learning disabilities, mental problems, or psychotic illnesses. Even severely physically disabled people can experience the liberating effects of dance.

*"**Mirroring**," based on the work of Rudolf Laban, is a method of understanding another person's physical and psychological condition. The aim is to reflect the person's movements and gestures.*

EVIDENCE & RESEARCH

There is a large body of research supporting the work of dance movement therapists. This is based on case histories, videotapes, and observational studies, and has been published since the 1970s in psychological and dance journals. Much of the research has focused on the relationship between personality and movement, and on movements that are characteristic of certain conditions.

MEDICAL OPINION

Most conventional doctors would regard dance movement therapy as a useful form of expression and exercise for people with a wide variety of conditions. Its benefits for those with physical disabilities, emotional problems, and mental illnesses are generally recognized.

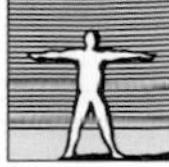

CONSULTING A PRACTITIONER

Dance movement therapy is practiced one-to-one and as group therapy. The number of sessions depends on the patient's needs, usually determined during a six-week assessment course: treatment for long-term conditions may last up to five years.

A session begins with a warm-up to ease joints, increase body awareness, and focus your attention on why you are there. Music is not always necessary – rhythm can be made with the hands, feet, or legs. What occurs next may evolve naturally from the warm-up or be helped along by suggestions from the practitioner. Participants often lie on the floor waiting for an impulse to move; they may, for example, decide to act out a dream. Gestures, mainly spontaneous and unchoreographed, can also include formal dance steps. Some practitioners move with you, mirroring and supporting your movements, others act as empathetic observers. Occasionally the practitioner might dance alone to reflect back her perceptions or to help the patient or group feel comfortable.

A way to end the sequence is found, and feelings raised by the therapy are discussed.

ONE-TO-ONE THERAPY

Individual sessions allow the practitioner to establish a deeply trusting relationship with the patient, which is vital if the patient is to feel safe expressing himself.

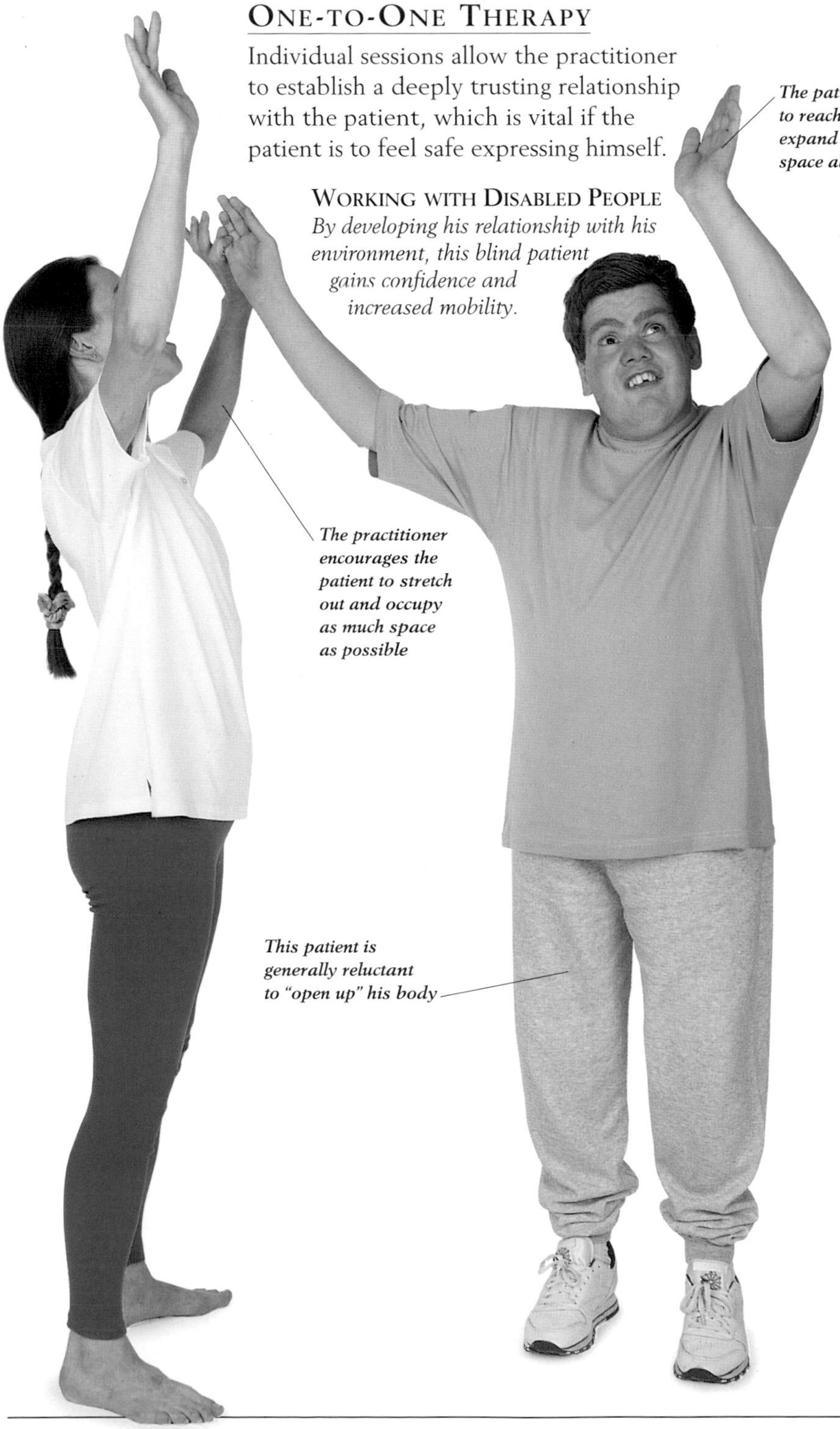

WORKING WITH DISABLED PEOPLE
By developing his relationship with his environment, this blind patient gains confidence and increased mobility.

The patient tries to reach up to expand into the space above him

The practitioner encourages the patient to stretch out and occupy as much space as possible

This patient is generally reluctant to "open up" his body

GROUP THERAPY

Working with a group enables the practitioner to assess how the participants relate to other people and work together, and how they react to different situations.

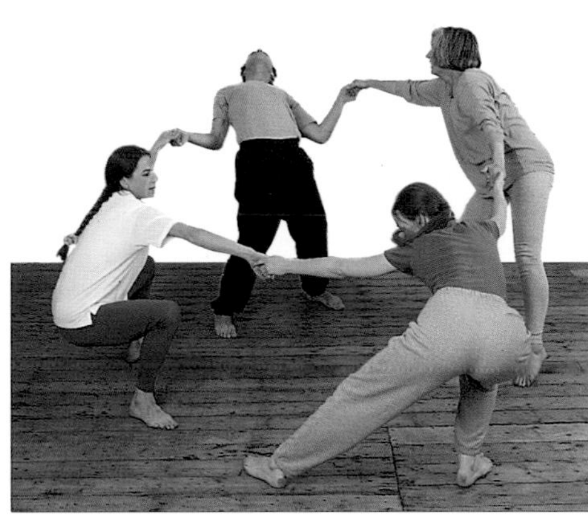

***Group participants** form a circle. Often used to begin or end a session, this technique supports the participants' movements, and encourages them to look at one another as they move.*

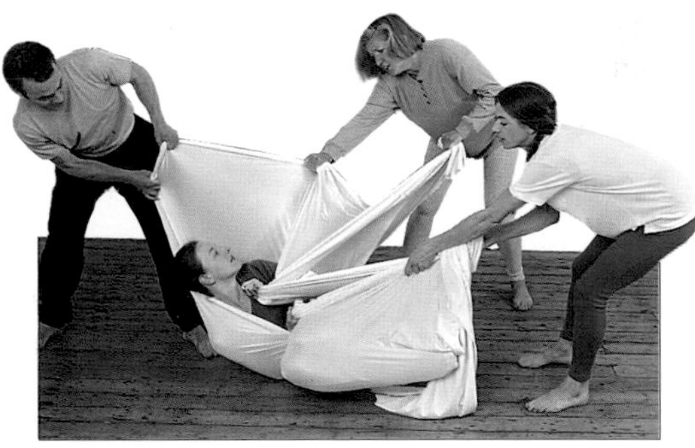

***Props are sometimes used** to explore a theme that emerges during a session. Balls, bean bags, stretch cloths, and other props can be catalysts for inspiration, or may simply help patients to express themselves with greater freedom and confidence.*

PRECAUTIONS

- Check with a doctor before embarking on vigorous exercise if you have back pain or high blood pressure.
- See also page 52.

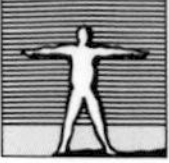

THE BATES METHOD

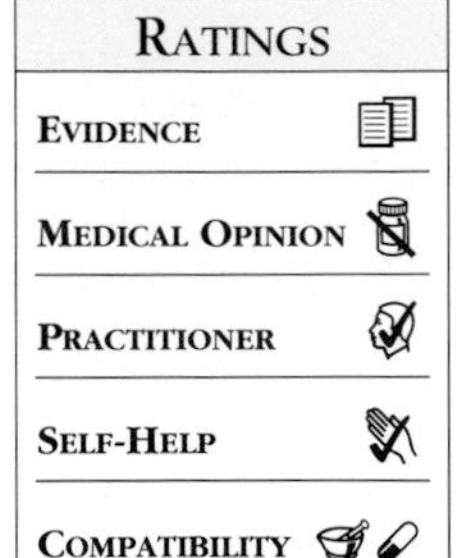

DEVISED AT THE BEGINNING of the 20th century by Dr. William H. Bates, an American ophthalmologist, the Bates method aims to enhance eyesight without the aid of lenses or surgery. Dr. Bates argued that perfect vision was the product of perfectly relaxed eyes, unconsciously controlled, and that misuse of the eyes accounted for many vision defects. He believed that eyes could be reeducated using a series of simple exercises. Practitioners of the Bates method, who can be found in countries around the world, claim that these exercises benefit people of all ages, however good or poor their eyesight.

MAIN USES

- All conditions for which glasses & contact lenses are prescribed, including nearsightedness and farsightedness, squints & astigmatism
- Coordination problems
- Learning difficulties

HISTORY

The Bates method of "vision education" was developed early in the 20th century by the New York ophthalmologist Dr. William H. Bates. He believed that bad habits and tension affecting the eye muscles and optic nerves accounted for many vision defects, which could be corrected with eye exercises. Although initially dismissed by doctors, Dr. Bates's theories attracted followers in the US, Europe, and India who continued his work after his death in 1931. Among these were Margaret Darst Corbett, the American ophthalmologist, and the British writer Aldous Huxley, who claimed amazing results. Today, practitioners of various complementary therapies use the Bates method, and it is best established in the US, UK, and India.

CONSULTING A PRACTITIONER

The practitioner assesses your eyesight and may suggest 6–10 weekly sessions. You are taught simple eye exercises, to be practiced daily. Dr. Bates argued that bad habits, such as staring, "switch off" the eyes' ability constantly to adjust and focus on an image (a process called "central fixation"). Exercises, he believed, could reeducate the eye and help achieve "optimum" central fixation. He taught patients to relax the optic nerve and eye muscles, and use the powers of memory and imagination to improve coordination between the eyes and the brain.

Advice on breathing, relaxation, diet, and exercise may also be given, since Dr. Bates claimed that lifestyle factors could affect vision capability. Artificial light and VDT screens, which encourage staring, are thought to worsen eyesight.

***Swinging**: To relax the eyes and help mobilize them, Dr. Bates recommended swaying gently from side to side with your eyes focused on a distant point. Do this 100 times daily, blinking at the left and the right as you sway. Blinking cleans and lubricates the eyes, and discourages staring, which strains the eyes.*

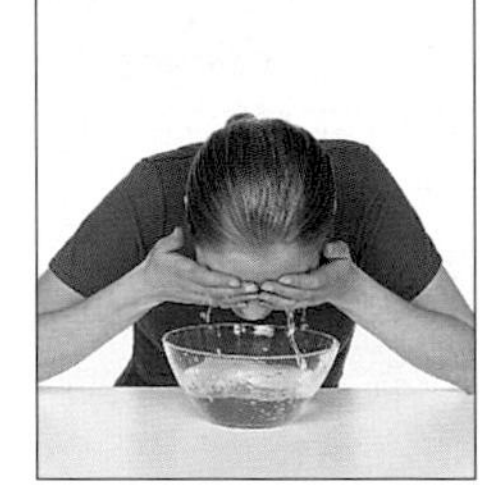

***Splashing**: To stimulate circulation, splash your closed eyes with warm, then cold, water 20 times each morning. Repeat at night, but using cold water first.*

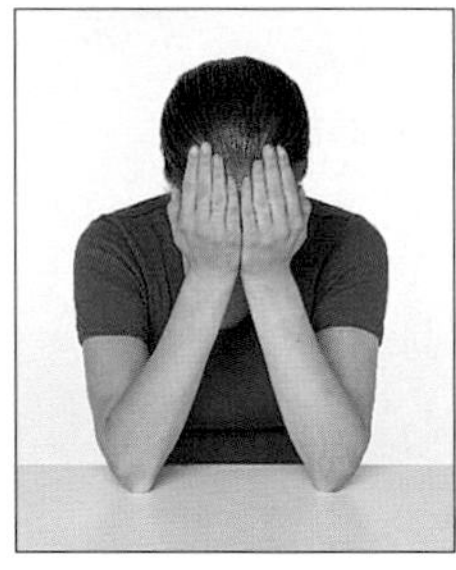

***Palming**: Covering your eyes with cupped palms relaxes them, shutting out light without pressing on the eyes. Don't daydream; listen to music or think of pleasant images while palming for 10 minutes, 2–3 times a day.*

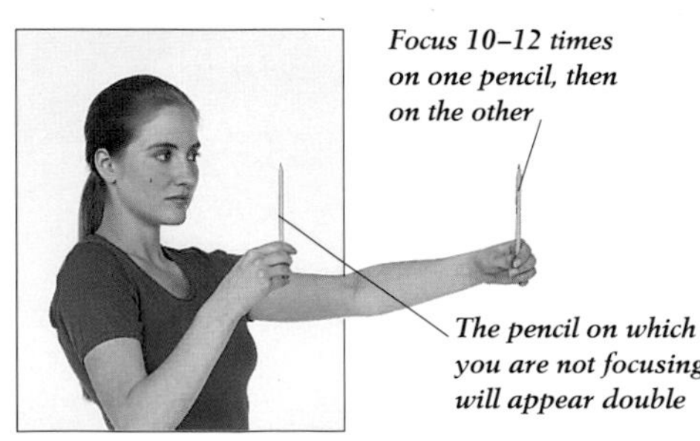

***Focusing**: To improve focusing, hold one pencil at arm's length and one 6 in (15 cm) in front of you. Focus on one, blink, then focus on the other.*

COMMON EYE PROBLEMS

NEARSIGHTEDNESS

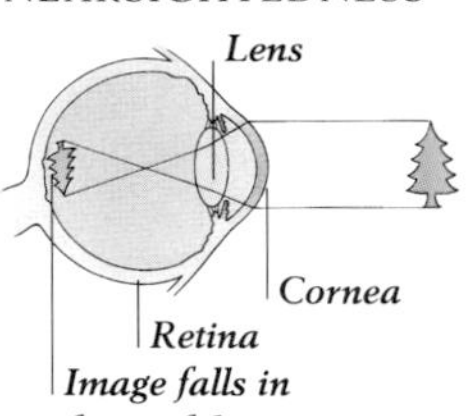

FARSIGHTEDNESS

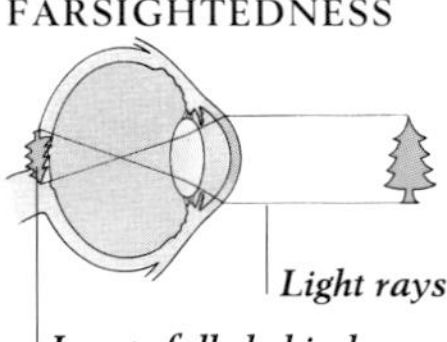

An object that is seen in perfect focus is refracted by the lens on the center of the retina, the fovea centralis, *where images are at their most precise. The eye makes constant tiny adjustments to keep the fovea trained on an image (called "central fixation"). If the eyeball is too short or too long, the image will be out of focus because it falls not on the retina, but behind or in front of it.*

EVIDENCE & RESEARCH

Most trials were carried out in the early 20th century by Dr. Bates. Anecdotal evidence suggests that the method can help to improve eyesight, but there have been no recent clinical trials.

MEDICAL OPINION

Doctors recognize that vision involves the use of eye muscles and instinctive visual skills, and acknowledge that eye exercises may sometimes improve sight. However, since the Bates method requires a certain amount of perseverance, and improvement may not be dramatic, it is not seen as a substitute for lenses or surgery.

PRECAUTIONS

- Consult a teacher if you have glaucoma or cataracts, and an ophthalmologist if your eyesight is fading.
- Do not perform eye exercises while wearing glasses or contact lenses.
- See also page 52.

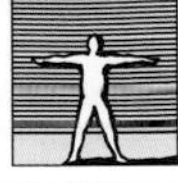

OTHER THERAPIES

THE BOWEN TECHNIQUE

This non-manipulative, hands-on technique was pioneered in Australia in the 1950s by a bodyworker (see glossary), Tom Bowen. He taught his method to an Australian osteopath, Dr. Ossie Rentsch, who continued Bowen's work after his death in 1982, training practitioners in Australasia, North America, and the UK. The Bowen technique is said to stimulate "energy flow," enabling the body's self-healing resources to restore harmony.

The therapy is carried out on a soft, low treatment table with the patient in loose clothing. The practitioner makes a series of light, rolling movements on the muscles and tendons with his fingers and thumbs. This is believed to encourage circulation, increase mobility, and promote lymphatic drainage of waste products. Often only 2–3 sessions are given, each of 30–40 minutes.

The technique claims to benefit any condition, especially back and joint pain, sports injuries, bronchitis, and menstrual problems. Most doctors who encounter it would probably find it slightly bemusing.

ZERO BALANCING

An American doctor, osteopath, and acupuncturist, Fritz Smith, developed this touch technique combining aspects of Western and Eastern medicine in 1975. It has a following today mainly in the US.

Zero Balancers believe that the body has an unseen energy field, which is related to the musculoskeletal system. Treatment aims to promote a smooth flow of energy through the body, improving posture and inducing a sense of harmony, which boosts the body's self-healing ability. Attention is paid to "foundation" joints, for example in the foot, that act as shock absorbers for the weight-bearing skeleton, and to breathing patterns, eye movements, and stomach rumbles (said to indicate energy flow).

The practitioner applies gentle finger pressure to stretch and hold you, while you lie fully clothed on a treatment table. Three sessions of 20–40 minutes each may be recommended, with more as required. The therapy claims to heal past emotional or physical traumas, and while doctors are skeptical, they generally feel it is harmless.

KAHUNA

An ancient system of massage originally practiced by Hawaiian *kahunas* (healers), kahuna aims to help patients accept their body and love themselves. Greater self-love is believed to encourage recognition of the beauty of the surrounding world. The practitioner massages you with sweeping, rhythmic strokes as you lie naked on a treatment table. Treatment takes two hours, with sessions every 2–3 months for as long as desired. Treatment is said to speed up the "vibrational rate" of body cells, but most doctors dismiss this claim.

CHAVUTTI THIRUMAL

Part of the Ayurvedic system of medicine (see page 144), this form of massage comes from southern India, reputedly developed to promote suppleness in Kathakali dancers and practitioners of *kalaripayattu*, a martial art. It is beginning to be practiced in the US and UK as a specialized form of massage to stimulate the circulation, lymphatic system, and digestion. You lie on the floor with body oiled, while the practitioner, hanging onto an overhead rope, uses his feet and toes to apply firm, continuous strokes, said to stimulate the body's *nadi* (energy lines). Sessions last 90 minutes, and are usually given every 2–3 months. Doctors generally consider it a curiosity.

INDIAN HEAD MASSAGE

This Ayurvedic (see page 144) head massage, traditionally used by Indian women to keep their hair lustrous and healthy, is said to relax the thin layer of muscle covering the head, improving blood flow, nourishing hair follicles, and alleviating anxiety and stress.

Practitioners massage the shoulders and head with alternate firm and gentle strokes, using warm oil (coconut, sesame, almond, or olive). Sessions last 20–30 minutes and are usually weekly. Most doctors consider the therapy to be harmless and relaxing.

SHEN THERAPY

This mind and body therapy was created in 1977 by an American bodyworker (see glossary), Richard R. Pavek. He believed that painful emotions, if repressed, stay in the body, affecting behavior and health. Love, sadness, and grief are said to affect the heart and chest; fear, excitement, and anger the digestive tract; and shame, inadequacy, and confidence the genitals. As you lie on a special table, the practitioner places her hands on your clothed body to direct natural "energy" through your key emotion centers in patterns designed to release repressed feelings. Ten weekly treatments may be recommended, with sessions of 60–90 minutes. Used for PMS and psychoemotional ailments like anorexia, SHEN is unknown to most doctors.

EUTONY

Eutony was developed in the 1930s by German-born Gerda Alexander, who observed through her involvement in dance that pupils tended to follow their teacher too closely. Better known in Canada and South America than in the US and UK, eutony is a form of movement therapy in which patients achieve self-knowledge by exploring their own movements, and is often practiced as part of psychotherapy. Sessions last 60–90 minutes, and length of treatment varies widely according to the individual. Eutony claims to treat musculo-skeletal disorders and conditions linked to psychological problems, and seems to be well regarded by doctors who know of it.

HAKOMI

Developed by an American psychotherapist, Ron Kurtz, in the 1970s, hakomi treats the patient mentally, physically, emotionally, and spiritually to promote self-healing. Practitioners help patients enter a state of "mindfulness" (awareness of the moment) to explore self-limiting attitudes that may be reflected in physical traits, such as posture or facial expression. Hakomi is used for any physical condition caused by emotional problems. It may be continued for years, with sessions lasting 60–90 minutes.

PRECAUTIONS

- Avoid Indian head massage if you have a severe scalp condition.
- See also page 52.

Medicinal Therapies

No matter what the healing method, people in every part of the world take medicine, and all cultures have a tradition that attributes therapeutic powers to particular plants, minerals, and parts of animals.

Complementary therapies have their roots in such traditional systems, in which the cause of illness is commonly attributed to an imbalance within an individual or to the influence of external factors.

The mouth is literally a gateway between the external and the internal world, and there is a certain magic in the way we feel hungry, eat, and are satisfied, and in which food provides energy and enables growth and repair. The primitive urge to eat extends to the way in which we regard food as a medicine and take medicinal substances to heal ourselves.

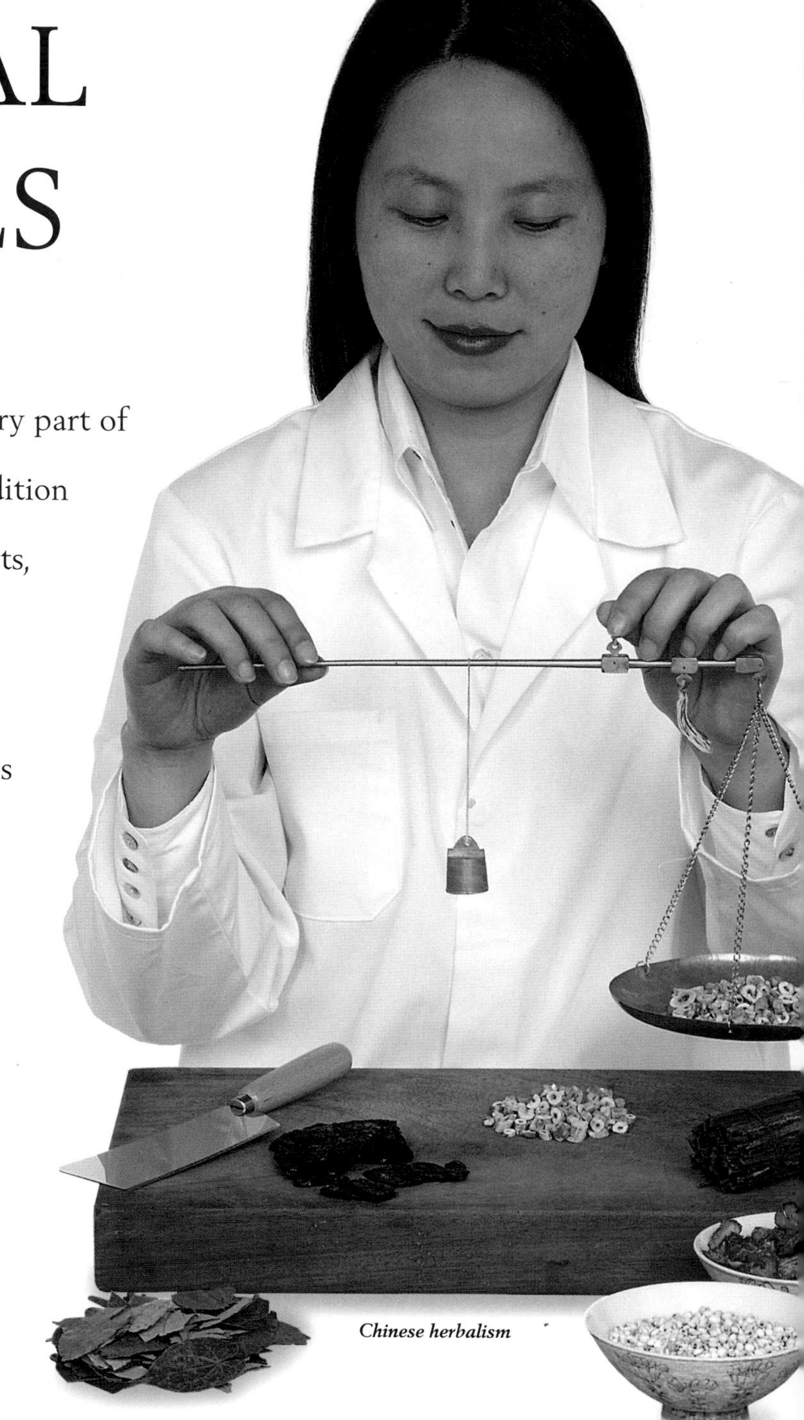

Chinese herbalism

Many medicinal therapies from around the world subscribe to a theory that the internal organs have a direct effect on health. They also share a consensus that when these organs are weak, overactive, or uncoordinated, illness can occur.

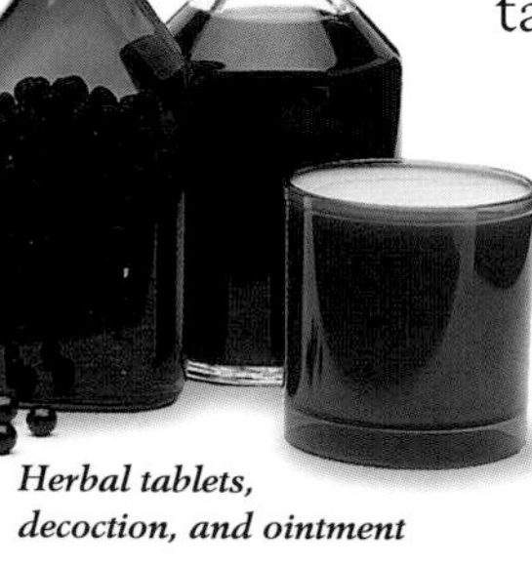

Herbal tablets, decoction, and ointment

There is a tremendous variety of ideas and different medicinal substances involved in this richly disparate group of therapies. Together, these treatment systems draw on experience from every part of the planet, from China to the Amazonian jungle. They are also enriched by a vast bank of knowledge, from the ancient traditions of Indian Ayurvedic medicine to the latest biochemical research into nutritional science carried out in the United States.

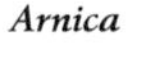

Arnica

The Therapies

Naturopathy *page 118* ◆ Hydrotherapy *page 122*

Anthroposophical Medicine *page 124*

Homeopathy *page 126* ◆ Biochemic Tissue Salts *page 131*

Bach Flower Remedies *page 132* ◆ Crystal Therapy *page 133*

Western Herbalism *page 134* ◆ Chinese Herbalism *page 140*

Ayurveda *page 144* ◆ Nutritional Therapies *page 148*

Orthomolecular Therapy *page 153* ◆ Clinical Ecology *page 154*

Magnetic Therapy *page 156* ◆ Other Therapies *page 157*

Crystals

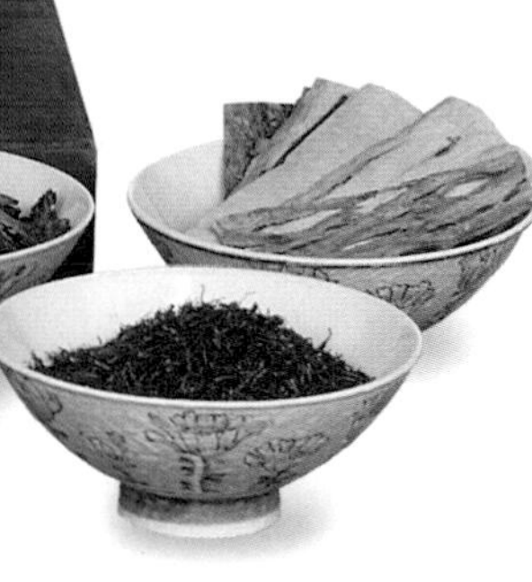

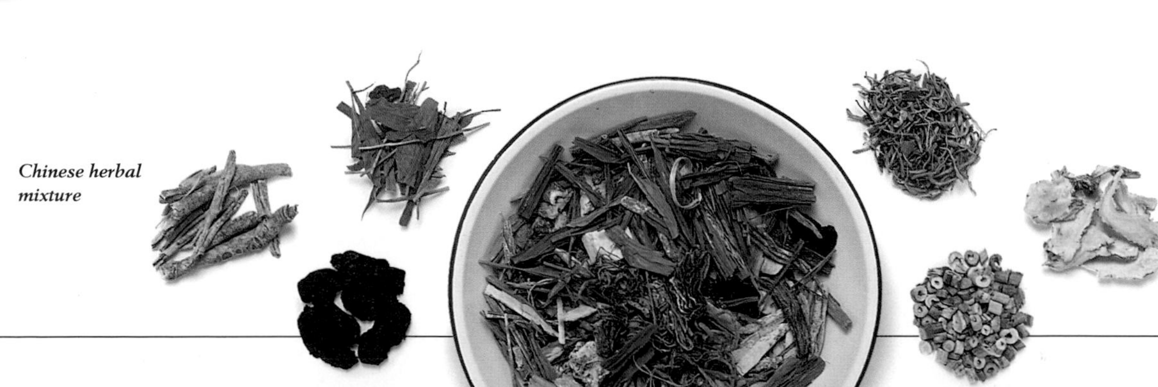

Chinese herbal mixture

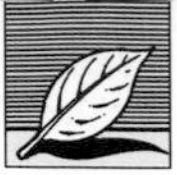

NATUROPATHY

RATINGS

EVIDENCE	
MEDICAL OPINION	
PRACTITIONER	
SELF-HELP	
COMPATIBILITY	

ALSO KNOWN AS "NATURAL MEDICINE" or "nature cure," naturopathy developed in the late 19th century, founded on an ancient belief in the power of the body to heal itself. Naturopaths believe that the body's natural state is one of equilibrium, which can be disturbed by an unhealthy lifestyle. They look for the underlying causes of a problem rather than treating symptoms alone, combining diet and noninvasive therapies where possible to stimulate the healing process. Naturopathy is practiced throughout the Western world and some of its principles have been adopted by conventional medicine.

MAIN USES

- Degenerative & long-term conditions, such as arthritis & asthma
- Rheumatoid arthritis
- Depression
- Fatigue, CFS
- High blood pressure, hardening of the arteries
- PMS
- Gastrointestinal problems, such as ulcers
- Skin conditions

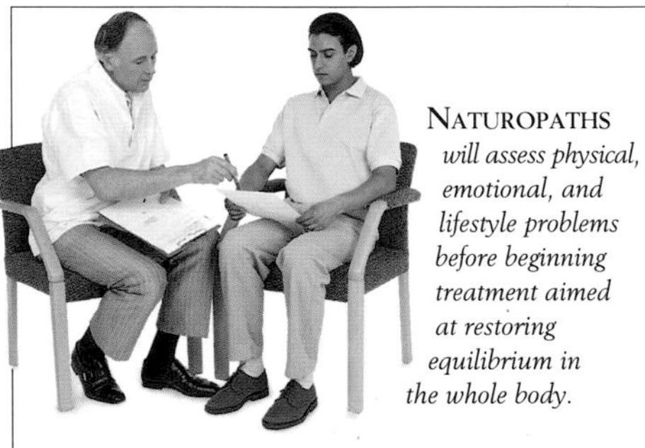

NATUROPATHS *will assess physical, emotional, and lifestyle problems before beginning treatment aimed at restoring equilibrium in the whole body.*

HISTORY

Some aspects of naturopathy have common ground with other ancient holistic health systems, such as Traditional Chinese Medicine (see page 140) and Ayurveda (see page 144), which share the belief that the body has an innate power to heal itself. In naturopathy this power is known as the "vital force." Many of the principles of naturopathy can be found in the work of the Greek physician Hippocrates. Writing in the 5th century B.C., he said that health could be maintained by a balance of rest, exercise, and plain food in moderation, while cures should be as natural as possible to stimulate the body's ability to heal itself.

The term "naturopathy" was coined in 1895 by Dr. John Scheel of New York, but the system grew out of the "nature cures" popular in 19th-century spa towns in Austria and Germany. These emphasized the benefits of hydrotherapy (see page 122), fresh air, sunlight, and exercise. Naturopathy was also influenced by the work of the French physiologist Claude Bernard in the 1850s. Bernard developed the concept of *le milieu interieur* (the body's internal environment), the equilibrium of which, he maintained, was vital for good health, or "homeostasis" (see opposite).

Naturopathy was introduced in the US in the 1890s by Benedict Lust, a follower of the German monk Father Sebastian Kneipp, who had established health spas in Europe. Lust founded the American School of Naturopathy in New York in 1896. The practice flourished in the US and in 1909 California became the first state to recognize it as a therapy. By the late 19th century, John Kellogg (famous for his breakfast cereals) was using natural therapies at his sanatorium in Battle Creek, Michigan. In 1918–19, the naturopath Henry Lindlahr set out the principles of naturopathy in his *Philosophy of Natural Therapeutics*. Advances in pharmaceuticals and surgery in the 1930s swept natural methods aside in the US, and it was not until the 1960s that interest revived.

Naturopathy is widely practiced in many countries. In Germany, there are several thousand state-licensed naturopaths, or *Heilpraktiker* (health practitioners), and, as in the US, Canada, the UK, Australia, and the Netherlands, they are reasonably autonomous. In some states, naturopaths are recognized as family practitioners. Italy, Spain, and Israel also have growing numbers of naturopaths.

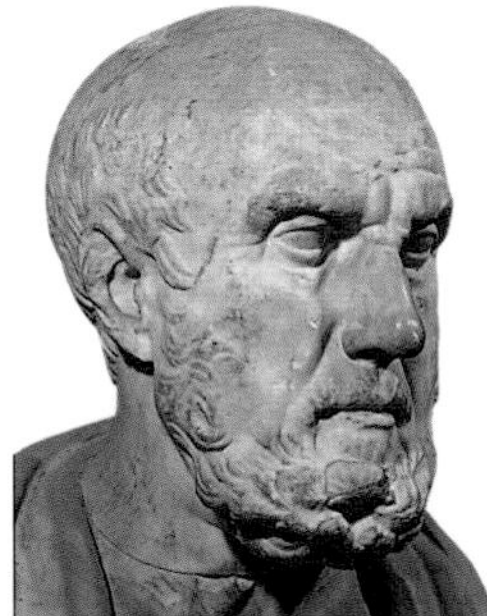

***Hippocrates**, known as the "father of medicine," expressed ideas over 2,000 years ago that were to become guiding principles for modern naturopaths.*

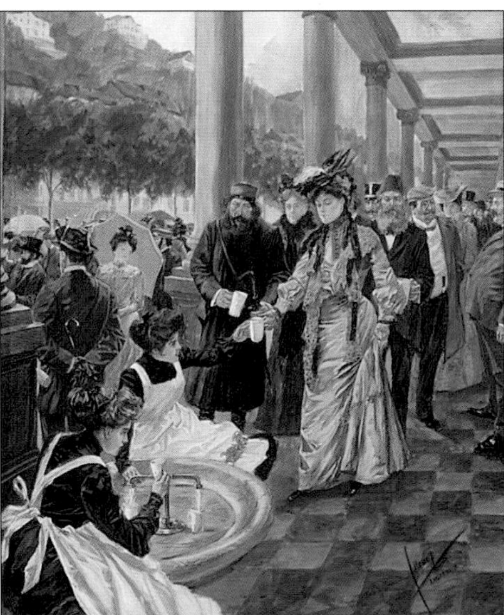

***Taking the waters** at Karlsbad, Germany, in 1900. Spas offering hydrotherapy, fresh air, and exercise were popular in 19th-century Europe.*

KEY PRINCIPLES

Modern naturopaths believe the body will always strive toward good health, or homeostasis (see opposite), and that the body is its own best healer. They maintain that many factors, such as an unhealthy diet, a lack of sleep, exercise, or fresh air, any emotional or physical stress, pollution in the environment, even negative attitudes, allow waste products and toxins to build up in the body and upset self-regulation. This in turn can overload the immune system and weaken the vital force, the body's innate ability to maintain good health. If this vital force is weakened, the body becomes susceptible to viruses, bacteria, and allergens.

Naturopaths believe that symptoms such as fever or inflammation are signs of

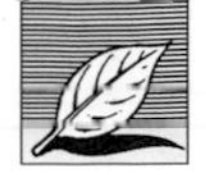

THE THEORY OF NATUROPATHY

Naturopathy is a multidisciplinary approach that uses the healing power of natural resources, such as whole foods, medicinal herbs, and fresh air and water, to allow the body to heal itself. Treatment is given to support what naturopaths term the "triad of health": the musculoskeletal structure of the body, its internal biochemistry, and emotional well-being.

HOMEOSTASIS

Naturopaths believe that self-healing depends on a "vital force," which helps the body fight disease and maintain equilibrium, known as homeostasis. An unhealthy lifestyle can throw this process off balance, weakening the vital force.

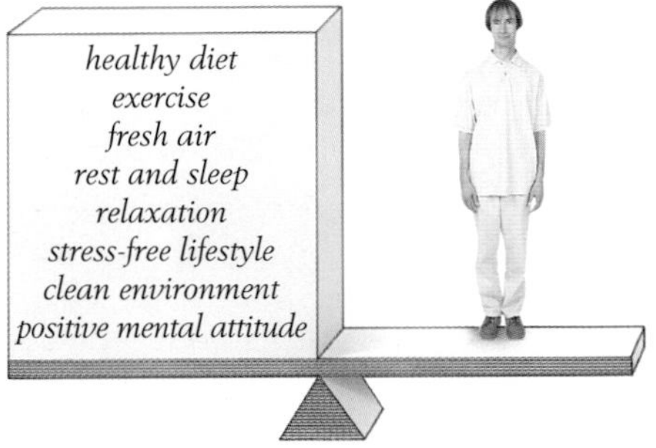

A balanced lifestyle *sustains homeostasis, strengthening the body's self-healing abilities and enhancing the immune system.*

unhealthy diet
lack of exercise
lack of fresh air
lack of sleep
emotional stress
physical stress
pollution
negative attitudes

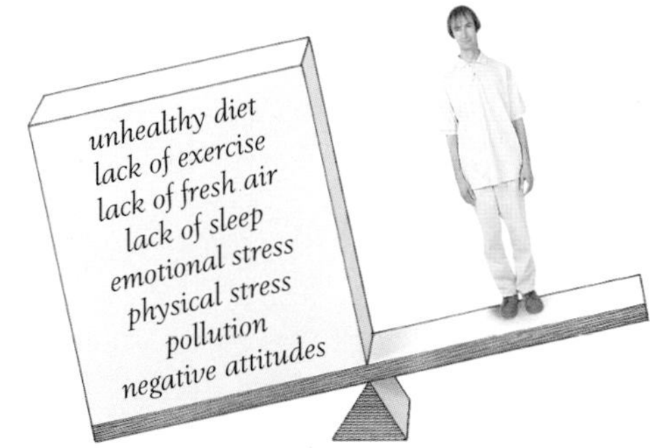

An unhealthy way of life *may overwhelm the body's natural ability to regulate itself, and can therefore lead to illness.*

NATUROPATHIC TREATMENT

Naturopathy uses a range of therapies to enhance the body's self-healing powers. These aim to work by improving digestion and circulation, increasing the elimination of waste products, and boosting the immune system.

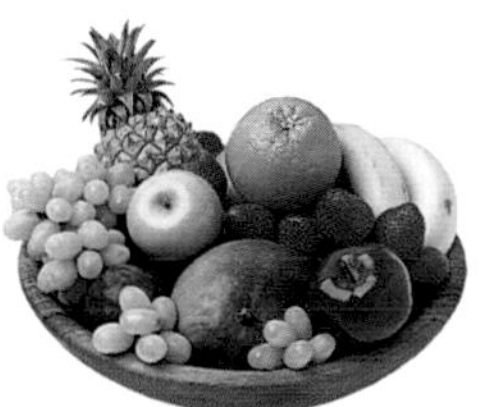

A whole-foods diet *rich in unrefined, preferably organic, fresh fruit and vegetables is recommended (see page 148).*

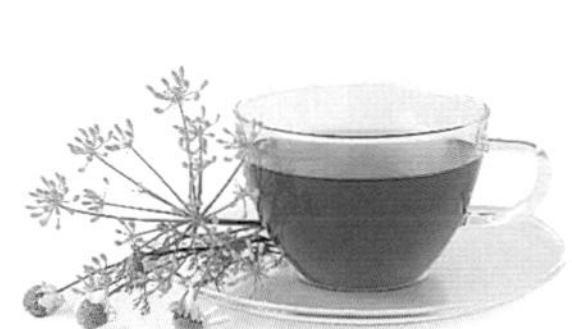

Herbal remedies *are prescribed to support the body's natural regenerative powers (see page 134).*

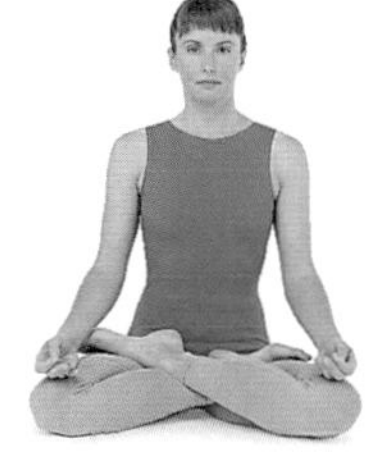

Yoga *postures and breathing develop physical flexibility and promote relaxation (see page 108).*

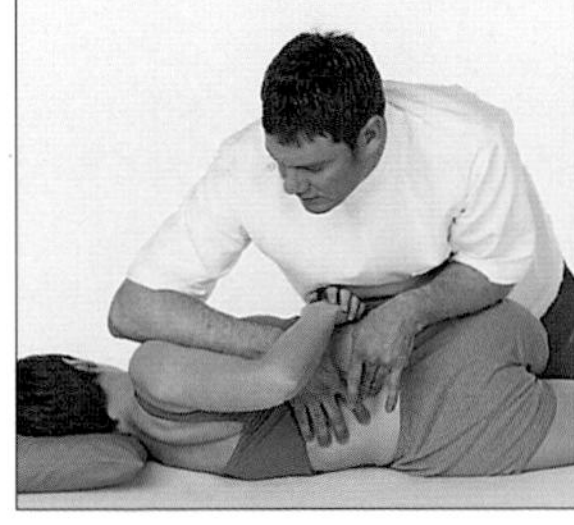

Osteopathy *is important in promoting a healthy body structure, considered essential for well-being (see page 70).*

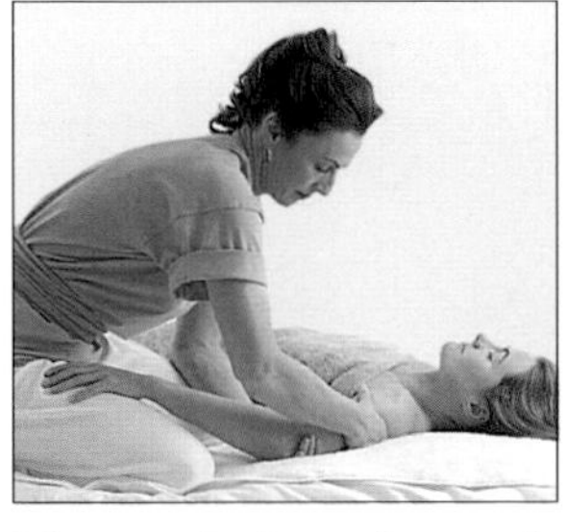

Massage *is often a feature of naturopathic programs. It relaxes taut muscles and helps circulation (see page 56).*

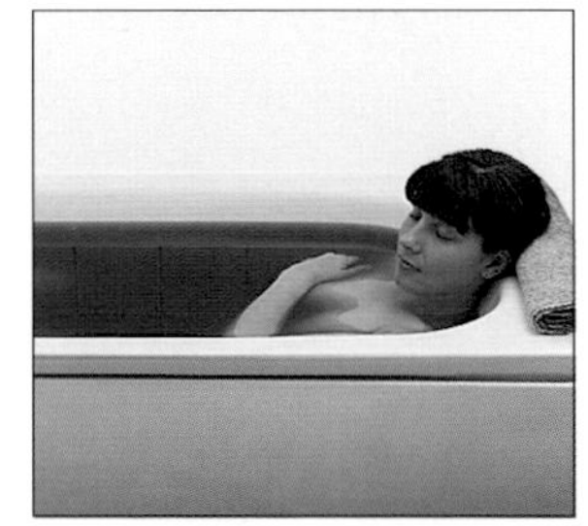

Hydrotherapy *is a traditional naturopathic remedy that improves circulation and boosts vitality (see page 122).*

the body's self-healing powers at work, and advise against suppressing such symptoms, since that can cause disorders to "go underground," becoming chronic and causing further degeneration. Rather than treating symptoms directly, naturopaths work to improve underlying health so that the patient is less susceptible to infection.

Naturopathic treatments are as non-invasive as possible. Some practitioners specialize in a particular approach, while others draw on a wide range of techniques. Some of the most commonly used treatments include clinical nutrition and fasting (diet is a very important part of naturopathic medicine); hydrotherapy; physical therapies, including osteopathy or chiropractic, massage, and physiotherapy; counseling and lifestyle modification; herbal medicine; homeopathy; Traditional Chinese Medicine; light therapy; touch therapies including massage, acupressure, shiatsu, and reflexology; and yoga.

EVIDENCE & RESEARCH

The therapeutic benefits of a whole-foods diet and other naturopathic practices, such as regular exercise, relaxation, and the use of massage for stress relief, have been endorsed by medical research.

In 1991, a study of ear infections in children, undertaken by the American Association of Naturopathic Physicians, claimed that naturopathy was an effective alternative to antibiotics and surgery. At the Bastyr University Clinic in Seattle, the Healing AIDS Research Project treated 16 HIV-positive patients along naturopathic lines for a year, using vitamin supplements, hydrotherapy, homeopathy, and herbal remedies. The results of their trial, published in 1992, revealed that 12 of the 16 reported improved well-being and none of the group developed AIDS.

MEDICAL OPINION

Many long-held naturopathic notions, such as the importance of a diet that is high in fiber and antioxidants, and low in salt and fat, have since been adopted by conventional medicine. Stress management and exercise, now accepted by doctors as important to health, have been stock-in-trade in naturopathy for most of the 20th century. Conventional preventive medicine, though it might not admit it, owes a lot to the naturopathic tradition.

CONSULTING A PRACTITIONER

The first visit to a naturopath may last up to an hour as he will want to build up a complete picture of your physical and emotional well-being. He will probably give you a routine medical examination, including tests on your blood pressure, lungs and heart, spinal joints, and reflexes. The practitioner may also arrange for X rays, blood, urine, and other tests. In addition, he may carry out nonconventional tests, examining your irises (see page 195), analyzing your sweat or hair (see below and page 194), or using kinesiology muscle tests (see page 196). A naturopath may diagnose your condition in terms unfamiliar to conventional doctors, such as "toxic accumulation" and "leaky gut."

Treatment falls into two broad categories. *Catabolic* (cleansing) treatment is given for conditions caused by a buildup of waste products, and may include fasting to assist detoxification. *Anabolic* (strengthening) treatment is aimed at building up a weakened constitution with nutritional supplements and changes in diet. The practitioner may give advice about breathing patterns, exercise, and relaxation. Some naturopaths are also trained in counseling skills and techniques such as hypnotherapy (see page 166). Advice is tailored to individual needs, and willing participation in treatments and a positive mental attitude are crucial. Your health should improve steadily, possibly with temporary relapses known as "healing crises" as detoxification takes effect.

By asking detailed questions *about your lifestyle and medical history, the naturopath aims to treat the causes of the illness, not just the symptoms.*

STANDARD TESTS

Naturopaths assess the patient's health with a wide range of tests to build up a complete picture.

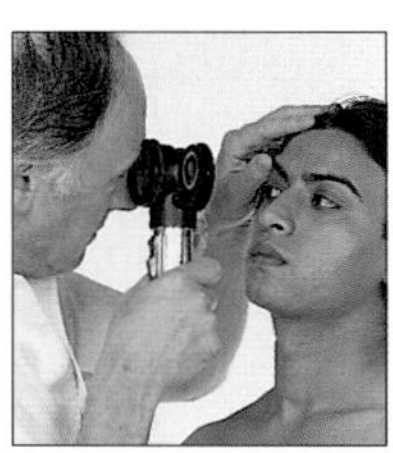

The irises *are said to indicate the state of internal organs.*

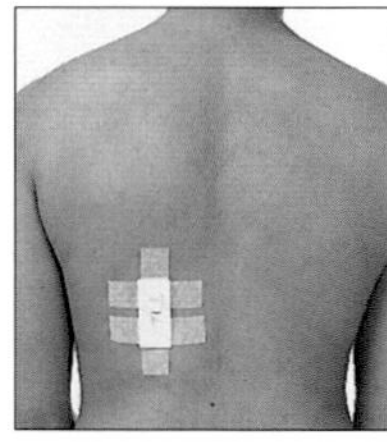

A sweat patch *can be applied to test for mineral imbalances.*

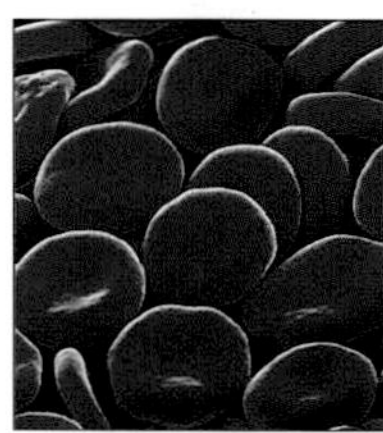

A blood test *may reveal anemia and food allergies.*

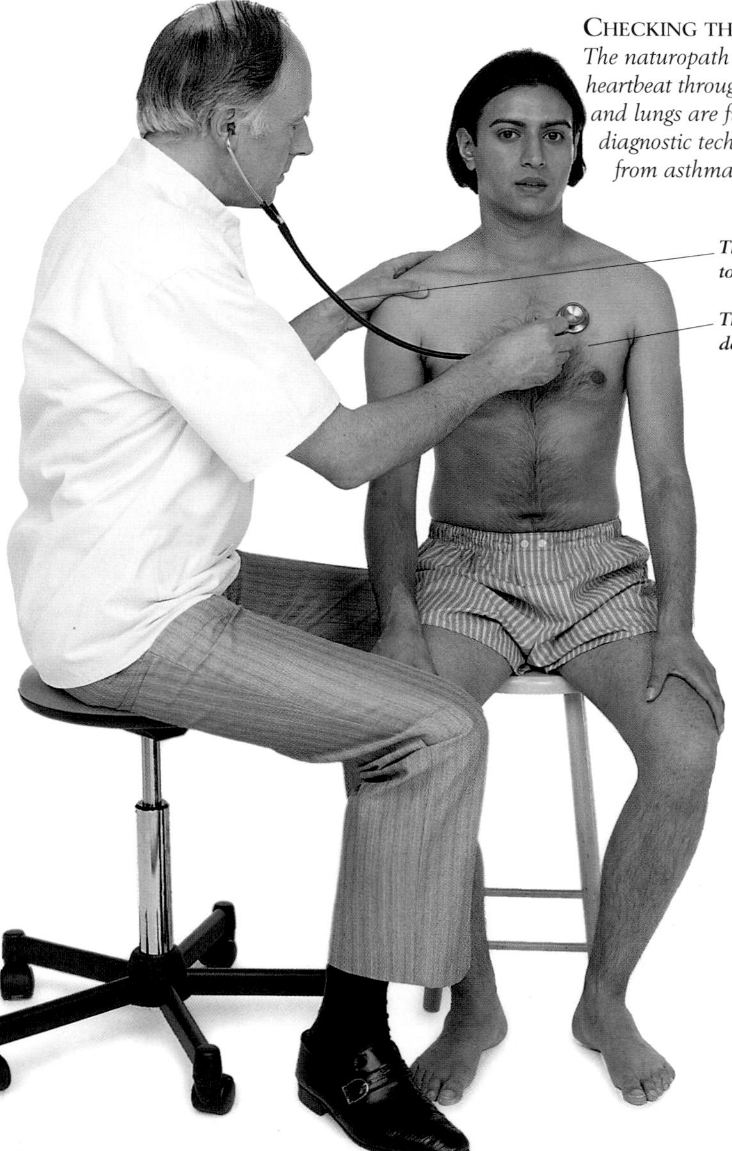

CHECKING THE HEART AND LUNGS

The naturopath listens to the breathing patterns and heartbeat through a stethoscope to check that the heart and lungs are functioning properly. This important diagnostic technique can reveal disorders ranging from asthma and emphysema to heart defects.

YOUR QUESTIONS

How long does a treatment session last?
The first session lasts about an hour; subsequent sessions last 20–40 minutes.

How many sessions will I need?
Between four and 30 weekly sessions, depending on the condition. A qualified naturopath will refer you to your doctor if he feels that your condition requires surgery or treatment beyond his expertise.

Will it be unpleasant?
The naturopath may ask you to give up some favorite foods for a time.

Will there be any aftereffects?
Symptoms may appear to worsen before improving as the body tries to eliminate toxins and return to a homeostatic state.

PRECAUTIONS

- Do not fast or follow a restricted diet without supervision by a qualified naturopath.
- See also page 52.

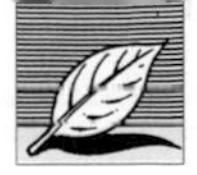

Treatment for Sinusitis

Sinusitis is an infection of the membranes lining the air-filled cavities (sinuses) in the bones around the nose, causing throbbing pain and fever. Naturopathic treatment for the condition will be tailored to the patient's individual needs, and will vary according to whether catabolic or anabolic principles are applied (see opposite).

The naturopath will first ask about the patient's lifestyle and take a detailed medical history. If the sinusitis is thought to have resulted from toxins in the body or from exposure to pollutants, catabolic treatments such as fasting may be recommended. On the other hand, if the patient's overall health is poor, and his self-healing powers are not strong enough to rid the body of infection, a health-promoting whole-foods diet and food supplements will be used, based on anabolic principles. Other options might include soft-tissue massage and cold compresses to stimulate the circulation.

***Lymphatic pumping**: The practitioner massages lightly around the lymph glands, stimulating the lymphatic system to help it expel toxins. Gently vibrating the muscles around the ribs "frees" the chest and helps the patient breathe more deeply.*

OVERHEAD VIEW

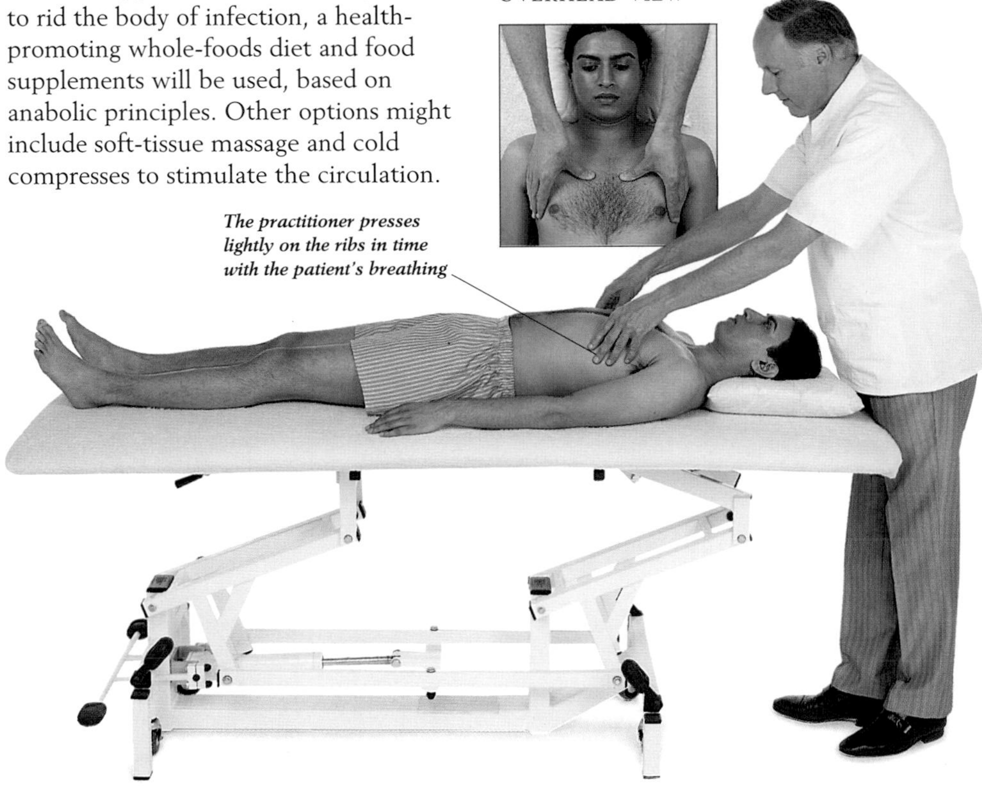

The practitioner presses lightly on the ribs in time with the patient's breathing

A Patient's Experience

Joan, a 31-year-old marketing executive, had "weakness" of the right side and extreme fatigue: "The naturopath believed it was chronic fatigue syndrome and put me on a very plain diet with lots of fruit, vegetable juices, and water. I was prescribed the herb echinacea to build up my immune system, and lots of supplements. She asked me to make some lifestyle changes – I had been driving to work through a tunnel full of exhaust fumes, so I traveled to work by train instead. After being sick for 18 months, within three or four weeks I was feeling much better."

Self-Help

One of the foundations of naturopathic medicine is diet, and you may be given a specific juice fast and diet to follow at home. The practitioner may prescribe nutritional supplements to complement the changes in your diet, and may also advocate hydrotherapy or self-massage.

General guidelines for leading a more healthy lifestyle include the following:

Mineral water: Drinking 2–8 glasses daily helps the body to eliminate waste products.
Supplements: There is no substitute for a healthy diet. However, vitamins B-complex, E, and C, and a multimineral preparation may help if you are in a stressful or polluted environment.
Breathing: Breathe deeply, from the bottom of the lungs, for two minutes twice a day.
Fresh air: Spend time outdoors in moderate sunshine to increase vitamin D production.
Skin-brushing: Using a loofah or special brush before a bath helps eliminate waste products and improve the circulation.

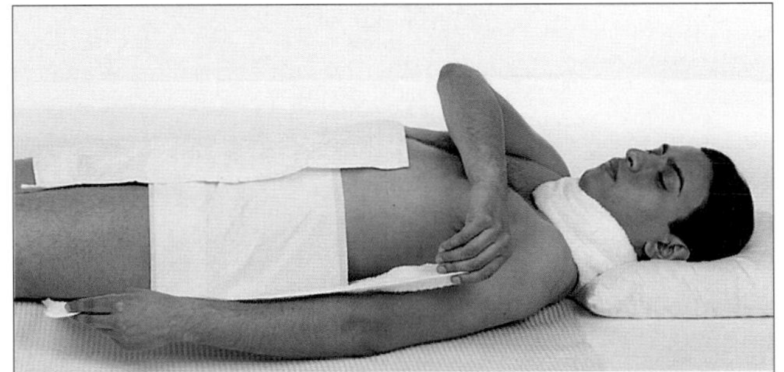

***Cold compresses**: Made from cotton cloth soaked in cold water, these can be left on the body for a few hours to promote sweating and detoxification (see page 122). For sinusitis, a compress should be wrapped around the throat, with another around the abdomen. Both should be covered with a towel, and sometimes also a blanket.*

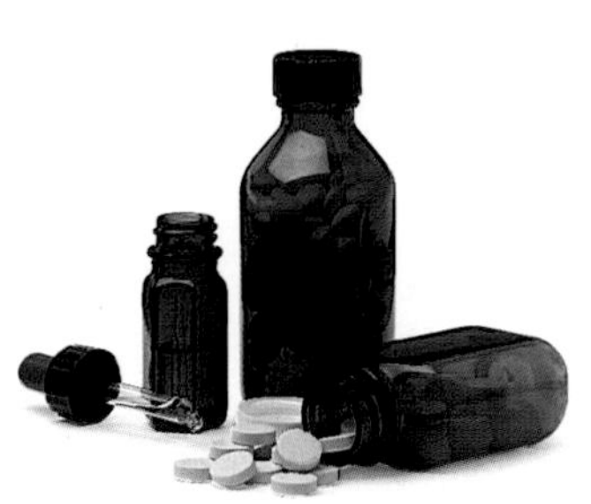

***Supplements**: Taking vitamin and mineral supplements when ill or stressed can boost the digestive system and help the elimination of waste products.*

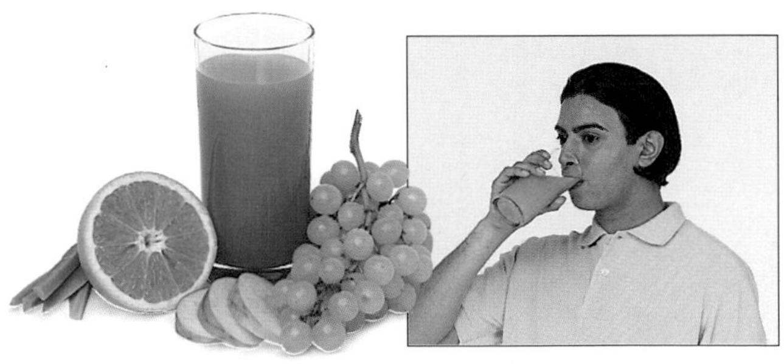

***Fresh juice**: Freshly squeezed juice is rich in vitamin C and potassium. For sinusitis, a juice combining apple, carrot, orange, and grape might be prescribed. Following a juice fast for three days, avoiding mucus-generating foods, such as dairy products, salt, and sugar, can encourage detoxification of body systems.*

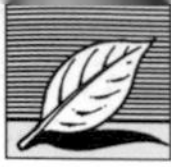

HYDROTHERAPY

RATINGS	
EVIDENCE	
MEDICAL OPINION	
PRACTITIONER	
SELF-HELP	
COMPATIBILITY	

THE ANCIENT GREEKS believed that water contained the essence of life and the secret of health. In hydrotherapy, water is used internally and externally in all its forms – hot and cold, as liquid, steam, or ice – to cleanse, revitalize, restore, and maintain health. Traditionally, hydrotherapy consisted of baths, saunas, and compresses, but in modern times, whirlpools and water jets have been introduced. An established part of conventional medicine until the beginning of the 20th century, hydrotherapy has long been practiced by naturopaths (see page 118), and is now enjoying a resurgence in popularity.

MAIN USES

- Muscle & joint pain, such as backache, muscle strains & sprains
- Circulatory problems
- Asthma, bronchitis
- Cystitis
- Menstrual problems
- Fevers
- Anxiety, stress
- Headaches, fatigue

HISTORY

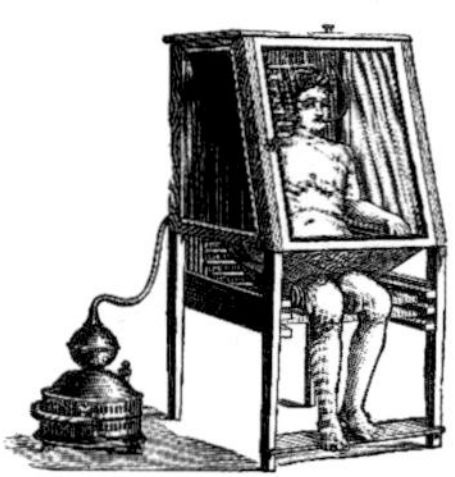

***Steam baths** became very popular in the 19th century, and are still used today. They make the body sweat, which is said to expel impurities through the pores of the skin.*

The therapeutic properties of water have been valued throughout history by societies around the world, from the Chinese to the Native Americans. In ancient Greece, temples to Asklepios, god of medicine, were built near hot springs. In New Zealand, natural hot springs have been used for centuries to improve health.

No Roman town was deemed complete without baths where citizens could enjoy hot, cold, and tepid immersions. In many towns, such as Baden-Baden in Germany, Spa in Belgium, and Bath in the UK, the practice of "taking the waters" at natural springs has continued to the present day. The first serious medical use of the therapy was probably made by Vincent Priessnitz, who opened a spa in the early 19th century at Grafenburg, Austria.

The true pioneer of hydrotherapy, however, was Father Sebastian Kneipp, a 19th-century Bavarian monk who claimed that water could cure disease by improving the elimination of waste products from the body. His patients followed a program of hot and cold baths and compresses, foot baths, sitz baths, steam baths, showers, and wraps – techniques still in use today.

In Germany and a number of eastern European countries, hydrotherapy is still widespread and is often subsidized by the government. It is an important part of naturopathy, which is popular in the US and Australia, and has gained a reputation as a cheap therapy with few side effects.

KEY PRINCIPLES

Water has a remarkable ability to alter the body's blood flow, and this can be manipulated by varying its temperature. Cold water is stimulating. It makes surface blood vessels constrict, restricting blood flow and inhibiting the biochemical reactions that cause inflammation. It sends blood toward the internal organs, helping them to function more efficiently. Hot water, conversely, is relaxing. It dilates blood vessels, which reduces blood pressure and increases blood flow to the skin and muscles, easing stiffness. The improved circulation boosts the immune system, helps remove waste products from the body, and sends more oxygen and nutrients to the tissues to repair damage.

Some therapies use hot and cold water alternately. This is said to stimulate the hormonal system, reduce circulatory congestion caused by muscle spasm, and relieve inflammation. Floating in warm water, unburdened by gravity, can also be mentally soothing (see page 177).

EVIDENCE & RESEARCH

European studies in 1995 found that warm underwater jet massage enhanced athletes' performances. American research in 1991 showed that hydrotherapy was helpful for varicose veins, while two studies in Israel indicated that mud and mineral baths were beneficial for rheumatoid arthritis. A 1986 study published in the *British Medical Journal* concluded that sitz baths were helpful in healing anal fissures.

MEDICAL OPINION

The effect of water as a vehicle for heat and cold is obvious. Recently, conventional medicine has expressed renewed interest in the ability of water temperature to affect body tissues, and in its buoyant and stimulating properties, as used in physiotherapy. Hydrotherapy is an example of a therapy that is not as far removed from conventional practice as it may appear.

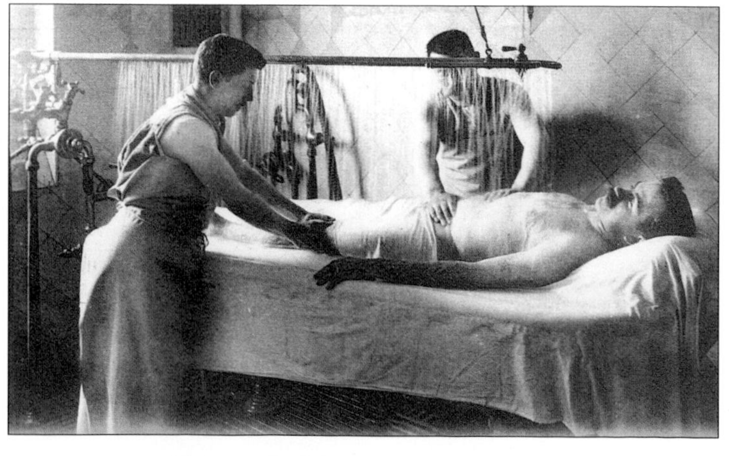

***Spas** have been popular since Roman times, both as a form of diversion and as a healing therapy. This 19th-century photograph shows a patient receiving a massage with mineral water in Vichy, France, where spa waters have long been taken both internally and externally.*

CONSULTING A PRACTITIONER

Hydrotherapy is usually practiced at health farms and spas, particularly those founded on naturopathic principles, and you are most likely to visit one if referred by a naturopath. Treatments are diverse and will depend on your condition. They may include some of the following:

High-powered jets: Hot or cold water is directed at your back for about 2–3 minutes as you face the wall, holding supports. Jets are said to stimulate the circulation and internal organs, and are used for anemia, amenorrhea, angina, arthritis, and asthma.

Whirlpool baths: Immersing the body in pressurized bubbles for about 15 minutes soothes and massages the body and is also believed to treat sores, infected wounds, swellings, and circulatory problems.

Sitz baths (see below): This treatment uses two hip baths, and may benefit hemorrhoids, menstrual problems, cystitis, incontinence, and prolapse.

Hot or warm baths: Soaking in hot water (about 100°F/38°C) for 20–30 minutes is believed to help arthritic conditions. Therapeutic herbs, oils (see page 65), and minerals can be added to a warm bath. These include Epsom salts to relieve swollen joints and relax muscles, finely blended oatmeal or bran (possibly added in a muslin bag) to soothe the skin, and mineral "muds" and extracts, such as Dead Sea salts, to nourish the skin.

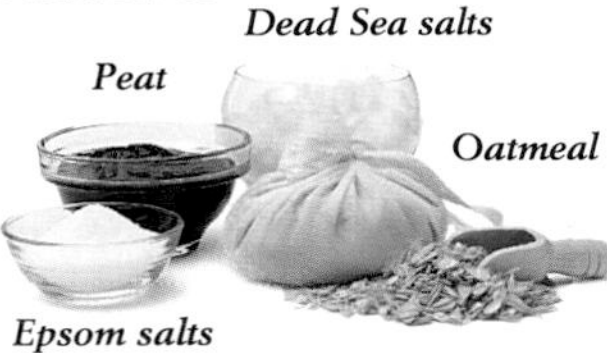

Seawater treatments ("thalassotherapy"): Seawater is said to have healing properties, and minerals in seaweed are believed to induce sweating, cleanse and tone the skin, and promote relaxation. Treatments may include seawater jets, seaweed wraps, or seawater or kelp (seaweed) baths.

Fresh seaweed

Seaweed powder

Wraps (see right): Cold, wet flannel sheets are wrapped around your body, then covered with dry towels and finally blankets. After the initial shock, the body warms up rapidly, drying the sheets. Wraps promote sweating, which is said to flush out waste products, and may be used for fevers, colds, bronchitis, back pain, and skin disorders.

Compresses: Towels are soaked in hot or cold water, wrung out and applied to the affected area of the body. Hot compresses increase blood flow, make the body sweat, and ease stiff muscles. Cold ones restrict circulation, reducing inflammation.

Turkish baths, steam rooms, and cabinets: Sitting in a hot, steamy room for about 20 minutes, or in a cabinet for up to 1 hour, induces sweating, eliminating impurities and relieving water retention.

Saunas (see right): These are similar to Turkish baths but generate dry rather than humid heat.

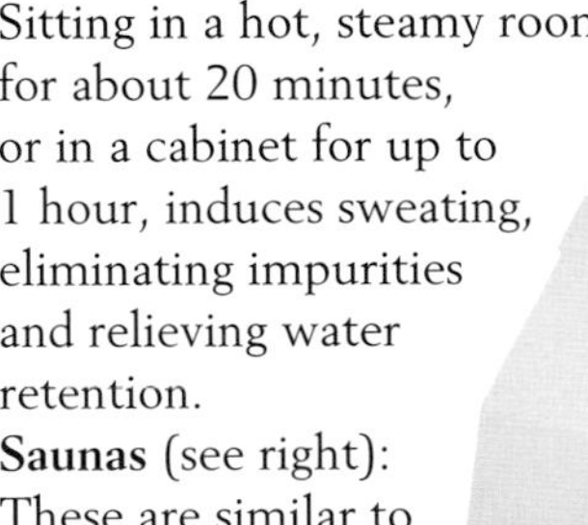
Steam cabinet

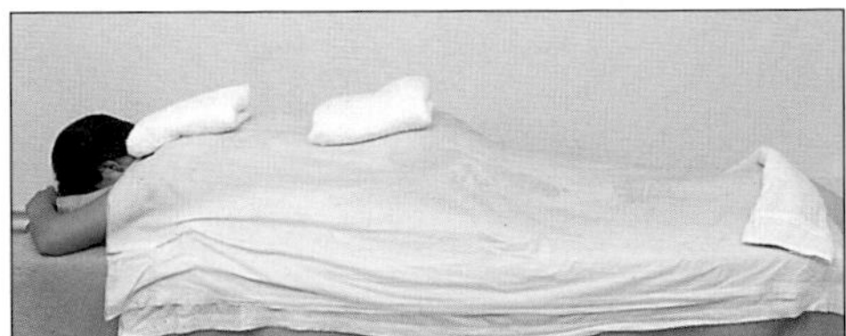

***Wraps**: A cold flannel sheet is wrapped around the body and hot or cold packs enveloped in towels are placed on top. The patient is then covered with a warm blanket and left for 30 minutes. This form of constitutional treatment is used to aid circulation and stimulate the immune system, to treat problems such as viral illnesses and long-term fatigue.*

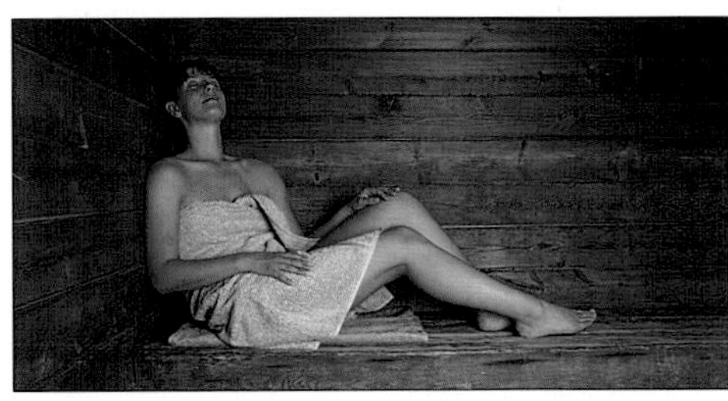

***Saunas**: A hot, dry environment (above 100°F /38°C) encourages sweating, which helps the body eliminate waste products. A dip into a plunge pool or a cold shower is advised every 5–10 minutes during the sauna and at the end of the sauna.*

PRECAUTIONS

- Avoid hot baths, steam baths, and saunas if you have high blood pressure, angina, or heart disease.
- Avoid steam baths or sitz baths in the first three months of pregnancy, and limit steam treatments to a maximum of 10 minutes for the remaining months.
- Avoid steam treatment if you are postoperative, epileptic, asthmatic, or have a history of thrombosis.
- Avoid seaweed if you are allergic to iodine, and do not add ingredients to a bath if you have an open wound.
- See also page 52.

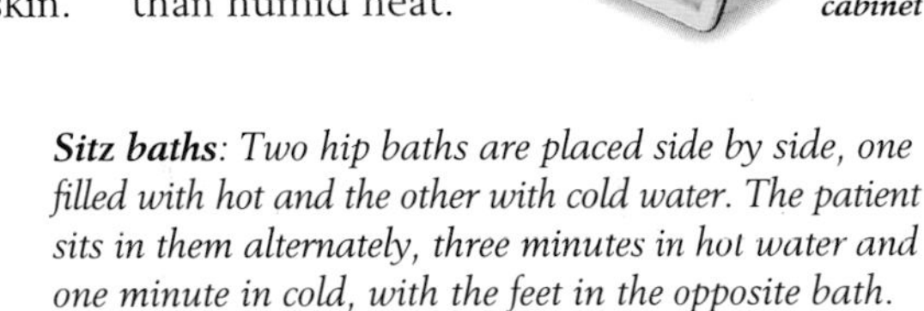
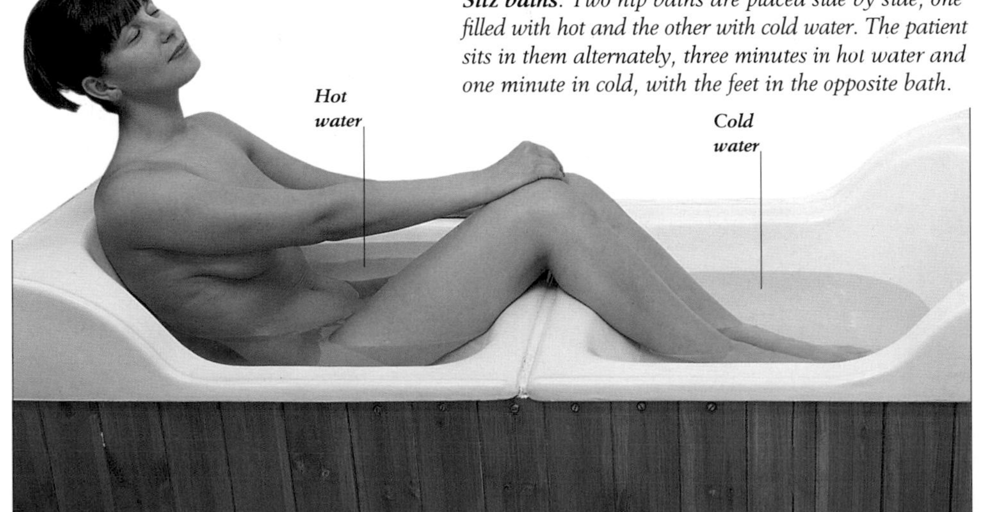

***Sitz baths**: Two hip baths are placed side by side, one filled with hot and the other with cold water. The patient sits in them alternately, three minutes in hot water and one minute in cold, with the feet in the opposite bath.*

SELF-HELP

Many treatments, such as compresses and ice packs, are simple to carry out at home.

A hot compress eases back or abdominal pain and muscle tension. Wring out a small towel in very hot water, fold it, and apply it to the affected area, alternating it with a cold compress, which restricts circulation and is useful for sprains and swollen joints. Use very cold water and leave for several hours, or overnight.

An ice pack relieves swelling and pain in emergencies. Place a towel or a drop of oil on the skin to avoid freezer burn, then apply ice, or even a package of frozen peas, wrapped in a cloth, to the affected area and leave for 10 minutes.

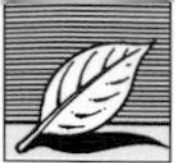

ANTHROPOSOPHICAL MEDICINE

RATINGS	
EVIDENCE	
MEDICAL OPINION	
PRACTITIONER	
SELF-HELP	
COMPATIBILITY	

THE PHILOSOPHY OF ANTHROPOSOPHY was founded early in the 1900s by an Austrian, Rudolf Steiner, in reaction to the contemporary scientific view of the body as a purely physical entity. According to Steiner, the natural world is guided by cosmic rhythms, and each human being is a unique individual for whom life has meaning and purpose. Claiming that the loss of this sense of self was reflected by a deterioration in well-being, he developed anthroposophical medicine as a holistic approach to health following his philosophy. Practitioners are trained as medical doctors and the practice is especially popular in Europe.

MAIN USES

- Practitioners are medically qualified and may treat any condition
- Childhood infections
- Hay fever & asthma
- Anxiety
- Depression
- Cancer
- Musculoskeletal problems
- Fatigue, CFS

HISTORY

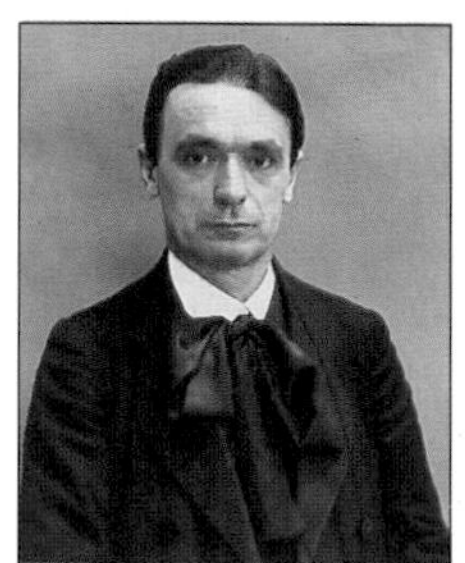

***Rudolf Steiner**, father of anthroposophy, was an Austrian scientist and philosopher. His work embraced not only medicine but education, art, drama, movement, agriculture, and architecture.*

Anthroposophical medicine is part of Rudolf Steiner's theory of anthroposophy, from the Greek *anthropos* (man) and *sophia* (wisdom). His holistic view of medicine stressed the need for an "awareness of man's humanity." With Dr. Ita Wegman, a Dutch doctor, Steiner developed his ideas to include a medical science. He established his headquarters at Dornach in Switzerland in 1913. In Europe, at least 10 hospitals and several hundred doctors practice anthroposophical medicine. Interest is growing in the US, the UK, and Australia. Over 170 schools worldwide teach children based on Steiner's theories.

KEY PRINCIPLES

Steiner's approach was based on Christian principles, although he worked initially with the Theosophical Society, a late 19th-century religious movement influenced by Hindu and Buddhist traditions. The Theosophist belief in reincarnation corresponds to Steiner's theory that health in this life reflects the *karma* or "load" carried over from past lives. He taught that illness, when appropriately treated, is an opportunity to bring renewed balance and greater wholeness into the patient's life. The anthroposophical medicines and therapeutic techniques Steiner developed were intended to stimulate the healing process from within.

In addition to a physical body, Steiner believed that humans, animals, and plants have an "etheric" body, which is the source of life and growth, and contributes to physical shape. Humans and animals are furthermore said to possess an "astral" body that governs the senses, impulses, and emotions, but only humans have a fourth component – an "ego," the consciousness of self. A patient is seen as an individual in whom all four of these bodies influence one another; thus illness in one body can cause disturbances in the other three.

The nature of illness is determined by Steiner's principle of polarity. The human organism, he said, consists of two "poles," with a system that links and harmonizes them. The upper "cephalic," or "head," pole includes the brain, nerves, and senses, and is associated with perception and thinking. Overactivity in this pole may lead to degenerative conditions, including tumors and osteoarthritis, that are associated with old age. The lower "metabolic" pole includes the limbs, movement, and metabolism, and is associated with action and will. Too much activity in this pole can result in inflammatory disorders, such as pneumonia and other feverish illnesses, which are common in childhood. Linking the two poles is the "rhythmic" system that includes the heart, lungs, respiration, and circulation, and is associated with states of mind and emotions. Practitioners employ anthroposophical medicines and a range

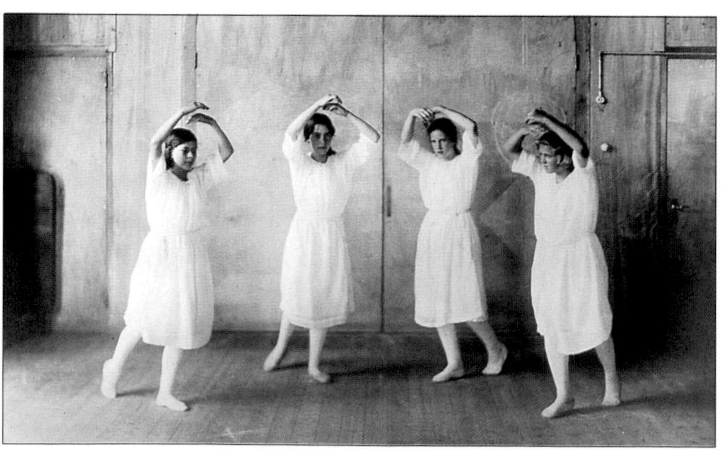

***Eurythmy** is a movement therapy developed by Steiner in the early 1900s to enhance the relationship between the ego and the physical body. Unlike dance steps and mime, eurythmic movements are choreographed to symbolize sounds, making speech and music "visible" in shapes, gestures, and color.*

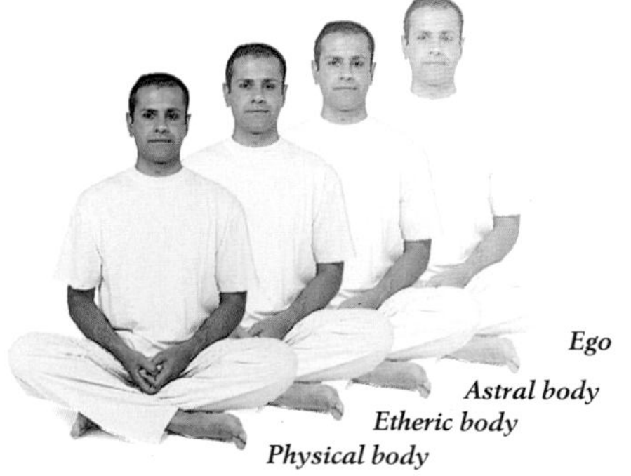

***Good health**, according to Steiner, depends on a harmonious relationship between the physical, etheric, and astral bodies, and the ego.*

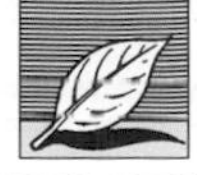

of therapies (see right) to integrate these components into a harmonious whole.

Anthroposophical medicines treat specific ailments and are made from animal, mineral, and plant substances, such as mistletoe, an extract of which, Iscador, is given by injection to treat cancer. Medicines are prepared by the homeopathic method of potentization (see page 126), but the plants used are grown according to a system of "biodynamic" agriculture, which takes into account cosmic influences on plant growth. Steiner believed that the seasons and the position of the sun, moon, and Earth affect everything in the natural world, including agriculture and the preparation of medicines, and at least one manufacturer of anthroposophical medicines does not prepare remedies in the two hours after midday, when cosmic influences are thought to render them less effective.

Mistletoe

EVIDENCE & RESEARCH

Many studies of anthroposophical medicines have been made by medical researchers in Europe. Iscador, for example, appeared in trials to stimulate all areas of the immune system, increase the production of white cells and antibodies, and to have a mild anticancer action. A 1995 study at the Royal London Homoeopathic Hospital found that a cancer care package that included Iscador enhanced patients' quality of life.

MEDICAL OPINION

Doctors are often unaware of the concepts behind Steiner's approach, but many of those who have studied anthroposophy have great respect for his ideas on the relationship between mind and body (he corresponded with Jung), and his psychological and educational theories (he knew Montessori). Doctors sometimes refer patients to anthroposophical doctors, although often this is at the patient's own request. Many doctors find it difficult to accept Steiner's belief in *karma* and homeopathic medicine. Nevertheless, his insights do seem more profound than the superficial theorizing that underpins some other complementary therapies.

CONSULTING A PRACTITIONER

An anthroposophical doctor will often spend more time than a conventional doctor (often as much as an hour) asking questions about your diet, lifestyle, and constitution, with an emphasis on your body's rhythms. For example, are your eating and sleeping patterns regular? If you are a woman, are your menstrual periods regular? The practitioner may also carry out standard medical tests, and will use the information to aid diagnosis, prescribing treatment to balance the poles and systems regulating your body. You will usually be prescribed anthroposophical medicines to treat physical conditions, in conjunction with conventional drugs if necessary.

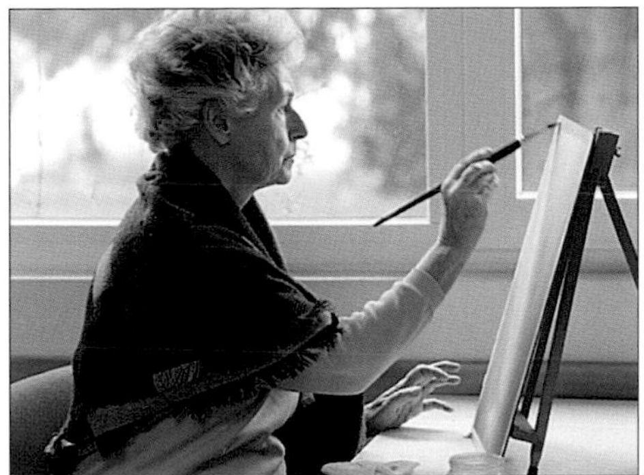

***Painting**: Using color to create a harmonious image may influence the astral body, or inner emotions, and indirectly affect physical health.*

Practitioners are fully qualified doctors, who make use of modern technology and medication as required – Steiner aimed to complement and develop medicine as it exists, rather than to set up an alternative system. Anthroposophical doctors believe that this approach gives them a fuller picture of an individual compared to conventional medicine, allowing them to take a broader view of illness and therapy.

A comprehensive treatment will often include artistic therapies (see below and page 182) to harmonize your emotional condition, and counseling (see page 163) to look at opportunities presented by the illness for developing your ego, or individual self. Massage, hydrotherapy (see page 122), and eurythmy (see opposite) may also be used for long-term problems. Many practitioners have a team of therapists attached to their practice, specializing in one or more of these areas.

Because anthroposophical medicine is a holistic system, aimed at harmonizing elements of the spiritual as well as the physical self, it is said by its followers to be of benefit in cases where a conventional cure cannot be achieved. According to Steiner's philosophy, even where therapy cannot be of help in the present life, it may be used to prepare for a future life.

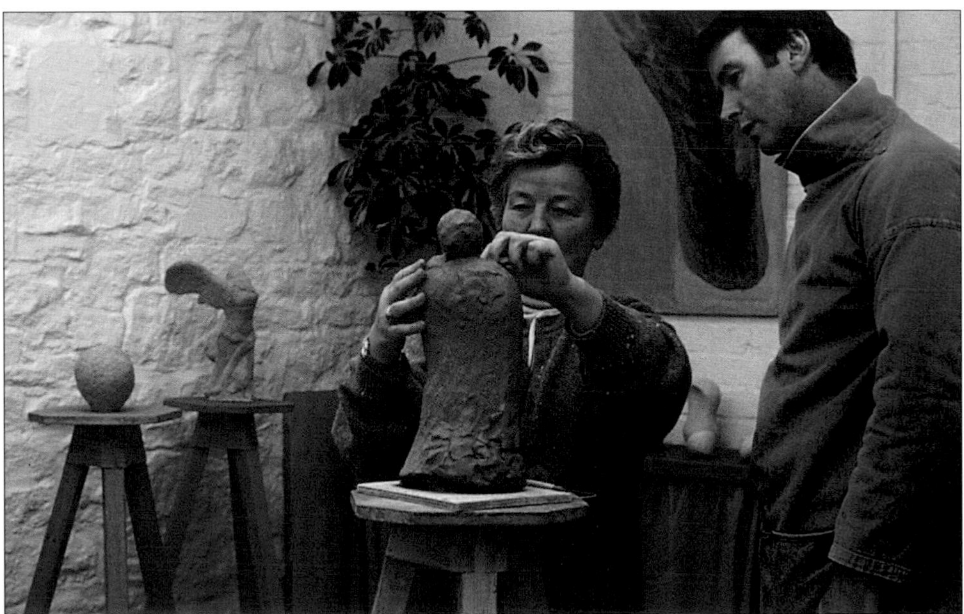

***Sculpture**: Modeling in clay can foster self-confidence through practical achievement and may also make the patient more aware of her body. The aim is to encourage closer union of the ego, or individual self, with the physical body.*

PRECAUTIONS

- See page 52.

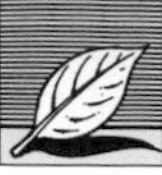

HOMEOPATHY

RATINGS	
EVIDENCE	
MEDICAL OPINION	
PRACTITIONER	
SELF-HELP	
COMPATIBILITY	

DEVELOPED IN 18TH-CENTURY GERMANY, homeopathy is a system of medicine based on the theory that "like cures like" – a poison that causes symptoms of illness in a healthy person can treat the same symptoms in one who is ill. The substances are diluted many times to make the remedy safe to use, yet homeopaths believe sufficient "likeness" remains between the remedy and the illness to stimulate the body's self-healing abilities. Homeopathy is one of the most popular complementary therapies. Well established in Europe, Australia, and India, it is undergoing a revival in the United States.

MAIN USES

- Long-term & relapsing disorders
- Asthma, allergies
- Anxiety, nervous tension, shock
- Eczema
- Menstrual & menopausal problems
- Problems in pregnancy, including morning sickness

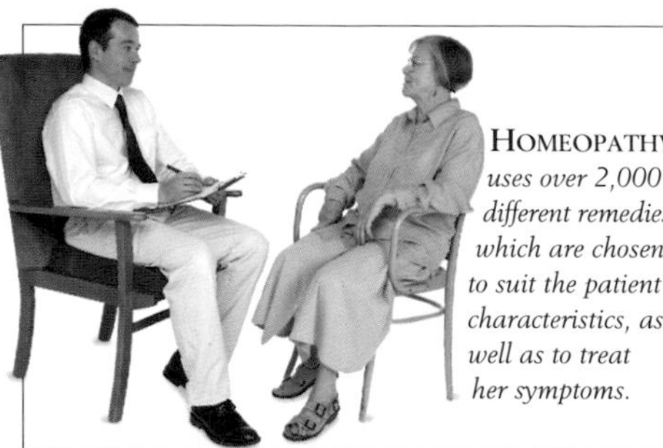

HOMEOPATHY *uses over 2,000 different remedies, which are chosen to suit the patient's characteristics, as well as to treat her symptoms.*

HISTORY

The principle of "like cures like" (see opposite) can be found in the writings of the "father of medicine," Hippocrates, which date from the 5th century B.C., and has been echoed through the ages in folk cures, such as rubbing frostbite with snow.

A German doctor, Samuel Hahnemann, rediscovered this principle in the late 18th century. Rejecting leeches, violent purges, and other severe medical practices of the day, he developed homeopathy, taking the name from the Greek *homoios* (same) and *pathos* (suffering). His starting point was the contemporary use of quinine to treat malaria, allegedly due to its bitter qualities. Using himself as a guinea pig, he took regular doses of quinine and developed malaria-like symptoms. He concluded that it was actually quinine's ability to cause a malaria-like reaction that made it effective against the disease. He then persuaded healthy people to test, or "prove," other substances, such as arsenic and belladonna, and began to use these "remedies" to treat illnesses whose symptoms resembled the effects the substances had produced.

Hahnemann's ideas quickly spread across Europe to Asia and the Americas. In the 1820s two American doctors expanded his theories: Dr. Constantine Hering developed the "laws of cure" (see right), which explain how disease is cured in homeopathy; Dr. James Tyler Kent introduced the concept of "constitutional types" (see page 129). The American Institute of Homeopathy was founded in 1844, but faced with the demand for "rational" modern medicine, homeopathy had almost disappeared in the US by the 1930s, reemerging only in the 1970s. Opposition persists in several states. In the UK, however, its popularity perhaps boosted by royal patronage, the practice was included as part of the National Health Service when this was founded in 1948.

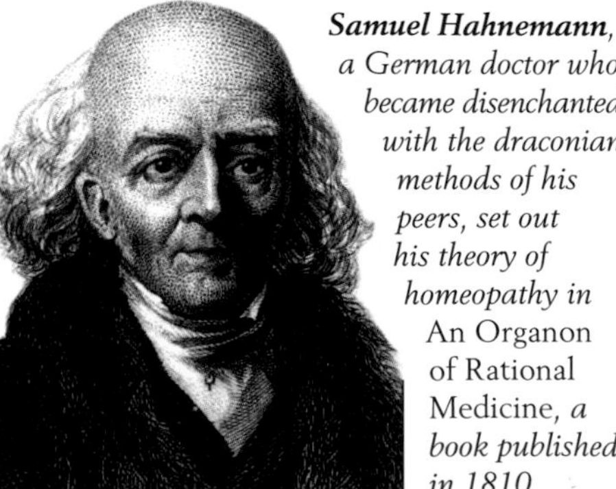

***Samuel Hahnemann**, a German doctor who became disenchanted with the draconian methods of his peers, set out his theory of homeopathy in* An Organon of Rational Medicine, *a book published in 1810.*

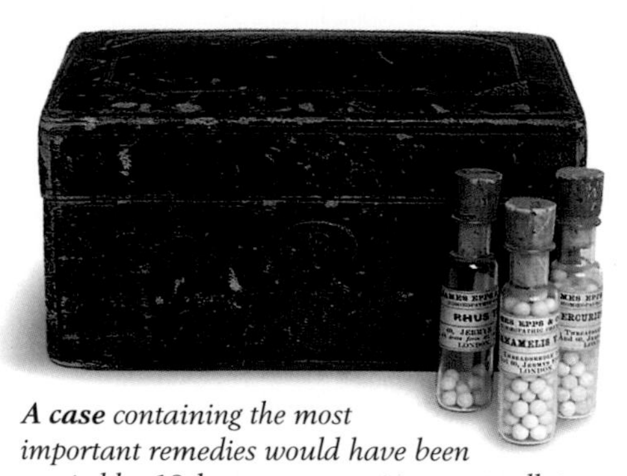

***A case** containing the most important remedies would have been carried by 19th-century practitioners at all times.*

KEY PRINCIPLES

"Vitalism" – the idea that a "vital force" regulates the body – was an important theory in 17th-century medicine. Symptoms of disease, such as fever or inflammation, were seen as signs that the vital force was fighting infection. Modern homeopaths still choose remedies according to the "law of similars" (see opposite) to stimulate the vital force.

Patients are classified according to their particular constitutional type, and symptoms are grouped, with unusual ones considered more significant than common ones. Treatment is said to work according to the three basic laws of cure: that symptoms move down from the top of the body, outward from the inside of the body, and from the most important organs to the least important, with long-standing complaints taking longer to disappear than those that developed more recently.

Hahnemann observed that the more a remedy was diluted, the more specific the effect seemed to be. From this he derived the law of potentization (see opposite).

"Nosodes" were homeopathic remedies devised by Hahnemann to counteract "miasms," which he alleged were inherited weaknesses that blocked a patient's response to treatment. He made them from body secretions linked with what he saw as the fundamental illness (scabies, for example, was treated with nosodes made from scabies sores). In modern practice nosodes are made from many body tissues.

Isopathic treatment uses remedies made from the substances that cause the ailments for which they are given. An example is *Mixed pollen 6c*, a hay fever remedy made by diluting a range of spring pollens.

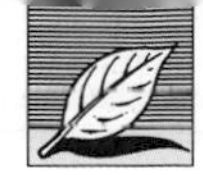

THE THEORY OF HOMEOPATHY

The body is said to be integrated by a "vital force," which maintains it in a state of health. If this force is put under strain, illness can result. Symptoms of illness are seen by homeopaths as signs that the body is using its natural powers of self-healing to fight back. Homeopathic treatment seeks to stimulate this self-healing process rather than to suppress symptoms.

THE LAW OF SIMILARS

According to the law of similars, or "like cures like," patients' symptoms are a reliable guide to the remedy needed to activate the self-healing power of their vital force. Hahnemann applied this principle to his homeopathic remedies; to stimulate the vital force to fight an illness, the remedies are derived from substances that induce symptoms similar to those of the illness. For instance, eyebright, an irritant herb, is used in a remedy to soothe sensitive eyes, while belladonna is used to treat scarlet fever, because the symptoms of belladonna poisoning are very similar to those of scarlet fever.

Eyebright

Belladonna

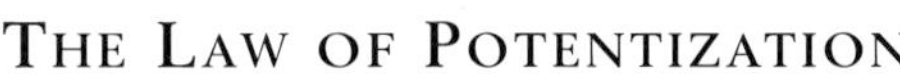

THE LAW OF POTENTIZATION

Diluting doses repeatedly limits their potential to cause side effects and helps to avoid so-called "aggravations," although these are still experienced by some patients. Hahnemann observed that the more a substance was diluted, the more potent it seemed to become. Remedies might even contain nothing of the original substance.

A remedy is "potentized" by diluting it on either the decimal scale (x) with a dilution factor of 1:10 or the centesimal scale (c) with a dilution factor of 1:100.

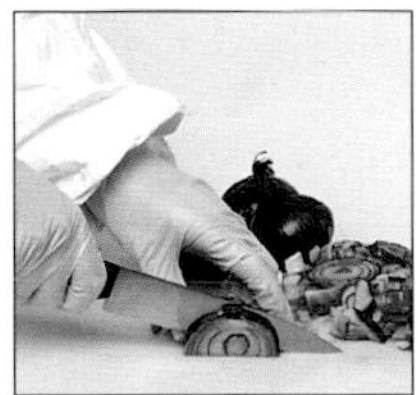

1 *Remedies are made from plant, animal, and mineral extracts. First the material is chopped or ground roughly.*

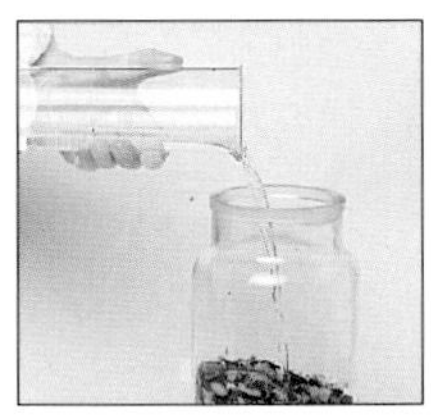

2 *The material is soaked in a mix of 90% alcohol and 10% distilled water and left to stand for 2–4 weeks.*

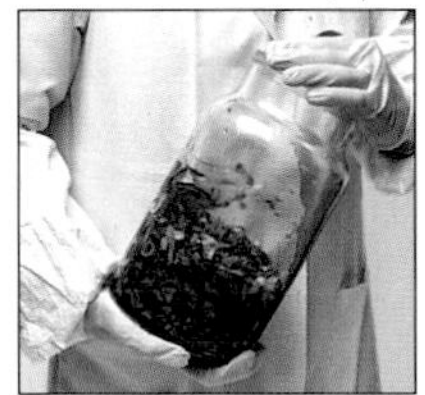

3 *The jar is sealed with an airtight lid and the mixture is shaken from time to time to dissolve the material.*

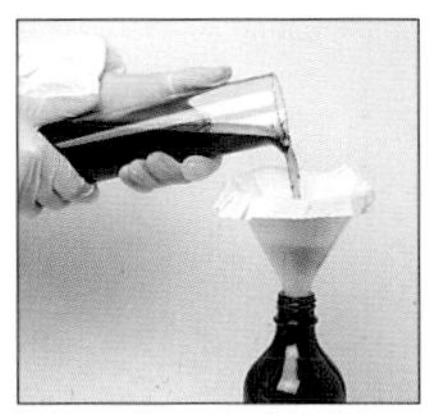

4 *The infused mixture is strained into a dark glass bottle, after which it is known as the "mother tincture."*

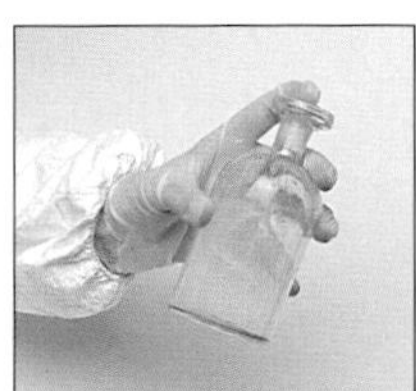

5 *One drop of the tincture is diluted in 99 drops of alcohol, then shaken rapidly – a process called "succussion."*

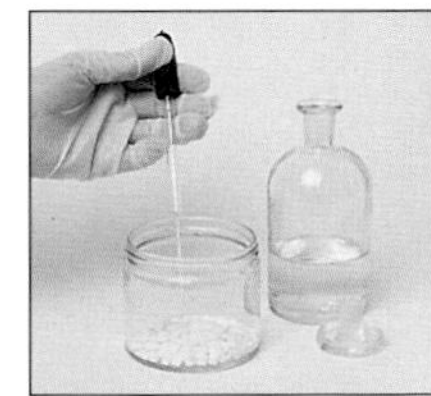

6 *After repeated dilution and succussion to the required potency, a few drops are added to lactose tablets.*

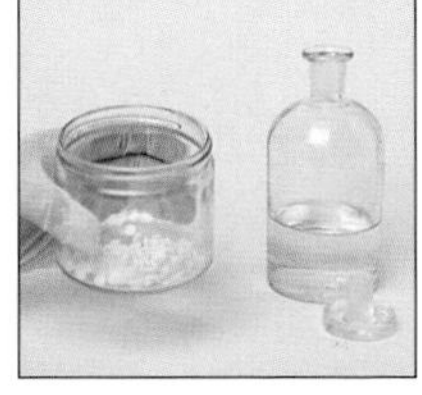

7 *The jar is then swirled gently to ensure that each tablet is properly impregnated with the potentized remedy.*

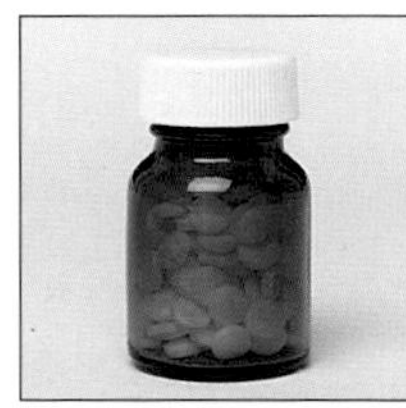

8 *The homeopathic tablets are placed in an airtight bottle made of dark glass, and stored away from direct sunlight.*

EVIDENCE & RESEARCH

A scientific study in support of homeopathy was published in *The Lancet* in 1994. Dr. David Reilly of Glasgow University carried out three separate clinical trials using the double-blind principle (neither doctors nor patients knew which patients were receiving medication; see page 16). These indicated that the homeopathic treatment was more successful than a placebo treatment in relieving hay fever and allergic asthma.

An American study, also in 1994, at the Cleveland Clinic Foundation, showed that zinc gluconate lozenges reduced the duration of colds by 42%, as well as greatly decreasing the frequency of symptoms. A 1991 survey in the *British Medical Journal* of 107 controlled trials concluded that the higher the methodological quality of the study, the more likely it was to be positive.

A survey of 73 homeopathic doctors in the UK, published in 1989 in the *Journal of the Royal College of General Practitioners*, claimed a 35% success rate for treatment using homeopathic remedies.

In 1988, French scientist Jacques Benveniste showed that extremely diluted substances still affected living cells in quite a different way than water. The findings are controversial; no other scientist has been able to repeat them.

MEDICAL OPINION

Current scientific understanding cannot explain homeopathy. While accepting that minute quantities of a substance can affect physiological processes, many doctors are skeptical of the efficacy of a substance that is so diluted that barely a molecule remains in the remedy. A 12c potency, for example, is said to be equivalent to a pinch of salt in the Atlantic Ocean.

The popular but controversial theory of "water memory," which needs further research, contends that even though molecules have been diluted away, they leave electromagnetic "footprints" in the solution, to which the body responds.

A growing number of doctors in the UK, Europe, and India practice homeopathy. However, more research is required to substantiate claims by homeopaths and to establish whether homeopathy can offer cures, especially in conditions where conventional medicine has none.

CONSULTING A PRACTITIONER

Practitioners may be homeopaths who are not medically qualified or conventional doctors who practice homeopathy. They may also be "classical" or "complex" homeopaths (see page 130).

The practitioner will ask about your medical history, diet, lifestyle, moods, likes, and dislikes. A classical homeopath will also identify your constitutional type (see opposite). Practitioners then draw up a "symptom picture" to pinpoint your strengths and weaknesses.

The practitioner will try to match your symptom picture with those cataloged in the homeopathic "repertories," which include 2,000–3,000 remedies, often stored on a computer database. The skill lies in prescribing the remedy that fits your individual type and condition. Advice about diet and lifestyle may also be given.

You will be asked to report any reactions and changes in symptoms at your next visit, and your prescription may be altered or adjusted as necessary. With self-limiting illnesses, such as colds, practitioners say that improvement should occur after the first few doses of the correct remedy. Long-term conditions that have developed gradually require longer treatment. Once signs of improvement show, the remedy dose may be tapered off and eventually discontinued. An awareness of the symptoms and their process of resolution is important to this tapering off.

PRECAUTIONS

- Check unexplained symptoms with a doctor if you are consulting a homeopath who is not medically qualified.
- Tell your practitioner if you are using essential oils; in certain cases they are thought to be incompatible with homeopathic remedies.
- Ask for lactose-free homeopathic tablets or liquids if you are allergic to milk-based products.
- See also page 52.

The patient's physical type, in addition to her emotional and intellectual traits, is assessed

The practitioner builds up a "picture" of the patient's symptoms

THE INITIAL CONSULTATION
A homeopathic practitioner might spend an hour or two asking questions to determine the patient's condition and the most appropriate remedy. In his diagnosis he will take into account factors such as food fads or unusual emotions that may accompany the illness.

TAKING THE REMEDIES

The practitioner may dispense a remedy himself or tell you what to buy from a health food store or pharmacy. The higher the remedy's dilution factor, the more diluted it is – and the more potent, according to homeopathic theory. Remedies should be taken apart from food and without strong flavors in the mouth; take no food or drink 10–15 minutes before or after the dose. The practitioner might advise you to avoid strong-tasting substances such as candies, tobacco, toothpaste, spicy food, and in some cases coffee, camphor, peppermint, alcohol, and menthol, which are believed by some to counteract the effect of remedies. He may also warn against the essential oils used in aromatherapy and herbal medicine.

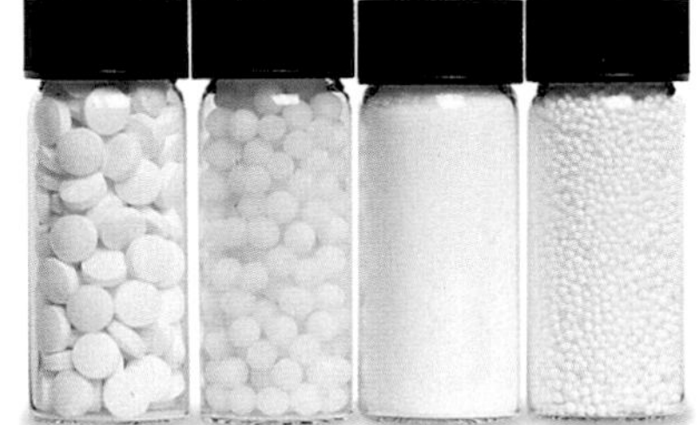

Remedies are made *in the form of lactose tablets, pills, powder, granules, or liquids.*

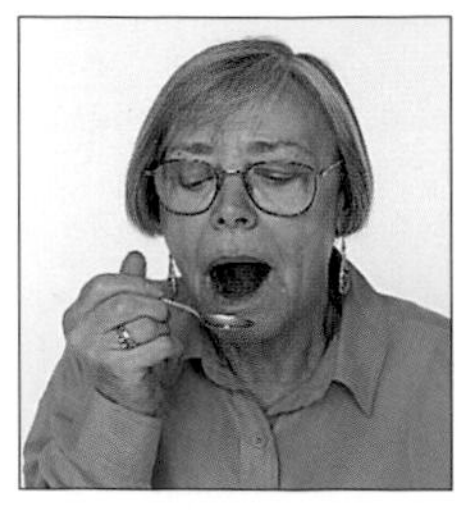

Patients should not *touch the remedies with their hands or fingers. The correct dose should be taken in a clean, dry teaspoon and allowed to dissolve slowly in the mouth.*

YOUR QUESTIONS

How long will treatment last?
The first consultation may last 1–2 hours, although subsequent visits are usually shorter.

How many sessions will I need?
Short-term conditions, such as colds, may improve after only one dose. Some long-term conditions, however, may require many months' treatment.

Will it taste unpleasant?
Most remedies taste mildly of sugar.

Will there be any aftereffects?
Symptoms may briefly worsen after treatment. Homeopaths claim that since the body is healed from the inside out, deep-seated conditions may be temporarily replaced by more superficial ones. For example, as asthma improves, eczema may flare up in its place.

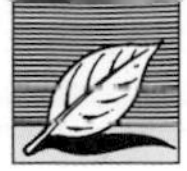

CONSTITUTIONAL TYPES

Practitioners believe that illness results from inner imbalance; the homeopath takes stock of all aspects of a person. To help do this, he classifies a patient as a constitutional type – some of the most common types are shown below. Different types are said to have certain physical, intellectual, and emotional traits. The practitioner considers appearance, symptoms, personality, and habits – such as dislikes, fears, food preferences and the way weather, seasons, and times of day affect the patient. He is very interested in what makes the patient feel better or worse, and in unusual symptoms that seem unrelated to the illness. Each type is associated with a specific remedy, and they share the same name. Different remedies will be used to treat the same illness. Homeopaths prescribe some remedies for the ailment and some to support the person's constitutional type.

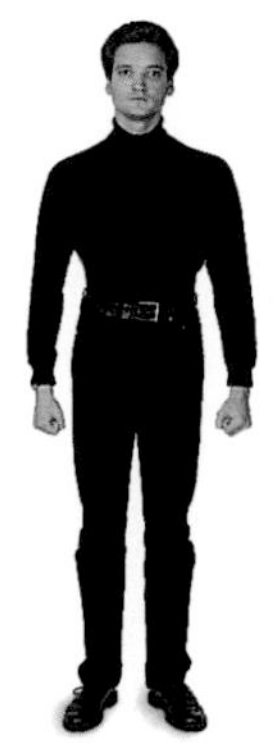

Argent. nit. *types may be quick-tempered, pale-skinned extroverts likely to suffer from nervous problems.*

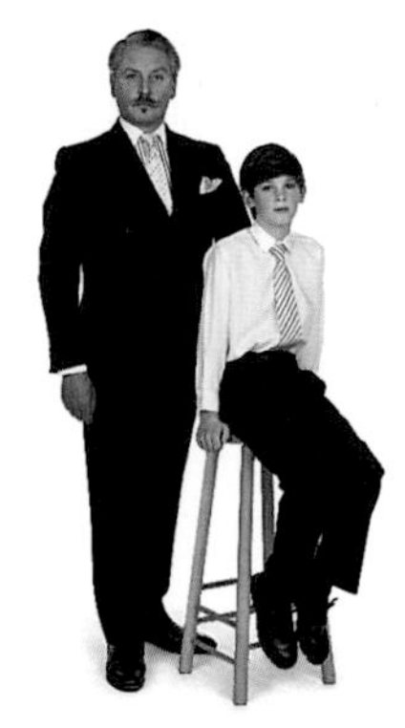

Arsen. alb. *types may be restless, ambitious perfectionists, well groomed, anxious, and insecure.*

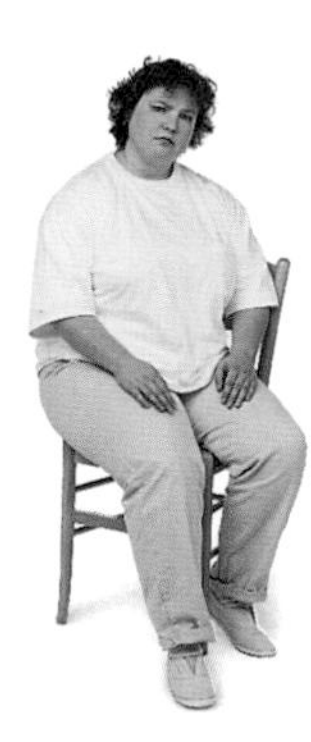

Calc. carb. *types may be quiet, cautious, obsessive, and often overweight. They tend to suffer from joint pain.*

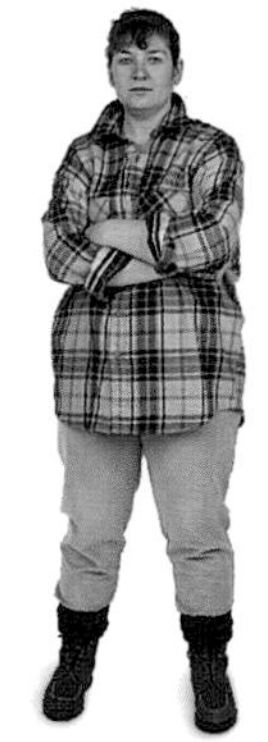

Graphites *types can be indecisive and mentally lazy. They are heavily built and inclined to skin complaints.*

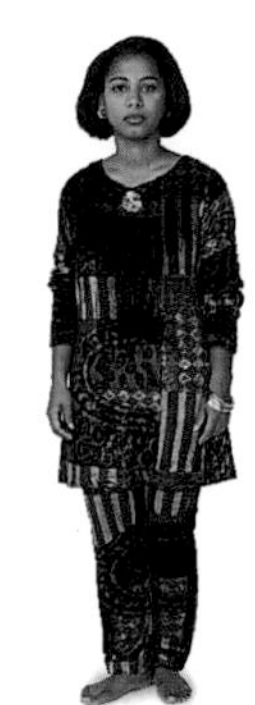

Ignacia *types are usually dark-haired women. Artistic and idealistic, they may be prone to emotional problems.*

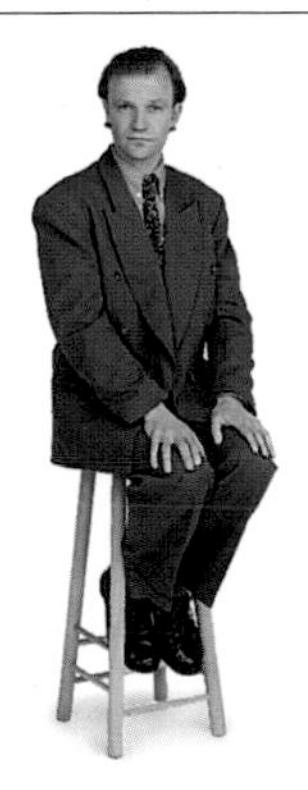

Lycopodium *types are often high achievers, but insecure. Intolerant of illness, they are prone to digestive problems.*

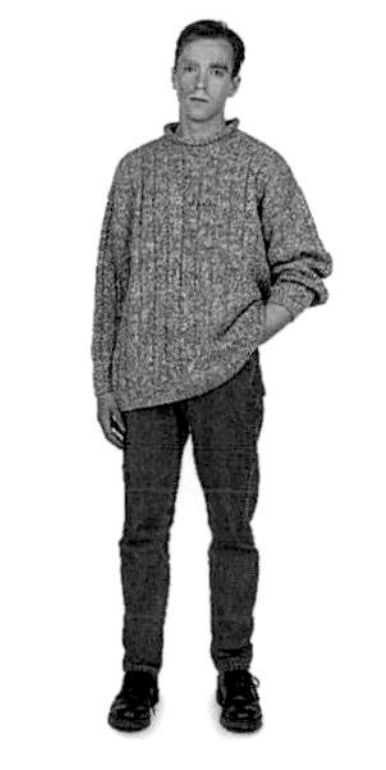

Merc. sol. *types may be easily offended, quick-tempered introverts, prone to respiratory complaints.*

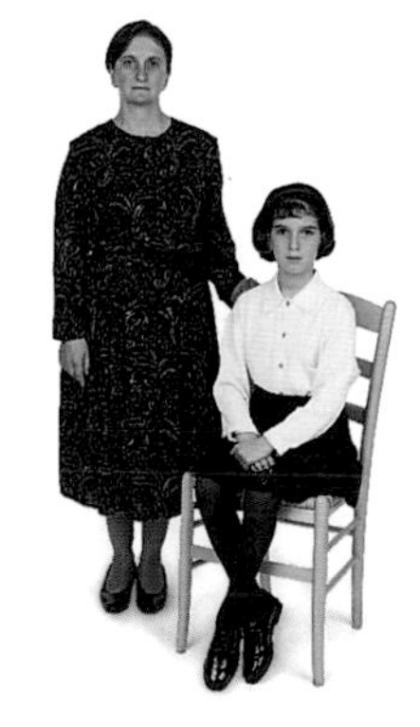

Natrum mur. *types may be serious, sensitive to criticism, introspective, and given to headaches and moodiness.*

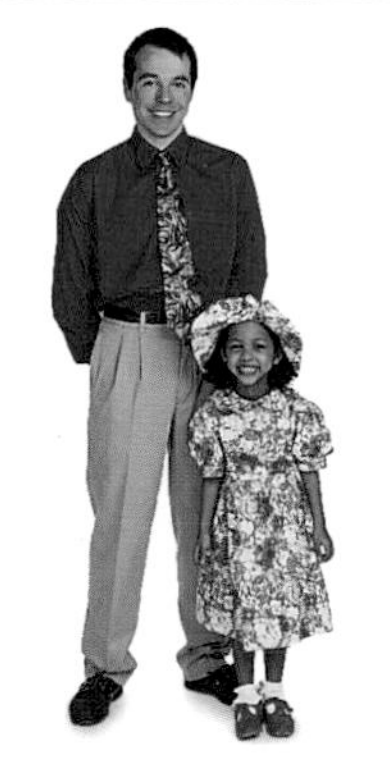

Phos. *types may be fun-loving and kind but do not cope well under pressure. They can be nervous and fidgety.*

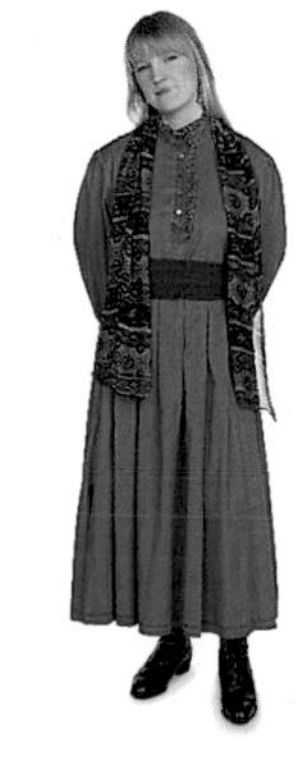

Pulsatilla *types, usually women, may be affectionate and gentle. They cry easily and are prone to colds and PMS.*

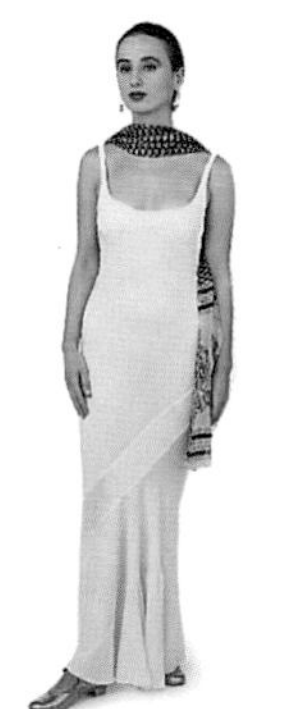

Sepia *types may be elegant, irritable extroverts. They tire quickly and tend to feel burdened by responsibility.*

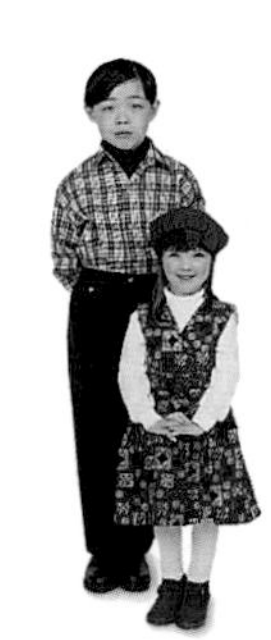

Silica *types may work hard but lack confidence. Likely to be thin and pale, they may succumb easily to colds.*

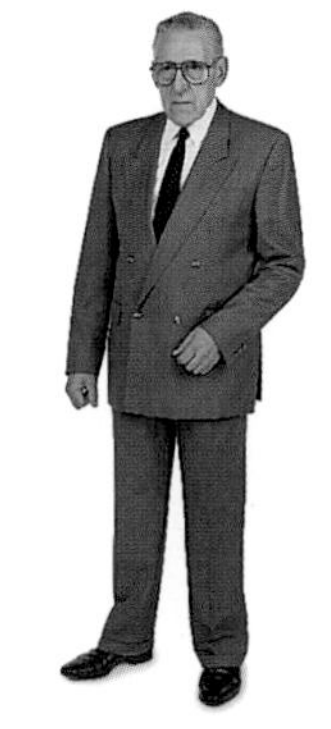

Nux vomica *types may be high-strung and impatient. Very competitive, they can become ill from overwork.*

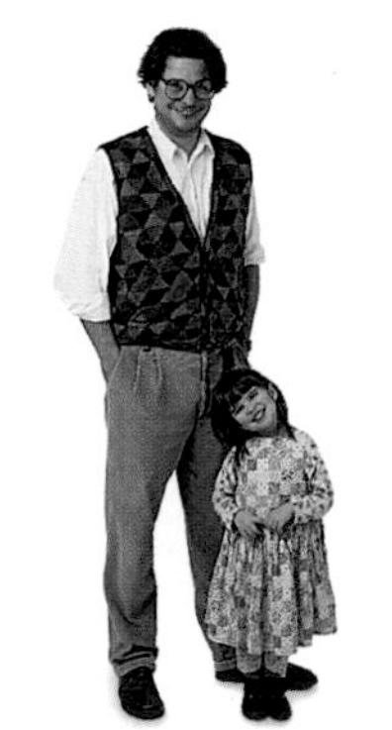

Sulfur *types are often very imaginative, intellectual, and messy. They are susceptible to dry, scaly skin.*

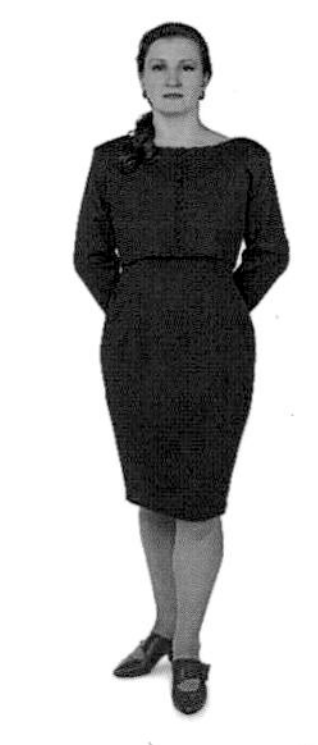

Lachesis *types may be creative but volatile, with behavioral or emotional problems and bad circulation.*

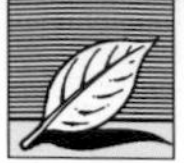

CLASSICAL & COMPLEX HOMEOPATHY

There are some differences between the complex and classical schools of homeopathy, although many practitioners use both systems, and practices may vary from one country to another.

Classical homeopaths prefer to find a single remedy that matches the patient's constitutional type and symptom picture, and will treat with single doses of that one remedy. This approach depends on identifying the *similimum* – the match – which may not happen on the first visit. Two or three remedies may be tried before the right one is found.

A British homeopath, Richard Hughes, extended what is known as "complex" homeopathy in the late 19th century. Hughes looked for organic causes of ailments to guide his prescription, instead of "temperament." Today, his followers still seek to treat sick organs, such as the liver or kidneys, rather than the constitutional type. Complex homeopaths tend to use low-potency remedies, often incorporating herbal extracts.

Hughes' method became popular in continental Europe, especially France and Germany, where it is still widely practiced. In the UK and Australia, homeopaths are more likely to use the classical system.

A Patient's Experience

When Yvonne's daughter Claire was four, she developed a constant cough and was diagnosed as asthmatic: "The doctor prescribed various conventional medicines to be taken three or four times a day, and was considering a nebulizer. I balked at all the medication, but my husband wanted medical supervision for Claire, so we tried homeopathy. The homeopath didn't stop the medication, but taught me to recognize and homeopathically treat an oncoming asthma attack. Claire's constitutional type was Natrum sulf. *It wasn't instant magic, but she gradually improved. Now, four years later, she hasn't used albuterol for the last six months."*

SELF-HELP

Basic, low-potency homeopathic remedies are available at health stores, some pharmacies, and even supermarkets for conditions such as coughs, colds, heartburn, nausea, and stress. These tablets, tinctures, and creams either contain a single remedy to be taken for various conditions, or combine ingredients in the hope that there will be something to suit everyone. For the use of any over-the-counter remedies, reputable manufacturers provide full instructions, which should be followed closely and supplemented with information from a good reference book.

BASIC HOME REMEDY KIT

A good homeopathic first-aid kit should contain about ten remedies, including ointments, tinctures, and tablets. Some remedies that are considered good for nonemergency conditions are described below. Long-standing complaints, such as arthritis or eczema, are best treated with remedies prescribed individually for the patient by a qualified homeopath.

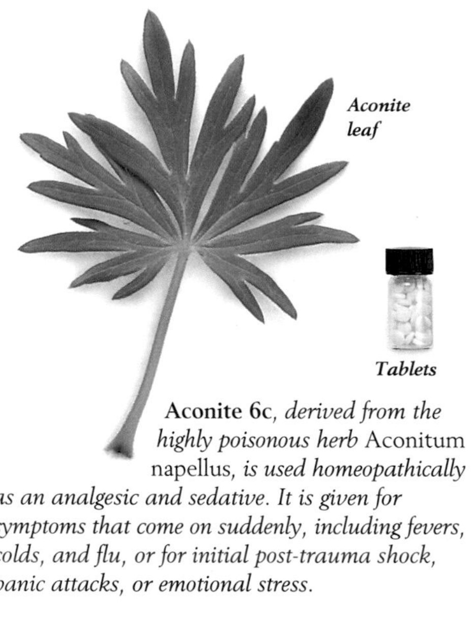

Aconite 6c, *derived from the highly poisonous herb* Aconitum napellus, *is used homeopathically as an analgesic and sedative. It is given for symptoms that come on suddenly, including fevers, colds, and flu, or for initial post-trauma shock, panic attacks, or emotional stress.*

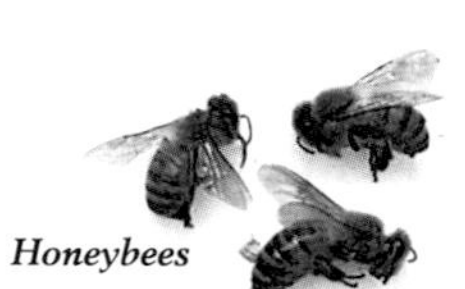

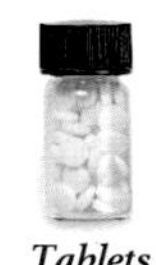

Apis 6c *is made from whole bees, including the stinger. It is used for inflammation that is accompanied by a burning, stinging pain, and for cystitis, hives, bites, and stings.*

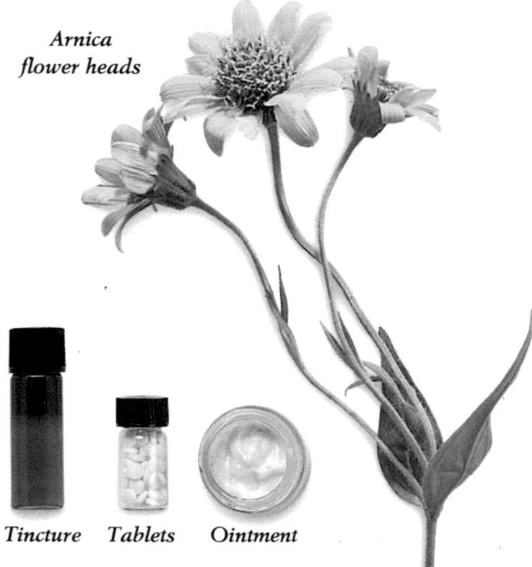

Arnica 6c, *made from the herb* Arnica montana, *is taken for shock, usually in the form of tablets. The tincture and ointment are used for bruises and to reduce swelling.*

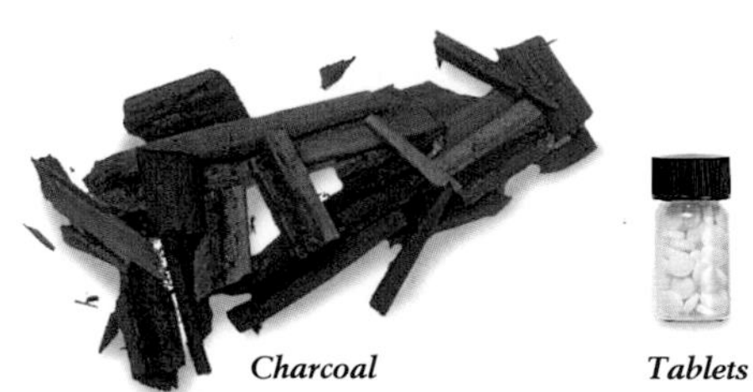

Carbo veg. 6c *originates in the charcoal made from silver birch, beech, or poplar trees. It is commonly given for digestive disorders such as gas, bloating, indigestion, and heartburn, or for headaches associated with overeating.*

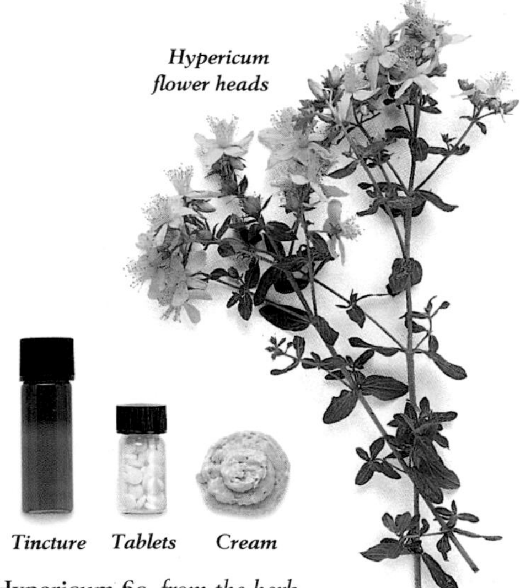

Hypericum 6c, *from the herb St. John's wort (*Hypericum perforatum*), is taken in the form of tablets for nerve pain. The cream or tincture is applied to grazes, painful wounds, or neuralgia, and the tablets are used for backache.*

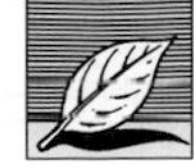

BIOCHEMIC TISSUE SALTS

RATINGS
EVIDENCE
MEDICAL OPINION
PRACTITIONER
SELF-HELP
COMPATIBILITY

ALSO KNOWN AS "SCHÜSSLER SALTS," biochemic tissue salts are homeopathically prepared from mineral sources, such as rock salt and quartz. They were developed in the 1870s by Dr. Wilhelm Schüssler, a German homeopathic doctor, to supplement deficiencies of vital minerals which, he believed, would otherwise leave the body weak and susceptible to disease. Biochemic tissue salts are commonly prescribed by homeopaths worldwide. They are often used as a self-help treatment for minor ailments with recognizable symptoms, and to supplement the dietary intake of minerals.

MAIN USES

- **Colds, phlegm, coughs, sore throats**
- **Hay fever**
- **Headaches**
- **Anxiety**
- **Indigestion, heartburn**
- **Cramps, neuralgia, muscle pain**
- **Minor skin conditions**

HISTORY

In 1873 Dr. Wilhelm Schüssler, a German homeopathic doctor, published a paper in which he claimed that many ailments were due to a lack of essential inorganic minerals in the body. To redress these deficiencies, he recommended nutritional supplements consisting of 12 mineral or "biochemic" tissue salts, to be taken either singly or in combination. Tissue salts are now available worldwide; related naturopathic minerals are popular in Australia.

CONSULTING A PRACTITIONER

Homeopaths, naturopaths, and herbalists will often recommend tissue salts as part of a nutritional program, but they are also frequently used as a self-help measure. Many health food stores and some pharmacies, especially homeopathic ones, stock tissue salts, and manufacturers usually provide dosage information.

The salts are homeopathic preparations that are highly diluted (or "potentized," see page 127). One part of the mineral salt is mixed with nine parts lactose (milk sugar) and this process is repeated six times. The salts are taken in the form of small tablets, dissolved under the tongue.

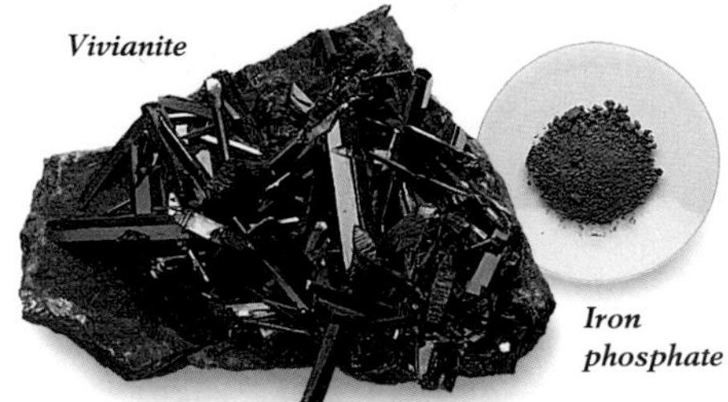

Ferrum phos. *is the name given to the tissue salt made from iron phosphate powder. Vivianite is a natural source of iron phosphate.*

EVIDENCE & RESEARCH

Some of Dr. Schüssler's theories have been verified by medical research. For example, it is now accepted that calcium deficiency can cause susceptibility to bone disorders and problems in absorbing nutrients. There is no evidence, however, that tissue salts redress this deficiency.

MEDICAL OPINION

Lack of research makes it impossible to reach scientific conclusions. In such tiny amounts the active ingredients are harmless.

PRECAUTIONS

- See homeopathy (page 128) and page 52.

THE 12 BIOCHEMIC TISSUE SALTS

NAME	SOURCE	MAIN USES
Calc. fluor.	Calcium fluoride	Hernias, prolapses, hemorrhoids, poor dental health, varicose veins, and other circulatory problems
Calc. phos.	Calcium phosphate	Bone deformities, poor teeth, frostbite, muscle cramps, colds, phlegm, poor digestion
Calc. sulf.	Calcium sulfate	Boils and abscesses, phlegm, dandruff, headaches, kidney problems, neuralgia, pimples
Ferrum phos.	Iron phosphate	Early stage of inflammatory conditions: coughs and colds, earaches; also rheumatism, hemorrhages
Kali mur.	Potassium chloride	Secondary stage of inflammatory conditions: phlegm, ear infections, tonsillitis, chicken pox, measles, mumps
Kali phos.	Potassium phosphate	Anxiety, emotional strain, phobias, sexual frigidity, shyness, incontinence, pus-filled discharge
Kali sulf.	Potassium sulfate	Asthma, bronchitis, dandruff, eczema, halitosis, headaches, menstrual disorders, palpitations
Mag. phos.	Magnesium phosphate	Constipation, enlarged prostate, gas, hiccups, colic, muscle cramps, menstrual pain, neuralgia
Nat. mur.	Sodium chloride	Anxiety, depression, runny colds, migraines, cold sores, canker sores, acne
Nat. phos.	Sodium phosphate	Acidity, heartburn, constipation, diarrhea, nausea, rheumatism, conjunctivitis
Nat. sulf.	Sodium sulfate	Asthma, bronchial phlegm, digestive problems, gas and colic, hay fever, nausea
Silica	Silicon dioxide	Colds and flu, ear infections, boils and pimples, chronic bronchitis, neurological disorders, lack of stamina

BACH FLOWER REMEDIES

RATINGS
EVIDENCE
MEDICAL OPINION
PRACTITIONER
SELF-HELP
COMPATIBILITY

DR. EDWARD BACH was an English doctor who concluded from studies of his patients that negative emotions could lead to physical illness. He was also convinced that flowers possessed healing properties, which could be used to treat emotional problems and so restore health and harmony to mind and body. In the 1930s, Dr. Bach began to produce his remedies, which are made by infusing or boiling plant material in springwater. Bach Flower Remedies and other flower essences are today popular around the world, and are often taken for self-help during times of emotional crisis or stress.

MAIN USES

- Negative emotional states, including fearfulness, uncertainty, disinterest, loneliness, oversensitivity, despair & excessive concern for other people
- Any physical symptoms arising from emotional problems

HISTORY

Early in the 20th century, a London doctor and homeopath, Dr. Edward Bach (pronounced "batch"), made a study of his patients and concluded that harmful emotions, such as despair or fearfulness, could lead to physical disease. Convinced that flowers could affect one's state of mind, and familiar with the homeopathic law of potentization (see page 127), Dr. Bach developed his Flower Remedies. He identified these by holding his hand over each flower in the belief that he could intuitively discern its healing properties. By 1936, Bach's remedies were being made commercially. They are now available from natural health outlets worldwide.

CONSULTING A PRACTITIONER

Although practitioners in other fields – for example, homeopathy, naturopathy, and aromatherapy – may prescribe Bach Flower Remedies in certain cases, Dr. Bach developed his remedies primarily for self-help use. Several remedies may be taken together, and the selection is generally based on the patient's assessment of his or her emotional state. However, some people select the individual remedies by holding a pendulum over each in turn (see page 198).

Oak

Bach remedies are not intended directly to relieve the physical symptoms of an ailment. Dr. Bach believed that harmful emotions were the main cause of disease, and he sought to treat moods such as fear, anger, guilt, and depression in order to restore the harmony of mind and body necessary for good health.

Dr. Bach classified the various moods into seven categories, which he then subdivided into 38 negative feelings, each one associated with a particular plant. He also developed a compound, Rescue Remedy, to be taken for shock, panic, and hysteria.

Gorse

Remedies are prepared by infusion, with flower heads placed on the surface of pure springwater and left to infuse in direct sunlight for three hours, or by boiling short lengths of twigs with flowers or catkins in pure springwater for 30 minutes. After either process the water is retained and preserved in brandy.

Bach remedies are sold in a concentrated form that should be diluted in fruit juice or mineral water, rubbed on the lips or behind the ears, or dropped directly on the tongue. The dose is usually four drops of solution, repeated four times a day. For immediate problems, the dose may be repeated every 3–5 minutes until symptoms subside.

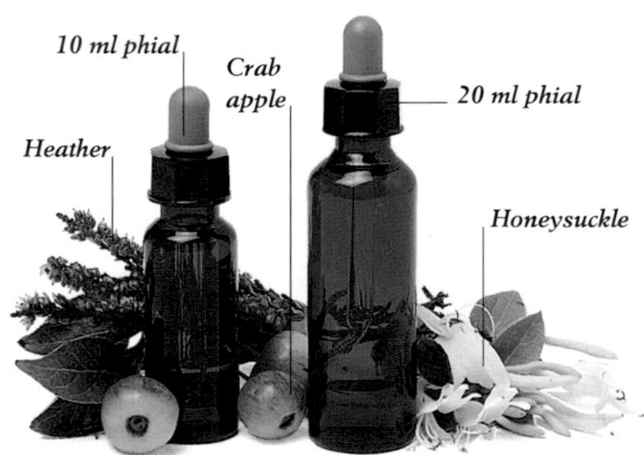

Bach Flower Remedies *are sold in 10 ml and 20 ml "stock" phials, containing individual remedies in a concentrated solution. Remedies should always be stored in a cool, dark place.*

EVIDENCE & RESEARCH

No clinical trials have been carried out on Bach Flower Remedies, and in chemical analysis only springwater and alcohol were detected. One theory attributes any effects to a kind of "molecular imprinting," but this is controversial (see page 126), and claims of efficacy are anecdotal.

MEDICAL OPINION

The unorthodox methods by which Dr. Bach identified and produced his remedies, together with stories of patients choosing their own remedies by dowsing, have not surprisingly left most doctors unimpressed by the claims made for Bach Flower Remedies. Doctors are likely to attribute any benefits derived from them to the placebo response (see page 17).

FLOWER & GEM ESSENCES

An extension of the work of Dr. Bach, 70 Californian flower essences were developed by an American, Richard Katz, in the 1970s, and are said to contain "vibrations of the sun's energy," absorbed by the petals of flowers infused in sun-warmed water. The remedies are taken in a similar way to Bach Flower Remedies, and are also organized by mood and designed to bring harmony to body and mind. Other essences have since been identified, notably from plants in the Himalayas and the Australian bush. Gem essences are also available, made in a similar way by steeping precious and semiprecious stones in springwater.

PRECAUTIONS

- See page 52.

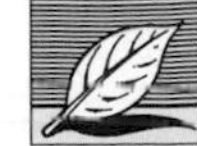

THE SEVEN EMOTIONAL GROUPS & THEIR BACH FLOWER REMEDIES

STATE OF MIND	BACH FLOWER REMEDY	
Fearfulness	◆ *Rock rose* for terror and nightmares ◆ *Mimulus* for known fears and shyness ◆ *Cherry plum* for uncontrollable rage and impulses	◆ *Aspen* for vague fears and apprehension ◆ *Red chestnut* for excessive fear on behalf of family and friends
Uncertainty	◆ *Cerato* for lack of confidence in making decisions ◆ *Scleranthus* for indecision and mood swings ◆ *Gentian* for hesitation, and for doubt and despondency due to past disappointments	◆ *Gorse* for despair and hopelessness ◆ *Hornbeam* for "Monday morning" tiredness and procrastination ◆ *Wild oat* for dissatisfaction and lack of motivation
Lack of interest in present circumstances	◆ *Clematis* for escapism and lack of concentration ◆ *Honeysuckle* for nostalgia and homesickness ◆ *Wild rose* for apathy and resignation ◆ *Olive* for sapped vitality and exhaustion	◆ *White chestnut* for preoccupation with worry ◆ *Mustard* for melancholy ◆ *Chestnut bud* for failure to learn from mistakes
Loneliness	◆ *Water violet* for aloofness and reserve ◆ *Impatiens* for impatience	◆ *Heather* for self-absorption, self-obsession, and excessive desire for companionship
Oversensitivity	◆ *Agrimony* for concealed problems ◆ *Centaury* for anxiety to please	◆ *Walnut* for periods of transition ◆ *Holly* for negative feelings such as hatred or envy
Despondency and despair	◆ *Larch* for lack of self-confidence ◆ *Pine* for guilt and self-reproach ◆ *Elm* for a sense of overwhelming responsibility ◆ *Sweet chestnut* for unbearable anguish	◆ *Star of Bethlehem* for shock and grief ◆ *Willow* for resentment and bitterness ◆ *Oak* for those losing the strength to fight ◆ *Crab apple* for those feeling ashamed or unclean
Overconcern for the welfare of others	◆ *Chicory* for possessiveness, selfishness, self-pity, and overprotectiveness toward others ◆ *Vervain* for the argumentative and overbearing	◆ *Vine* for the ruthless and dictatorial ◆ *Beech* for the critical and intolerant ◆ *Rock water* for self-denial and narrowmindedness

CRYSTAL THERAPY

RATINGS

- EVIDENCE
- MEDICAL OPINION
- PRACTITIONER
- SELF-HELP
- COMPATIBILITY

FROM THE INUIT of the Arctic to the Indians of the Amazon, shamanistic cultures throughout the world have valued precious and semiprecious gems for the magical and therapeutic qualities attributed to them. Crystals, particularly quartz crystals such as amethyst and rose quartz, are believed to possess healing "life energy," storing and discharging this rather like a battery. Despite the skepticism of the conventional medical profession, such theories have been widely adopted by New Age spiritual healers, who use crystals to treat all kinds of physical and emotional problems.

MAIN USES

- Used to enhance the process of healing in the treatment of any physical or emotional condition

Rose quartz

Topaz

Garnet

Among the many gemstones *said to possess healing energy are topaz (for high blood pressure), rose quartz (for stress), and garnet (for depression).*

CONSULTING A PRACTITIONER

While a proportion of practitioners work only with crystals, others use them in conjunction with theories such as the *chakras* (see page 109), acupoints (see page 91), or auras (see page 104). Methods vary widely, but all are said to tap healing energy stored within the crystals.

Practitioners often work by holding a crystal in one hand and resting the other on the part of your body that requires healing. Alternatively, crystals may be placed on the part of your body that needs healing, or on *chakra* or acupoint sites on the body. You may be asked to visualize healing energy channeling through the crystals or be given a crystal to carry, wear around your neck, or place in your room.

MEDICAL OPINION

With no scientific evidence, and diverse philosophies underlying the use of crystals, doctors are generally skeptical. However, a patient's belief may help speed recovery due to the placebo response (see page 17).

PRECAUTIONS

- See page 52.

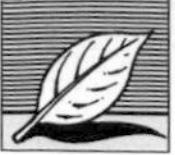

WESTERN HERBALISM

RATINGS	
EVIDENCE	
MEDICAL OPINION	
PRACTITIONER	
SELF-HELP	
COMPATIBILITY	

OVER 80% OF THE WORLD'S population relies on herbs for health. Diverse cultures use herbal remedies to treat disease and promote well-being. Many laboratory-produced drugs are derived from plants, but herbal remedies differ from conventional medicine in using parts of the whole plant rather than isolating single active ingredients. In the past 200 years, plant species from North America, Africa, and Australasia have become part of Western herbalism, and today herbs from other cultures are being introduced as herbal medicine experiences a resurgence in popularity.

MAIN USES

- Most illnesses, including persistent conditions, such as migraines & arthritis
- Respiratory, digestive & circulatory problems
- Skin conditions
- Mild depression
- Insomnia
- Cystitis, PMS & menopausal problems

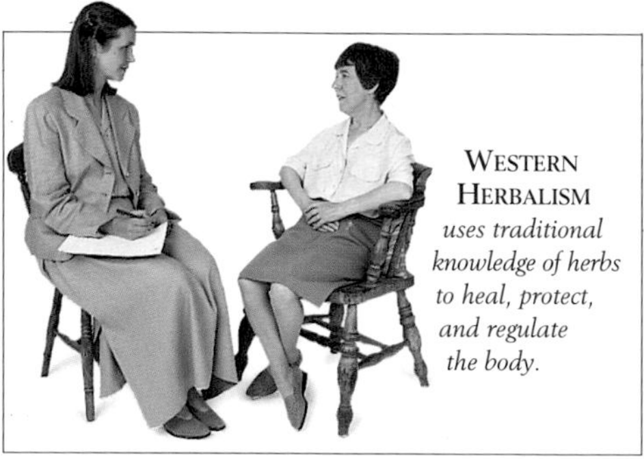

WESTERN HERBALISM *uses traditional knowledge of herbs to heal, protect, and regulate the body.*

HISTORY

Some of the earliest records of medical herbalism can be found in Egyptian papyri dating from 1500 B.C., which refer to many remedies still in use today. Ancient civilizations in China (see page 140), Persia, India (see page 144), and the Americas also relied on medicinal herbs. It was the writings of classical physicians, however, that expanded the knowledge of Western herbalism. Texts on herbal medicine, such as *De Materia Medica* (1st century A.D.) by Dioscorides, an army doctor who traveled throughout the Roman Empire, and *De Simplicibus* (2nd century A.D.) by Galen, were used by Islamic physicians right up to the Middle Ages. This learning filtered back to Europe with the Crusaders, and the texts were translated into Latin again.

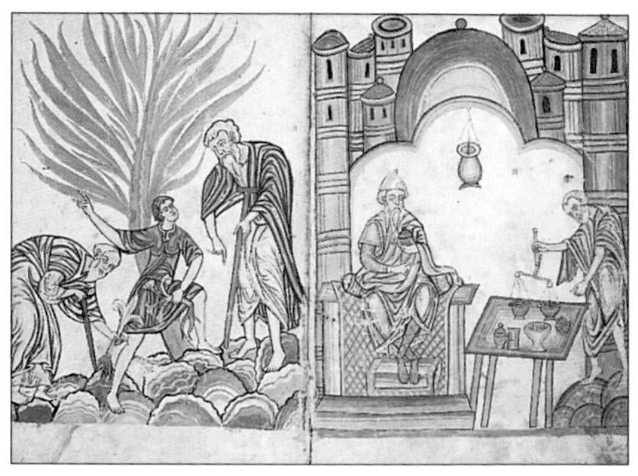

***Illustrated manuscripts**, such as this Latin work by Dioscorides, were the only source of herbal lore until 15th-century developments in printing.*

Herbal folklore was the medicine of the people, part of an oral tradition in Europe, while Greek and Arab herbal lore was the prerogative of monks practicing in monasteries. Only upon the invention of the printing press in the 15th century did this knowledge become available to anyone who could read, and herbalism flourished for the next 200 years. The 16th-century scientist Paracelsus advocated the "doctrine of signatures," an ancient theory that a plant's appearance gave clues as to the ailments it treated. His work influenced John Gerard, whose *Herball* appeared in 1597, and Nicholas Culpeper, author of *The English Physitian* (1653).

With the growth of science in the 18th century, herbal medicine began to decline in Europe, although New World settlers retained their allegiance to herbal lore and also adopted indigenous remedies. Samuel Thomson, a descendant of the Pilgrim fathers, set up herbal schools in the US in the early 19th century. His ideas were taken back to Europe in 1830, and led to a revival of herbalism in the UK.

Conventional medicine remained dazzled by pharmaceutical breakthroughs until the 1970s, but a World Health Organization report concluded that herbal remedies could fulfill an important role in modern health care. Medical herbalism is now well established in continental Europe and can be studied at British universities. In the US, laws restricting the sale of herbal remedies were relaxed in 1994.

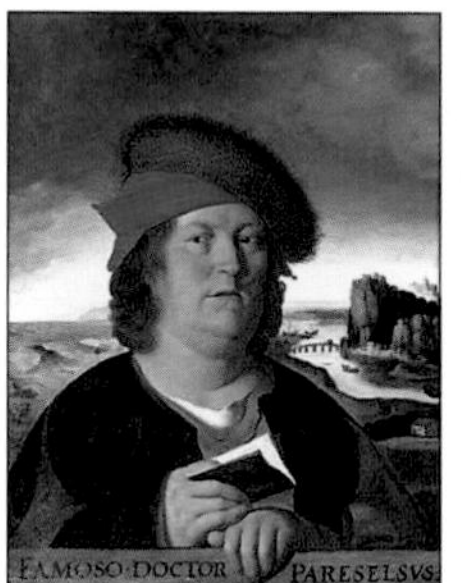

***Paracelsus**, the "father of chemistry," advised an approach to herbal medicine based on close observation and exact dosage.*

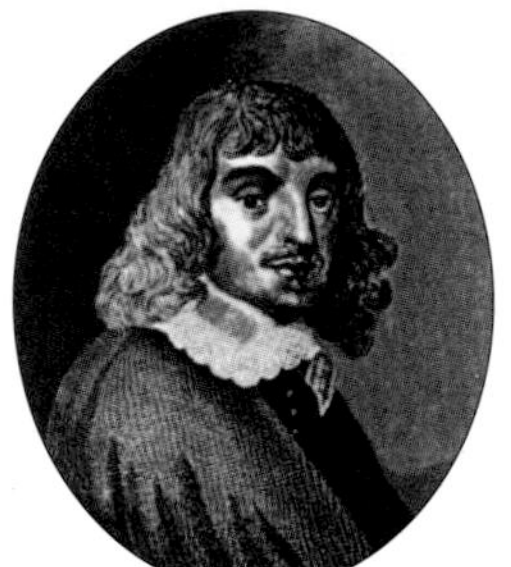

***Nicholas Culpeper** based his popular 17th-century herbal,* The English Physitian, *on personal and practical experience.*

KEY PRINCIPLES

Herbalism is a holistic medical system that seeks to restore the body's self-healing mechanism, or "vital force," and prescribes remedies tailored to the patient, not the symptoms. Rather than treating symptoms in isolation, herbalists look for the cause of illness, such as poor diet, an unhealthy lifestyle, or excessive stress, which may have overburdened the body's fine balance. Herbalists attribute disease to disturbances in the body's self-regulating state of harmony ("homeostasis": see page 26). Remedies promote healing by supporting the efforts of the body's vital force to restore homeostasis. Much of the herbalist's skill lies in knowing the actions of different plants on specific body systems; for example, a plant may stimulate the circulation or calm the digestive system.

Herbal "synergy" (see right) is a key factor in medical herbalism. According to this theory, parts of whole plants are more effective than the isolated constituents used in drugs that are made synthetically.

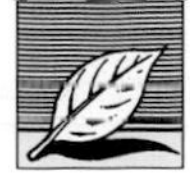

THE THEORY OF SYNERGY

Herbal remedies are extracted from leaves, flowers, and other parts of a whole plant, which contain a complex mix of active ingredients that produce the plant's medicinal effects. Herbalists believe that this mix creates "synergy," where the therapeutic effect of ingredients is greater when used together rather than separately. This is the major difference between herbal remedies and pharmaceutical drugs based on isolated plant extracts.

HERBAL SYNERGY

Pharmaceutical companies often isolate and synthesize the active ingredients of plants. An example is digoxin, manufactured for cardiac drugs, and found naturally in foxglove, which is traditionally used to treat heart disorders. Herbalists, on the other hand, claim that the mix of ingredients in a plant is necessary to make each one safe and enhance its actions. Meadowsweet (*Spirea*), for instance, which is used to treat digestive disorders, contains salicylic acid, the basis of the drug aspirin. However, while aspirin can cause internal bleeding in those with sensitive stomach linings, meadowsweet contains tannin and mucilage, which protect the stomach.

Meadowsweet

Foxglove

PROCESSING PLANT MATERIAL

Different parts of the same plant, for example the flowers and seeds, can have quite different actions, and it is essential that the correct medicinal part of the plant is processed. To ensure a high concentration of active constituents, herbs are processed as quickly as possible after harvesting (see page 137).

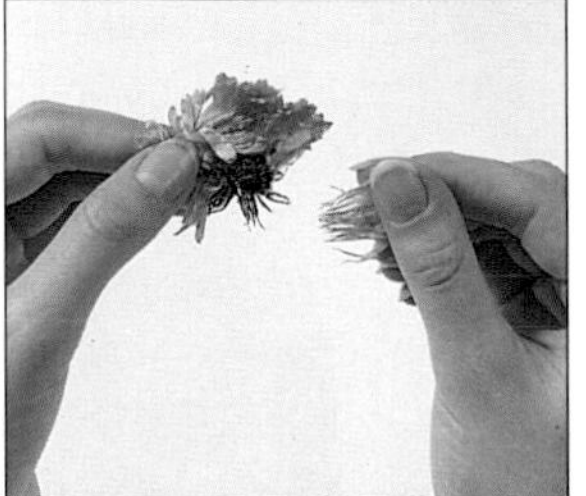

***Petals** of plants with large flowers, such as calendula, are picked from the dried flower heads before being stored.*

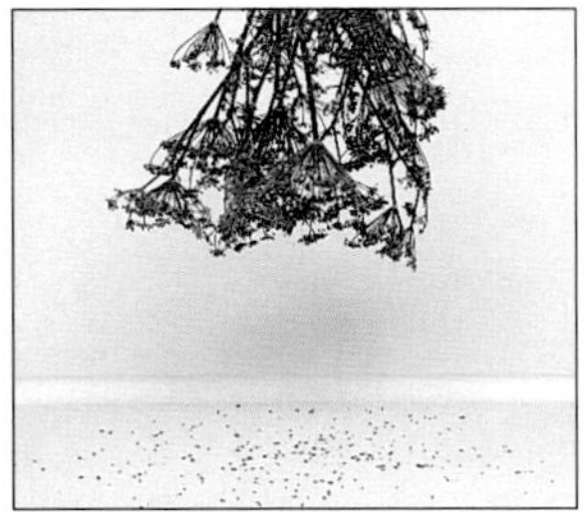

***Seeds** are separated by drying bunches of seed heads upside down and then gently shaking them over a paper-lined tray.*

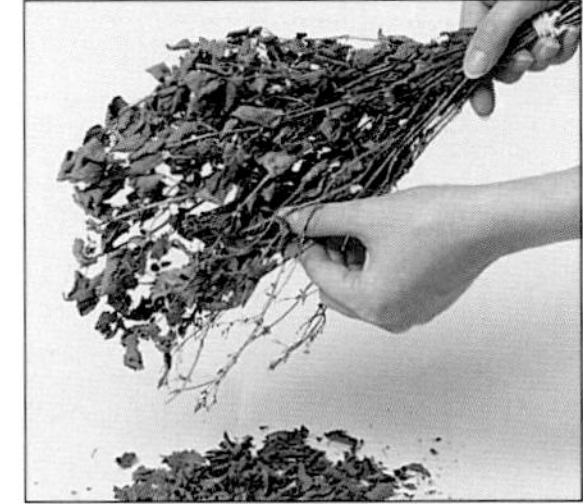

***Aerial parts**, such as leaves, flowers, and seeds, are dried in bunches and removed by rubbing over a sheet of paper.*

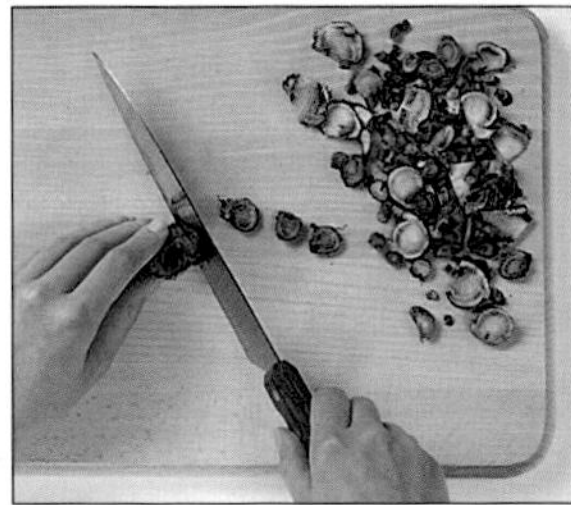

***Root parts** are chopped into small pieces and left to dry for a few hours in a warmed oven with the door slightly open.*

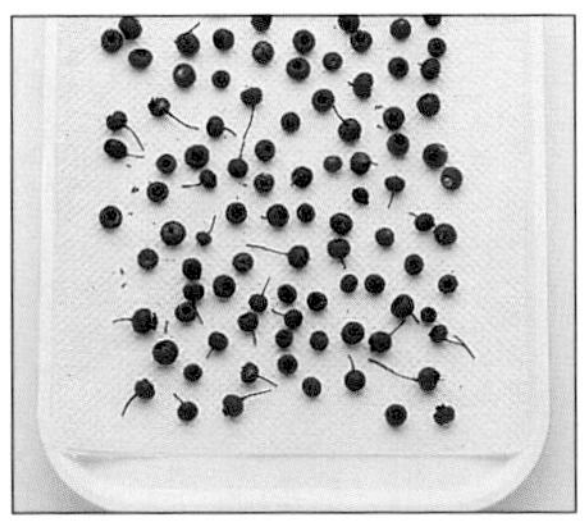

***Berries or fruit** are placed on absorbent paper and dried in a gently warmed oven with the door ajar for a few hours.*

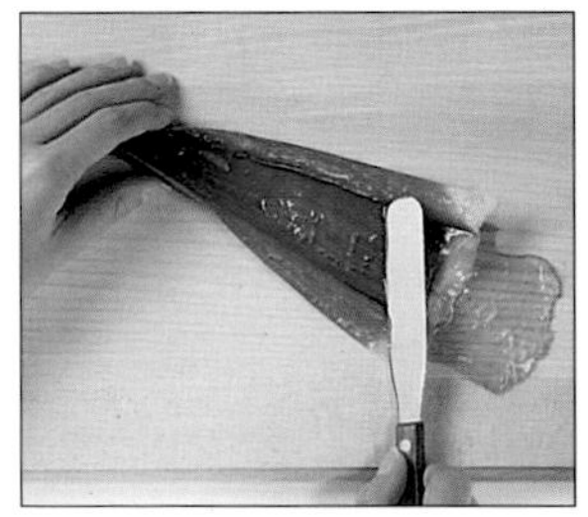

***Gel** is collected from plants such as aloe vera by scraping along the inside of the leaf. It must be used immediately.*

EVIDENCE & RESEARCH

Evidence to support herbal medicine is growing fast, and can be as strong as that for pharmaceutical drugs. In Europe and Australia, herbal products need to be backed by scientific evidence before they are allowed to make medicinal claims. This provides incentive for research.

In the US, it is illegal to state therapeutic uses for herbal products on the label. Clinical research supports the claims made for many herbs, including:

Echinacea: Traditionally used by Native Americans, this herb appears to stimulate the immune system and prevent infections by increasing the flow of white blood cells. It is being investigated as a treatment for HIV and AIDS, and in Germany is an approved treatment for many disorders, including multiple sclerosis.

Garlic: The subject of over 1,000 research papers, garlic lowers blood cholesterol and fat levels, and reduces blood pressure. Research since the 1980s, especially in the US, Germany, and Japan, has verified its antibiotic and antiseptic actions and its ability to fight certain cancers.

Ginger: In 1990 a British study showed ginger to be of benefit in relieving nausea in postoperative patients.

Ginkgo: One of the oldest living plant species, ginkgo is the best-selling herbal medicine in France and Germany. Research carried out in France in 1986 provided evidence of its effectiveness in treating tinnitus, while a study published in *The Lancet* in 1992 showed that it improved blood circulation.

St. John's wort: A study published in *The Lancet* in 1996 showed this herb can treat depression as effectively as synthetic anti-depressants, and without side effects.

MEDICAL OPINION

Many doctors view herbalism as an outdated tradition, although they realize that plants are the source of many synthetic drugs. However, doctors stress that not all herbs are safe, that their consituents are difficult to standardize, and that herbal medicines should only be taken with expert advice. If the evidence for herbal treatment of diseases were more widely known, doctors might be more willing to use them, especially now that they are being mass-produced in tablet form and made more widely available.

Consulting a Practitioner

Practitioners have some knowledge of biology, anatomy, and physiology, as well as plant pharmacology, but their approach to treating illness is holistic and they will consider all aspects of your life before prescribing treatment. Your first consultation will usually last an hour, during which the practitioner will take an extensive medical history. She will ask you about your lifestyle – focusing on areas of stress – and about your diet, work, mental and emotional state, and recent life events. Details of any conventional medication you are taking will also be recorded to ensure compatibility with the herbal remedies prescribed.

The practitioner will carry out some simple tests (see below) or give you a physical examination, for which you may need to undress. Based on her conclusions, she will prescribe one or more herbal remedies, which can normally be made up on the spot. Treatment may also include advice on diet and exercise. You will probably be asked to return in a week or two, or earlier if your condition is acute. If appropriate, the herbalist may suggest that you see a conventional doctor.

Herbal remedies usually take longer to work than conventional medicine, and should generally be taken for a week or two after symptoms disappear.

Your Questions

How long does a treatment session last?
The first consultation may last an hour and subsequent sessions 15–30 minutes.

How many sessions will I need?
You may need only one or two sessions for minor ailments, but for a long-term condition, you can expect approximately one month of treatment for every year the condition has lasted.

Will remedies taste unpleasant?
Although licorice or honey is often used to disguise the flavor of herbs, many remedies are fairly unappealing.

Will there be any aftereffects?
Used sensibly and under the supervision of a professional, herbal medicine is usually free from aftereffects.

Standard Tests

Practitioners may carry out some of the same diagnostic tests as those used by a conventional doctor.

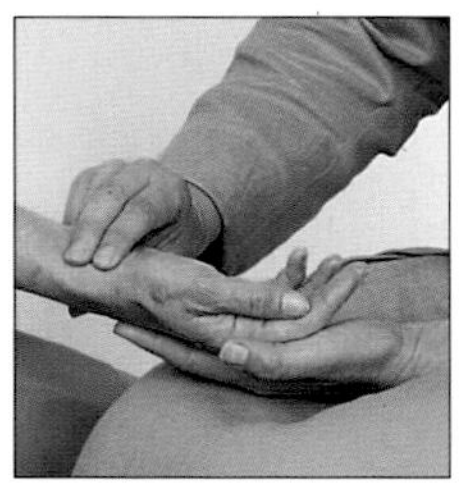

Pulse *is taken to check the rate at which blood pumps from the heart.*

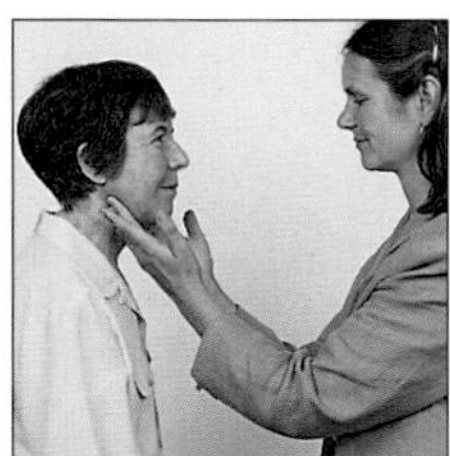

Glands *in the neck are examined for signs of swelling.*

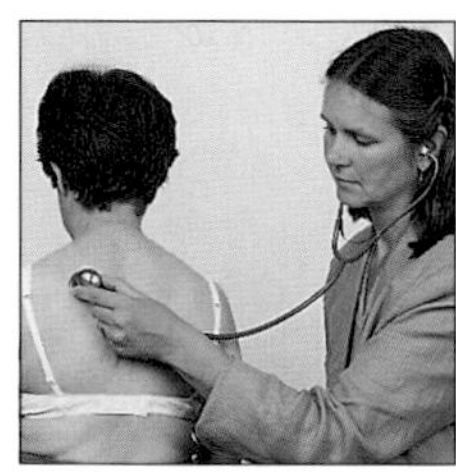

Lungs *and heart are checked by listening with a stethoscope.*

Diagnosis

A medical herbalist will make a diagnosis on the basis of her examination of the body systems, focusing on digestion, circulation, respiration, and elimination of waste products, to identify weaknesses that may be at root of the problem. Herbal remedies are prescribed to stimulate the affected body system to fight illness.

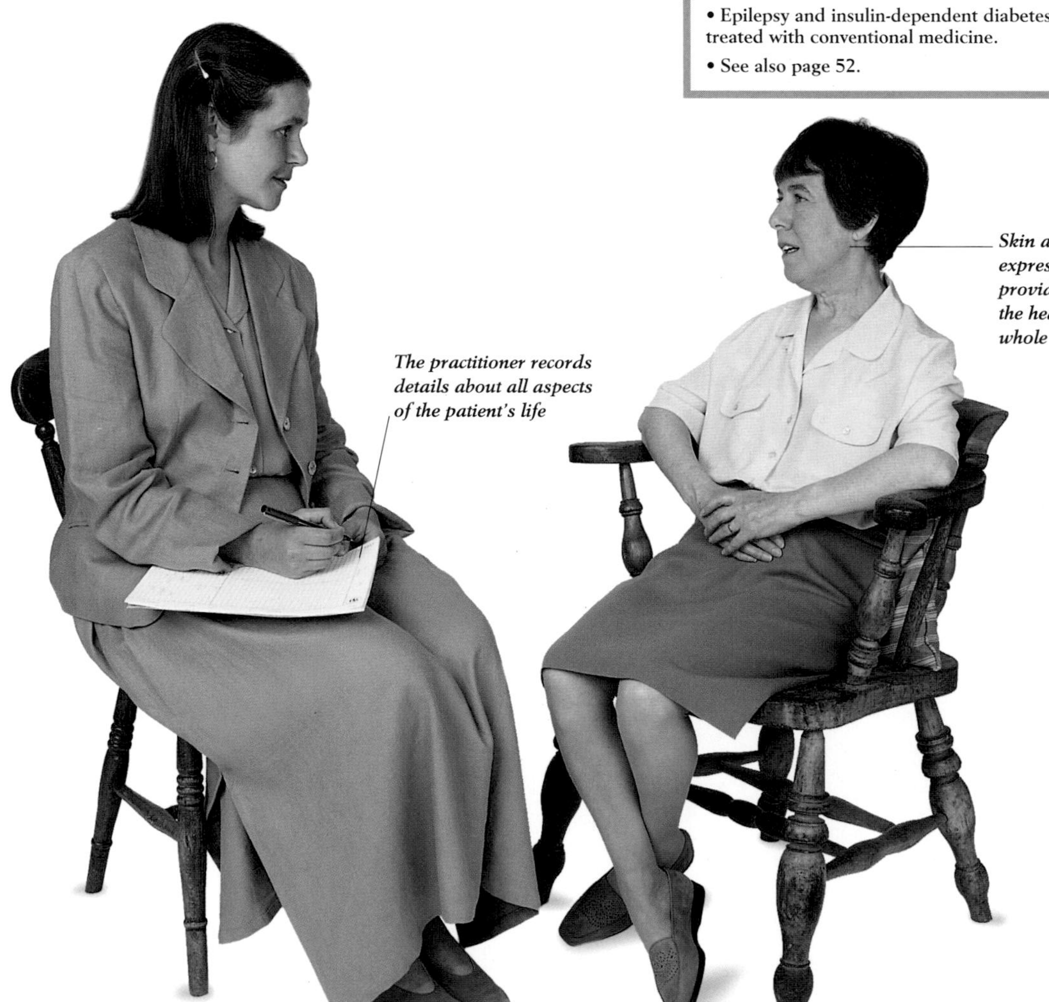

The practitioner records details about all aspects of the patient's life

Skin and facial expression may provide clues to the health of the whole body

Precautions

- Consult a qualified herbalist before taking an herb if you are taking prescribed medication, and do not discontinue a medicine without telling your doctor.
- Consult a qualified herbalist before taking herbal medicine if you are pregnant, or if you have heart disease, hypertension, high blood pressure, or glaucoma.
- Epilepsy and insulin-dependent diabetes are best treated with conventional medicine.
- See also page 52.

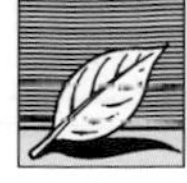

How Herbal Remedies Are Made

The medicinal parts of plants can be made into a wide variety of herbal preparations, the most common of which are shown below.

Infusions and decoctions should be consumed within about a day of making, while tinctures can be stored for up to two years, and infused oils, creams, and ointments for several months.

DECOCTIONS

Tough plant materials, such as bark, roots, and berries, are boiled in water to extract the active ingredients. Herbs may be boiled fresh or dried, and singly or in combination. Decoctions can be taken hot or cold.

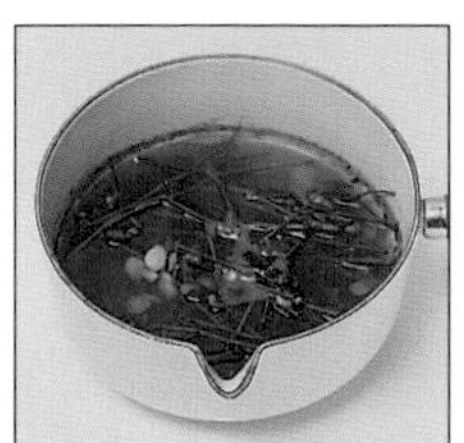

1 Herbs are placed in a saucepan, covered with cold water, and brought to a boil. They are then simmered until the liquid has reduced by about one-third.

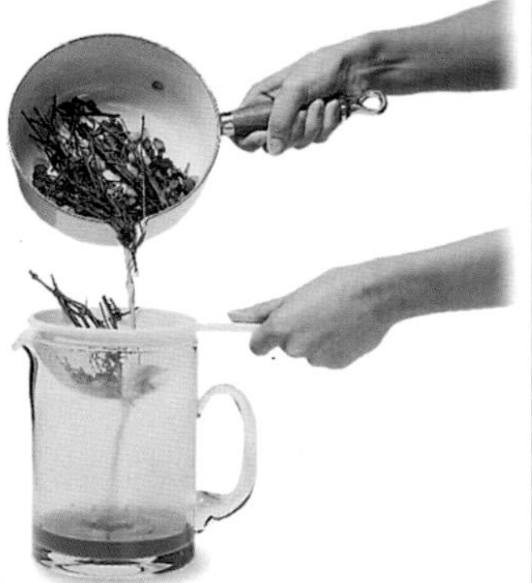

2 The liquid is strained into a jug, which can then be covered and stored in a cool place.

TINCTURES

A tincture is made by soaking an herb in alcohol and water, which help extract its active ingredients and act as a preservative. Tinctures of more than one herb can be combined and are usually taken with water.

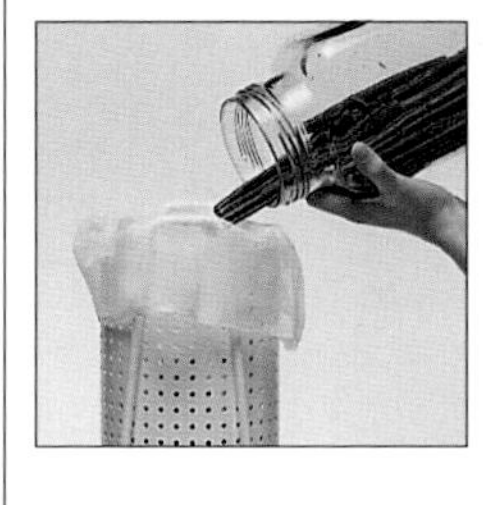

1 Herbs are steeped in alcohol and water for two weeks, then poured through a muslin-lined wine press.

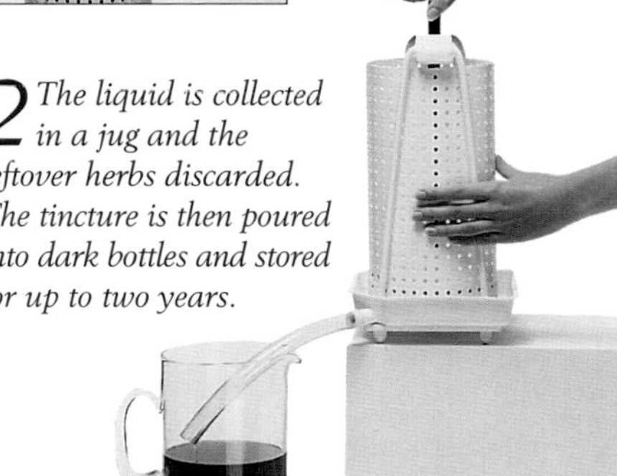

2 The liquid is collected in a jug and the leftover herbs discarded. The tincture is then poured into dark bottles and stored for up to two years.

INFUSIONS

Made in a similar way to tea, an infusion is a simple way to prepare the leaves and flowers of plants. It can be made with one or more herbs and is taken hot or cold, either as a medicine or as a pleasant drink.

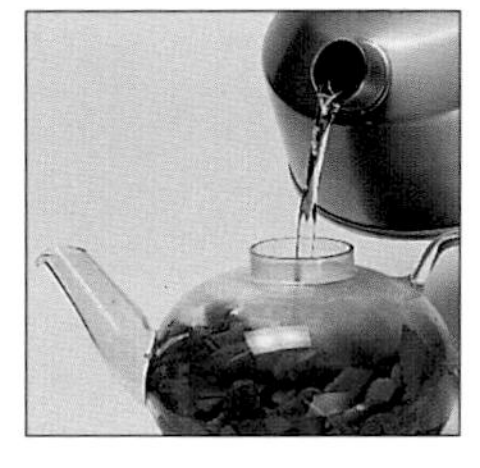

1 Herbs are placed in a teapot and covered with hot water that has just boiled. The lid of the teapot is replaced and the herbs are left to infuse for about 10 minutes.

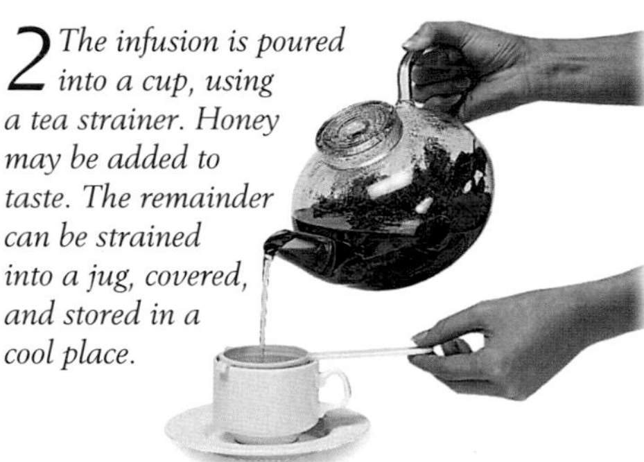

2 The infusion is poured into a cup, using a tea strainer. Honey may be added to taste. The remainder can be strained into a jug, covered, and stored in a cool place.

INFUSED OILS

Herbs are infused in oil to extract their fat-soluble ingredients. Hot infused oils are made by simmering; cold infused oils are simply infused in sunlight. Both can be used for massage, or in creams and ointments.

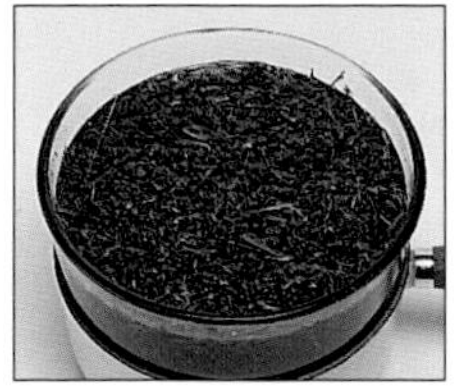

1 Hot infused oils are made by placing chopped herbs and oil in a glass bowl, which is set in a pan of boiling water and simmered gently for 2–3 hours.

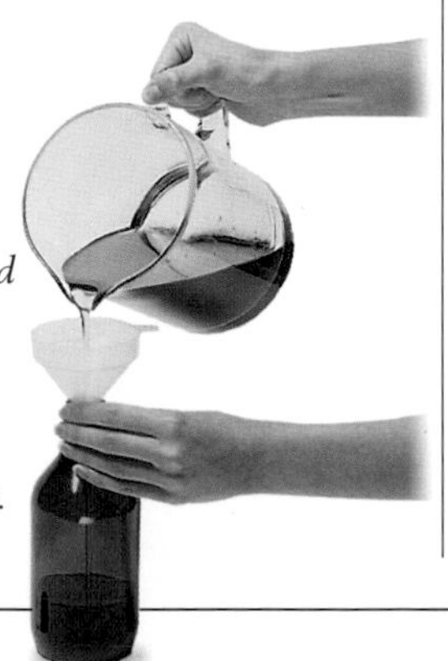

2 The mixture is removed from the heat, cooled, and strained through a wine press. The infused oil is then poured into dark glass bottles, using a funnel, and sealed. The oil can be stored for up to a year.

CREAMS

Water is slowly combined with oil or fat to make cream. Unlike ointments, creams blend with the skin, allowing it to breathe. They deteriorate quickly and are best stored in airtight jars in a refrigerator.

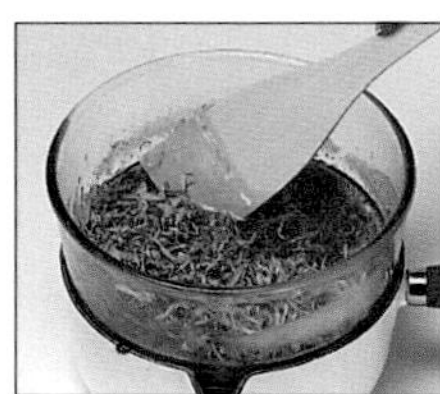

1 Emulsifying wax is melted in a glass bowl set in a pan of boiling water. Herbs, glycerine, and water are stirred in and simmered for about three hours.

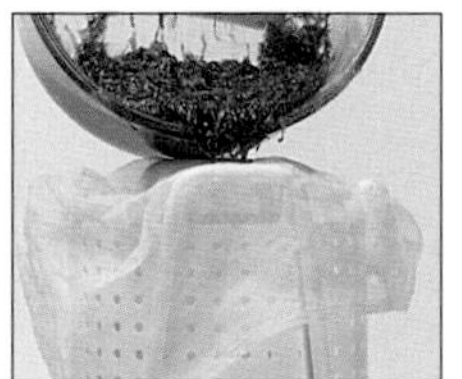

2 The herb mixture is strained through a wine press or cheesecloth and stirred until it cools and sets.

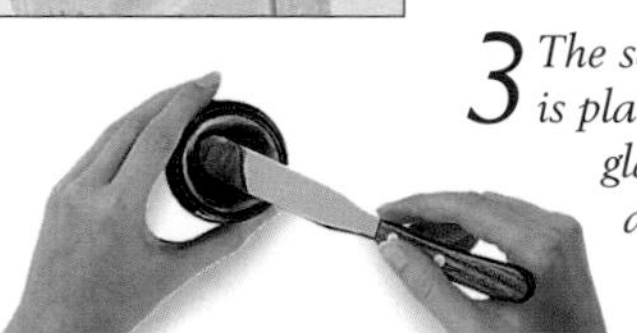

3 The set cream is placed in dark glass jars with a spatula, and the lids are secured.

OINTMENTS

Made by heating oil or fat with herbs, ointments form a protective layer over the skin. They are useful in conditions where the skin needs protection from moisture, such as chapped lips.

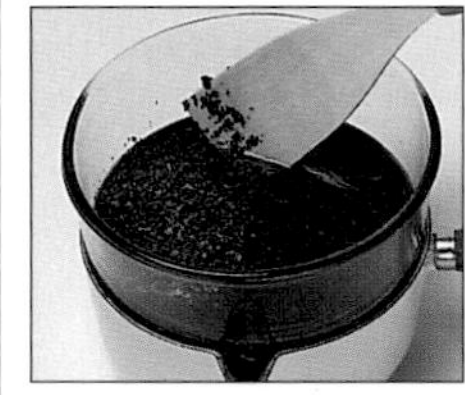

1 Olive oil and beeswax are placed in a glass bowl set in a pan of boiling water. Chopped herbs are added and the mixture is simmered.

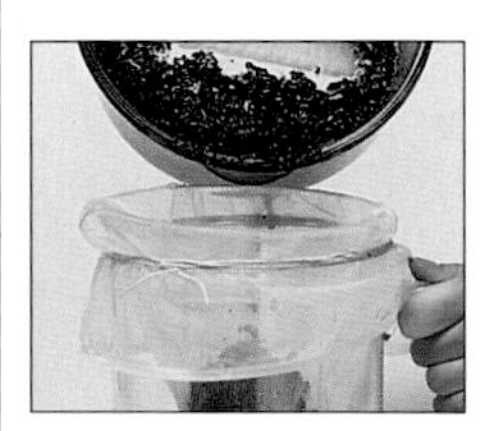

2 A cheesecloth is secured to the rim of a jug to strain the herb mixture and collect the liquid.

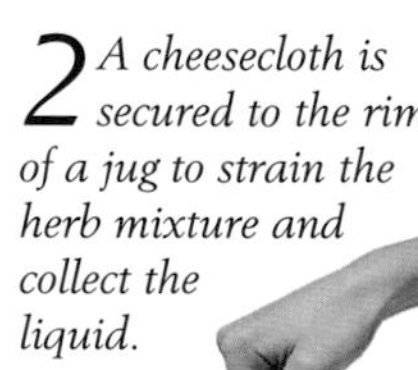

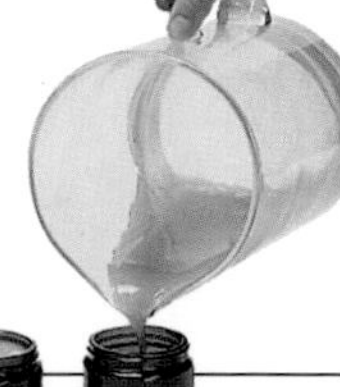

3 The molten herbal ointment is quickly poured into dark glass jars and left to cool and set. The lids are then fastened.

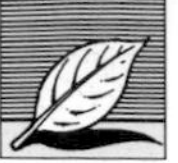

Dispensing Herbs

Most practitioners of herbal medicine have a dispensary where they make up prescriptions tailored to the needs of individual patients. These may contain a single herb or a combination of herbs. Herbs are commonly dispensed as tinctures, made by steeping herbs in alcohol (see below). Other remedies taken internally include tablets, infusions, and decoctions. Creams, lotions, oils, and ointments are prescribed for external use.

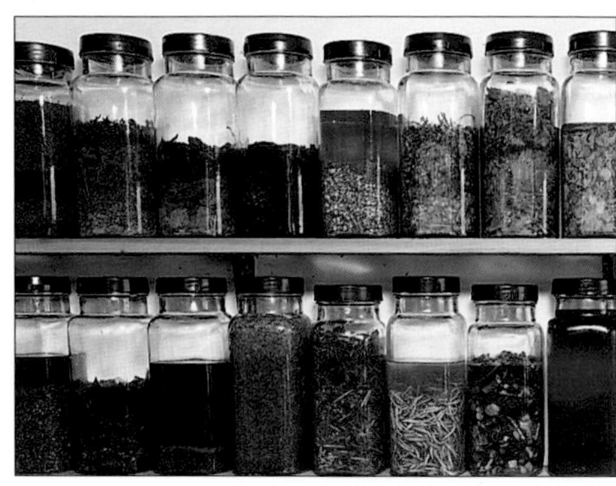

***Tinctures are prepared** by placing fresh or dried herbs in jars of alcohol and allowing the active constituents to dissolve. The jars are stored in a cool, dark place for about 14 days before extracting the tincture and discarding the herbs.*

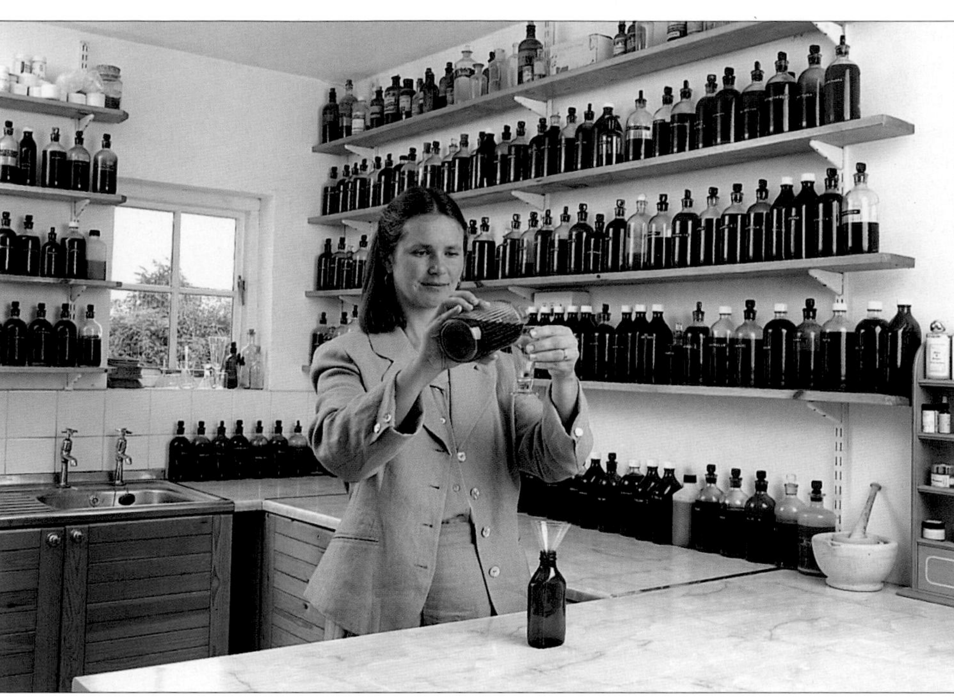

***Once extracted, tinctures** are stored in sterilized, dark glass bottles for up to two years. Here, the practitioner measures out the required dosage of a tincture for a patient. It is possible to make your own tinctures (see page 137).*

Treatment for Arthritis

A painful condition characterized by stiffness and inflammation of the joints, arthritis is attributed to aging, or to poor digestion and inefficient elimination of waste products. Applying a poultice of cabbage leaves to swellings and painful joints is a traditional remedy for arthritis still used by some practitioners of herbal medicine today. The leaves of the plant are blanched and softened in hot water, then squeezed out to remove excess liquid, and bandaged onto the affected area with gauze or cotton strips. The poultice is reapplied every 2–4 hours.

The practitioner may also prescribe an internal remedy, such as an infusion or tincture. Useful detoxifying herbs include those with a diuretic action, such as celery seeds, and bitter herbs, such as devil's claw, which stimulate the digestion.

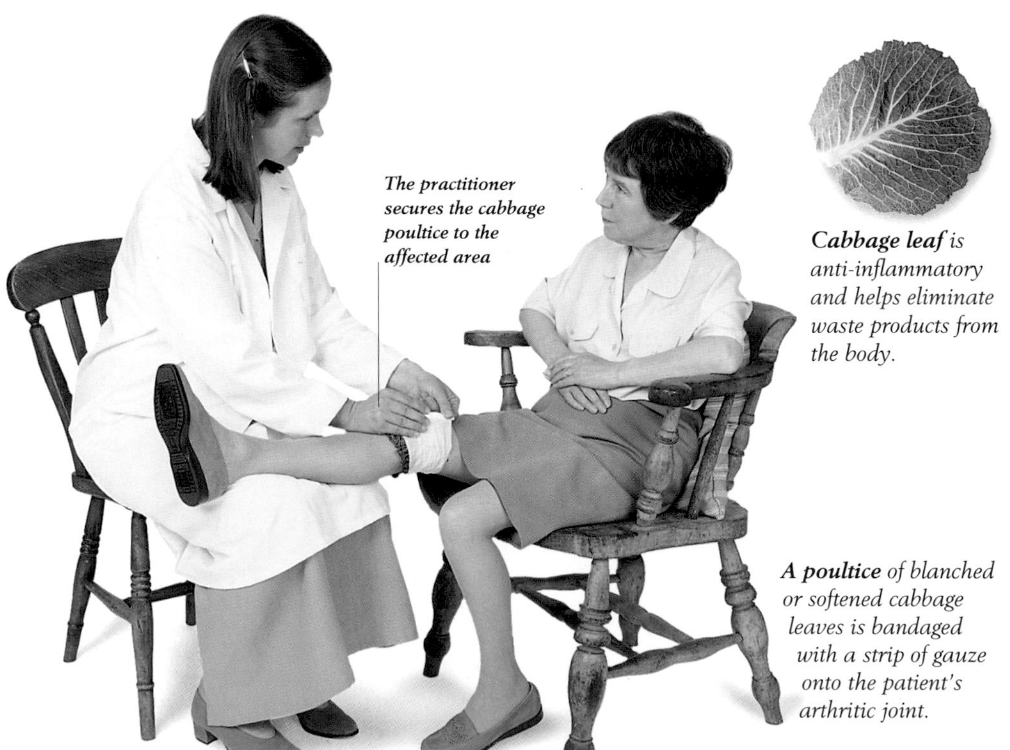

The practitioner secures the cabbage poultice to the affected area

***Cabbage leaf** is anti-inflammatory and helps eliminate waste products from the body.*

***A poultice** of blanched or softened cabbage leaves is bandaged with a strip of gauze onto the patient's arthritic joint.*

A Patient's Experience

Marilyn, 48, first saw a practitioner of herbal medicine when her periods became erratic: "She helped me out then, so when I started having hot flashes and palpitations four years later, I went back. I'd feel myself burning and perspiring at work and was waking up several times a night in a panic. I was also generally tired and depressed. The herbalist gave me a remedy which I took for three weeks, but I was still getting flashes, so she adjusted it and since then the flashes have improved. It contains sage, motherwort, licorice, and St. John's wort, and tastes revolting, but I'm glad not to be pumping synthetic hormones into my body."

SELF-HELP

Complex or potent herbal prescriptions should only be prepared by professional herbalists, but there are many over-the-counter herbal products, such as tinctures, oils, ointments, creams, tablets, capsules, and teas, that are useful for the self-treatment of common ailments. Modern mass-production methods and standardization techniques ensure that these preparations have consistent levels of active ingredients. They are available from health food stores, pharmacies, and mail-order companies. Choose products from reputable suppliers and always follow the instructions on the label.

For self-treatment to work effectively, a holistic approach to health is important, and diet, lifestyle, and exercise are all important considerations.

ARTHRITIS REMEDIES

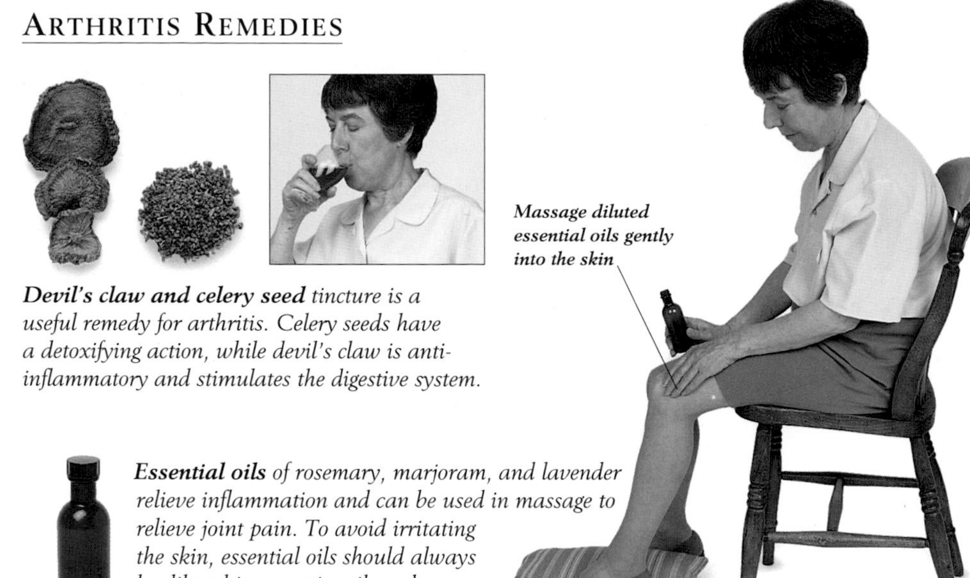

Devil's claw and celery seed *tincture is a useful remedy for arthritis. Celery seeds have a detoxifying action, while devil's claw is anti-inflammatory and stimulates the digestive system.*

Essential oils *of rosemary, marjoram, and lavender relieve inflammation and can be used in massage to relieve joint pain. To avoid irritating the skin, essential oils should always be diluted in a carrier oil, such as sunflower or almond oil, before use.*

HERBAL FIRST AID

Herbal remedies are claimed to be as effective as their pharmaceutical counterparts for minor injuries and illnesses. The following herbs and remedies are particularly valuable in a first-aid kit, and can be found in some pharmacies, health food stores, and herbal shops. Check the recommended dosage and any cautions on the label before you use an herbal remedy. Other useful herbal preparations include feverfew capsules to prevent migraines, slippery elm tablets for stomach upsets, myrrh tincture for sore throats, and tea tree essential oil for cuts, boils, pimples, and insect bites.

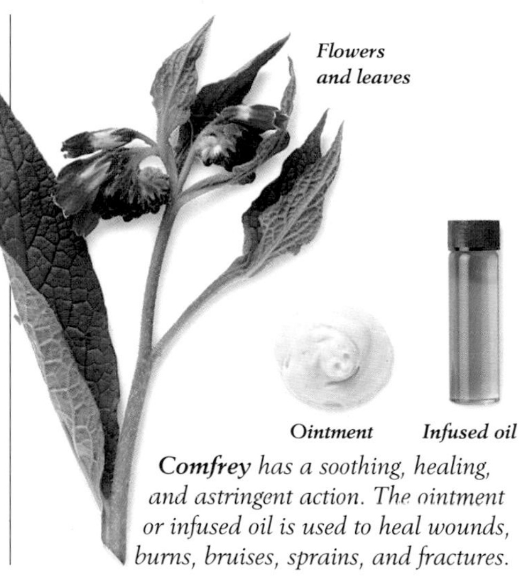

Comfrey *has a soothing, healing, and astringent action. The ointment or infused oil is used to heal wounds, burns, bruises, sprains, and fractures.*

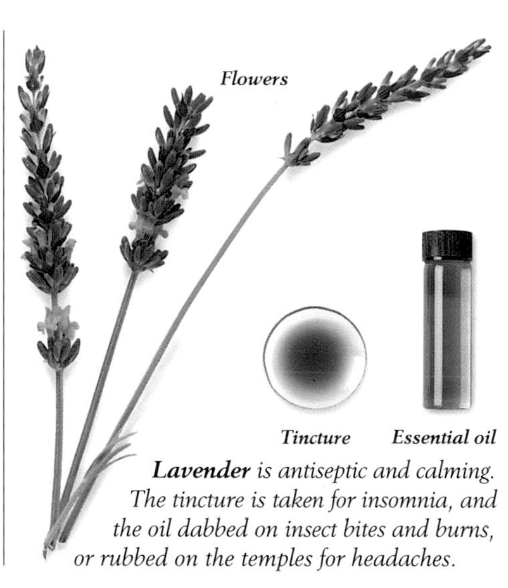

Lavender *is antiseptic and calming. The tincture is taken for insomnia, and the oil dabbed on insect bites and burns, or rubbed on the temples for headaches.*

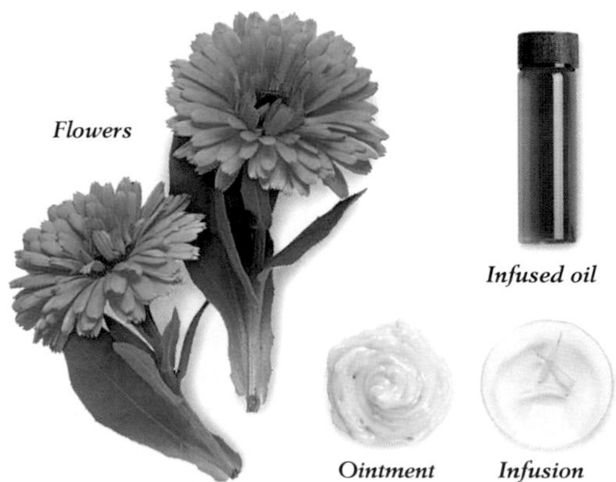

Calendula *is antiseptic and healing. The infused oil and ointment soothe inflamed skin conditions, bruises, scalds, cuts, and grazes, while the infusion can be used for digestive disorders and infections.*

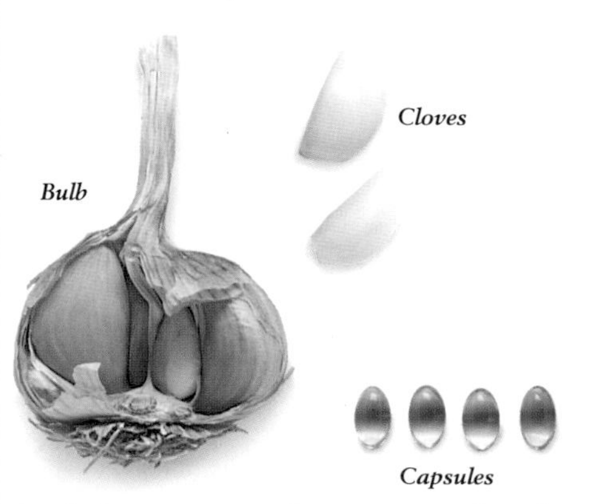

Garlic *has a strong antibiotic action and is taken, often as capsules, for colds, coughs, sinusitis, and digestive disorders. Garlic cloves can be rubbed on acne, or used infused in olive oil to relieve earache.*

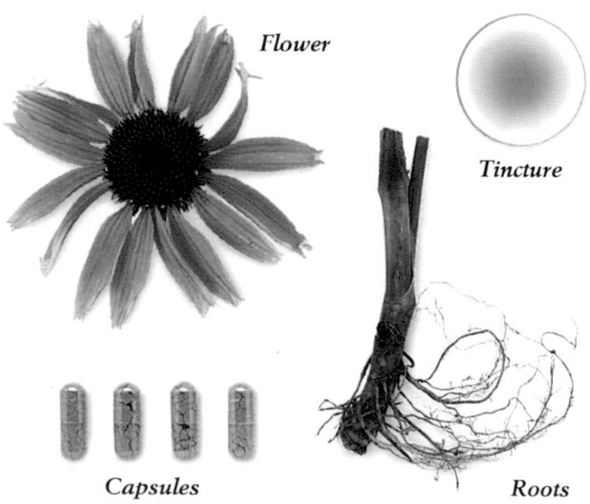

Echinacea *is antibiotic and stimulates the immune system. Preparations made from the root are used to treat infections of all kinds, and are excellent for colds, flu, and sore throats.*

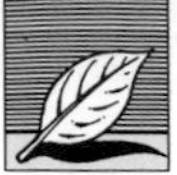

CHINESE HERBALISM

RATINGS	
EVIDENCE	
MEDICAL OPINION	
PRACTITIONER	
SELF-HELP	
COMPATIBILITY	

TRADITIONAL CHINESE MEDICINE (TCM) is an ancient system of healing that bases diagnosis on an individual's pattern of symptoms rather than looking for a named disease – an approach very different from that of Western medicine. Chinese herbalism is one element of TCM, the predominant form of Asian medicine worldwide, which covers a vast range of therapies from acupuncture (see page 90) to herbal remedies. Acupuncture is better known in the West, but herbal medicine is much more important in China, and practitioners of Chinese herbalism can now be found all over the world.

MAIN USES

- Eczema, psoriasis & other skin conditions
- Migraines
- Women's health, including PMS
- Vague aches & pains
- Fatigue, CFS
- Digestive disorders, such as irritable bowel syndrome

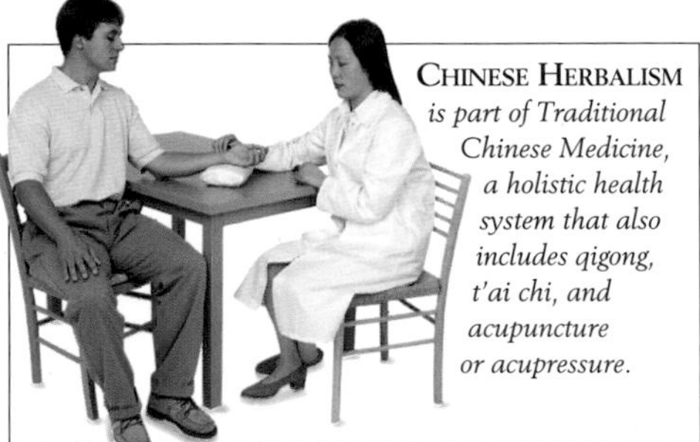

CHINESE HERBALISM *is part of Traditional Chinese Medicine, a holistic health system that also includes qigong, t'ai chi, and acupuncture or acupressure.*

HISTORY

The *Nei Jing* (*The Yellow Emperor's Classic of Internal Medicine*), dating to *c.* 200 B.C.–A.D. 100, is the earliest known document to set out the principles that underlie Traditional Chinese Medicine to this day. This important text takes the form of dialogues between the Yellow Emperor, considered to be the father of Traditional Chinese Medicine, and his follower, Ji Buo. It emphasizes the ideals of moderation, balance, and harmony, which are central to the ancient Chinese philosophy of Taoism.

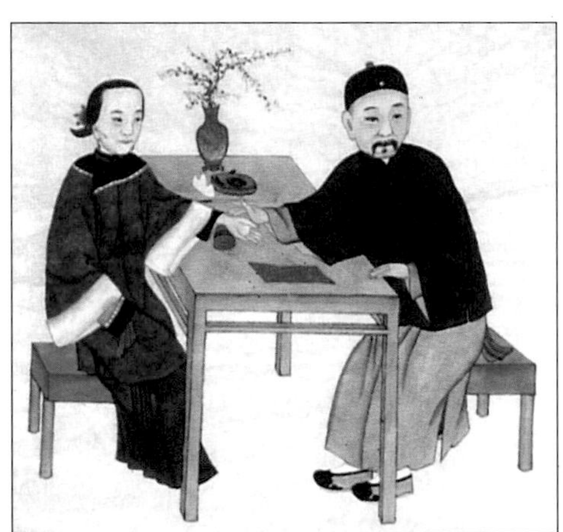

***Pulse-taking** has been vital to TCM diagnosis for centuries, and notions of decency formerly limited doctors' touch to only the wrists of female patients.*

Compendiums such as the 3rd-century *Shen Nong Bencaojing* (*Classic of Roots and Herbs of Shen Nong*) provided some of the earliest written descriptions of herbal remedies. The first comprehensive encyclopedia of Chinese herbs, the *Bencao Gangmu* (*Outlines of Roots and Herbs Studies*), was compiled by Li Shizhen in the 16th century. Around this time, less scholarly reference works for home use also began to be published.

Western medicine, introduced to China by 16th-century missionaries, gradually threatened to overtake traditional healing. However, the establishment of the People's Republic in 1949 led to a revival of herbalism, acupuncture, and other ancient medicinal skills, known collectively as Traditional Chinese Medicine. In China, TCM is now taught at universities and practiced in all hospitals alongside Western methods. Its popularity is growing fast in countries with a large Chinese community, such as the US, the UK, and Australia.

KEY PRINCIPLES

The concepts of holism, of *yin* and *yang*, and of the "five elements" are the three most important principles of TCM.

TCM views the body holistically, as an integrated whole, so problems in one area affect other areas, just as treating specific problems benefits the system as a whole. Running through the body are meridians, a network of channels carrying *qi*, or "life energy" (see page 91). The organs of the body are nourished by the so-called "vital substances": *qi*, blood, body fluids, and "Kidney essence"; all govern growth and sexuality, and determine the general constitution of each individual. *Yin* ("moon" or "overcast") and *yang* ("sun" or "sunshine")

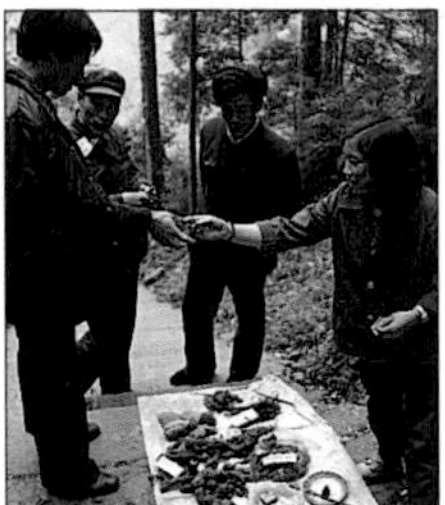

***Herbal remedies** in China are often dispensed in hospitals or street pharmacies. A few animal and mineral substances are included under the general heading of medicinal "herbs."*

symbolize opposing but complementary forces in nature (see opposite and page 91). Each continually changes into its converse, just as day turns into night, and one helps define the other; without day, we would not know what night was. When the dynamic of *yin* and *yang* in the body is disturbed and either one becomes excessive, disease or emotional problems follow. Factors that may provoke a disturbance include infection, accidents, emotional states, poor diet, pollution, even the time of year and weather conditions.

Yin and *yang* can be further divided into interior (*yin*) / exterior (*yang*), deficiency (*yin*) / excess (*yang*), and cold (*yin*) / hot (*yang*). Together, these categories form the eight principle patterns of potential disharmony, a diagnostic framework used to categorize symptoms. For example, a slow pulse is a "cold" symptom. The treatment principle is to "scatter the cold," bringing *yin* and *yang* into balance.

Another key concept in TCM is that of the five elements or five phases – fire, earth, metal, water, and wood (see opposite). The qualities represented by the five elements can be ascribed to all things in the universe, including the body's internal organs. The Chinese concept of an organ is broader and less literal than its Western equivalent. Just as one element will support or inhibit the

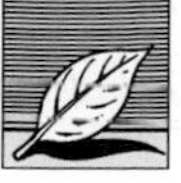

THE THEORY OF CHINESE MEDICINE

While Western doctors start with a symptom, then look for a specific cause, Traditional Chinese Medicine regards the symptom as part of a "pattern of disharmony." *Yin/yang* and the five elements theory are used both to classify the pattern and to determine an effective herbal cure.

YIN & YANG

Yang organs (below left) are thought to "channel" energy – acute pain, spasms, and headaches indicate excess *yang*. *Yin* organs (below right) "hold" energy – dull aches and pains, chilliness, and fatigue are signs of excess *yin*. Most people show a mixture of *yin/yang* symptoms; the skill of the practitioner lies in discerning the pattern and prescribing the correct remedy. *Yin* and *yang* are traditionally represented as broken and solid lines in symbols known as trigrams (see below).

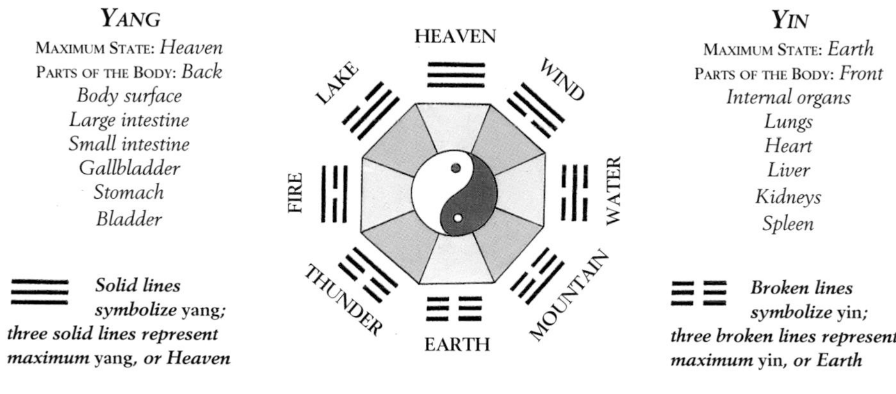

THE FIVE ELEMENTS

Each element has a *yin* organ and a *yang* organ, plus specific tastes, emotions, and seasons of the year. Qualities belonging to the same element are said to support one another. So, to treat a liver disorder, a *yin* organ with the element wood, a Chinese doctor might use sour-tasting herbs, since sour is associated with wood.

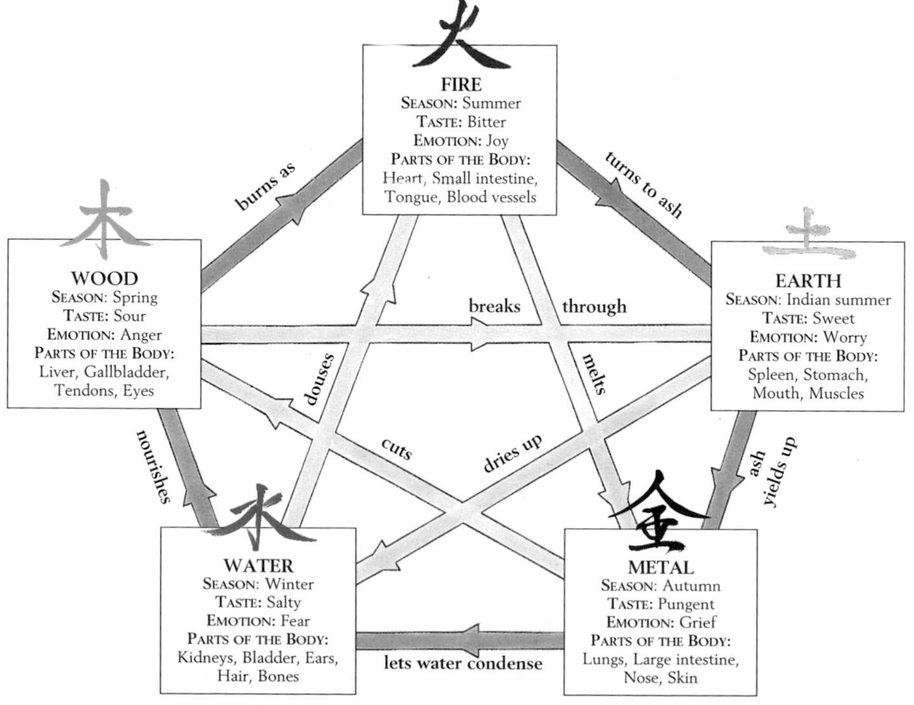

function of another (water dowses fire; fire melts metal), so one organ affects another. The kidneys (water) control the heart (fire); the heart controls the lungs (metal).

Herbal remedies are used to rebalance these forces within the body. Herbs are classified under the five elements according to taste, each of which denotes a medicinal action: sweet, sour, bitter, pungent, and salty. The opposing *yin/yang* qualities of hot and cold are also linked with the action of specific herbs. Baical skullcap (*huang quin*), for example, is a bitter, "cold" herb, used to lower fever. Each herb is said to work in specific organs and related meridians, and with "tendencies of action": floating and sinking, ascending and descending. An herb with an "upward" action would be used to treat a "sinking" disorder, such as diarrhea.

EVIDENCE & RESEARCH

Extensive clinical trials of various herbs and formulas have been carried out in China. Most persuasive for Westerners, however, has been the recent success of Chinese herbs in treating eczema, described in the *British Journal of Dermatology* in 1992. Dr. David Atherton and Dr. Mary Sheehan, consultants in dermatology at the Hospital for Sick Children, London, undertook a study of 47 children with severe atopic eczema (see glossary). Dr. Ding Ho and another Chinese herbalist, Dr. Guang Xu, devised the standardized herbal formulas prescribed. Most children's eczema showed a 60% improvement within four weeks, with no side effects (despite concern that certain herbs could cause liver damage). Interestingly, some children who did not respond to the standardized remedy proved to be responsive when their formulas were individually adjusted.

A further trial with adult atopic dermatitis at the Royal Free Hospital, London, published in *The Lancet* in 1992, supports these findings.

MEDICAL OPINION

While interest has been sparked by studies such as those described above, the focus of conventional medicine on the physiological causes and symptoms of illness makes it difficult for doctors to understand concepts such as *yin*, *yang*, and *qi*. Drug companies are seeking to exploit some Chinese herbs, but many doctors are concerned about the possible side effects of certain remedies (see page 142).

CONSULTING A PRACTITIONER

The initial consultation may take as long as an hour. Your health is assessed by means of the "Four Examinations" of TCM:
Looking: The practitioner observes all the visible evidence of your state of health, particularly your tongue (see right and page 193), the tone of your skin and hair, and the way you move.
Listening and smelling: The sound of your voice and breathing is noted, as is any distinctive body odor.
Asking: The practitioner asks about your family history, habits, body functions, and any symptoms of poor health.
Pulse-taking and touching: The pulse is checked for quality, rhythm, and strength (see also page 192). Areas of discomfort or pain are examined by touch (see right).

The diagnosis hinges on your unique pattern of disharmony. While a Western doctor might diagnose many people as suffering from high blood pressure, the TCM practitioner would take into account particular factors such your pulse rate, the condition of your tongue, teeth, and urine, and how well you eat and sleep. On the basis of the diagnosis, she will prescribe an herbal remedy tailored to your individual pattern of disharmony, possibly supplemented with acupuncture.

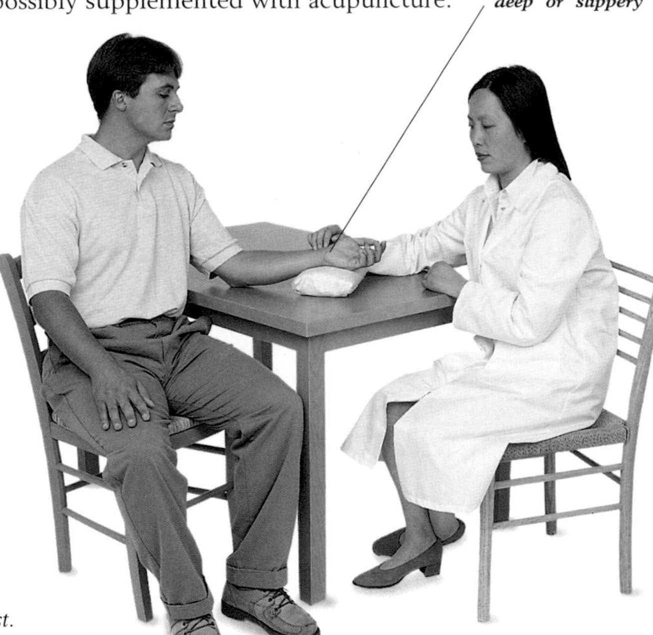

***Touch alone** determines up to 28 pulse types, such as "deep" or "slippery"*

TAKING THE PULSE
TCM identifies three different pulse points on each wrist. The locations are related to meridian pathways, said to channel the life energy known as qi *through the body (see page 91).*

STANDARD TESTS

When you first consult a TCM practitioner, you are assessed according to four diagnostic methods, two of which are illustrated below.

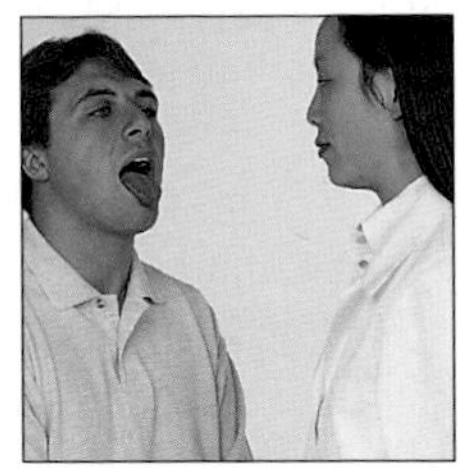

***The tongue** reveals vital clues about your pattern of symptoms.*

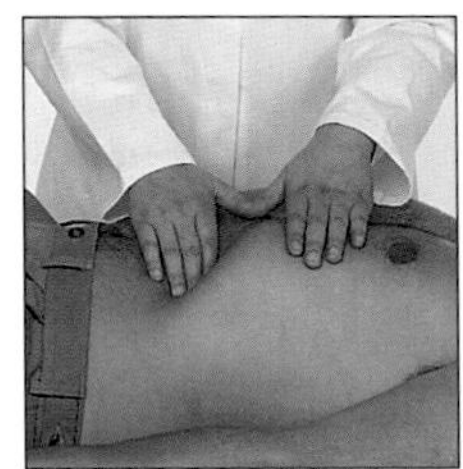

***Touch** detects hard and tender areas, keys to yin/yang balance.*

USING CHINESE HERBS

In TCM, herbs are rarely prescribed singly, but are generally taken as a formula – a standard prescription may have 10–15 herbs with a history of treating a particular pattern of disharmony. Each herb in the formula has a different role, and each is classified according to its taste and temperature (see page 141). Practitioners often adapt a basic formula, adding other herbs to suit the patient's age, constitution, and pattern of disharmony (see above).

Remedies are usually taken as herbal teas, prepared in daily doses, but herbs may also be prescribed as pills, powders, pastes, ointments, creams, and lotions.

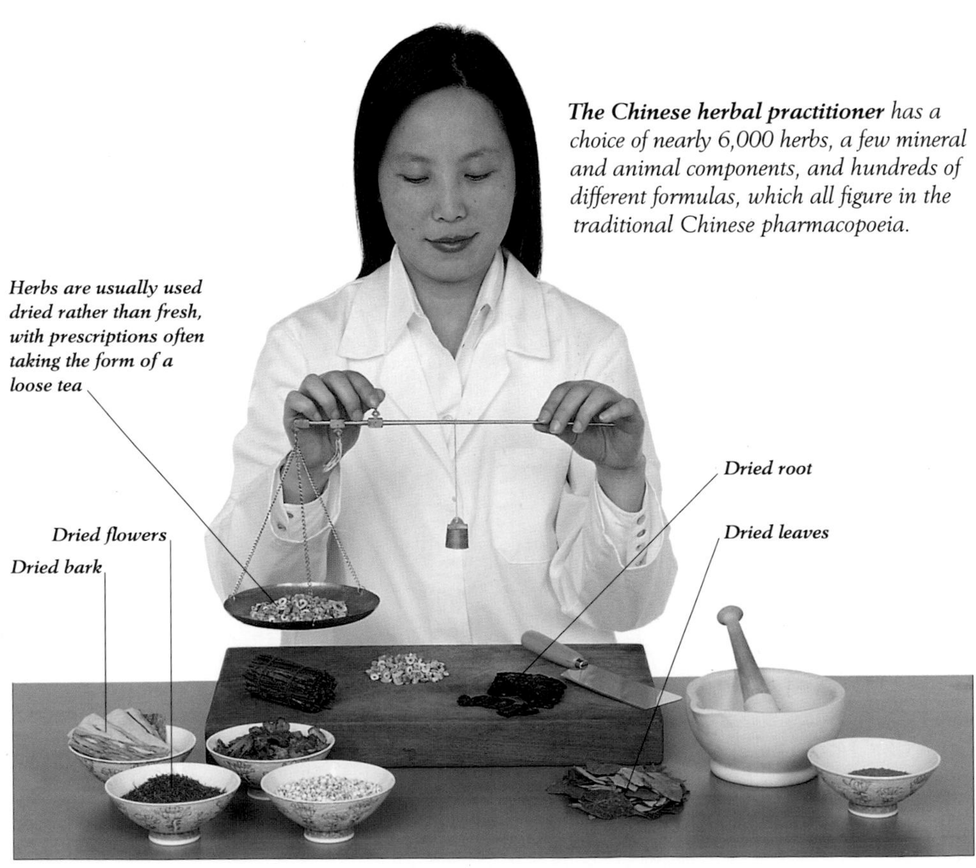

***The Chinese herbal practitioner** has a choice of nearly 6,000 herbs, a few mineral and animal components, and hundreds of different formulas, which all figure in the traditional Chinese pharmacopoeia.*

Herbs are usually used dried rather than fresh, with prescriptions often taking the form of a loose tea

PRECAUTIONS

- Always consult a licensed practitioner who is fully qualified to prescribe herbal remedies.
- Seek medical advice before taking herbs if you are pregnant, or if you have ever had hepatitis or other liver diseases.
- See also Western herbalism (page 136) and page 52.

TREATING ECZEMA

In TCM, eczema is believed to indicate an imbalance resulting from excess "heat" (*yang*). In order to restore harmony, the practitioner would prescribe treatment with "cooling" (*yin*) herbs – such as dittany (*bai xian pi*), bamboo leaf, and white barley – in the form of pills, powders, and a decoction of dried plants. Dry, flaky eczema is specifically categorized as an excess of "wind heat" (wind, cold, fire, dampness, dryness, and summer heat being the "six pernicious influences" – environmental factors that play upon disease). Ointment for home treatment would also be prescribed. For weeping eczema (indicating "damp heat"), an herbal compress would be applied.

With both manifestations of the condition, the practitioner would advise against spicy foods, alcohol, and "heating" foods, such as beef and lamb, and recommend "cooling" foods, such as melon, cucumber, and freshwater fish.

Eczema treatments *are formulated as pills, powders, decoctions, ointments, and washes.*

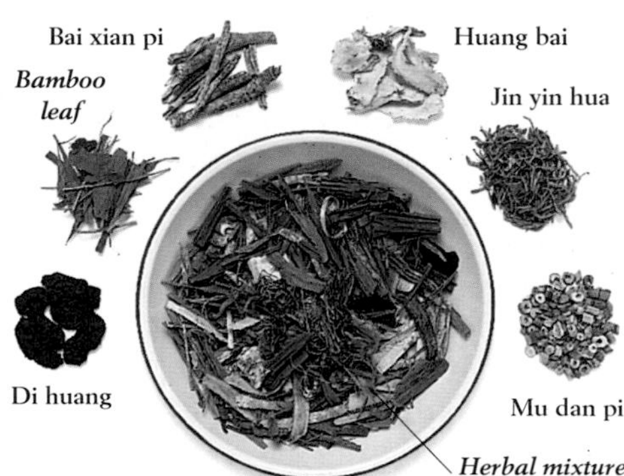

An herbal remedy *to treat eczema might include the ingredients above. Practitioners of TCM often start with a fixed formula, adding or deleting herbs according to the symptoms and the individual.*

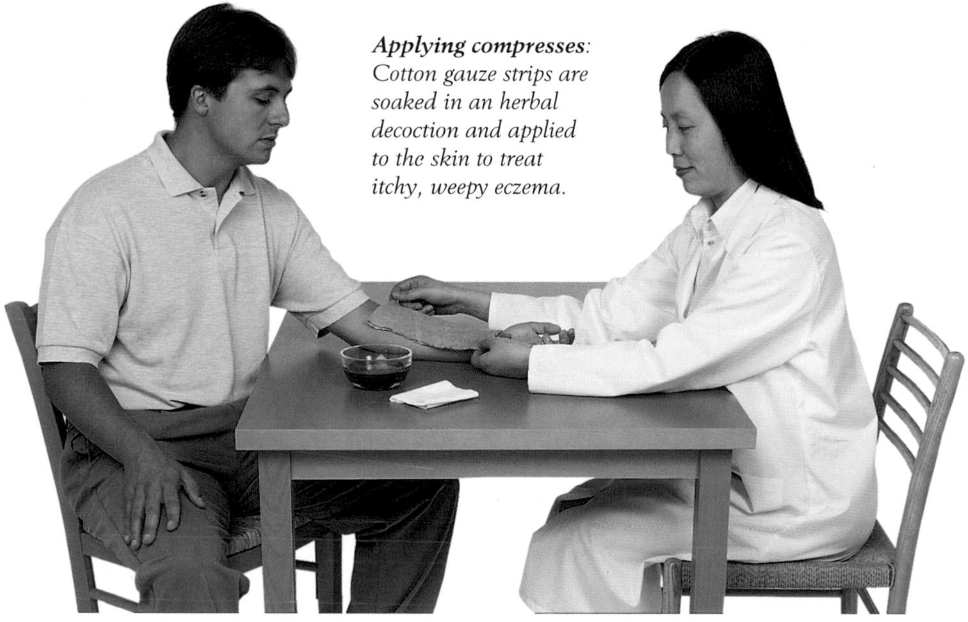

Applying compresses: *Cotton gauze strips are soaked in an herbal decoction and applied to the skin to treat itchy, weepy eczema.*

YOUR QUESTIONS

How long does a treatment session last?
The initial consultation lasts about an hour and subsequent sessions 30 minutes.

How many sessions will I need?
Some conditions, especially chronic (long-standing) complaints, may require several months of treatment, with consultations every 4–6 weeks. Others may respond favorably after one session. Practitioners also recommend regular checkups.

Will remedies taste unpleasant?
Chinese herbal teas can be notoriously unpalatable to Western tastes.

Will there be any aftereffects?
Allergic reactions may occur in rare cases. If you have nausea, diarrhea, or flulike symptoms after taking an herbal remedy, call your practitioner immediately.

A Patient's Experience

Anya, 48, suffered from migraines and had recently had surgery, chemotherapy, and radiation therapy for breast cancer: "The cancer had gone, and I wanted to clear my system of chemicals. Arthritis was a side effect of treatment that even physiotherapy didn't help. The Chinese doctor worked bit by bit, adjusting the herbs each week. It's not instant relief – the first thing I noticed was that headaches were less frequent. Three months ago I felt 80% better. Now, a year later, it's 99.9%. She gives me a week's supply of herbs – 20 or 30 ingredients – and she's very strict about how I take them. The taste isn't too bad, a bit bitter or sour but no worse than some cough medicine. When I drink it I really feel something is happening. Now that the arthritis is relieved, she's working on my immune system so I can fight infection better."

SELF-HELP

Herbal teas, pills, ointments, and tinctures that use Chinese "tonic" herbs, such as ginseng, for minor conditions like fatigue, can be purchased over the counter from reputable herbal suppliers, pharmacies, and health food stores. They may be less effective than those prescribed by a practitioner who will make an individualized diagnosis.

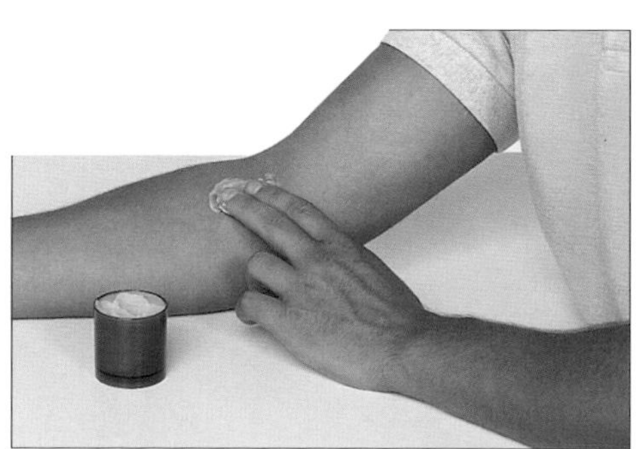

Creams and ointments *that contain a ready-made blend of herbs may be effective for minor skin problems. For persistent conditions, however, always consult a doctor.*

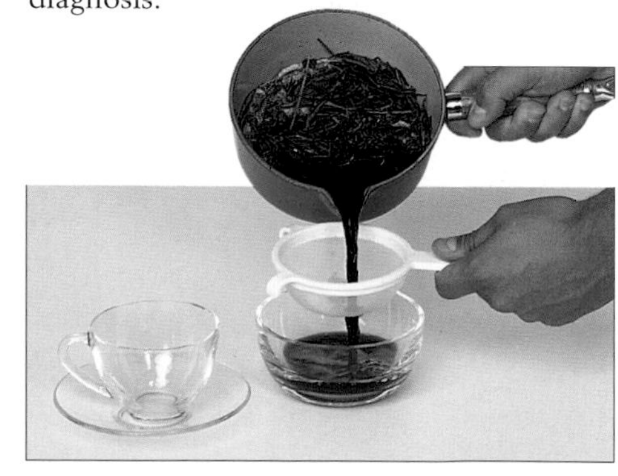

Herbal teas *containing standard formulas of herbs are available for a wide range of conditions. Adjusting the amounts of heating and cooling foods in your diet may also help.*

AYURVEDA

RATINGS	
EVIDENCE	
MEDICAL OPINION	
PRACTITIONER	
SELF-HELP	
COMPATIBILITY	

THE MAJOR TRADITIONAL holistic healing system of the Indian subcontinent, Ayurveda covers all aspects of health, encouraging physical, mental, emotional, and spiritual well-being. Practitioners believe well-being is affected by three doshas, *or "vital energies," which constantly fluctuate. Treatment aims to restore health, or* doshic *balance, through purifying techniques, diet, yoga postures and breathing exercises (see page 108), massage, and herbal remedies. Ayurveda is currently undergoing a government-sponsored revival in India, and is attracting much interest in the West, particularly in the United States.*

MAIN USES

- Digestive problems, such as stomach ulcers
- Heart disease
- Rheumatoid arthritis
- Allergies, asthma
- Eczema, psoriasis & other skin conditions
- Anxiety, insomnia
- Wound healing
- Viral infections, especially hepatitis

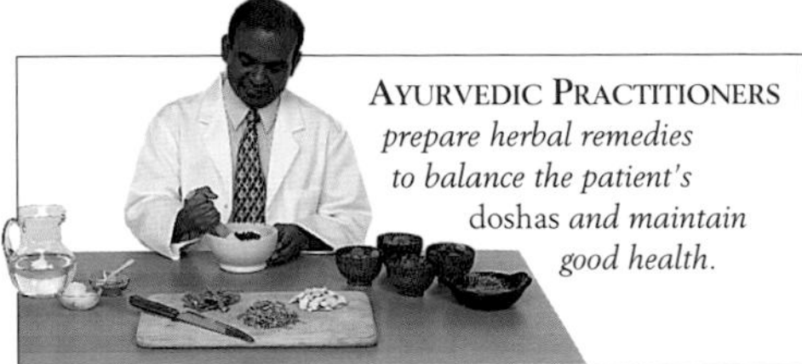

AYURVEDIC PRACTITIONERS *prepare herbal remedies to balance the patient's* doshas *and maintain good health.*

HISTORY

Ayurveda (Sanskrit for "science of life") has been used on the Indian subcontinent since about 2500 B.C. Derived from the *Vedas*, ancient Hindu texts by *rishis*, or holy men, it is a sophisticated, comprehensive health system, and has similarities with Traditional Chinese Medicine (see page 140).

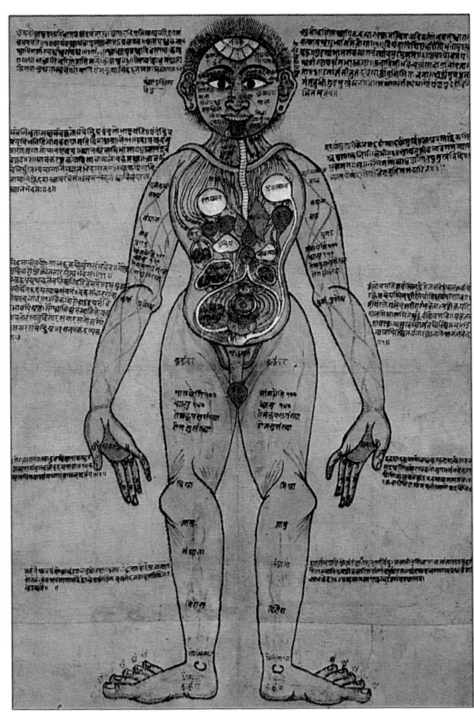

***This anatomical guide**, annotated in Sanskrit, was used by doctors in Nepal, where Ayurveda has been practiced for thousands of years.*

For thousands of years Ayurveda was a well-regulated oral tradition. It remained the most accessible form of health care for Indians until the 19th century, when the British Raj attempted to stamp it out, resulting in a proliferation of poorly trained practitioners. Following Indian independence in 1947, Ayurveda underwent a revival. A Central Council now monitors training and practice, with colleges offering a degree course that includes a basic study of Western medicine. In the US, Ayurveda is mainly practiced as part of "Maharishi Ayur-Ved," a system set up by followers of the yogi Maharishi Mahesh (see page 174), and the health guru and writer Dr. Deepak Chopra has also focused attention on Ayurveda.

KEY PRINCIPLES

Ayurveda teaches that there are five great elements – ether, air, fire, water, and earth – which underlie all living systems and are constantly changing and interacting. They can be simplified into three *doshas*, or vital energies (see opposite), existing in ever-changing proportions throughout nature.

In the human body, the levels of the *doshas* are believed to rise and fall daily, affected by factors such as different foods, time of day, season, levels of stress, and repressed emotions. Imbalances in the *doshas* are thought to disrupt the flow of *prana*, the "life energy" that enters the body through food and breath (see page 109), and to impede *agni*, the body's "digestive fire," which processes food and experiences. If *agni* is low, toxic substances called *ama*, said to be a major source of illness, are produced. Ayurveda therefore places great importance on diet and detoxification techniques designed to purge *ama* by means of sweat, urine, and feces – known as the three *malas*. Herbal remedies, yoga, massage, and meditation are also believed to balance the *doshas* and increase *prana*, and are all practiced as part of Ayurveda.

EVIDENCE & RESEARCH

Much research into Ayurvedic medicine has been carried out in India. In clinical trials at the Government Medical College, Jammu, in the 1980s, 122 out of 175 rheumatoid arthritis patients improved after treatment with *Boswellia serrata*, an herb commonly used in Ayurveda. In a 1990 study at Ohio State University, a Maharishi Ayur-Ved herbal remedy (see left) that appeared to contain antioxidants was shown to reduce tumors in rats. A study by the Federation of American Societies of Experimental Biology indicated in 1993 that *panchakarma* (see page 147) reduced cholesterol and anxiety levels in patients with heart disease. In the US, the National Institutes of Health has funded some research on Ayurveda and its compatibility with other therapies.

MEDICAL OPINION

Many Western doctors accept that they cannot discount the medical systems of other cultures. Ayurvedic herbal remedies have been tried and tested by centuries of use, but their quality and efficacy cannot be guaranteed, since very few scientific tests have been carried out. Doctors find Ayurveda's emphasis on health promotion, and its belief that illness is caused by factors such as diet and lifestyle, easier to accept than some of its treatments. Most would consider that anyone with a critical illness is better off with conventional medicine.

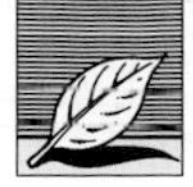

THE THEORY OF THE *DOSHAS*

The *doshas* are three constantly fluctuating energy qualities that define all things on Earth. Each is made up of a combination of two of the five great elements of Ayurveda: *vata* is formed from air and ether, *pitta* from fire and water, and *kapha* from water and earth. Although the *doshas* cannot physically be measured or experienced, each has distinctive attributes that can be recognized in human beings and in the environment.

CONSTITUTIONAL TYPES

Every individual has a unique combination of *doshas*, known as *prakriti*, determined by the *doshas* of his or her parents at the time of conception. Physiological strengths and weaknesses, intellectual capacity, and personality are governed by one or, in some people, two dominant *doshas*.

BALANCING THE *DOSHAS*

Ayurvedic practitioners believe that good health depends on "pacifying" excesses in the *doshas* and keeping fluctuations to a minimum. Each *dosha* has a "seat" in the body that is able to absorb and eliminate small excesses, but disease can result if the seat cannot cope with larger imbalances.

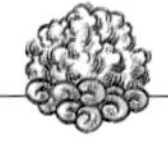

VATA

- Vata ***types*** *are either tall or short and of slight build; they are creative, with quick, nervous movements, but tend to waste energy*
- ***Dominant element****: air, then ether*
- ***Seat of*** vata*: colon*
- ***Shared quality*** *with* kapha*: coldness*
- ***Tastes that increase*** vata*: pungent, bitter, astringent;* vata *types should avoid raw foods*
- ***Tastes that pacify*** vata*: sweet, sour, salty; moist, warming foods, such as casseroles; cooked root vegetables*

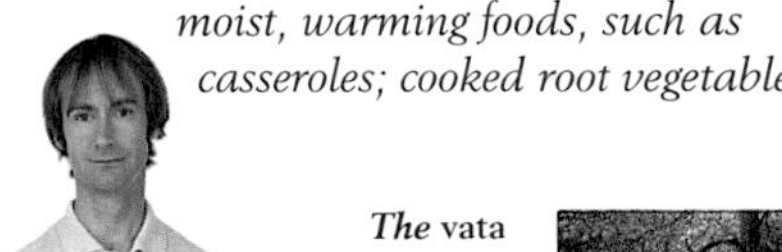

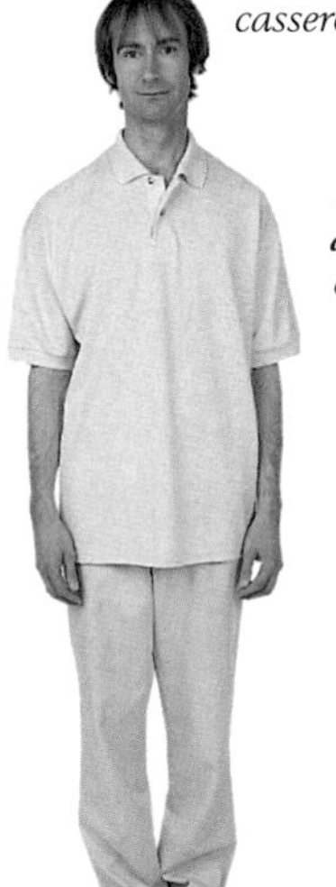

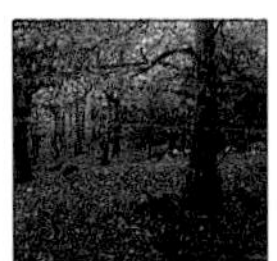

The vata *seasons are autumn and early winter*

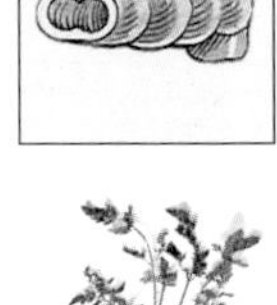

The seat of vata *is the colon*

Carrots pacify excess vata

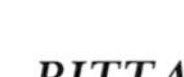

PITTA

- Pitta ***types*** *are evenly proportioned and of average height; confident and ambitious, they can be aggressively competitive*
- ***Dominant element****: fire, then water*
- ***Seat of*** pitta*: stomach and small intestine*
- ***Shared quality*** *with* vata*: lightness*
- ***Tastes that increase*** pitta*: sour, salty, pungent;* pitta *types should avoid red meat*
- ***Tastes that pacify*** pitta*: sweet, astringent, bitter; cooling foods, especially salads; also fish, chicken, tofu, and mushrooms*

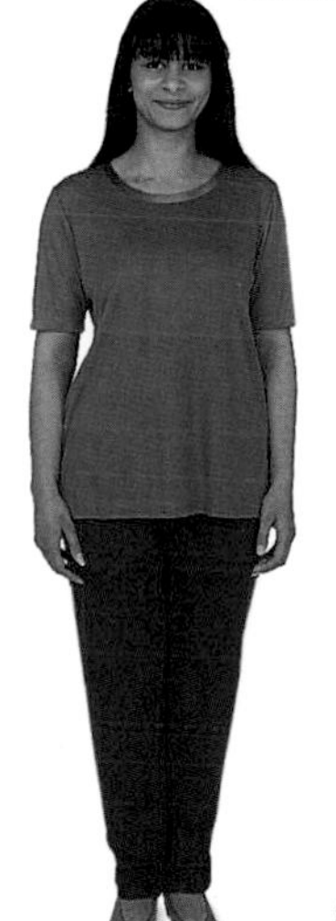

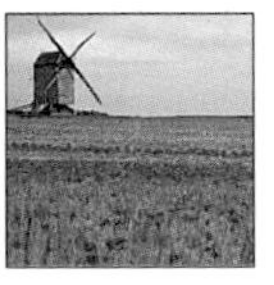

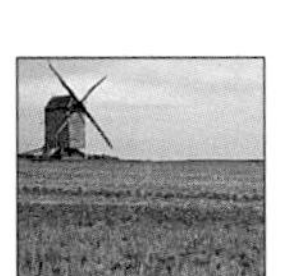

The pitta *season is summer*

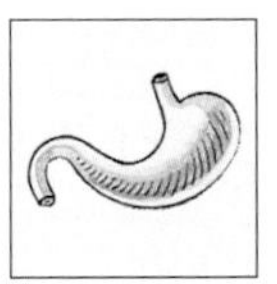

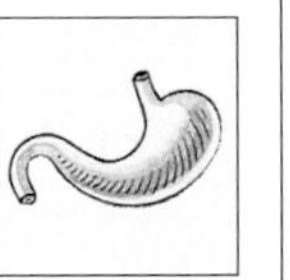

The seat of pitta *is the stomach*

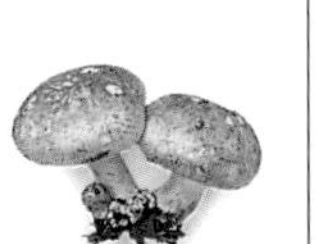

Mushrooms pacify excess pitta

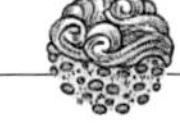

KAPHA

- Kapha ***types*** *are heavily built, slow-moving, and physically strong; they are stable and patient, but inclined to possessiveness*
- ***Dominant element****: water, then earth*
- ***Seat of*** kapha*: stomach and lungs*
- ***Shared quality*** *with* pitta*: oiliness*
- ***Tastes that increase*** kapha*: sweet, sour, salty;* kapha *types should avoid dairy products*
- ***Tastes that pacify*** kapha*: pungent, bitter, astringent; hot and spicy foods; apples and pears; also leafy vegetables, beans, and lentils*

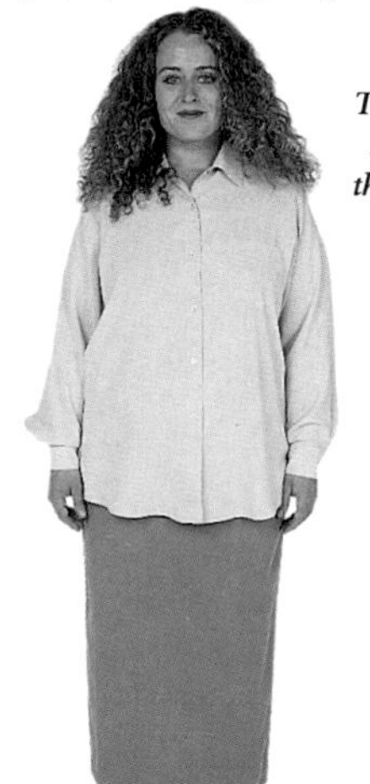

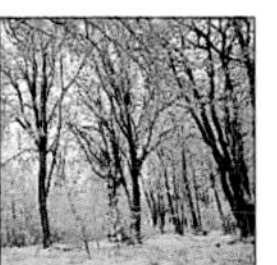

The kapha *season is the middle of winter*

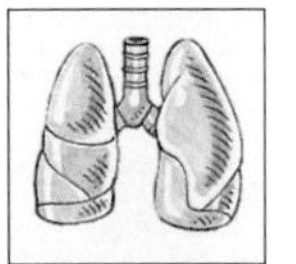

The seat of kapha *is the lungs*

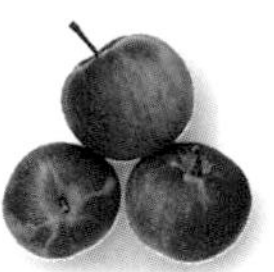

Apples pacify excess kapha

DAILY PATTERN OF THE *DOSHAS*

Vata, pitta, *and* kapha *are said to exert their greatest influence at dawn, at midday, and in the evening respectively; each* dosha *also has a second, weaker period of influence. Healing foods and herbal remedies should be taken at the correct time of day to pacify the* dosha *that is causing the imbalance. For example, a* vata*-related illness may flare up in the early morning and can be alleviated by taking calming remedies at night, when* kapha *– which promotes rest – is in the ascendant.*

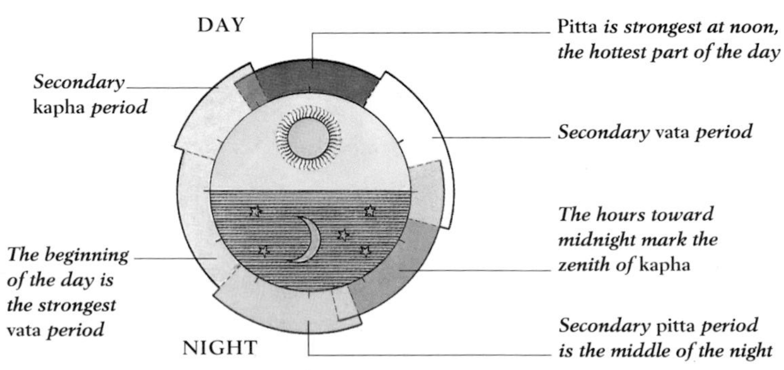

Secondary kapha *period*

Pitta *is strongest at noon, the hottest part of the day*

Secondary vata *period*

The hours toward midnight mark the zenith of kapha

The beginning of the day is the strongest vata *period*

Secondary pitta *period is the middle of the night*

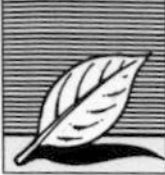

CONSULTING A PRACTITIONER

At the first consultation the practitioner identifies your *doshic* constitution (*tridosha*) and any imbalances in it. He asks detailed questions about your personal and family history and about your lifestyle, from eating and bowel habits to relationships at work. As in Traditional Chinese Medicine, taking the pulse is an important part of diagnosis. The practitioner checks the pulse at three points on both wrists, each thought to correspond to one of the *doshas* and to reflect the condition of specific internal organs (see page 192). You may also be asked for a sample of urine, taken in midstream early in the morning; its color and odor will be noted.

Your practitioner will recommend dietary changes to rebalance your *doshas*. He will advise you to eat at certain times of day, depending on your age and condition, your *doshic* type, and the season of the year.

If your practitioner is qualified to prescribe medicinal remedies, he will also treat you with herbs or minerals according to your constitution and particular *doshic* imbalance (see opposite). This is part of a program known as *shaman*, which aims to pacify and calm the *doshas*.

If the practitioner considers you strong enough, he may begin treatment with a cleansing and detoxifying regime called *shodan*, which takes the form of enemas, laxatives, therapeutic vomiting, and washing out the nasal passages, collectively known as *panchakarma* (see opposite). Saunas may also be used in preparation for detoxification. Some practitioners offer Ayurvedic massage with oils. This lasts about an hour and is carried out by two masseurs, who work together on either side of you, stimulating your body's *marma* points (similar to acupoints; see page 91) to encourage the flow of *prana*. Or you may receive *chavutti thirumal*, a massage given with the feet (see page 115).

Finally, the practitioner may suggest *rasayana*, a rejuvenating regime that may include herbal remedies, yoga, chanting, meditation (*satvajaya*), and sunbathing.

STANDARD TESTS

The practitioner may listen to your internal organs and use other diagnostic techniques shown below.

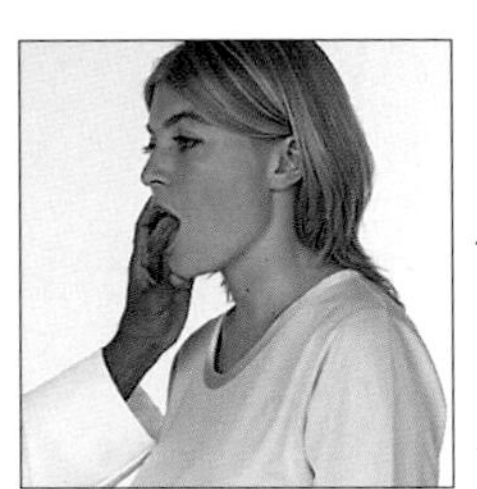

***The tongue** is examined for signs of toxins in the body.*

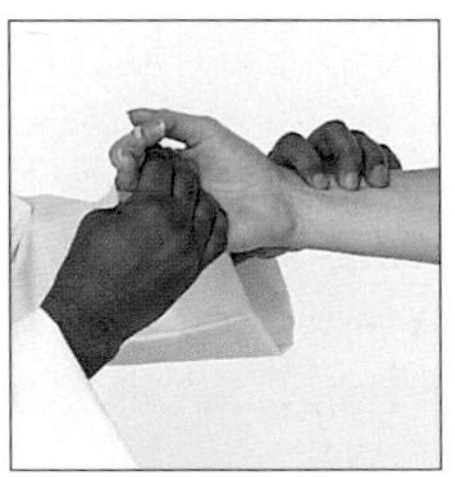

***The pulse** is taken to reveal the* doshic *state of related body organs.*

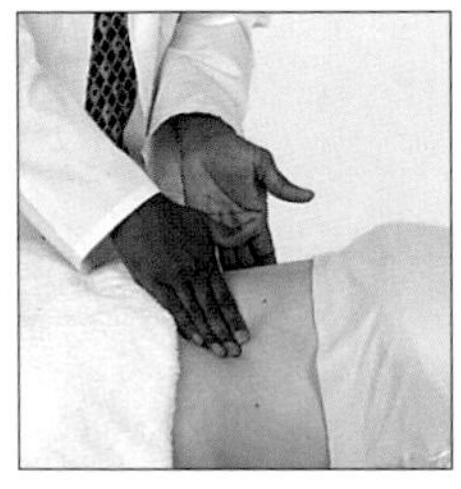

***Palpating** or feeling the abdomen may reveal* doshic *imbalances.*

ASSESSING THE STATE OF THE *DOSHAS*

The patient's physical appearance and the way she moves are closely examined as aids to diagnosis. The eyes and nails can be important indications of doshic *constitution.* Pitta *types, for example, tend to have bright, sparkling eyes.*

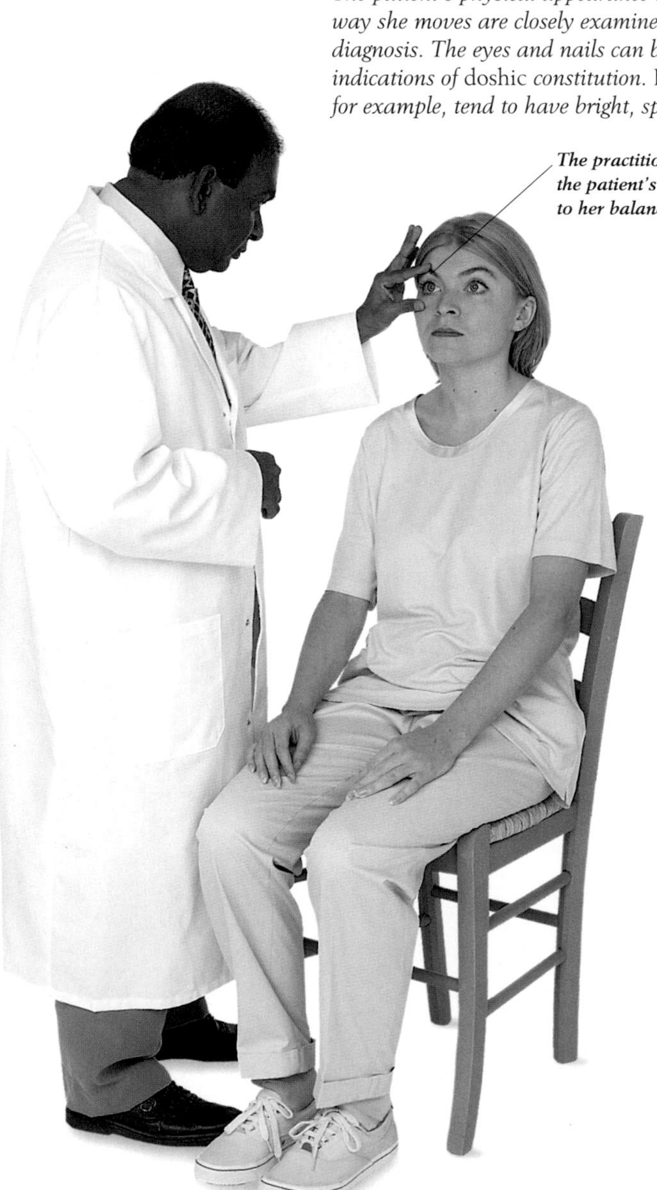

The practitioner examines the patient's eyes for clues to her balance of doshas

YOUR QUESTIONS

How long does a treatment session last?
An initial consultation may take up to an hour; later sessions last 15–30 minutes.

How many sessions will I need?
Minor ailments may require only two or three sessions; long-standing disorders may need weekly appointments over several months.

Will it be unpleasant?
Powerful cleansing treatments, such as enemas or induced vomiting, may cause temporary discomfort.

Will there be any aftereffects?
When used under the supervision of a qualified practitioner, Ayurvedic therapies should not cause aftereffects.

PRECAUTIONS

- Make sure that your practitioner is fully qualified to prescribe herbal remedies, and that long-term treatment with herbs is carefully monitored.
- Avoid enemas and other purgative treatments if you are pregnant or elderly, or if you have heart disease. Enemas are not suitable for the very young.
- See Western herbalism (page 136) and page 52.

MEDICINAL REMEDIES

Ayurvedic remedies are made from up to 20 different herbs, minerals, and vegetables, and should be prescribed by a qualified practitioner. Each prescription will vary according to environment, season, the patient's constitutional type, and his or her current *doshic* imbalance. Remedies may be administered orally, anally, through the nose, or rubbed into the skin as oils to avoid being broken down by enzymes in the digestive tract.

Remedies may be given in powder form, or as dried herbs, pills, or pastes. Medicinal wines and jams are sometimes prescribed. If a powder is to be taken internally, the practitioner may recommend that it is mixed in food with a "carrier," usually water, honey, or ghee (clarified butter). Dried herbs may be boiled in water to make a tea or decoction. Traditionally, practitioners repeat a suitable mantra over the mixture as it is prepared; this is thought to increase its potency.

A Patient's Experience

Karen, a 29-year-old actress, was troubled by insomnia: "I've always been a nervous person and my career has meant that my life has little routine. The practitioner asked lots of questions about my lifestyle and took my pulse. I am a typical vata *type and the insomnia was due to excess* vata *energy, made worse by a run of bad luck in my career. She suggested I eat cooked vegetables, dairy food, and fish, with hot cereal for breakfast. At bedtime, I should give myself an oil massage – preferably with sesame oil, but grapeseed will do – and drink warm milk with ginger, cinnamon, or cardamom. I haven't had a real problem sleeping since."*

Ghee
Licorice
Nutmeg
Long pepper

***The practitioner mixes** a remedy to suit the patient's individual type. An Ayurvedic prescription is likely to include at least ten different herbs.*

PANCHAKARMA

Panchakarma, which means "five actions," is a purification process to remove *ama*, or impurities, in the body, and rebalance the *doshas*. Treatment requires physical strength, and should always be carefully monitored by a trained practitioner. Traditionally, *panchakarma* is performed in three stages after a restricted diet or fast. Massage with medicated oils is followed by induced sweating, said to return the *doshas* to their seats in the body (see page 145). The main purging process is achieved with herbal or oil enemas, herbal laxatives, or induced vomiting. *Panchakarma* aims to restore the mind as well as the body; a treatment called *shirodhara* may be given for this (see below). *Rasayana*, in the form of herbal remedies or lifestyle changes, helps the body to recuperate. In India, *panchakarma* may take a month, but in the West it often lasts only 3–5 days.

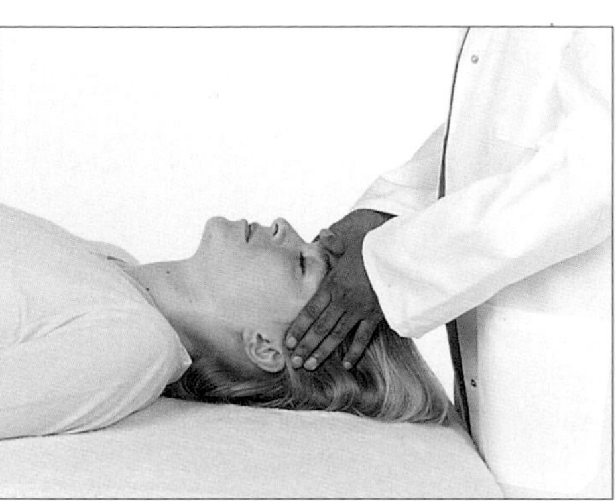

***In a head massage** (see page 115), the* marma *points (similar to acupoints) on the patient's head are stimulated to promote the flow of* prana.

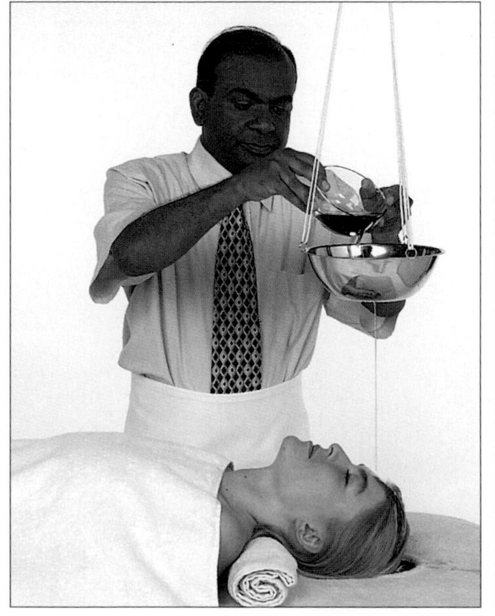

Shirodhara *is a relaxation technique often used as part of* panchakarma. *After a head massage, warm sesame oil is poured over the patient's forehead in a continuous, soothing stream for up to an hour.*

SELF-HELP

Ayurveda is a holistic system of health care and a way of life for millions of people in the Indian subcontinent. Therapeutic practices such as yoga or special diets can easily form part of a daily routine, and some herbal remedies, such as teas, can be made in the home. Replacing one regular cup of tea or coffee with an Ayurvedic tea, such as ginger, will help detoxify the body and support the digestive system.

Minor conditions may be treated in the home using widely available herbs and spices. In India, ripe bananas and fried cumin powder are taken for insomnia, while turmeric in milk is taken to relieve flu symptoms.

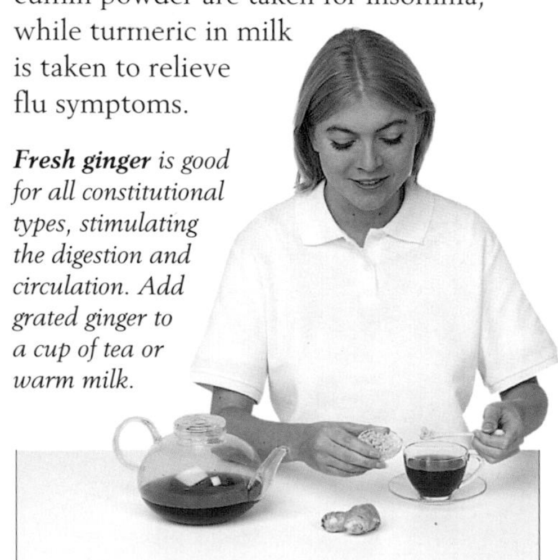

***Fresh ginger** is good for all constitutional types, stimulating the digestion and circulation. Add grated ginger to a cup of tea or warm milk.*

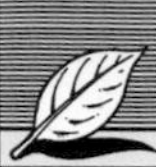

NUTRITIONAL THERAPIES

RATINGS	
EVIDENCE	
MEDICAL OPINION	
PRACTITIONER	
SELF-HELP	
COMPATIBILITY	

ARE WE WHAT WE EAT? All health systems, complementary and conventional, include dietary advice. Research into the effects of diet on the human body began early in the 20th century, and led to the recognition of the importance of vitamins and minerals in maintaining health. Embracing a wide range of approaches, nutrition-based complementary therapies seek to alleviate physical and psychological disorders through special diets and food supplements. Conventional doctors acknowledge the benefits of a balanced diet, but tend to be skeptical about the power of specific dietary regimes to treat disease.

MAIN USES

- Headaches, migraines
- Fatigue, CFS
- Irritable bowel syndrome, bloating
- Digestive disorders
- Arthritis
- High blood pressure
- Circulatory disorders
- Menstrual problems
- Asthma, eczema
- Allergies

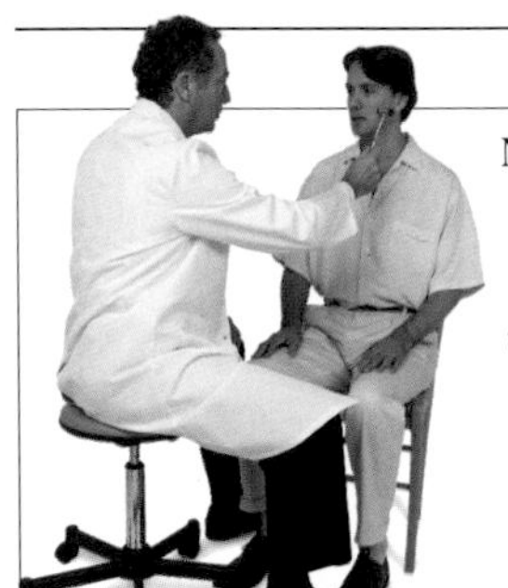

NUTRITIONAL THERAPISTS *use supplements and diets to boost health and maintain well-being.*

HISTORY

Food and diet have had an important role in health care for millennia. Garlic, for example, was used to treat a wide variety of health problems throughout ancient Egypt and Greece. Modern clinical trials have since demonstrated garlic's ability to lower blood pressure and cholesterol levels and confirmed its antibacterial and antiviral properties. In the 18th century, the British navy prevented scurvy in sailors by feeding them limes and lemons, although the preventive agent, vitamin C, was not identified until 1928.

In the 19th century, proponents of the "nature cure" (a practice later known as naturopathy; see page 118) claimed that food could be used as medicine. Advances in biochemistry in the 20th century led to a greater understanding of the need for a balanced diet containing nutrients that included vitamins and minerals. The term "vitamines" or "vital amines" was coined by a Polish biochemist, Casimir Funk, working in London. In 1912 he suggested that minute quantities of substances found in various foods were essential for health. Within a few years, investigators discovered that pellagra, a disease whose psychological symptoms resembled schizophrenia, could be cured with large doses of niacin (vitamin B_3). Further research isolated the fat-soluble vitamins A, D, E, and K, and the water-soluble vitamins C and B complex.

The role of antioxidants (see page 37) in maintaining health, preventing and treating disease, and delaying the aging process has only recently become well understood. Other nutritional topics making headlines in the 1980s and 1990s include the importance of dietary fiber in digestion, the detrimental effects of food additives, cholesterol and other fats, and pesticides on the body (see pages 34–37), and the discovery of natural estrogens, or phytoestrogens, in soy. Public health bodies worldwide now recognize the value of diet in maintaining a healthy population and reducing the burden on health services.

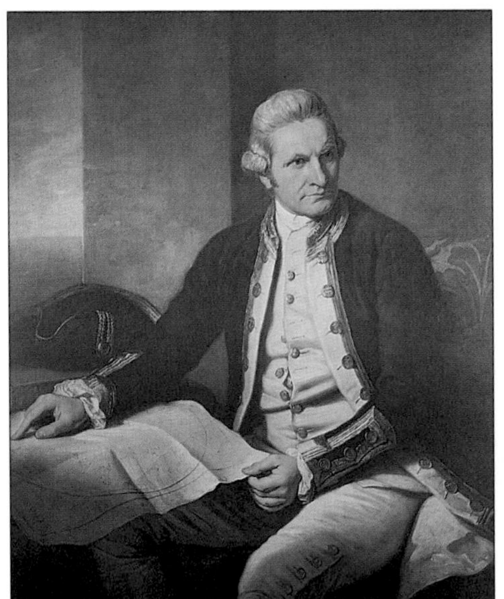

***By issuing citrus fruit** to his crew, the 18th-century British explorer Captain James Cook warded off scurvy, a disease that had always plagued sailors on long sea voyages.*

KEY PRINCIPLES

The links between disease and poor diet have long been recognized, and some medical doctors specialize in nutrition. Together with nutritional therapists, who are not medically qualified, they use diet and nutritional supplements to prevent and treat disease. All practitioners believe that good health is directly related to the quality of the food eaten by the individual. For example, food grown in poor soil will lack nutrients, crops sprayed with pesticides could contain toxic chemicals, and antibiotics given to livestock may find their way into the human bloodstream. Although there is an overabundance of fresh food in the West, many people prefer to eat highly processed "junk" foods, from which nutrients have been stripped, and as a result their diets may become deficient in essential vitamins and minerals.

Both medically qualified nutritionists and practitioners of nutritional therapy seek to explore every avenue by which a patient's nutrition can be improved to promote maximum health. In general, treatment is said to improve the patient's mood, fitness, and well-being, and delay aging. Practitioners look for nutritional deficiencies, for allergies or intolerances to food (see pages 302–303), and for environmental factors, which can cause poor digestion or absorption in the stomach and intestines, preventing nutrients from reaching the bloodstream. Other factors are said to include "toxic overload" from an excess of heavy metals (see glossary) or environmental chemicals (see page 154), and problems with the balance of gut flora (see right), which complementary practitioners often refer to as "dysbiosis."

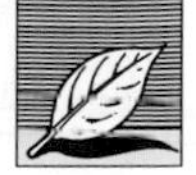

THE THEORY OF HEALTH & DIGESTION

The digestion of food and the elimination of waste products are cornerstones of well-being. If impaired, the body may be deprived of essential nutrients and become overloaded with toxins. A balanced diet and low stress levels are vital to the healthy functioning of the digestive and excretory systems.

THE DIGESTIVE SYSTEM

***Food passes** through the digestive system, where it is broken down by enzymes and acids to be absorbed through the small intestine into the bloodstream. The waste products are processed, and excreted as feces (see page 230) and via the kidneys as urine.*

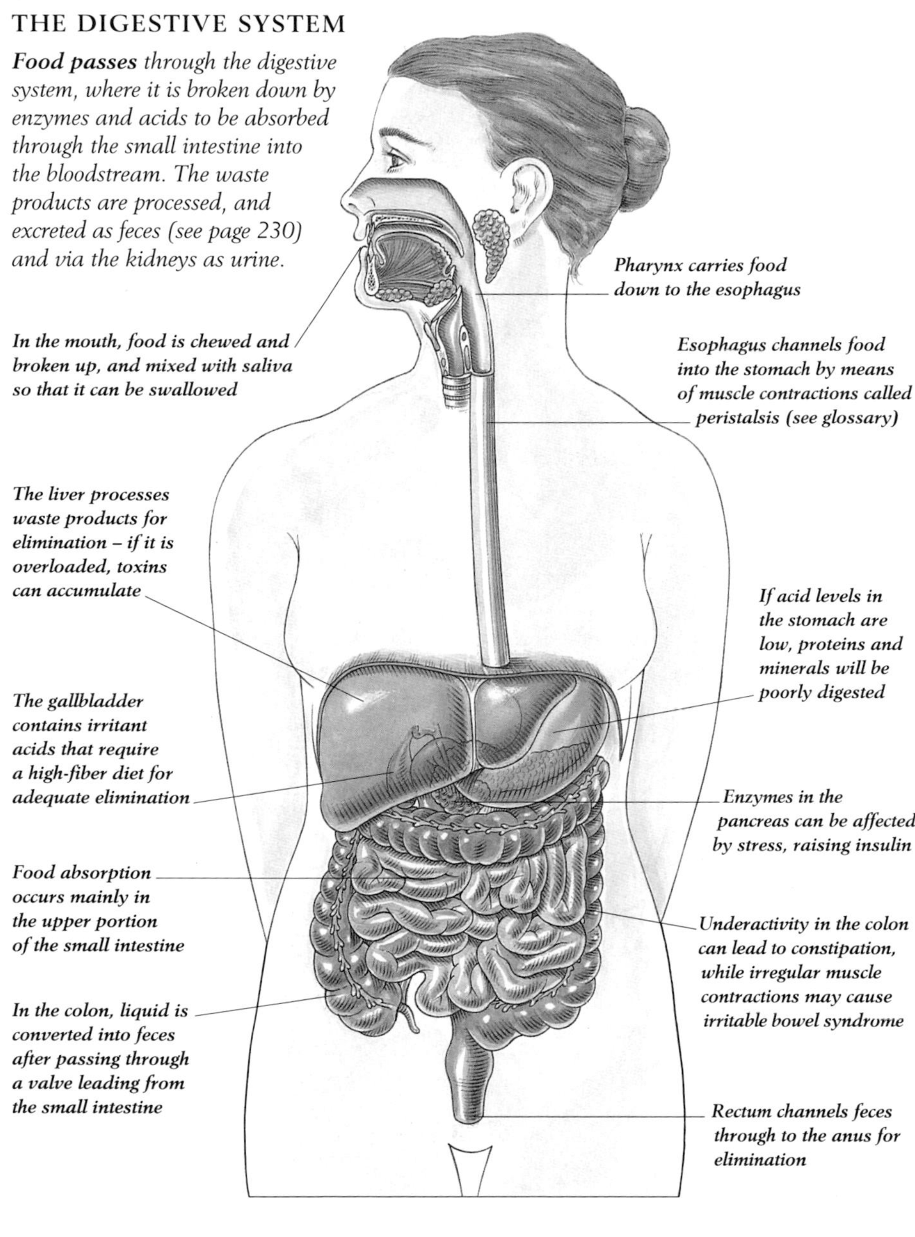

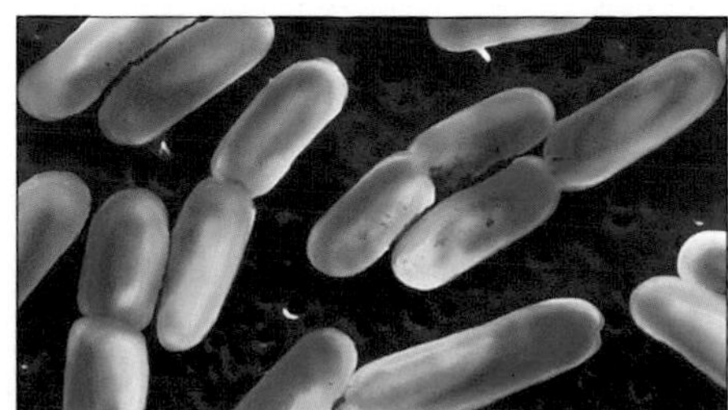

GUT FLORA

***An entire ecosystem** of bacteria, known as the gut flora, inhabits the intestines, protecting the gut lining and maintaining its delicate chemical balance. This balance can be disrupted by illness and medication – particularly antibiotics – leading to a condition that nutritional therapists call dysbiosis (see food intolerances, page 303).*

EVIDENCE & RESEARCH

Research linking nutrition and health is substantial. Many studies associate excessive fat intake with cancers of the breast, prostate, colon, and rectum, and colon cancer in particular is linked with a diet that is too low in fiber.

In a study at the University of Cambridge and Papworth Hospital in the UK, reported in *The Lancet* in 1996, large supplements of vitamin E, an antioxidant, slowed down the process of underlying arterial disease in angina patients.

A study reported in *The Lancet* in 1994 found that the "Cretan Mediterranean diet" reduced the incidence of secondary heart attacks by 70%. This diet is low in saturated fats and red meat, and high in plant foods, olive oil (which lowers harmful cholesterol levels), and oily fish (containing an essential fatty acid).

Antioxidants given to 30,000 people in Linxian province in China over a five-year period resulted in a 20% drop in stomach and esophageal cancer, according to research published in the *Journal of the National Cancer Institute* in 1993.

A study at Epsom District Hospital in Surrey, in the UK, published in 1993 in the *British Journal of Rheumatology*, indicated a possible link between rheumatoid arthritis and food intolerances.

Other dietary supplements with strong clinical support include folic acid (taken by pregnant women to help prevent neural tube defects and reduce the risk of cleft palate in babies), magnesium (shown to alleviate pre-eclampsia in pregnancy, a condition characterized by high blood pressure and fluid retention), and vitamin B_6 (helpful in treating PMS).

MEDICAL OPINION

Most doctors are open-minded about the role of nutrition in preventing illness, although there is much interest in the potential of certain diets to reduce the risk of cancer. Doctors are more skeptical about the effectiveness of nutrition as *treatment* for illness, except in the case of specific conditions, such as gout, diabetes, high blood cholesterol, and to a lesser extent, migraines, irritable bowel syndrome, and eczema. There is widespread acceptance among doctors of the benefits of the Cretan Mediterranean diet, which can help prevent heart disease (see above).

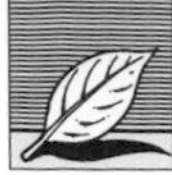

CONSULTING A PRACTITIONER

Some doctors specialize in using nutritional approaches to the treatment of illness, often as one aspect of their interest in clinical ecology (see page 154). Non-medically qualified nutritional therapists will usually be trained in nutrition, physiology, biochemistry, pathology, naturopathic techniques, and the principles of clinical ecology. You may decide to consult a nutritional therapist if you have unexplained, long-term symptoms for which conventional medicine finds no cause – for example, fatigue, headaches, bloating, and skin or digestive problems.

Nutritional therapists believe that you can be lacking in essential nutrients even if your diet is healthy. Before beginning treatment, the practitioner may ask you to complete a questionnaire about your current diet, medical history, and symptoms. You may be asked how much you drink or smoke, and about your exercise habits, your emotional state, and any medication you are currently taking. He may also request that you keep a diary of typical food intake over approximately three days.

The practitioner also examines the condition of your skin, hands, and other features; these can provide important clues about nutritional intake. Nutritional therapists (and some medically qualified nutritionists) often use other diagnostic techniques to determine nutritional deficiencies and food allergies. These may include tests on samples of your hair (see page 194), urine, and sweat, and muscle testing, or applied kinesiology (see page 196). You may be required to follow an exclusion or elimination diet, cutting out suspect foods progressively over a period of several weeks until a food allergy or intolerance is detected (see page 199). Some nutritional therapists use Vega testing, in which you are connected to an electrical device that is designed to indicate the presence of allergens (see page 200).

Using the test results, and taking into account factors such as your age and sex, the practitioner develops a dietary regime tailored to your needs (see opposite).

PRECAUTIONS

- Check with your doctor before beginning a course of nutrient supplements if you are taking medication; they may be incompatible.
- Excessive doses of vitamins A, D, E, and B_6 and zinc may have toxic side effects. Do not take high doses of vitamins or minerals without consulting your doctor or a nutritionist who is also a doctor.
- Do not follow a strict diet for long periods without the supervision of your doctor or a nutritionist who is also a doctor.
- See also page 52.

STANDARD TESTS

Physical symptoms are assessed, and laboratory tests carried out if necessary.

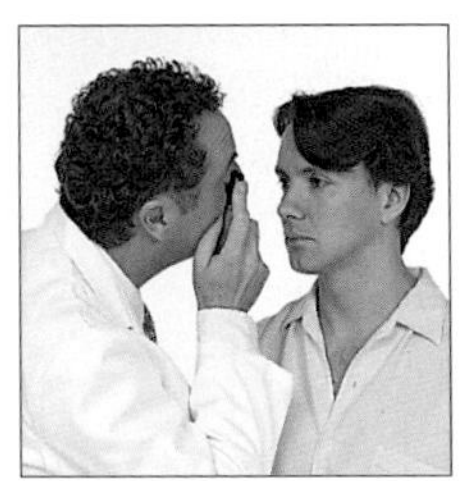

The cornea *is examined for signs of vitamin A deficiency.*

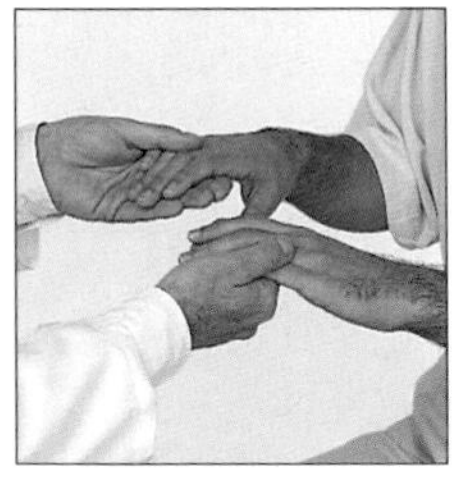

Nails *with white spots may indicate low dietary levels of zinc.*

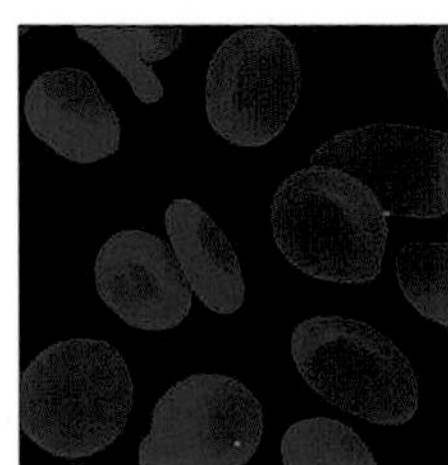

Blood tests *can reveal nutritional deficiencies.*

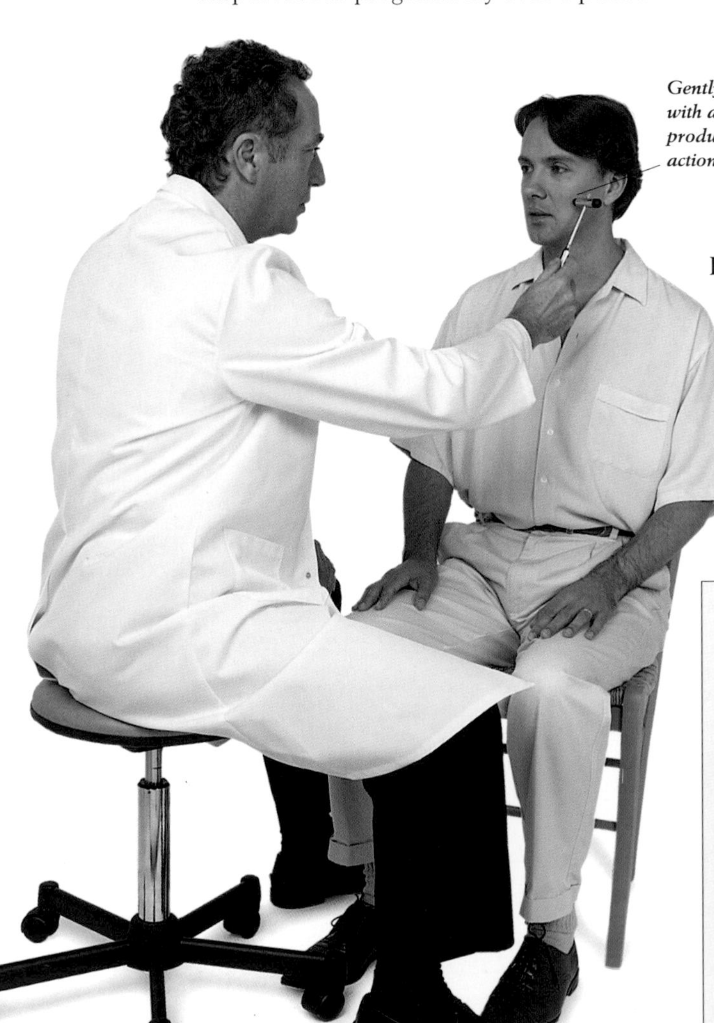

Gently tapping the jaw with a tendon hammer produces a slight reflex action in a healthy person

REFLEX TESTING

The practitioner tests the patient's jaw reflex with a tendon hammer. An increased reflex may indicate a magnesium deficiency, preventing the transmission of nerve impulses.

YOUR QUESTIONS

How long does a treatment session last?
The first consultation lasts about an hour and subsequent sessions 15–20 minutes.

How many sessions will I need?
Several sessions are usually required. The number and timing will depend on the condition and how long you have had it.

Will remedies taste unpleasant?
Most nutritional supplements are in tablet or capsule form and are quite palatable.

Will there be any aftereffects?
You may experience a worsening of your symptoms when following an elimination or detoxification diet. Expect a coated tongue and a headache, especially if you usually drink a lot of tea and coffee.

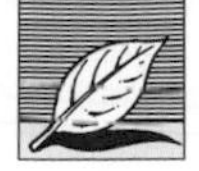

TREATMENT

The nutritional therapist will prescribe a course of treatment based on his analysis of your condition. If he believes you have a nutritional deficiency, he will probably recommend and monitor one of various diets (see page 152). He may further supplement the diet with enzymes, herbal remedies, and vitamins or minerals (see below), which are usually taken with meals in the form of tablets, capsules, powders, and liquids (some practitioners also give injections). At the end of the course of treatment, the practitioner will help you establish a balanced diet to maintain health, and may suggest that you get more exercise. He may also advise other lifestyle changes or further treatment with another form of complementary therapy.

***Recording** dietary intake and any resulting effects is an important part of therapy.*

Many practitioners believe that even if you eat a balanced diet and have an otherwise healthy metabolism, you may be adversely affected by toxins. Due to industrialization and the increasing number of cars on the road, the environment now contains higher levels of lead, cadmium, mercury, and aluminum than at any time in human evolution. Coping with these can put a strain on the body, and practitioners are convinced this causes problems ranging from frequent infections and vague aches and pains, to serious conditions, including chronic fatigue syndrome (CFS), depression, developmental abnormalities, kidney disease, high blood pressure, and cancer.

The practitioner will recommend minimizing the effects of toxins by eating plenty of fiber and organically grown fruits and vegetables, and avoiding foods bought from roadside stands, which may be exposed to leaded exhaust fumes. Suggestions may include avoiding food that has been cooked in unsuitable utensils, such as aluminum, plastic, or synthetic nonstick lining, and reducing exposure to exhaust fumes and tobacco smoke.

A Patient's Experience

Wendy, 35, saw a nutritional therapist after suffering from depression and other symptoms for 18 months: "I had hot flashes, palpitations, blurred vision, and wanted to sleep all the time – I thought it was an early menopause. My doctor wanted to give me antidepressants but I felt the cause was physical, not mental. The nutritional therapist diagnosed candida. He prescribed vitamin and mineral supplements and a strict diet – no sweeteners, vinegar, alcohol, or cow's milk products. Cooked food had to be eaten within 12 hours and fresh food within 24 hours. It was three months before I saw signs of improvement, but gradually I felt less tired, and later the other symptoms cleared."

DEFICIENCIES & SUPPLEMENTS

Believing that people can be nutritionally deficient even on a healthy diet, nutritional therapists prescribe vitamin and mineral supplements to treat a wide range of conditions. The recommended daily allowance (RDA) of supplements is indicated on package labeling. However, every country sets its own levels, and practitioners insist that the RDA may not be reliable, since individuals need different amounts of nutrients, and have different rates of absorption. Prescriptions are therefore tailored to the patient's individual requirements.

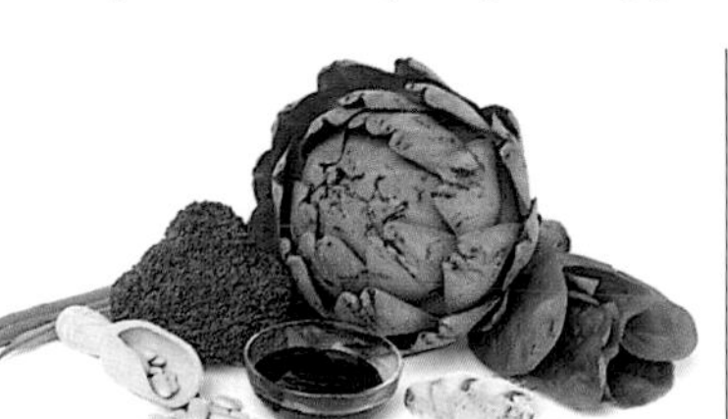

***Vitamin B** can be found in green vegetables, beans, mushrooms, cereal grains, and yeast extract. Deficiencies are often linked to heavy smoking and drinking and may cause depression.*

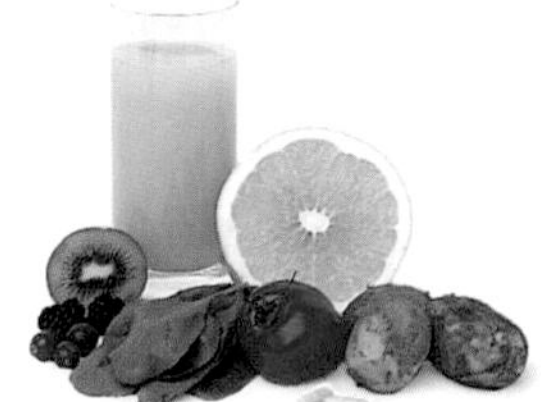

***Vitamin C** is found in citrus fruits, berries, tomatoes, leafy greens, and potatoes. Deficiency weakens the immune system, and leads to skin, bone, and connective tissue problems.*

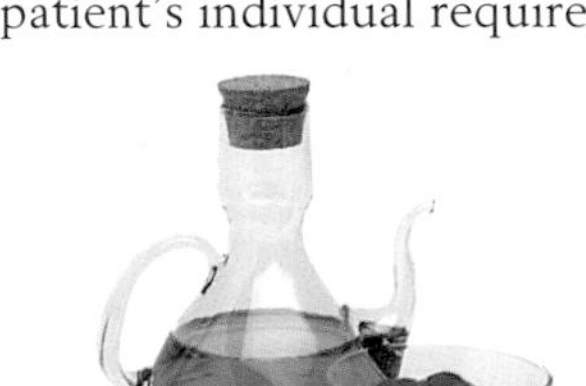

***Vitamin E** sources include cold-pressed vegetable oils, nuts, cereal grains, and liver. Deficiency is rare, but this important antioxidant protects against degenerative disease.*

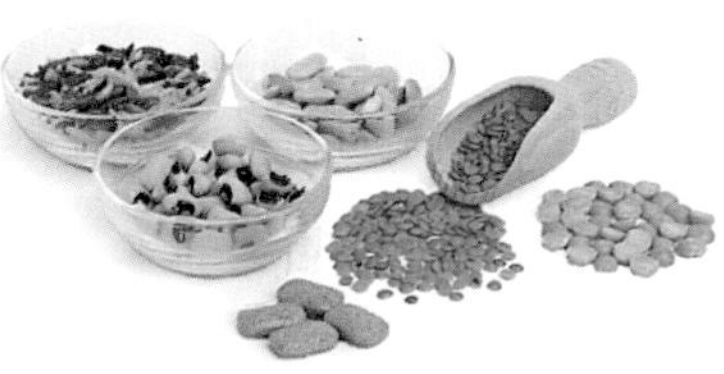

***Fiber** is found in whole grains and legumes. Eating fiber adds bulk to the feces, retains water, and improves bowel efficiency. Deficiency causes constipation.*

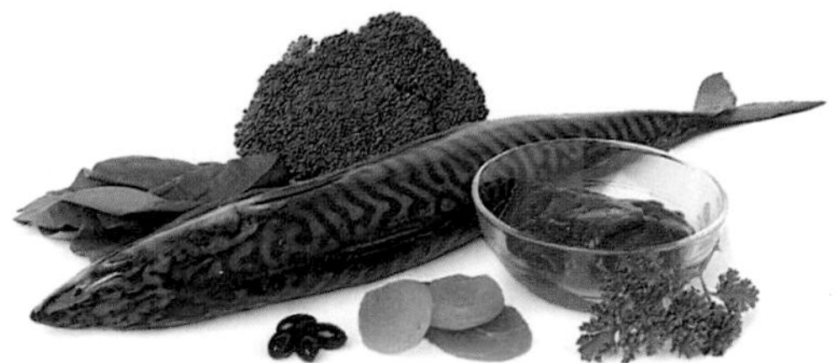

***Iron** is found in liver, oily fish, green vegetables, parsley, and dried apricots. This mineral is vital for the body's production of hemoglobin, which is essential for transporting oxygen to the cells of the body. Deficiency may lead to anemia, and is common in pregnant women.*

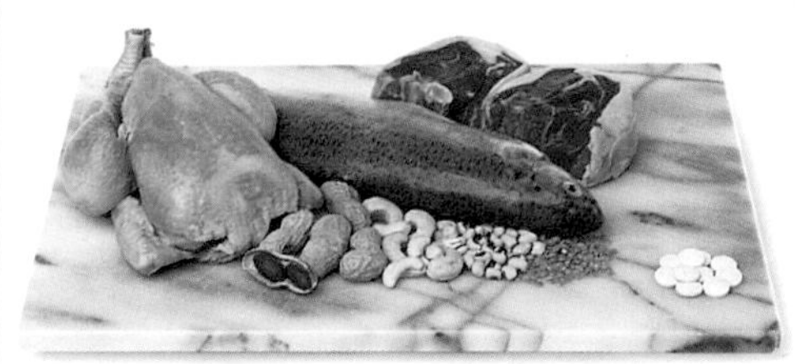

***Zinc** can be found in meat, fish, poultry, legumes, and nuts such as cashews and peanuts. Deficiency is common in old people, heavy drinkers, and convalescents. It leads to an impaired sense of taste and smell, and a weakened immune system.*

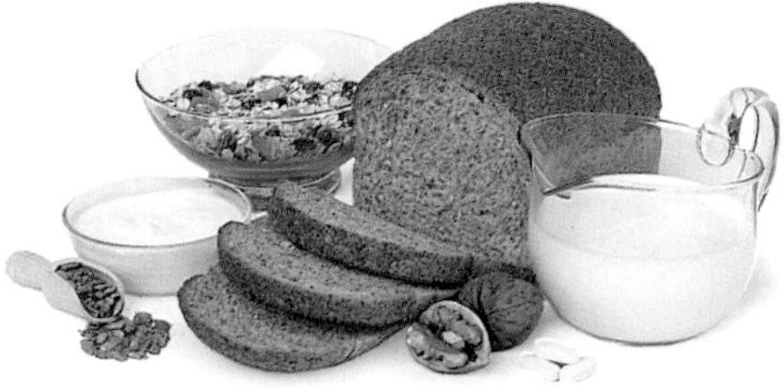

***Magnesium** is found in whole-grain cereals, dried fruits, non- and low-fat milk, yogurt, nuts, and seeds. Deficiency may contribute to persistent fatigue and also to muscle weakness and cramps, since magnesium is essential for the transmission of nerve impulses that cause muscles to contract.*

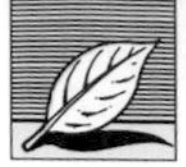

DIET THERAPIES

Medical research today confirms what nutritional therapists and naturopaths have said for years: a diet low in fat, animal protein, and processed food, and high in fruits, vegetables, fiber, and complex carbohydrates, benefits health. Concern about drugs such as antibiotics given to animals reared for consumption, and misgivings about the treatment of animals, has led an increasing number of people to give up meat entirely. There are, however, a wide range of philosophies and theories advocating different diets. Proponents of more extreme diets claim that these can have even greater health benefits than eating a standard balance of nutrients.

Some regimes target particular complaints, such as heart disease and cancer. Others may also involve fasting. Strict diets and long periods of fasting can lead to malnutrition and other problems, so professional supervision is advisable, particularly for children, pregnant women, and elderly people.

VEGETARIAN DIET

Fish and meat are excluded from this diet, but dairy products and eggs are allowed. Studies show that vegetarianism can reduce the risk of heart disease, gallbladder problems, diabetes, high blood pressure, osteoporosis, colon cancer, and diverticular disease (see page 34).

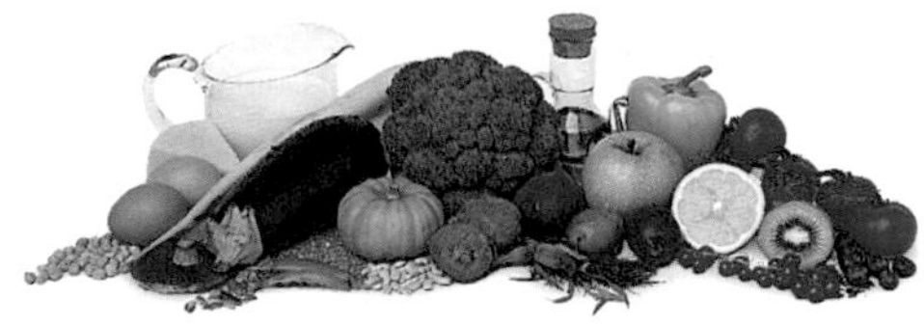

RAW FOODS DIET

Developed by Swiss doctor Max Bircher-Benner in the late 19th century, this diet consists of 70% raw fruits and vegetables and 30% grains, nuts, dairy products, and meat. Uncooked food is said to maintain its "chemical activity," benefiting the digestive system and increasing longevity.

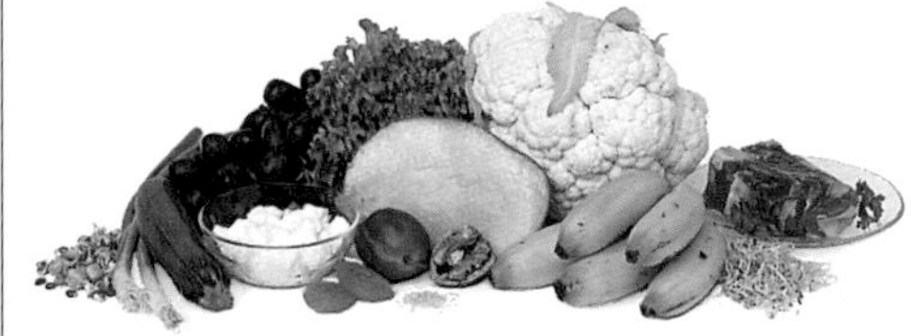

MACROBIOTIC DIET

In an approach devised by the Japanese practitioner George Osawa in the 1950s, foods are chosen for their *yin* or *yang* properties (see page 140). *Yin* foods, said to be calming, include green vegetables, fruits, and nuts. Fish, root vegetables, and cereal grains are strengthening *yang* foods.

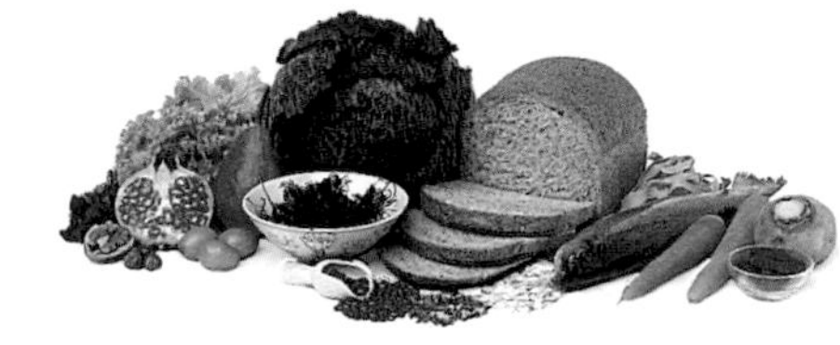

VEGAN DIET

The ultimate conclusion of vegetarianism, this diet also excludes eggs, dairy products, and honey. Protein is supplied by legumes, nuts, grains, and seeds. High blood pressure, angina, rheumatoid arthritis, and asthma have been treated with a vegan diet, but vegans may be deficient in vitamin B_{12}.

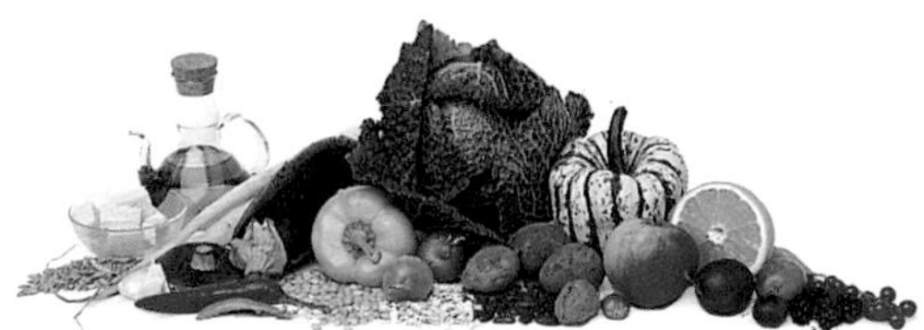

DETOXIFICATION DIET

Nutritional therapists recommend diets of fruits, raw vegetables, water, and yogurt to eliminate toxins caused by poor excretion of waste products, poor digestion, or absorbed from the environment. Detoxification is said to help headaches, allergies, arthritis, and respiratory and hormone problems.

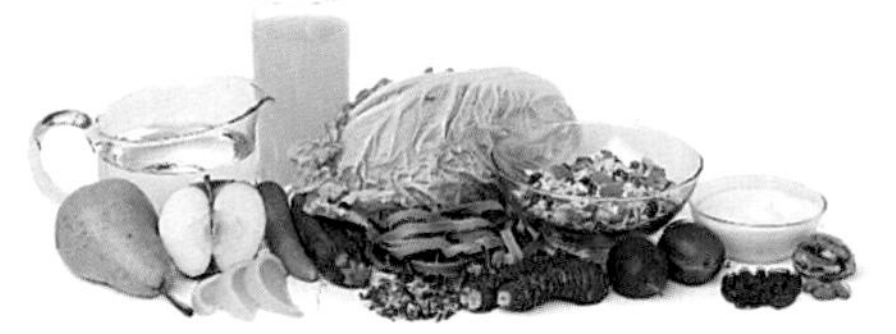

GERSON THERAPY

This controversial anticancer regime (see page 307) was developed in the 1920s by Dr. Max Gerson, a German-born American doctor. It is based on a low-salt, organic vegan diet, supplemented with vegetable and fruit juice hourly, and coffee enemas. The aim is to increase the alkaline level of body tissues.

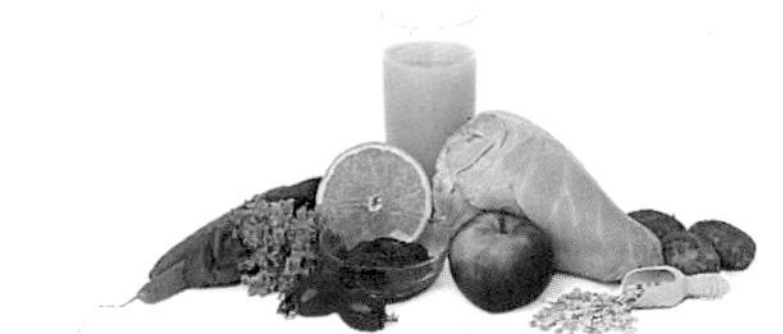

PRITIKIN DIET

Adopted in the 1980s by Dr. Dean Ornish, this diet is high in fiber and carbohydrates, but low in fat and cholesterol, excluding oils and animal products apart from non-fat milk and yogurt. With exercise, yoga, meditation, and support groups, the diet is part of the American doctor's program to reverse heart disease (see page 243).

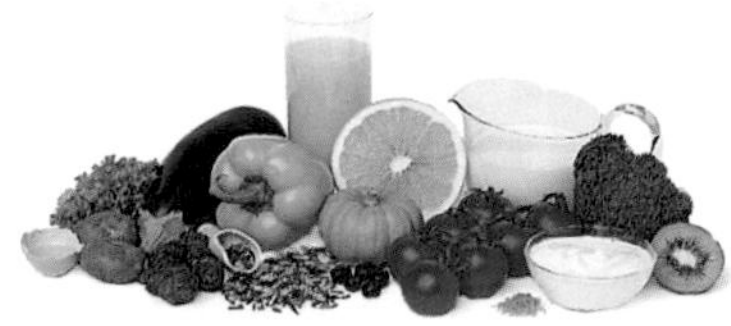

HAY DIET

William Hay, an American doctor, developed this "food-combining" diet in the early 1900s. He believed that carbohydrates and proteins are "foods that fight" and should not be eaten in the same meal, since proteins (above) cause the stomach to produce acid, and carbohydrates (left) must be digested in an alkaline environment. "Neutral" foods (below) are said to combine with either group. The Hay diet has many followers, but no scientific basis. The digestion should cope with any food mixture, and most plants contain both proteins and carbohydrates.

Proteins

Carbohydrates

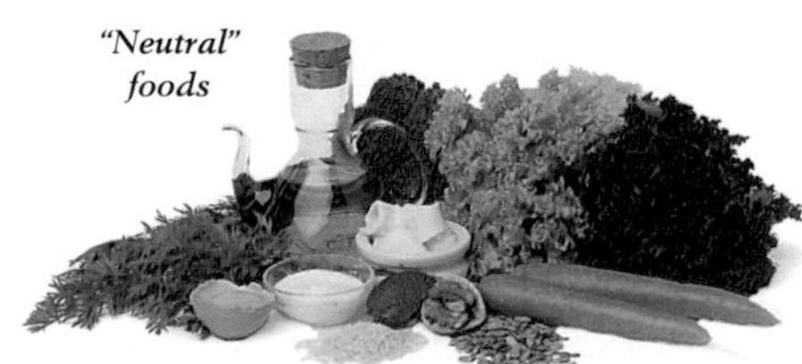

"Neutral" foods

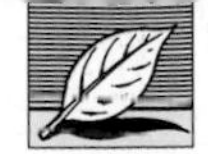

ORTHOMOLECULAR THERAPY

RATINGS	
EVIDENCE	
MEDICAL OPINION	
PRACTITIONER	
SELF-HELP	
COMPATIBILITY	

ORTHOMOLECULAR THERAPY also known as megavitamin therapy, involves the prescription of large doses of vitamins, minerals, and amino acids to treat physical illnesses and psychiatric disorders. Practitioners believe that because each individual is biochemically unique, nutritional deficiencies affect some people more than others. They seek to restore health by using a wide variety of supplements to treat each individual at a biochemical level. The therapy, named by American scientist Dr. Linus Pauling in the 1970s, is now relatively well established in the US and, to a lesser extent, in the UK and Australia.

MAIN USES

- Anxiety, depression
- Schizophrenia
- Anemia
- Heart disease, including angina
- High blood pressure
- Cancer

HISTORY

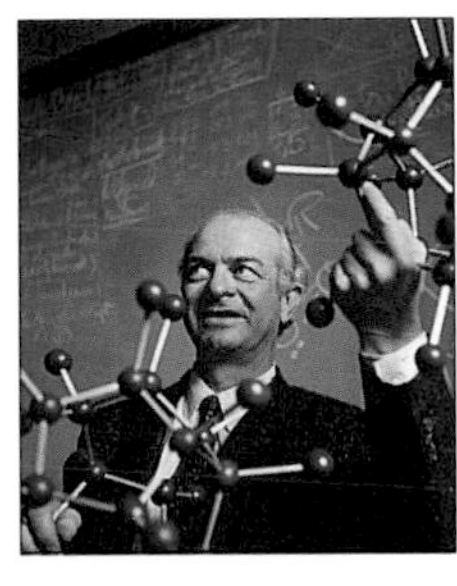

Dr. Linus Pauling's *research into molecular bonds, for which he won a Nobel prize, led him to study the role of vitamin C in preventing common colds and boosting the immune system.*

In the 1950s, psychiatrists Dr. Abram Hoffer and Dr. Humphrey Osmond, working in Canada, began to use high doses of vitamin B_3 (niacin) to treat schizophrenia. Dr. Osmond hypothesized that schizophrenics inadequately absorb sufficient amounts of certain nutrients, leading to a failure to break down substances such as epinephrine, and resulting in severe psychological instability.

High-dose vitamin therapy was popularized in the US in the 1960s by the American nutritionist Adele Davis, but it was biochemist Dr. Linus Pauling who coined the term "orthomolecular" (from the Greek "ortho," or "correct"). In 1970 he published the book *Vitamin C and the Common Cold,* in which he advocated using megadoses of this vitamin (see page 225). Despite skepticism from the medical profession, Dr. Pauling went on to become involved in the controversial area of using vitamin C therapy to treat cancer. Today, this therapy is used mainly in the US. Many practitioners are also medical doctors.

CONSULTING A PRACTITIONER

Orthomolecular therapy uses vitamins as medication and not as food supplements, as in nutritional therapy (see page 148). Practitioners stress the need for antioxidant vitamins, such as vitamin C, which are said to mop up the free-radical molecules that cause cell damage (see glossary). They believe that some people may need far higher levels of certain nutrients than the recommended daily allowances (RDAs; see page 151) might suggest, and prescribe doses of vitamins and minerals that are hundreds of times higher than the RDA, for heart disease, cancer, and other ailments.

Practitioners take a medical history, give you a physical examination, and arrange for blood, urine, and tissue tests. Supplements prescribed are tailored to your individual requirements, and are taken several times a day at levels well above the norm: 5,000–20,000 mg of vitamin C per day, for example, or 25,000 iu (international units) of beta-carotene (vitamin A). Nutrients may also be given by injection or intravenous drip to speed up the process. If there are side effects, the practitioner reduces the dose until symptoms subside.

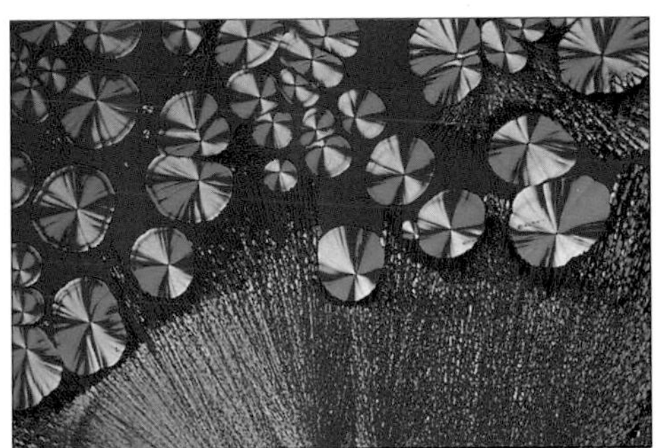

Pantothenic acid*, a B complex vitamin, viewed as a polarized light micrograph: vitamin B has been given in large doses to treat mental illness.*

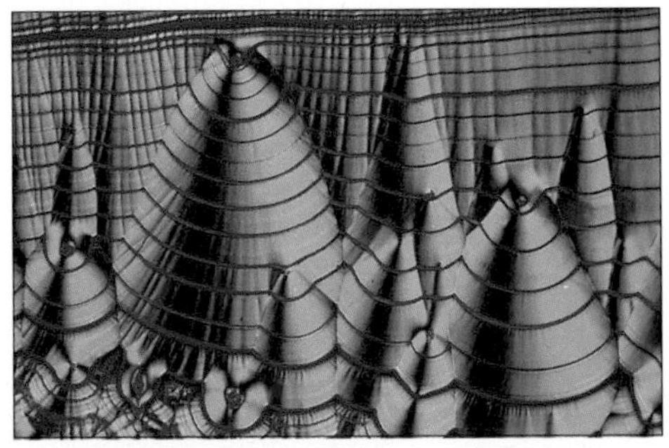

Vitamin C crystals *viewed as a polarized light micrograph: cancer patients who have undergone chemotherapy may be prescribed vitamin C.*

EVIDENCE & RESEARCH

While there is little scientific evidence for the therapeutic effects of orthomolecular megadoses, studies indicate that doses higher than the RDA may be required for some supplements to be effective. A study published in *The Lancet* in 1992 concluded that patients who had suffered heart attacks recovered faster when given injections of high doses of magnesium sulfate. In the early 1990s, research by Dr. Pauling showed that high doses of vitamin C could help reverse atherosclerosis (a major cause of heart attacks).

MEDICAL OPINION

The discovery of the role of antioxidant nutrients in the body lends credence to orthomolecular theories, but side effects associated with high doses of vitamins, and the lack of research into this therapy make conventional doctors uneasy.

PRECAUTIONS

- Do not self-prescribe; megadoses of certain vitamins can cause toxic reactions.
- See also nutritional therapies (page 150) and page 52.

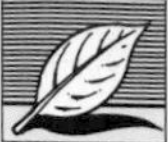

CLINICAL ECOLOGY

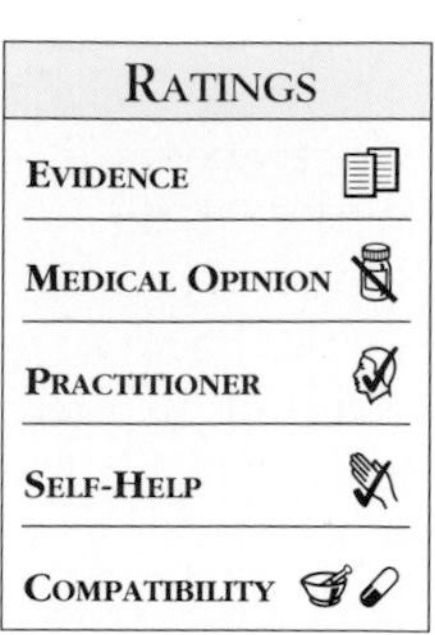

BASED ON THE IDEA that the environment can affect health, clinical ecology, sometimes called environmental medicine, developed from early 20th-century research into allergies. Practitioners claim that many disorders may be caused by environmental factors, including certain foods, pollen, dust, exhaust fumes, and pesticides; rather than causing full-blown allergic reactions, these lead to milder symptoms known as "intolerances" or "sensitivities." Treatment aims to identify irritants with tests and then minimize exposure. Clinical ecology is growing in the West as concern about pollution increases.

MAIN USES

- Asthma, hay fever
- Headaches, migraines
- Digestive disorders
- Fluid retention
- Rapid weight fluctuation
- Depression
- Fatigue, CFS
- Rheumatoid arthritis
- Eczema, psoriasis
- Recurrent infections

HISTORY

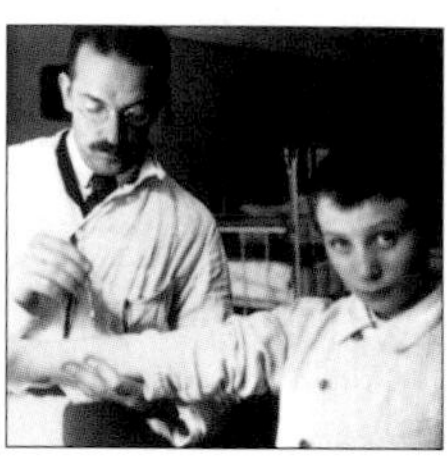

***Baron Clemens von Pirquet** studied patients' abnormal responses to environmental factors and defined the term allergy as "altered reactivity."*

Abnormal reactions to food were recorded in ancient Greece by Hippocrates, the "father of medicine," but only in 1906 was the term "allergy" coined, by the Viennese pediatrician Baron Clemens von Pirquet. He had realized that some of his patients reacted to certain foods, pollen, or insect stings, and used the term to describe any unusual response to the environment. Allergies came to be defined as reactions within the immune system, identified by a positive skin-prick test (see opposite).

From the 1920s, several American doctors studied "delayed" or "hidden" food allergies. Reactions took longer to appear than other allergies, were less acute, and provoked no skin-test response. Most doctors rejected these ideas about food "intolerances," or sensitivities, and there was little research within mainstream medicine.

In the late 1940s, American allergist Dr. Theron G. Randolph claimed that sensitivity to common foods could cause symptoms such as headaches and arthritis, and that environmental chemicals could have profound negative effects. The best-seller *Silent Spring*, a 1962 book by American biologist Rachel Carson, alerted the world to the dangers of insecticides.

At this time, the term "clinical ecology" began to be used to describe this field of medicine. The system gained ground in the UK during the 1970s and is practiced today throughout the Western world by qualified doctors and complementary therapists.

KEY PRINCIPLES

Clinical ecologists believe that foods are the most likely environmental carriers of "toxins", and claim that anyone drinking unfiltered tap water and eating a typical Western diet is likely to ingest 100 synthetic chemicals daily. These include pesticides and herbicides sprayed on vegetables and fruits, residues of drugs fed to animals prior to slaughter, and preservatives in processed foods. Air pollution, cleaning agents, and house dust are other potential hazards.

The body usually maintains health despite an onslaught of environmental toxins. For some people, particularly those susceptible to allergies, or those who have an infection or a diet deficient in antioxidant vitamins and minerals (see page 35), it can become more difficult to cope. According to clinical ecologists, these people are more prone to developing inflammatory reactions, or even changes in brain chemistry, which can alter their mood and vitality. Practitioners use various tests to identify the substances causing trouble so that they can be avoided or limited. They may also try to "desensitize" the patient to the irritant (see opposite).

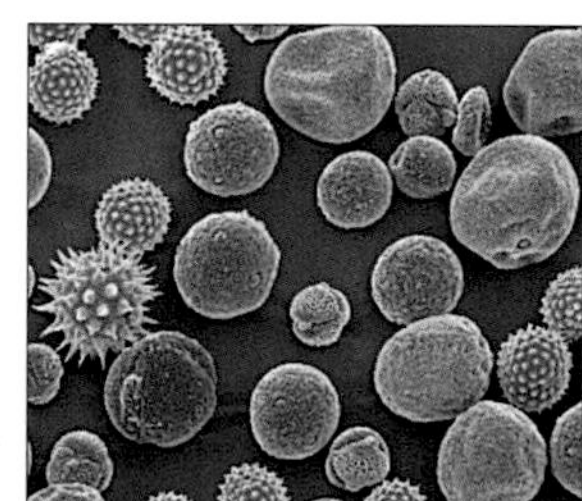

***A sample of air** contains different plant pollens, any of which may prompt an allergic reaction when inhaled.*

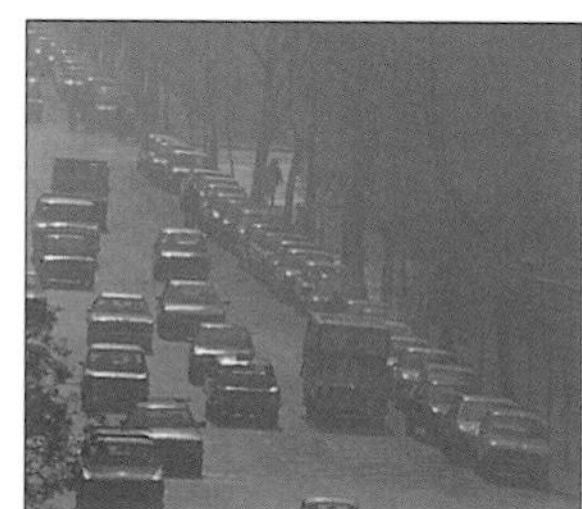

***Soaring levels** of chemicals found in exhaust fumes are thought to overload some people's capacity to deal with allergens and pollutants.*

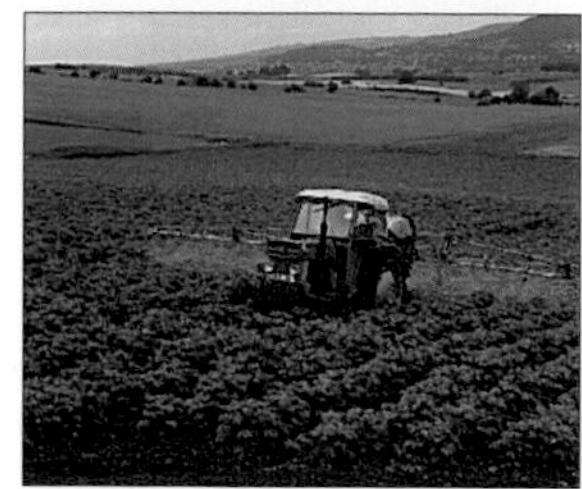

***Pesticides** and herbicides sprayed on crops are known to have a damaging effect on health.*

EVIDENCE & RESEARCH

The scientific basis for clinical ecology has not been well established, and the associated diagnostic tests are considered unreliable. However, the detrimental effects of environmental pollution on health are becoming more apparent, and further research is needed. True allergies, like asthma, are already strongly linked to environmental factors, such as air pollution.

MEDICAL OPINION

The premise that environmental irritants can affect health makes sense, but many doctors would question the effectiveness of clinical ecology in pinpointing them. The idea that diagnostic tests can distinguish between stress-related and environmental factors belies the complexity of patients' problems, and it is too easy to jump to an environment-linked conclusion.

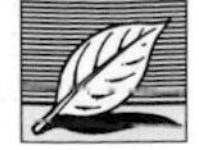

CONSULTING A PRACTITIONER

The practitioner asks about your medical history, diet, and lifestyle, to see if there is any evidence of exposure to irritants. He then checks for signs of sensitivity, such as swollen glands. A hair or blood test may be taken to determine mineral and nutritional factors thought to relate to the strength of the immune system. Other tests include:
Skin-prick test: Tiny samples of the diluted suspect substances are applied to an area of scratched skin or injected under your skin. Any subsequent inflammation or itchiness indicates an allergy or sensitivity.
Pulse test: A change in pulse rate after eating a certain food is said to be a sign that you are sensitive to it. Some practitioners use the *auriculocardiac reflex method* (see page 192), placing suspect substances next to the ear and noting any sudden increase in pulse rate.

SIGNS OF SENSITIVITY
The practitioner may check for pale skin, shadows under the eyes, and swollen glands.

PRECAUTIONS

- Check symptoms with a doctor if consulting a clinical ecologist who is not medically qualified.
- Carry out elimination diets only under qualified supervision to ensure adequate nutrition.
- See also page 52.

Muscle test: A solution of a suspected irritant is placed on your tongue or body. An inability to resist pressure then directed against a limb is seen to suggest intolerance (see page 196).
RAST **(Radio Allergo Sorbent Test)**: This conventional blood test shows whether immunoglobulin E has been made by your body, indicating an allergic reaction.

Cytotoxic test: A blood sample is taken and mixed with extracts of the possible irritant. Damage to the white blood cells is said to suggest sensitivity (see page 199).
Sublingual drop test: After five days of taking fluids only, a drop of a solution containing the suspect irritant is placed under the tongue and reactions noted.
Elimination diet: After a diet of "neutral" foods, possible irritants are gradually re-introduced (see page 199).
Vega test: Not approved in the US. The Vega machine generates a low-voltage current applied to the skin; this is said to reveal "sensitivities" to suspect substances. (see page 200).

Swollen glands may indicate sensitivity to certain substances

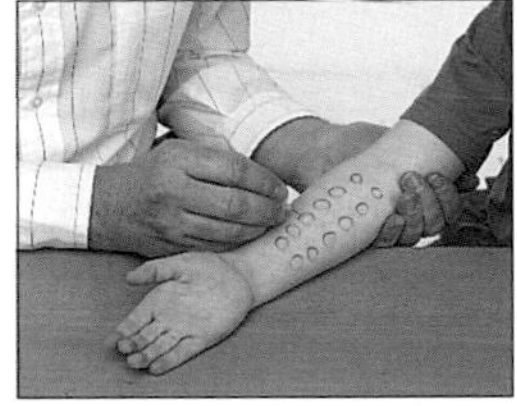

***In a skin-prick test** a dilution of the suspect substance is placed on an area of scratched skin.*

TREATMENT

The simplest treatment is to avoid any irritants identified, but this is not always practical. Your practitioner may opt to "desensitize" you using the following techniques so that the body can withstand limited exposure to the irritant.
Exclusion or elimination diets: Suspect foods, commonly dairy products, wheat, sugar, citrus fruits, nuts, eggs, or coffee, are excluded for 10–14 days in the hope that symptoms will disappear. Alternatively, food intake is reduced to one or two items for five days; individual foods are then reintroduced until symptoms are triggered.

***The practitioner** may recommend keeping a written record of when reactions take place, and in what circumstances, to help build up a complete picture of the problem.*

The culprit food is eliminated and added a week later to see if symptoms return.
Enzyme-potentiated desensitization: The diluted irritant is mixed with an enzyme and kept next to the skin for several days.
Provocation neutralization: Decreasing concentrations of the irritant are injected or given as drops under the tongue. The neutralizing dose is identified at the point at which no reaction occurs. This is then used as a vaccine once or twice a day.

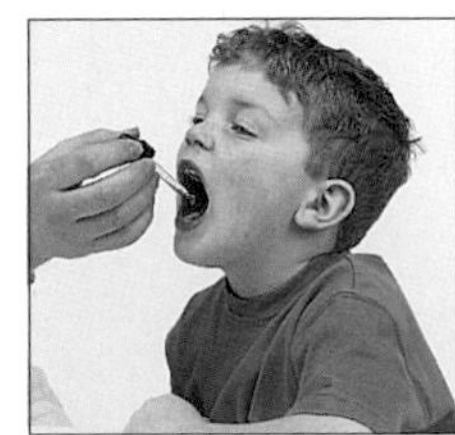

***In provocation neutralization**, drops of up to nine different dilutions of an irritant are placed in turn under the tongue, using a pipette.*

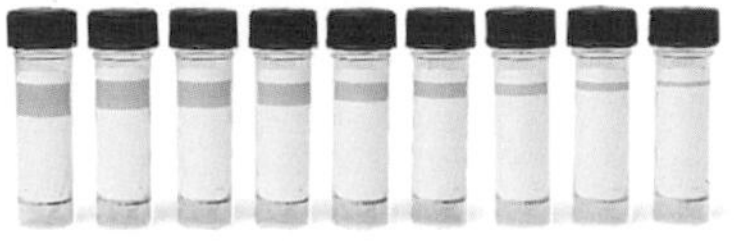

Standard nine dilutions

SELF-HELP

Your practitioner may suggest ways of changing your lifestyle to avoid exposure to irritants such as house dust, pollen, exhaust fumes, disinfectants, and chemicals in food and tap water. To avoid dust mites, air your bedding regularly and invest in a good vacuum cleaner. Keep windows open for ventilation or use an air filter. Mild forms of chemical sensitivity may respond to antioxidant supplements, especially vitamins C and E, zinc, and selenium.

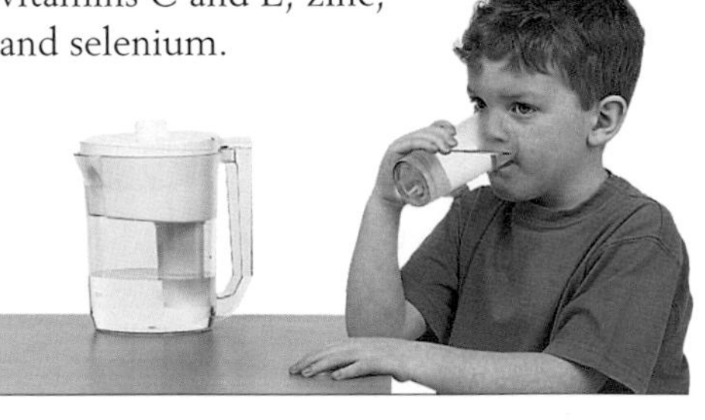

***Drinking filtered tap water** is a simple and effective way of reducing the amount of impurities absorbed by the body every day.*

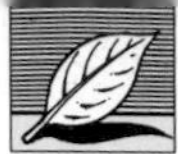

MAGNETIC THERAPY

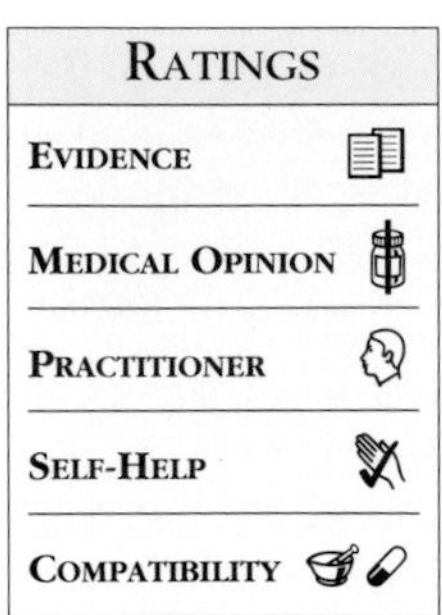

ELECTROMAGNETIC FIELDS (EMFs) are constantly present. The earth has its own magnetic field, aligned to the North and South poles, and even human body cells have subtle magnetic forces. Conventional medicine utilizes electrical equipment to generate EMFs that influence the body's natural electrical currents to promote healing. Complementary practitioners claim that ordinary magnets can also do this, and use devices such as magnetic wrist bands and beds to treat illness, particularly bone disorders. Magnetic therapy is not yet well established in the West, but is popular in Japan and eastern Europe.

MAIN USES

- Bone disorders, including fractures & osteoporosis
- Arthritis, inflamed joints & sprains
- Back & neck pain
- Insomnia, fatigue
- Headaches, migraines
- Hormonal imbalances
- Circulation problems
- Wound healing

HISTORY

The therapeutic benefits of magnets are said to have been known to ancient Greek, Egyptian, and Chinese doctors; Cleopatra allegedly wore a magnet on her head to retain her beauty. Aspects of the modern therapy can be traced to the work of the 18th-century Viennese physician Franz Anton Mesmer (see page 168), who argued that magnets could enhance "animal magnetism," a universal force that he claimed permeated the body. Mesmer's methods, such as holding a metal wand over his patients, were dubious, but his ideas about magnetic poles were influential.

Magnetic therapy, also known as magnetotherapy or biomagnetic therapy, is popular today in Japan and eastern Europe. So far, it has not become well established in the West. However, strong EMFs, generated by electrical devices, are now being used in conventional medical practice in the US, UK, and Australia, for example by orthopedic surgeons to heal fractures. Magnetic resonance imaging (see glossary), which uses EMFs in diagnosis, is considered superior to and safer than X rays.

CONSULTING A PRACTITIONER

According to practitioners, iron atoms in the red corpuscles of the blood respond to magnetism. When a magnet is placed on the patient's body, blood flow through the area is enhanced. This is said to improve the supply of oxygen to cells, stimulate the metabolism, and help in the elimination of waste products.

The therapy is more often practiced as a self-help treatment, using ordinary "static" magnets with weak EMFs. Products such as magnetic shoe insoles, straps, mattresses, pillows, and car-seat covers are available. The practitioner may show you how to use them, or you may receive instruction from the equipment manufacturer or supplier. A practitioner would try to choose the most suitable treatment for your needs. "Supermagnets," for example, are supposed to emit a higher magnetic force, and should be positioned on specific parts of the body, often over lymph nodes or acupuncture points (see page 90). Practitioners may also suggest electrical devices that emit pulsating fields at specific frequencies to target particular areas of body tissue. Such devices include beds, special belts, and cylinder-shaped machines in which you sit.

The length of a treatment session varies according to the type of magnetic device used and can be anything from a few minutes to several hours.

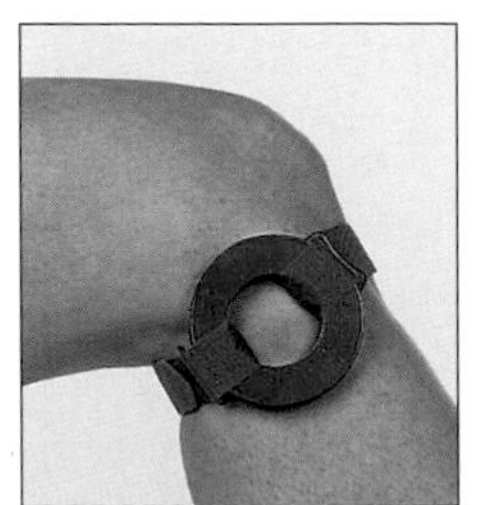

Magnetic straps *may be worn on the knees, elbows, ankles, or wrists. They are thought to ease muscular pain and benefit those with arthritis and rheumatoid arthritis.*

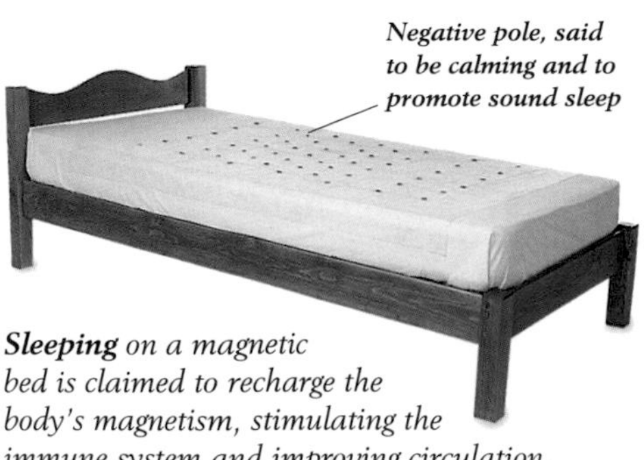

Sleeping *on a magnetic bed is claimed to recharge the body's magnetism, stimulating the immune system and improving circulation.*

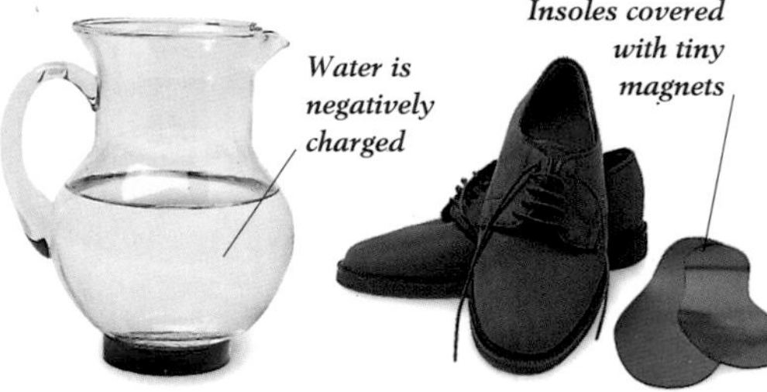

Magnetized water, *made by placing a jug of water on a magnet's negative pole for up to 24 hours, can be taken to aid digestion.*

Magnetic insoles *emit a small magnetic charge to the feet and are said to improve circulation, energy, and endurance.*

EVIDENCE & RESEARCH

Clinical research on the benefits of certain types of EMF is growing. A 1996 study in *The Lancet* found magnetic stimulation of the brain helped treat depression. In 1959, American surgeons discovered how to regenerate severed amphibian limbs using EMFs and developed this to heal human bone fractures. A 1990 University of Hawaii study found EMFs helpful in treating osteoporosis. Surgeons in the US and UK use EMFs to treat fractured bones, nonhealing wounds, edema, and deep vein thrombosis.

MEDICAL OPINION

Conventional medicine recognizes the potential of strong EMFs, but with no evidence that weak magnetic fields can treat disease, doctors feel that magnetic devices are mostly little more than placebos.

PRECAUTIONS

- Avoid magnetic therapy if you have a pacemaker, or are pregnant or trying to conceive.
- See also page 52.

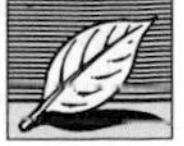

OTHER THERAPIES

CHELATION THERAPY

Chelation therapy was first used in the 1940s by the US Navy to treat lead poisoning, and is still practiced principally in the US, albeit controversially. It involves the administration of a synthetic form of the amino acid EDTA (see glossary) to "chelate," or chemically remove, heavy metals (see glossary) and toxins from the bloodstream, and break down calcium deposits or plaque from the artery walls.

The patient is hooked up to an intravenous drip containing a solution of EDTA, vitamins, and minerals. Treatment is carried out by a qualified doctor, and tests on circulation and blood pressure, cholesterol and blood sugar levels, and kidney and organ function are taken throughout the treatment. A session lasts about three hours, 1–3 times per week, and 20–30 sessions are recommended.

Chelation therapy is used to treat circulatory disorders, and is also practiced preventively to maintain a healthy bloodstream. Many studies have been carried out on it, but few of these have been scientifically controlled.

OXYGEN/OZONE THERAPY

Doctors began to treat infection using oxygen over a century ago; the first recorded use of oxygen therapy was in 1879 by a French physician, Dr. J. A. Fontaine. The treatment is popular today in Russia and Germany, but does not have official approval in the US, and is almost unknown in the UK and Australia.

Oxygen/ozone therapy covers a wide range of practices, all of which involve administering oxygen as a gas or in water to help body cells and tissues function efficiently. Ozone therapy is said to oxygenate cells and trigger chemical reactions that destroy viruses and bacteria.

Treatment is carried out by medically qualified therapists, and is given through an artery or intravenously, by mouth, via the rectum or vagina, by inhalation or absorption, or by injection into the joints or muscles. Treatment could comprise 2–3 sessions for a minor infection or 30–40 sessions for more serious conditions.

Oxygen therapy is claimed to kill cancer cells; it has also been used to treat strokes, arthritis, multiple sclerosis, and allergies. Ozone therapy has been used to heal wounds and treat bacterial and viral diseases (it is a controversial AIDS treatment).

COLONIC HYDROTHERAPY

This detoxification process, also called colonic irrigation or colon therapy, was reputedly known in ancient Egypt, China, and India, but the method that is popular in the West today has its origins in 19th-century European spas. Practitioners claim that fecal matter can cling to the wall of the large bowel (colon) and may be reabsorbed into the bloodstream. They aim to remove this waste material by flushing it away with purified water.

The patient lies on a treatment table, wearing a gown with an opening at the back. A tube is inserted into the rectum, and filtered water (possibly with added substances) is administered under gentle pressure. The patient holds the water in the colon for about two minutes. Then the pressure is released, and the water and any dislodged waste matter flows away. This process may be repeated several times. Treatment often consists of 4–8 sessions, each lasting 40–50 minutes.

The therapy is used to treat conditions such as digestive disorders, headaches, chronic fatigue, skin problems, fibroids, and backache. Medical opinion is divided toward colonic hydrotherapy.

TIBETAN MEDICINE

Dating back to the 7th century, this system of medicine is based on similar principles to Ayurveda (see page 144) and Traditional Chinese Medicine (see page 140). It is not well known in the West but is attracting increasing interest.

Practitioners believe that all body functions are governed by three "humors" (air, bile, and phlegm), and use pulse and tongue testing (see pages 192–93), urine analysis, and observation to diagnose illness. Treatment includes herbal remedies, dietary and lifestyle advice, massage, and acupuncture (see page 90). Religious ritual also forms a major part of treatment. Sessions last 60–90 minutes, and the number required depends on the condition and the methods used. Tibetan medicine claims to treat any condition.

RADIONICS

This form of distant healing (see page 105) was pioneered in the early 1900s by US neurologist Dr. Albert Abrams. There was opposition to his work from the medical establishment in the US, where radionics is still illegal, but in 1924 a UK medical committee found his diagnostic methods could be surprisingly accurate.

Radionics practitioners aim to tap into the "vibrational frequencies" of a patient's "bioenergy" to analyze the cause of illness. Patients might not meet their practitioner. They complete a questionnaire on their medical history and supply a drop of blood or hair sample (known as the "witness"). The practitioner places the witness on a radionic "black box," which has frequency settings "tuned" to the vibrational levels of various disorders. He may also dowse the patient's questionnaire with a pendulum (see page 198). After diagnosis, the practitioner uses the machine to "broadcast" healing energy to the patient, and may also suggest homeopathic or Bach Flower Remedies, or color therapy (see pages 126, 132, and 186). In theory, radionics can treat any condition, although most doctors are extremely skeptical.

PSIONICS

Developed in 1968, psionics resembles radionics, and is said to work by detecting and counteracting disruptions in a patient's "bioenergy." Practitioners dowse the patient to diagnose illness, for which homeopathic and anthroposophical remedies (see pages 126 and 124) are prescribed.

PRECAUTIONS

- Chelation therapy may cause weakness or dizziness due to low blood sugar levels.
- Oxygen/ozone therapy may cause breathlessness, chest pain, fainting, gas bubbles in the bloodstream, or inflammation of the lower intestine.
- Seek medical advice before using colonic hydrotherapy if you have a bowel disease.
- See also page 52.

MIND & EMOTION THERAPIES

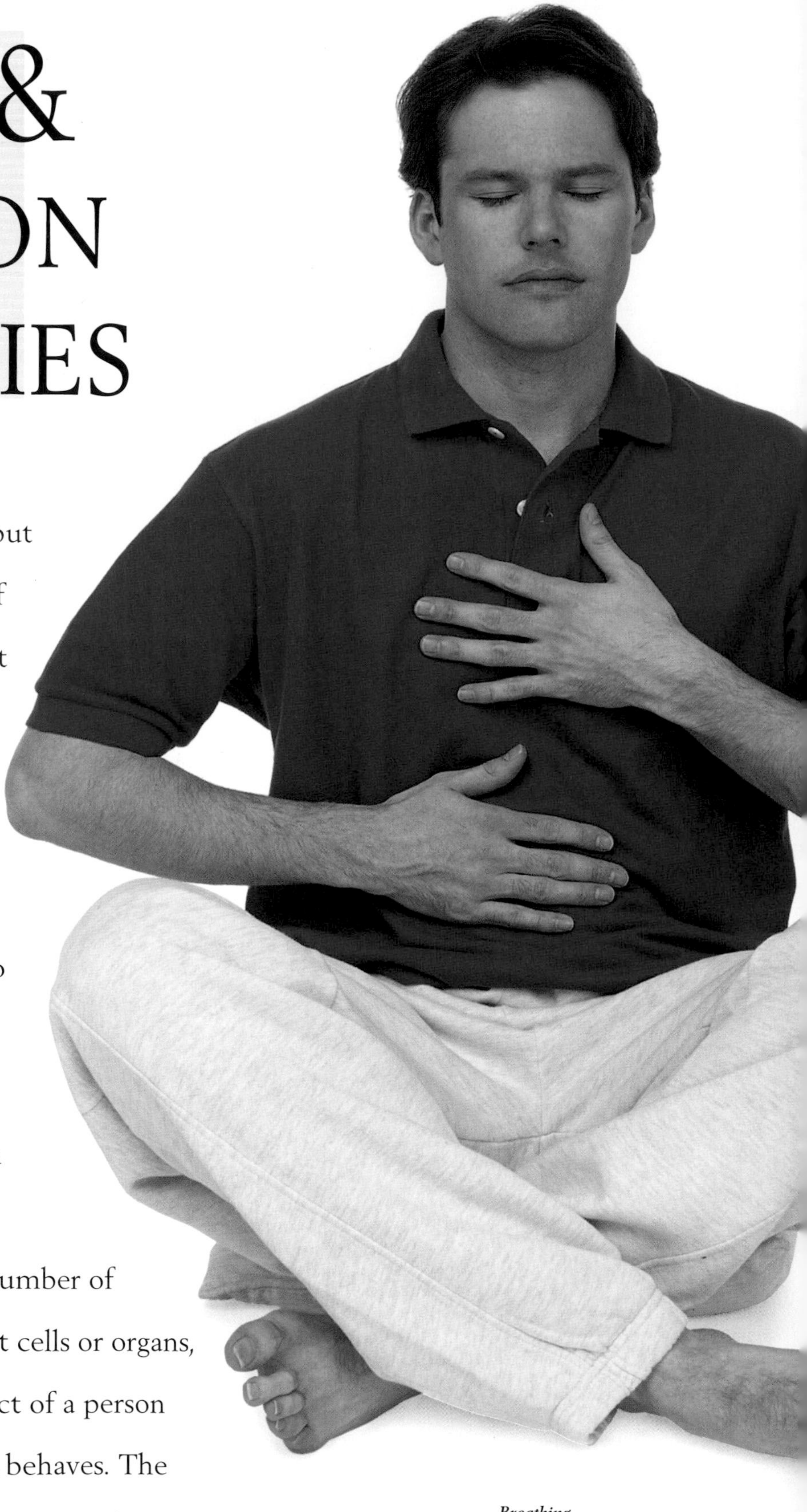

In 1637, the French philosopher Descartes put forward the view that the body was a kind of machine, separate from the mind – a concept that hugely influenced the future development of Western medicine. Yet, over three hundred years later, research has provided conclusive evidence that mind and body are intricately interwoven. There is also a renewed interest in "holism" – the notion that mind and body are indivisible, and that to treat illness, the whole person, rather than isolated parts, must be taken into account.

It is becoming clear to an increasing number of medical practitioners that it is people, not just cells or organs, who have diseases, and that an essential aspect of a person is the way he or she thinks, feels, relates, and behaves. The various treatments categorized as mind and emotion therapies aim to harness the power of thoughts, feelings, imagination, and actions in order to influence the

Breathing exercise

biological and structural processes of an individual. Until recently, Western scientists and conventional medical practitioners rarely probed into the nature of consciousness, or questioned its impact on the individual. Frustrated by this situation, many people interested in the subject have begun to turn to the East, where philosophers and physicians have been examining such questions for thousands of years. The fact that Western science and medicine are now beginning to study these traditions promises a rich future for mind/body medicine.

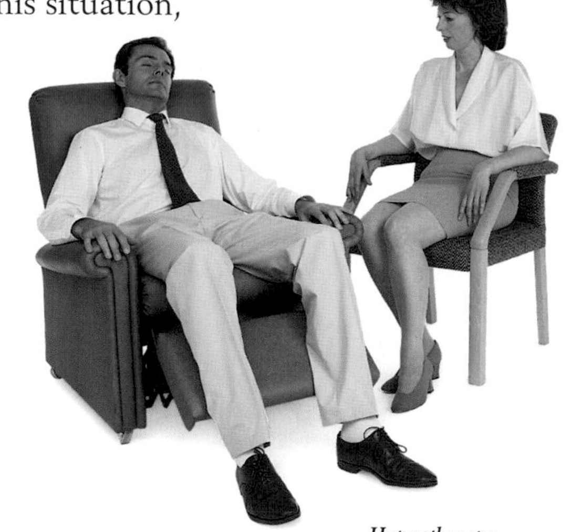

Hypnotherapy

The Therapies

Psychotherapy & Counseling *page 160* ◆ Hypnotherapy *page 166*

Autogenic Training *page 168* ◆ Biofeedback *page 169*

Relaxation & Breathing *page 170* ◆ Meditation *page 174*

Flotation Therapy *page 177* ◆ Visualization *page 178*

Sound Therapy *page 180* ◆ Music Therapy *page 181*

Art Therapy *page 182* ◆ Feng Shui *page 184* ◆ Geomancy *page 185*

Color Therapy *page 186* ◆ Light Therapy *page 188*

Biorhythms *page 189* ◆ Other Therapies *page 190*

Psychotherapy treatment

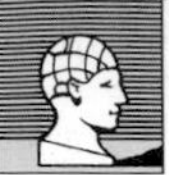

PSYCHOTHERAPY & COUNSELING

RATINGS
EVIDENCE
MEDICAL OPINION
PRACTITIONER
SELF-HELP
COMPATIBILITY

COVERING A WIDE RANGE of techniques used to ease psychological suffering, psychotherapy and counseling owe much to the work of Austrian psychiatrist Sigmund Freud at the turn of the 20th century. Whether treating mental and emotional disorders or promoting self-awareness, these therapies offer the chance to understand and resolve difficult thoughts, feelings, and situations by talking about them with a skilled listener. Many hospitals and doctors' practices now employ psychologists and psychotherapists, and many other practitioners offer a range of less mainstream therapies in the same field.

MAIN USES

- Stress, anxiety, depression
- Phobias, obsessions, compulsions
- Eating disorders
- Bereavement, grief
- Relationship problems
- Sexual problems
- Emotional instability
- Psychosomatic illness
- Personal development

HISTORY

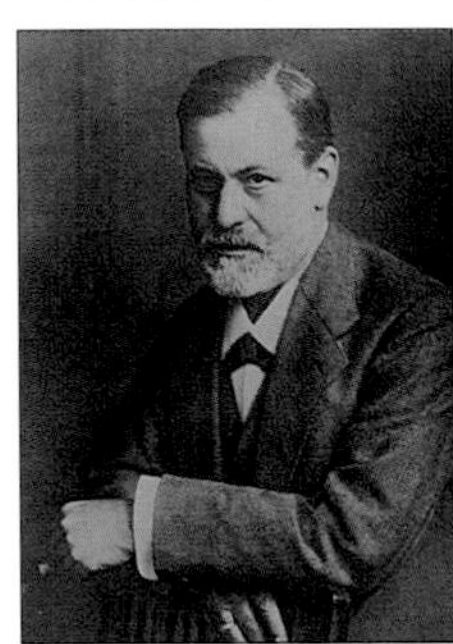

***Sigmund Freud** was the father of psychoanalysis, the forerunner of psychotherapy. He believed that sexuality, hunger, and other drives experienced unconsciously at an early age shape emotional responses throughout life.*

The origins of psychotherapy as we know it today can unquestionably be traced to the work of Sigmund Freud, who practiced psychoanalysis in Vienna from the 1880s to the 1930s. He introduced the idea of the unconscious mind, and tried to uncover buried motives for the disturbed thoughts, feelings, and actions of his patients by allowing them to talk freely.

In around 1914, a pupil of Freud, Carl Jung, broke away from his mentor to develop his own brand of analytic psychotherapy, based on the idea of a human drive toward an inner world of wholeness.

Another influential psychoanalyst was Melanie Klein. Between World Wars I and II, she carried out research into infant behavior, believing that young children's relationships with the outside world are at least as formative as their struggles to come to terms with their own bodies. Klein's theories about how children learn to think influenced many psychoanalysts.

During the first half of the 20th century, "behavioral" psychologists, such as John Watson and Burrhus Frederic Skinner, criticized the psychoanalysts' emphasis on the unconscious. They claimed that such unconscious states of mind, which could not be measured, were irrelevant, while hunger and other biological triggers "conditioned" predictable behavior that could be unlearned or corrected by therapy.

In reaction to the behaviorists' theories of negative "conditioning" and the clinical nature of Freudian psychoanalysis, psychologists Abraham Maslow, Carl Rogers, Fritz Perls, and others developed a "humanistic" approach to therapy, focusing on the positive, rather than the dysfunctional, aspects of behavior. By the 1960s, techniques such as encounter groups (see page 165) were being used to encourage "personal growth" and help people realize their "human potential."

While psychoanalysis remained popular in central Europe and on the East Coast of the US, the "personal growth movement" burgeoned on the West Coast, and the work of therapists such as Virginia Satir and Milton Erickson proved to be a major influence on developing techniques for brief psychotherapy. By the 1970s, psychotherapy and its sister therapy, counseling, were becoming established outside the US. Today many doctors refer patients to various types of psychotherapists and counselors, or even employ them in their practices.

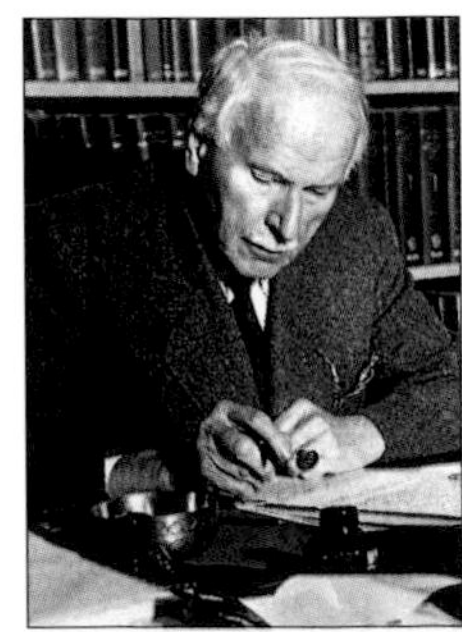

***Carl Jung**, a Swiss psychoanalyst and originally one of Freud's disciples, developed his own theories about man's search for his "essential self," and the existence of a "collective unconscious" shared by all human beings.*

KEY PRINCIPLES

For many people, the existence of the "unconscious" remains controversial. Analytic and psychodynamic therapies are based on the theory that memories and feelings become "repressed," or forgotten, and therefore disturb the mind and body. These approaches usually involve encouraging clients to talk about their experiences and vent emotions that have been repressed, while congnitive and behavioral therapies do not deal with the unconscious at all. The client usually initiates the dialogue and decides what is talked about.

Trained practitioners should be able to identify the importance not only of what clients say, but what they do *not* say, and suggest links between present behavior and past events. Most practitioners will have undergone therapy as part of their training, and even when qualified they should receive regular supervision from another practitioner. While the distinctions between practitioners may be blurred (particularly in the case of psychotherapists and counselors), they can usually be categorized as one of the following:

Psychoanalysts: Practitioners train for 5–7 years at a recognized institution, following the teachings of Sigmund Freud, Carl Jung, or Melanie Klein. Some may also have a medical degree (see page 162).

Psychologists: After taking a science-based university degree, studying the mind and behavior, practitioners choose a branch of psychology in which to specialize. Personal therapy is not part of their training. Clinical psychologists often use cognitive and behavioral methods directed by the practitioner (see page 164).

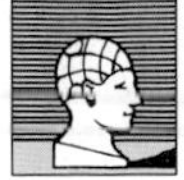

Psychotherapists: Practitioners usually train for four years with a recognized organization, but do not necessarily have a degree. They may specialize in a variety of techniques (see pages 162–65).
Counselors: While some counselors may receive only a weekend's training, the better ones have 2–3 years' training (see page 163) and work under supervision.

Both psychotherapists and counselors may use a variety of approaches, including psychodynamic as well as humanistic.

EVIDENCE & RESEARCH

Psychological therapies are difficult to research. Not only are the methods diverse but they rely on theories about the human condition that are impossible to prove scientifically. Often it is the skill of the practitioner, rather than the type of therapy, that determines a successful outcome. Behavioral and cognitive therapies have been widely evaluated – for example, studies published in the *Journal of Consulting and Clinical Psychology* in the 1990s – have been shown to be effective for anxiety, phobias, mild to moderate depression, relationship problems, and sexual dysfunctions.

In 1994, the *British Journal of Psychiatry* published research suggesting that cognitive therapy was more effective for panic attacks than either conventional medication or relaxation techniques. When the results of such studies are compared, clients are generally found to have benefited from treatment in the long term, although no technique seems more effective than another. Less research evidence is available for longer-term psychoanalytic therapies, but some studies indicate that there is little change even after the third year of treatment.

MEDICAL OPINION

Doctors do not doubt the value of good listening skills and communication, particularly where there has been loss or trauma. Giving patients the emotional help they need can be distressing for practitioners and patients alike, and most doctors stress the need for formal training. Many doctors use trained counselors in their practices, and forms of brief psychotherapy are widely available. The medical profession, however, is skeptical of more extreme theories and therapies.

CONSULTING A PRACTITIONER

There are many reasons why you may consult a psychotherapist or counselor: a life event may have triggered powerful emotions, or you may be distressed for reasons that you do not comprehend. The inability to make a major decision may be affecting your life, or you may have a history of relationship problems and wish to understand why.

It can be difficult to decide which type of therapy to choose, particularly as many practitioners adapt a range of approaches. Try to be as clear as possible about what you want to be doing differently at the end of treatment.

The initial consultation is a chance to see if you feel comfortable with the type of therapy and the practitioner. You will be asked to explain why you think you need help, and the practitioner will decide whether she can help you. Some practitioners offer the first consultation without charge, particularly if therapy is likely to be long term. It is important to be able to talk freely to your practitioner, so if you cannot do so on your first visit, do not hesitate to find someone else. Always ask how long therapy is likely to last, and if there will be regular progress reviews.

PRECAUTIONS

- When choosing a practitioner ask about training and qualifications, and whether he or she belongs to a professional body (see page 318).
- It is essential to trust your practitioner. Remember that you are paying for treatment and are entitled to stop therapy whenever you wish.
- Avoid psychoanalysis, psychotherapy, or counseling if you have any psychotic illness, such as schizophrenia or manic depression.
- See also page 52.

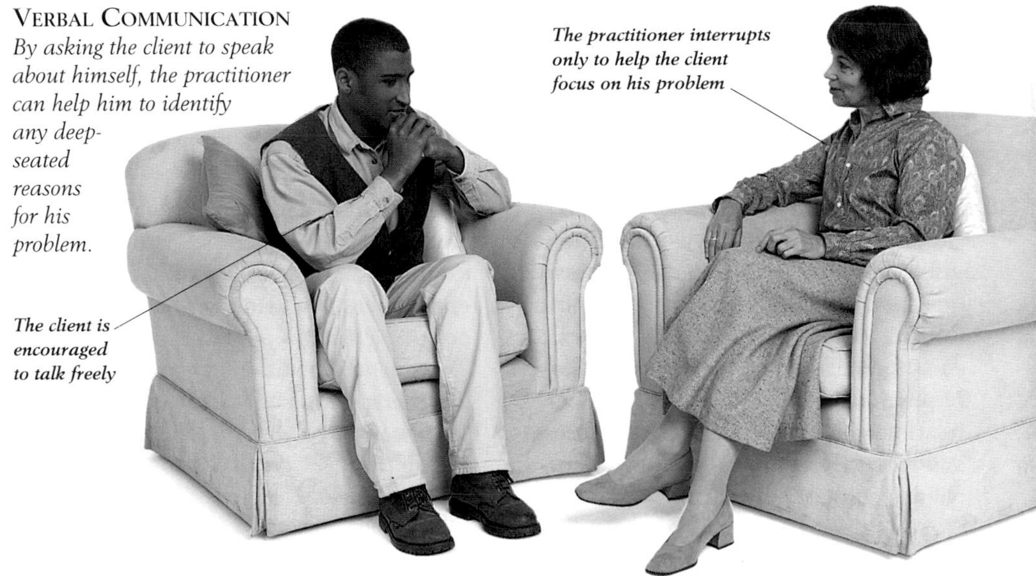

VERBAL COMMUNICATION
By asking the client to speak about himself, the practitioner can help him to identify any deep-seated reasons for his problem.

The client is encouraged to talk freely

The practitioner interrupts only to help the client focus on his problem

YOUR QUESTIONS

How long does a treatment session last?
The usual length is 50–60 minutes.

How many sessions will I need?
Sessions are usually held at least once a week. The length of treatment varies widely, from a few months to several years or more, depending on the approach.

Will it be distressing?
Therapy may release disturbing emotions. Your practitioner must be trained to help you work through these.

Will there be any aftereffects?
Provided your practitioner has been fully trained by a recognized institution and long-term treatment is properly reviewed, there should be no negative aftereffects.

A Client's Experience

Agnes, 34, saw a psychotherapist because of her bad relationship with an ex-boss: "The therapist would wait for me to speak and there was no social chitchat. I thought my problems were tied up with my boss, but once I started talking about my childhood, I realized my father was a similar man. He was always shouting at me, and I never answered him back. Talking to the therapist, I found myself crying in anger. Because my boss had unconsciously reminded me of my dad, I couldn't stand up to him and had to leave the job. Knowing why now makes a difference, and I feel stronger when I see my father."

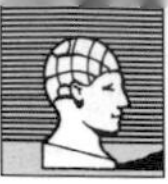

HYPNOTHERAPY

RATINGS	
EVIDENCE	
MEDICAL OPINION	
PRACTITIONER	
SELF-HELP	
COMPATIBILITY	

FOR CENTURIES, DIFFERENT CULTURES have experimented with inducing trance-like states by hypnosis, to promote healing. The founder of modern hypnosis was Franz Anton Mesmer, whose treatment of patients in the 18th century gave his name to "mesmerism." Practitioners induce a state of consciousness akin to deep daydreaming, in which the patient is deeply relaxed and open to suggestion and can be desensitized to fears, phobias, or pain. Hypnotherapy has moved away from earlier associations with quackery and gained respect within the medical establishment, but has yet to be incorporated into mainstream practice.

MAIN USES

- Pain relief
- Fears, phobias
- Stress, anxiety
- Depression
- Insomnia
- Digestive disorders
- Addictions
- Weight problems
- Menstrual problems
- Asthma, allergies
- Skin conditions

HISTORY

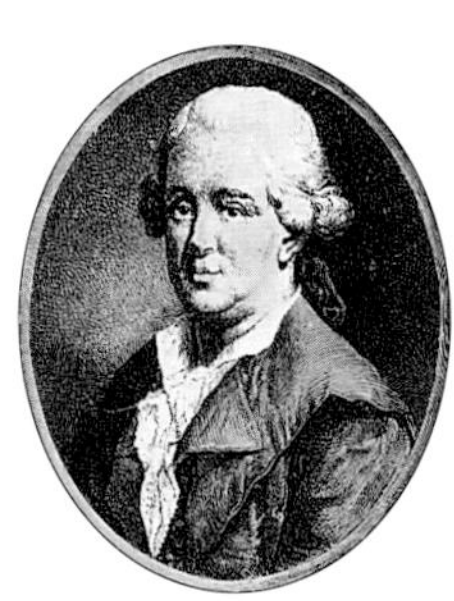

***Franz Anton Mesmer** practiced a form of hypnosis using magnets to balance the so-called "animal magnetism" in the human body. Mesmer's techniques were controversial, but interest in "mesmerism" has never faded.*

The ancient Egyptians and Greeks are said to have used healing trances, and tribal cultures in Africa and the Americas have long used dancing and drumming to hypnotic effect. Hypnotherapy, however, is generally understood to have evolved from the work of 18th-century Austrian doctor Franz Anton Mesmer. He was eventually branded a charlatan and "mesmerism" was denounced, but in 1843 a Scottish surgeon, James Braid, attempted to explain trances in scientific terms. Surgery was performed under what Braid termed "hypnosis," but the medical establishment remained uninterested, especially after the discovery of the anesthetic properties of ether in the 1840s. In the 1890s, the publication of Braid's papers in both French and German sparked new interest, and a "school of hypnotism" was founded in Nancy, France.

Sigmund Freud used hypnosis in his early work, but later preferred to work with the patient fully conscious (see page 162). In the 1950s and 1960s an American psychotherapist, Milton H. Erickson, developed the modern form of hypnotherapy, which is widely used in the West. Although the US and UK medical authorities recommend its inclusion in doctors' training, medical students rarely receive such teaching.

KEY PRINCIPLES

Practitioners believe that the mind has different levels of consciousness. Under hypnosis, the conscious, rational part of the brain is temporarily bypassed, making the subconscious part, which influences mental and physical functions, extremely receptive to suggestion. Although hypnosis may be light, medium, or deep, a medium trance is usually used, during which metabolism, breathing, and heartbeat slow and the brain produces alpha waves (see page 175).

It is claimed that 90% of the population is capable of entering a hypnotic state. Of these, 10% are highly hypnotizable and can be taken into a deep trance, in which minor operations may be performed without anesthesia. Imaginative people who are easily absorbed in what they are doing make the best subjects, but much depends on a willingness to be hypnotized and on a good rapport with the practitioner. Hypnotherapists claim that it is impossible to hypnotize an unwilling person, since the subconscious mind is extremely unlikely to accept unreasonable suggestions.

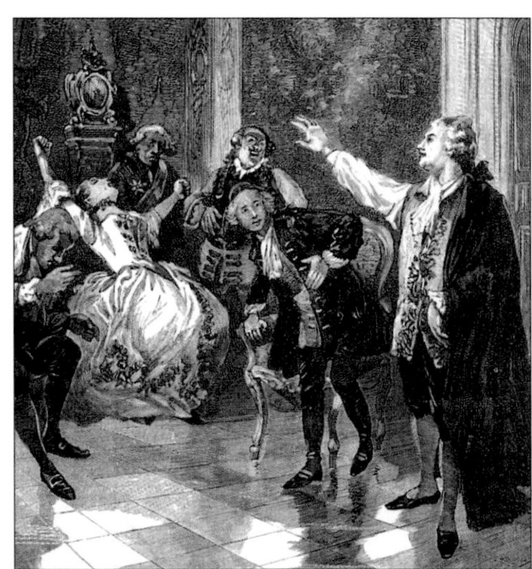

***Mesmer often treated patients** by sending them into therapeutic "crises" of shaking, coughing, and convulsions, after which they felt better.*

EVIDENCE & RESEARCH

There is no doubt that hypnosis works, but how is still a mystery. Some researchers claim that patients "allow" themselves to be hypnotized, and that the relationship between practitioner and patient is the key.

The Laboratory of Hypnosis Research was established at Stanford University in California in the 1960s and similar projects were set up elsewhere in the US, Canada, Europe, and Australia.

Studies published in *The Lancet* in 1989 showed hypnosis to be successful at relieving irritable bowel syndrome. In 1984, an Australian study found that anxiety levels could be controlled with hypnosis, while research in the US revealed that it enabled patients to relax during dental surgery.

Two trials published in the 1960s in the *British Medical Journal* showed hypnosis to be an effective treatment for asthma. In 1953, a study conducted by the British Medical Association concluded that it was helpful for psychosomatic and psychoneurotic disorders, and for pain relief in surgery, dentistry, and obstetrics.

MEDICAL OPINION

Despite being tainted by the exploits of showmen, hypnotherapy is supported by more scientific evidence than any other complementary therapy. Most doctors would support the use of self-hypnosis (see opposite) as a relaxation technique.

Consulting a Practitioner

Treatment usually consists of one-hour weekly sessions, the number of which varies according to the problem. The practitioner asks you about your physical and mental health, and your motivation to resolve any problem. Hypnosis may not begin until the second session. There are several different schools of hyponotherapy: **Classical induction**: You lie on a reclining chair or couch and the practitioner talks to you in a slow and soothing voice. You may be asked to visualize a walk down a country road, to stare at a light or pencil, or to listen to a series of monotonous statements. The practitioner will usually suggest that you feel heavy and relaxed, and that your eyes are closing. To take you deeper, she may count down from ten to zero or ask you to imagine descending in an elevator. As if in a relaxed daydream, you will still be aware of your surroundings.

"Ericksonian" hypnotherapy: "Ericksonian" hypnotherapists tend not to use classical induction techniques, preferring to use suggestions "strategically" during the "everyday trance" of a patient's daydreams and imagination.

Suggestion hypnotherapy: This is often used to treat addictions. The practitioner tries to "implant" positive suggestions – for example, that a symptom will disappear or a certain pattern of behavior will change.

Analytical hypnotherapy: A practitioner trained in this approach will "regress" you by asking you to recall any buried memories or emotions that might be at the root of your problem.

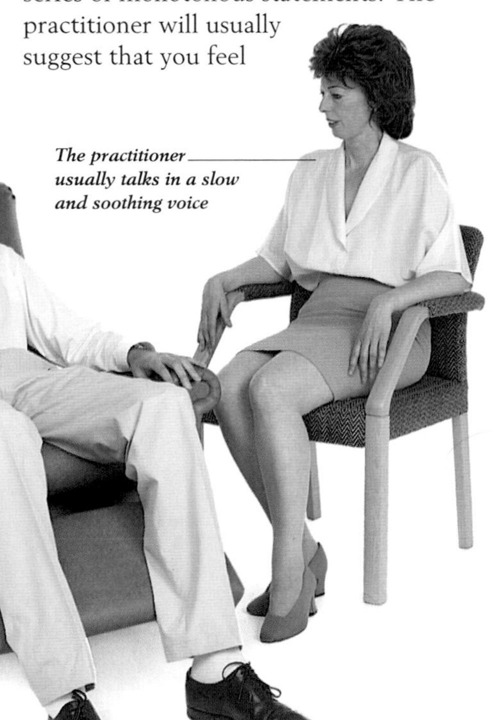

The practitioner usually talks in a slow and soothing voice

Eyes remain closed, as if in a daydream

Limbs feel heavy and breathing is slow

UNDER HYPNOSIS

The practitioner may ask about past experiences to establish reasons for current problems. Alternatively, she may feed suggestions to the patient's subconscious mind, aimed at overcoming specific problems, such as a lack of self-confidence or an addiction to smoking.

PRECAUTIONS

- **It is vital that you choose a trustworthy, qualified practitioner. Follow the checklist on page 318.**
- **Avoid hypnotherapy or self-hypnosis if you have severe depression, psychosis, or epilepsy.**
- **See also page 52.**

Self-Help

Most people can learn to induce hypnosis for themselves. Self-hypnosis may be used to alleviate pain, foster self-confidence and other positive attitudes, and even ease conditions such as asthma and bronchitis. Although the technique can be learned with books and tapes, it may be useful to consult a hypnotherapist first. Many practitioners teach patients to hypnotize themselves as a follow-up to treatment.

It is important to be clear about what you want to achieve from self-hypnosis. For example, if you want to be more confident, ask yourself what makes you nervous. Then try to empty your mind of distracting thoughts by repeating a simple statement such as "Every day, in every way, I am getting better and better." Known as *autosuggestion*, this technique was introduced in the 1920s by a French pharmacist, Emile Coué, whose work has since been incorporated into therapies such as visualization (see page 178).

Self-Hypnosis

1 *Be prepared to spend at least 20–30 minutes every day practicing self-hypnosis. Lie or sit in a quiet, comfortable place where you are unlikely to be disturbed. Relax and release any tension in your body.*

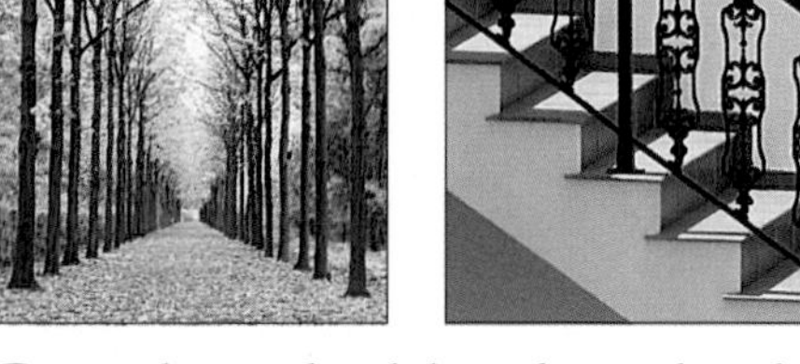

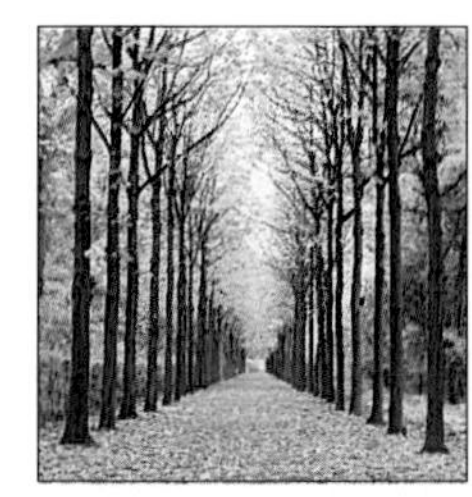

2 *To induce a relaxed, focused state of mind, imagine yourself walking down a long path, or descending a staircase, counting from ten to zero.*

3 *Repeat to yourself key statements that describe what you want to be. Use positive wording; say, "I feel confident" – for example, not "I will not be afraid," or try listening to an audio-tape on which you have previously recorded such messages.*

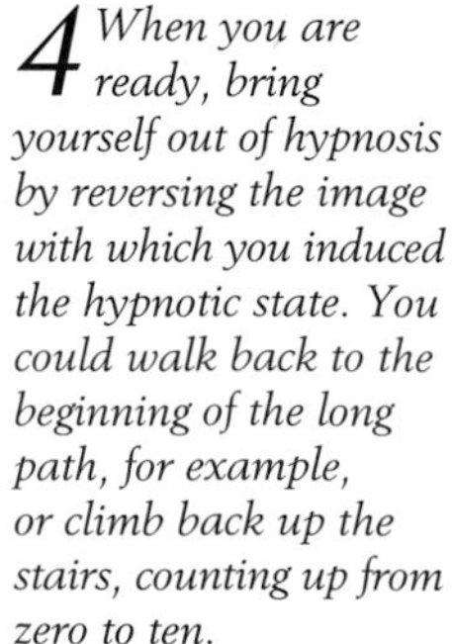

4 *When you are ready, bring yourself out of hypnosis by reversing the image with which you induced the hypnotic state. You could walk back to the beginning of the long path, for example, or climb back up the stairs, counting up from zero to ten.*

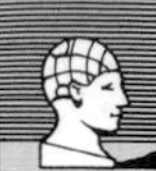

Autogenic Training

Ratings

- Evidence
- Medical Opinion
- Practitioner
- Self-Help
- Compatibility

Developed in Berlin in the 1920s, autogenic training (AT) claims to alleviate physical and mental problems, as well as improve work performance, creativity, and personal relationships. It consists of a series of six mental exercises that allow the mind to calm itself by switching off the "fight-or-flight" stress responses of the body (see page 170). The therapy offers a rational, organized way to relax at will and mobilize the body's self-healing powers. A useful self-help treatment for stress-related conditions, AT became more established in the 1970s and is now practiced worldwide.

Main Uses

- Stress-related conditions, such as high blood pressure, eczema, migraines, insomnia, depression, nervous tension, irritable bowel syndrome, ulcers
- PMS
- Addiction
- Alleviation of the symptoms of AIDS

History

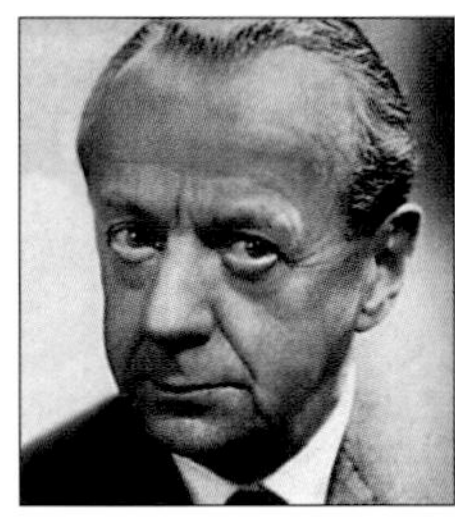

***Dr. Schultz**, founder of autogenic training, was influenced by 19th-century studies in which patients practicing self-hypnosis reported improved well-being and relief from tension and fatigue.*

Autogenic training was developed in the 1920s by Dr. Johannes Schultz, a German neurologist and psychiatrist. The word autogenic means "generated from within" in Greek. Dr. Schultz devised six silent verbal exercises for the mind which were further developed in Canada by his colleague, Dr. Wolfgang Luthe. Now available worldwide, AT is used in some corporate staff-training programs.

Standard Positions

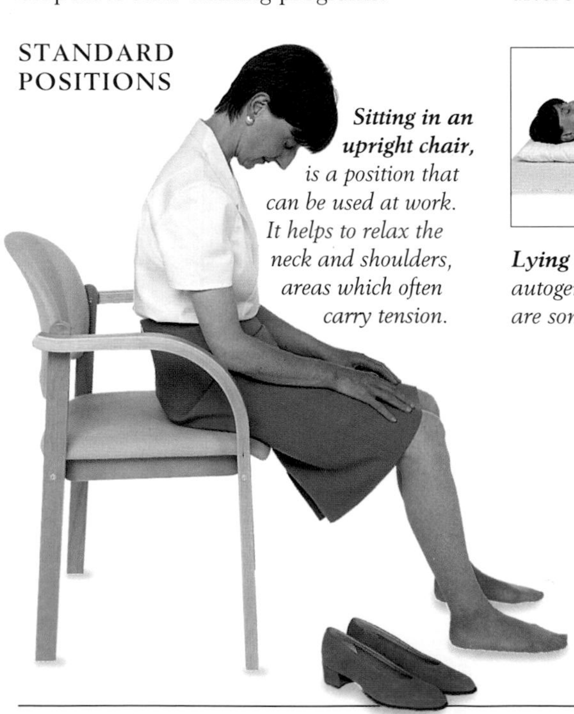

***Sitting in an upright chair,** is a position that can be used at work. It helps to relax the neck and shoulders, areas which often carry tension.*

Consulting a Practitioner

Autogenic training is usually taught in groups of 6–8 patients, or on a one-to-one basis, in eight 90-minute weekly sessions.

Before instruction, your medical history will be taken, and your physical and psychological suitability evaluated. The six exercises taught by the practitioner are done sitting or lying down, so comfortable clothes should be worn. Each exercise aims to induce relaxation in different areas of the body: heaviness in the limbs, neck and shoulders; warmth in the limbs; a calm heartbeat; relaxed breathing; warmth in the stomach; and coolness in the forehead. Throughout the sequence, you will be asked to repeat set phrases, such as "my right arm is heavy," and, with practice, you should be able to reach an altered state of consciousness known as "passive concentration." This is similar to meditation (see page 174) and boosts the body's self-healing processes.

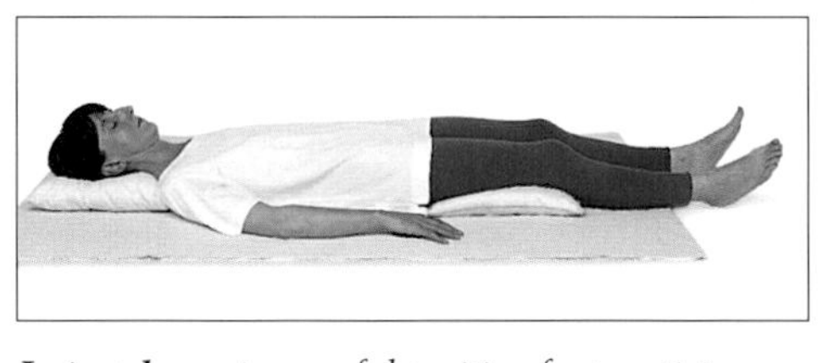

***Lying down** is a useful position for practicing autogenic exercises when going to sleep. Pillows are sometimes placed under the head and knees.*

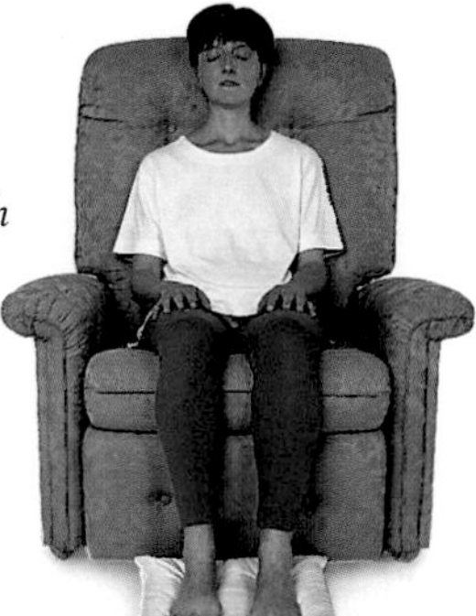

***Sitting in an armchair** is a comfortable position, which can easily be adapted for practicing AT in a bus, train, or plane.*

At a more advanced level, "autogenic modification" involves adopting formulas that focus on specific issues; someone with asthma, for example, may use the phrase "my sinuses are cool, my chest is warm."

Your practitioner can also teach you ways to cope with grief, anger, or anxiety, since repressed emotions ("autogenic discharges") may arise during treatment.

It is essential that you practice autogenic exercises between classes, about 15 minutes, three times a day, noting your responses for the next session. Once taught, you can use AT as self-treatment.

Evidence & Research

The therapeutic effects of AT are reported in more than 3,000 scientific papers. Many examples of physiological and brain-wave changes have been noted, which, when measured, resemble those produced in meditation. The Schultz Institute in Berlin and the Oskar Vogt Institute in Japan are leading research centers.

Medical Opinion

Autogenic training's structured approach has become relatively well-established as a relaxation technique, and a few doctors are beginning to refer patients for AT.

Precautions

- Check with your doctor if you have psychiatric problems.
- Advise the practitioner if you are pregnant or have a heart condition or diabetes.
- See also page 52.

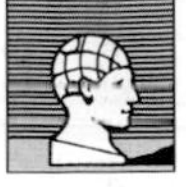

BIOFEEDBACK

RATINGS

EVIDENCE	
MEDICAL OPINION	
PRACTITIONER	
SELF-HELP	
COMPATIBILITY	

IN THE 1960S, AMERICAN SCIENTISTS began training people to control heart rate and other subconscious biological functions by using electronic "biofeedback" instruments that monitored subtle physical responses. Electrodes or probes are used to attach patients to the biofeedback device, and signals, such as electronic beeps, flashes, or needles on a dial, "feed back" information about changes in the body. By responding to these signals, patients can learn to self-regulate body functions. The technique is often used to treat stress-related ailments, and is practiced in North America, the UK, and Australasia.

MAIN USES

- Stress-related conditions, such as high blood pressure, anxiety, insomnia, headaches, migraines, asthma, irritable bowel syndrome
- Muscle disorders & weakness after surgery
- Incontinence
- Raynaud's disease

HISTORY

In the early 1940s US and UK scientists developed electronic devices to detect minute physical responses. At first, publicity focused on obtaining electrical signals from the brain, but the work of American scientists in the 1960s confirmed biofeedback's therapeutic value. Drs. Elmer and Alyce Green of the Menninger Foundation in Kansas used the method to study states of mind during yoga meditation; by the 1980s stress management courses using biofeedback were introduced to American primary schools. In the 1990s, better computer technology prompted further research.

CONSULTING A PRACTITIONER

The practitioner will show you how to use the biofeedback device, of which there are several types: a *skin temperature* (ST) gauge registers heat changes in the skin, a *galvanic skin response* (GSR) sensor measures the skin's electrical conductivity by the amount of sweat produced under stress, *electromyographs* (EMGs) use auditory or visual signals to indicate muscle tension, *electroencephalographs* (EEGs) show brain-wave activity, and *electro-cardiographs* (ECGs) monitor heart rate. Once the sensors are in place, you are taught to recognize signals that suggest relaxation. Techniques such as breathing and muscle relaxation (see page 170) help achieve the desired response (reduced blood pressure, for example). A state of relaxation is indicated by warm skin, low sweat gland activity, high levels of alpha waves from the brain, and a slow, even heart rate. Biofeedback takes practice; at least six half-hour sessions may be needed.

GSR sensor

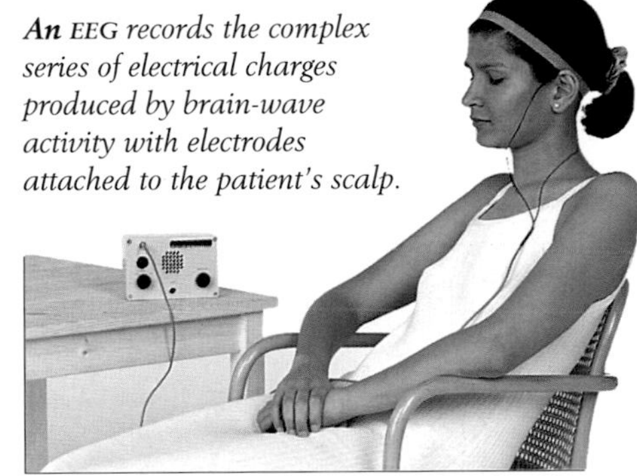

An EEG records the complex series of electrical charges produced by brain-wave activity with electrodes attached to the patient's scalp.

EVIDENCE & RESEARCH

An extensive body of clinical research exists to support the claims of biofeedback. A 1996 study in the US showed that using biofeedback to relax shoulder muscles could ease tension headaches. A 1992 American study showed that muscular pain in the lower back responded to biofeedback, and a US government report in 1992 found patients could control incontinence with the technique. It is also being used at Yale University to control heart rate and blood pressure, and some American doctors use it to treat epilepsy.

MEDICAL OPINION

Few doctors would have once believed that people could learn to influence blood pressure, let alone brain waves. Today, the evidence is conclusive and biofeedback's entry into the medical mainstream seems inevitable, although doctors question its reliability as a form of treatment.

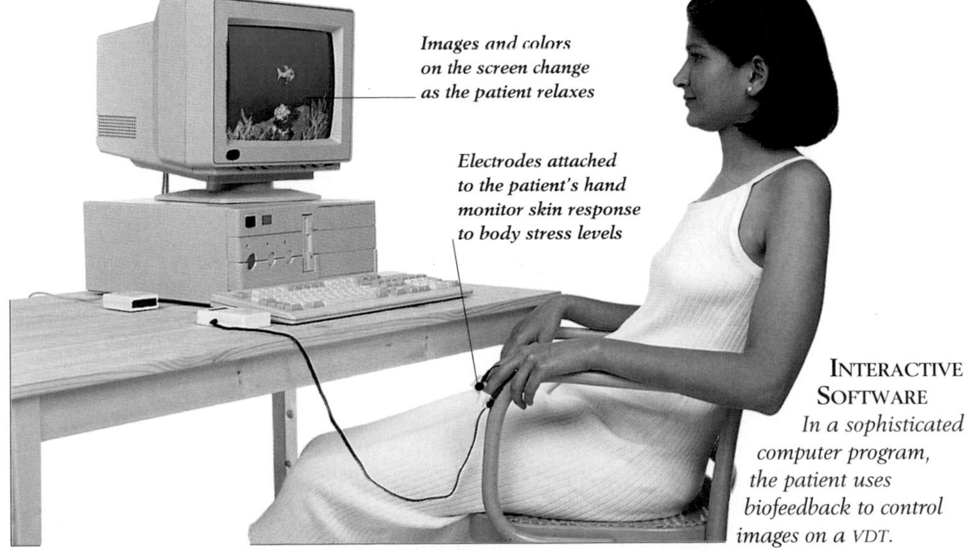

Images and colors on the screen change as the patient relaxes

Electrodes attached to the patient's hand monitor skin response to body stress levels

INTERACTIVE SOFTWARE
In a sophisticated computer program, the patient uses biofeedback to control images on a VDT.

PRECAUTIONS

- Do not change the dosage of any medication you are taking during biofeedback treatment without consulting a doctor.
- See also page 52.

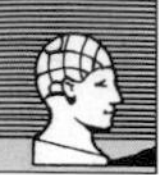

RELAXATION & BREATHING

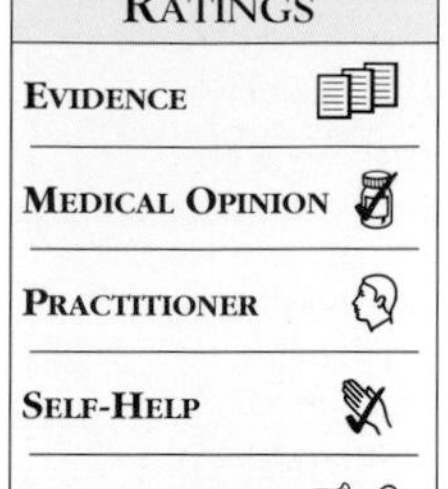

CONTROLLED BREATHING and the ability to relax at will are essential aspects of managing stress, and their importance is recognized by many complementary practitioners, particularly those working with Eastern approaches. Simple breathing exercises and muscle relaxation techniques can be practiced to reduce the physical and mental effects of stress, bringing therapeutic benefits such as lower heart rate, reduced blood pressure, and lower levels of stress hormones. Relaxation techniques are increasingly valued by conventional doctors in the West, and are often taught in hospitals and health centers.

MAIN USES

- **Anxiety, depression**
- **High blood pressure**
- **Insomnia, fatigue**
- **Phobias, panic attacks**
- **Asthma, eczema**
- **Pain relief**
- **Irritable bowel syndrome**
- **PMS, menopausal problems**

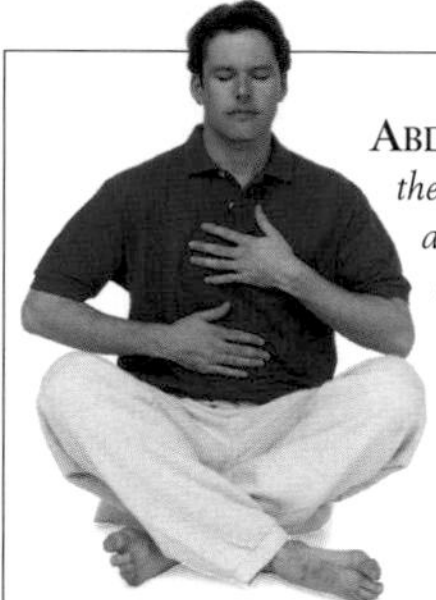

ABDOMINAL BREATHING *is the key to relaxation. It ensures an optimum balance of oxygen and carbon dioxide in the bloodstream and helps the body to release mental and physical tension.*

HISTORY

In Eastern health systems, techniques for breathing efficiently and maintaining a body and mind able to cope with stress have been used for thousands of years. In Western medicine, one of the earliest relaxation techniques was developed in the 1930s by American physiologist Dr. Edmund Jacobson, and is known as "progressive muscle relaxation" (see page 173). In the 1960s, Dr. Herbert Benson of Harvard Medical School researched the therapeutic effects of Transcendental Meditation (see page 174). Similar studies took place at the University of California at Irvine. All the results confirmed that simply sitting in a quiet environment and focusing the mind could affect major physiological systems and reverse the effects of stress. Dr. Benson identified this mental state as the "relaxation response."

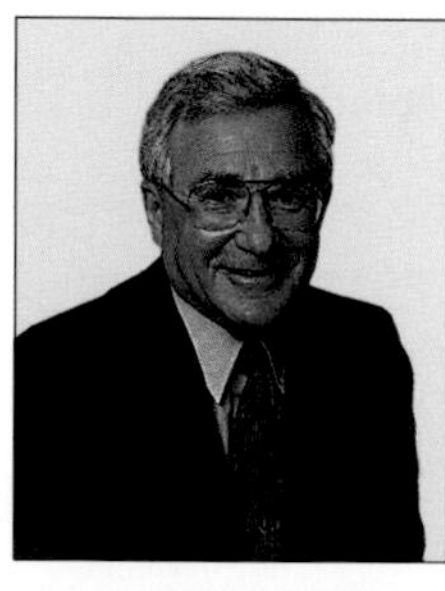

***Dr. Herbert Benson** carried out important research into relaxation after being approached by a group practicing Transcendental Meditation, who claimed they could use the technique to lower blood pressure.*

Many complementary practitioners use relaxation and breathing methods, and a number of hospitals in the US, Europe, and Australia teach progressive muscle relaxation and the relaxation response.

KEY PRINCIPLES

Breathing is involuntary and automatic, but since it can also be consciously controlled, it forms a bridge between mind and body. In Traditional Chinese Medicine (see page 141), good health is said to depend on the harmonious interaction of *qi* ("life energy") in the air with *qi* in the body, through the medium of the lungs. Therapies such as qigong (see page 99) involve breathing exercises to control *qi*. Indian yogis practice *pranayama* to steady the breathing and calm the body and mind (see page 108).

Conventional medicine does not recognize the concept of "life energy," but does acknowledge the important role of efficient breathing in dealing with stress. When stress triggers the body's "fight-or-flight" response (see opposite), breathing becomes quick and shallow, reinforcing the messages of alarm being sent to the brain. If this "overbreathing" continues, too much carbon dioxide is removed from the blood, which then loses its proper acidity. This directly affects the nerves and muscles, prompting symptoms such as faintness, palpitations, and panic attacks (see page 288). Conditions such as these may be alleviated by slow, abdominal breathing, often practiced in conjunction with muscle relaxation and visualization (see page 178). These techniques calm both body and mind, and help to "turn off" the fight-or-flight response, so enhancing well-being throughout the whole body.

EVIDENCE & RESEARCH

According to studies conducted since the 1970s at the Mind/Body Medical Institute of Harvard Medical School (founded by Dr. Herbert Benson), relaxation-response techniques coupled with nutritional advice and exercise helped stress-related conditions. UK researchers looking at children with asthma reported that relaxation techniques significantly reduced the incidence of attacks; their findings were published in the *Journal of Psychosomatic Research* in 1993. In a 1992 study published in the *American Journal of Occupational Therapy*, eight out of ten children with persistent headaches who had relaxation training found that their condition improved. In 1986, the *British Journal of Psychiatry* included a study showing that relaxation helped treat anxiety. An American study published in *Psychological Reports* in 1985 revealed that progressive muscle relaxation reduced epileptic seizures by 30%.

Other studies are more ambiguous. In a 1990 report in the *British Medical Journal*, relaxation techniques had no effect on patients with high blood pressure when they were monitored over 24 hours.

MEDICAL OPINION

Teaching patients to relax, especially in cases of persistent or relapsing illness, does no harm and often helps alleviate feelings of distress and helplessness. However, doctors do not consider that relaxation and breathing techniques offer a total solution to stress-related conditions. There may be psychological issues to consider, and practitioners should take into account *why* a patient has lost the ability to relax.

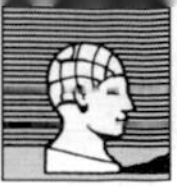

THE THEORY OF RELAXATION & BREATHING

With each breath, oxygen is absorbed into the blood, enabling production of the energy that fuels every body function. Under stress, breathing tends to be rapid, using the top half of the lungs. This causes a drop in blood levels of carbon dioxide, which is needed to maintain blood acidity. This can lead to tiredness and anxiety and create tension in the upper back, shoulders, and neck. Abdominal breathing, which allows the lungs to expand fully, is a more efficient and calm way to breathe, and has the potential to benefit both physical and mental health.

ABDOMINAL BREATHING

Abdominal, or diaphragmatic, breathing *uses the diaphragm – the sheet of muscle that forms the floor of the chest cavity and the ceiling of the abdomen. On breathing in, the diaphragm contracts and moves downward a bit like the piston of a bicycle pump. At the same time, the abdomen rises and the chest expands slightly as air is drawn in. On breathing out, the diaphragm relaxes and rises, making the space inside the chest cavity smaller and expelling air from the lungs.*

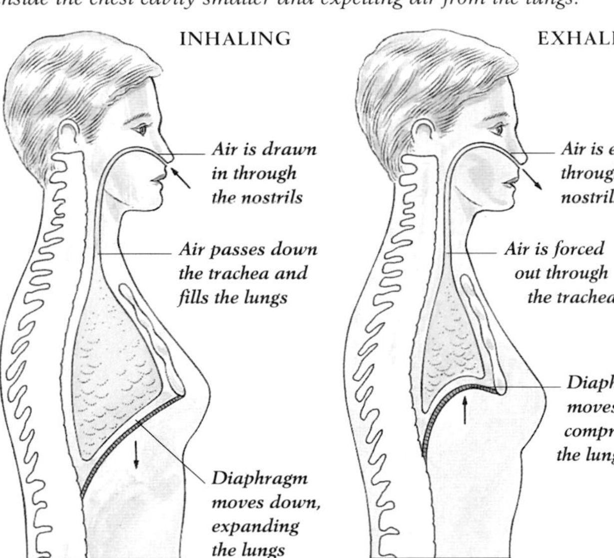

HOW OXYGEN REACHES THE BLOODSTREAM

As air is drawn *into the lungs, alveoli (air sacs) transfer oxygen into the bloodstream and remove carbon dioxide from it.*

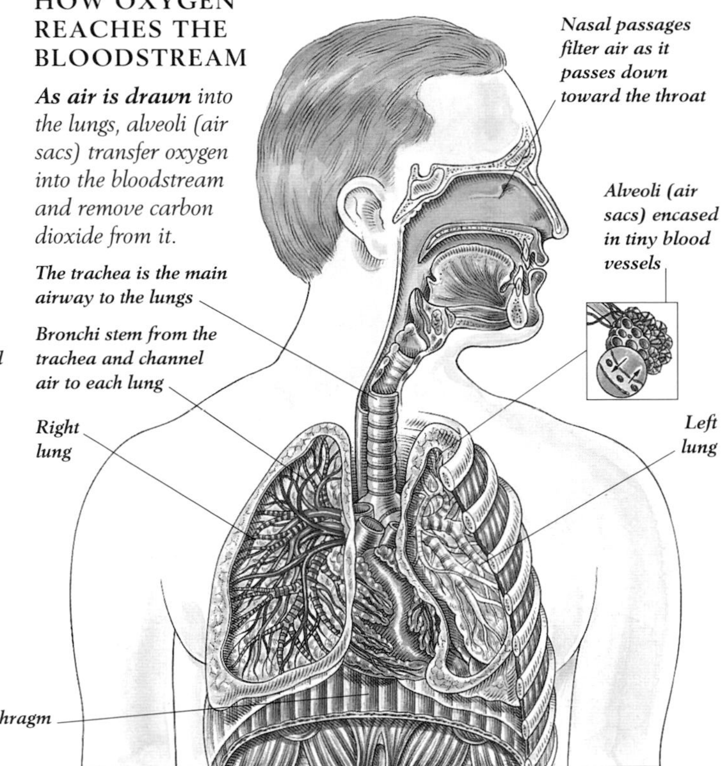

PHYSIOLOGICAL EFFECTS OF STRESS & RELAXATION

Stressful situations trigger the body's fight-or-flight response to stress (see below left and page 38). If stress persists, mental and physical health are undermined, partly because the stress hormones epinephrine and cortisol interfere with functioning of the circulatory and immune systems (see below center and page 27). Relaxation combats many of these effects (see below right).

RESPONSE TO STRESS	LONG-TERM EFFECTS OF STRESS	RESPONSE TO RELAXATION
Epinephrine is released into bloodstream, heart-rate and blood pressure increase	High blood pressure, anxiety, insomnia, irritability	Decreased epinephrine levels, lower blood pressure, less stress on cardiovascular system
Liver releases energy stored as glycogen, blood-sugar and cholesterol levels increase	High cholesterol levels	Decreased blood-sugar and cholesterol levels
Faster breathing, increased metabolic rate	Breathlessness, hyperventilation, palpitations	Slower breathing, improved lung function and metabolic rate
Muscular tension, increased production of lactic acid	Muscular aches and pains, including headaches and back pain	Relaxed muscles, less lactic acid in muscles
Gastric acid increases or decreases, digestive enzymes and peristalsis inhibited	Nausea, indigestion, constipation, ulcers, food intolerances	Improved digestive process
Perspiration increases	Skin rashes, eczema	Improved physiological stability
Increased levels of cortisol, immune system inhibited	Raised cortisol levels increase the risk of problems in the immune system	Increased activity of immune system, less susceptibility to illness
Emotional tension as attention focused on emergency reaction	Emotional outbursts, depression	Emotional calm, increased alertness and energy

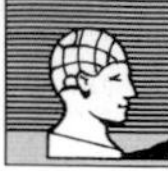

CONSULTING A PRACTITIONER

You may find it difficult to begin a relaxation program on your own, and it is worth consulting a practitioner who can guide you through the exercises on a one-to-one basis or in a group session, and can provide a quiet, calm environment.

On your first visit, the practitioner asks you about your medical history and any lifestyle factors that may be causing stress or anxiety. Depending on the relaxation method used, you will be asked to sit in a chair, or lie on a firm bed or on a mat on the floor. Speaking in a quiet, calm voice, the practitioner will talk you through techniques such as those shown on these pages. At the end, the practitioner will suggest exercises to do at home, and may give you an audio- or videotape with a relaxation program to follow.

You may be taught relaxation exercises while practicing therapies such as yoga or visualization (see pages 108 and 178).

YOUR QUESTIONS

How long does a session last?
A session that includes a consultation may last up to 60 minutes.

How many sessions will I need?
Depending on your commitment and willingness to practice, you can learn most techniques in 5–10 sessions.

Will it be uncomfortable?
Some people have extremely tense diaphragms and may at first find it hard to breathe in this way. Techniques such as yoga (see page 108) can help.

Are there any aftereffects?
Relaxation techniques may provoke the release of repressed emotions, such as anger or grief. The practitioner will be trained to offer support and guidance.

BREATHING

The first exercise the practitioner may help you to master is abdominal, or diaphragmatic, breathing. This is a gentle, relaxing technique, not necessarily "deep" breathing, which allows the lungs to fill and empty with minimal effort. Once learned, it can be practiced daily, and should take around 10–15 minutes to complete. If you feel faint and dizzy at any time during the exercise, you are probably overexerting yourself. Stop and breathe in your usual way for a few minutes until the sensation passes.

Abdominal breathing forms part of many complementary therapies, but a conventional doctor can also advise you on breathing techniques for relaxation.

PRECAUTIONS

- See page 52.

BREATHING EXERCISE

1 Remove your shoes and loosen any tight clothing. Sit in a comfortable position with your back supported. A cross-legged position suits some people; alternatively, you may prefer to sit on a chair, or lie on a mat or a firm bed, with a small pillow to support your head. If you want to, close your eyes.

2 Place one hand on your upper chest and the other on your abdomen just below your breastbone. Notice which hand moves when you breathe. If the hand on your chest moves more than the one on your abdomen, then your breathing is mainly in the upper chest. Try to breathe so that only your lower hand is moving.

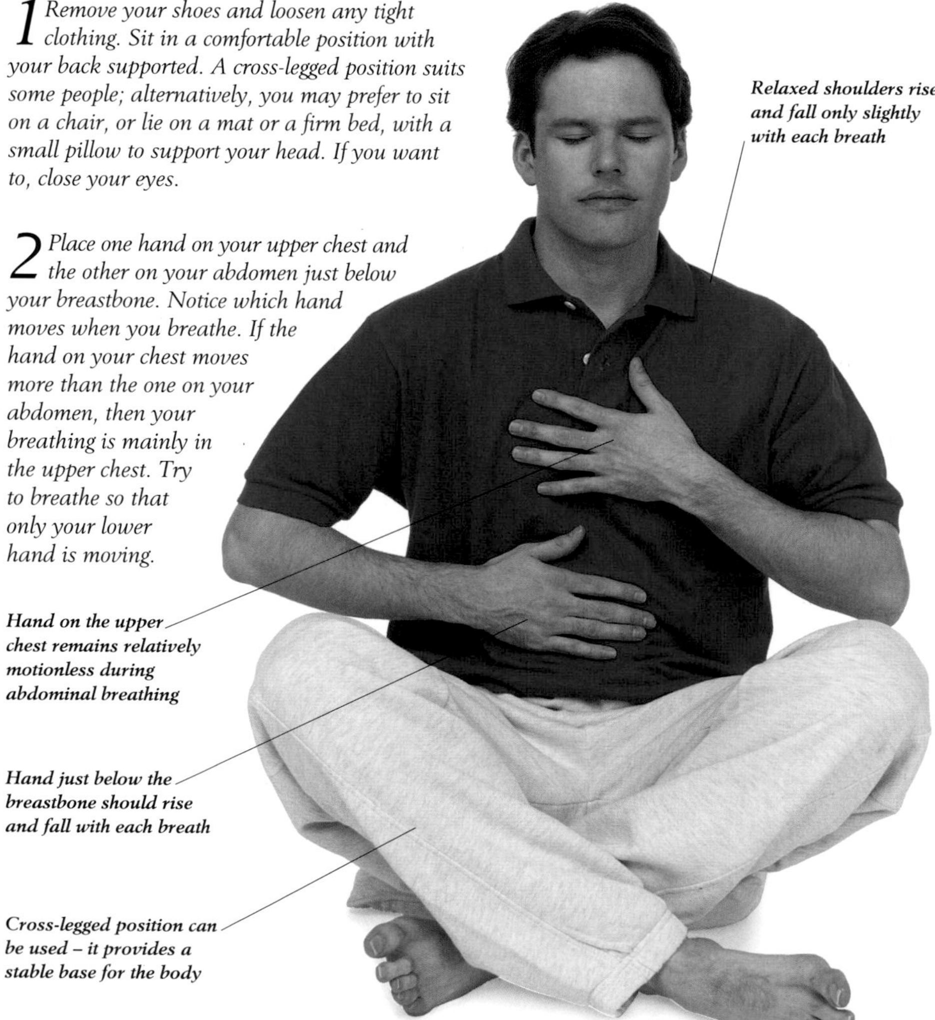

Relaxed shoulders rise and fall only slightly with each breath

Hand on the upper chest remains relatively motionless during abdominal breathing

Hand just below the breastbone should rise and fall with each breath

Cross-legged position can be used – it provides a stable base for the body

3 Place both hands on your abdomen below the ribs. Breathe in slowly through your nose, allowing your abdomen to rise as your diaphragm moves down.

Fingers move up and apart when breathing in

4 Pause for a few seconds between breaths, then breathe out slowly through your nose, feeling your abdomen fall as your diaphragm relaxes. Let as much air out of your lungs as possible.

5 Repeat three or four times. Throughout the exercise, try to relax your muscles and concentrate on your breathing, not on any thoughts that come to you. As you breathe, notice whether your chest is moving up and down with each breath. It should be relatively still if your abdomen is doing the work.

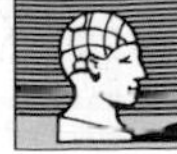

RELAXATION

When body and mind are under pressure, muscles become tense, resulting in aches and pains and fatigue (see page 26). A practitioner trained in a therapy such as massage (see page 56) or osteopathy (see page 76) can help you to become aware of any tension patterns in your body through touch and manipulation. Physical exercise classes often include stretching techniques designed to free muscular tension.

The muscle relaxation exercise below involves systematically tensing and releasing all the major muscle groups in the body, and is often taught in relaxation classes. Remove your shoes and loosen any tight clothing. Lie on a mat on the floor, or on a firm bed, your head supported by a small pillow. Your head, torso, and legs should be in a straight line, with your feet apart and hands by your sides.

Throughout the exercise, you will be asked to feel the difference between tension and relaxation. The practitioner may suggest that you repeat a phrase to yourself as you release each muscle, such as "Relax and let go." At first, you may find it difficult to relax for very long, but with practice you should be able to do the exercise while sitting on a train or at a desk; at bedtime, it will encourage sleep. Try to practice for 10–15 minutes daily.

A Patient's Experience

Arnold, 45, runs a small construction company: "I was waking up tired and finding it hard to concentrate. I had tingling fingers and toes, numbness in my hands and arms, and heart palpitations. My doctor said I was breathing too rapidly – a sign of stress. She showed me how to breathe with my diaphragm, but I found it difficult until I saw an osteopath, who now supervises me. Listening to a relaxation tape helps me release tension and I've followed advice on setting goals and making time for myself. My symptoms are better, but they return if I'm overworked, so then I have to pay extra attention to breathing and relaxation techniques."

PROGRESSIVE MUSCLE RELAXATION

1 Close your eyes and be aware of the weight of your body. Focus on the rhythm of your breathing and the rise and fall of your abdomen. Try to breathe more slowly than usual, emphasizing the out-breath and pausing before you breathe in again.

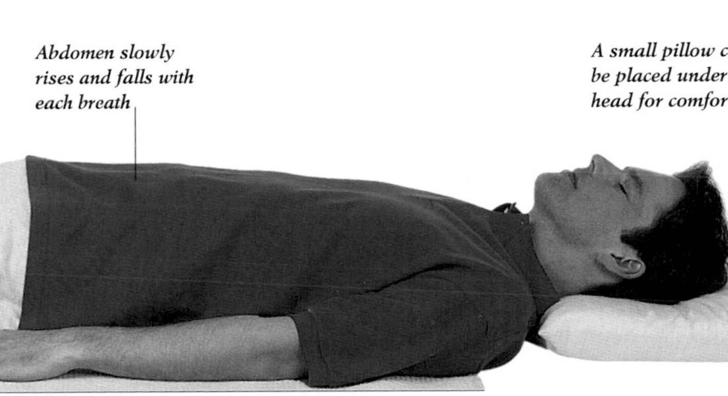

Abdomen slowly rises and falls with each breath

A small pillow can be placed under the head for comfort

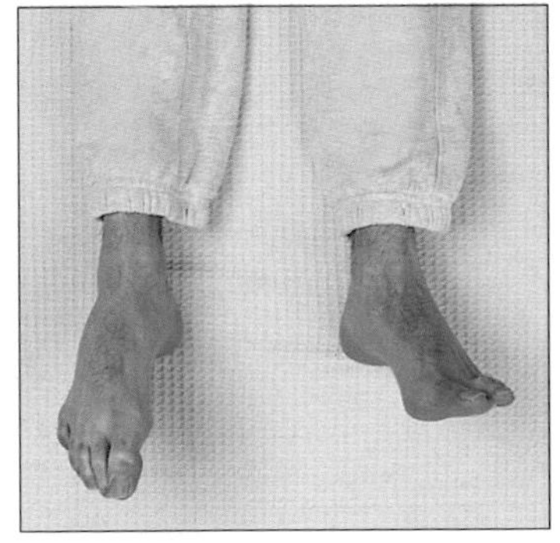

2 Tense the muscles in your right foot, hold for a few seconds, then release. Tense and release the calf, then the thigh muscles. Repeat the process with the left foot and leg.

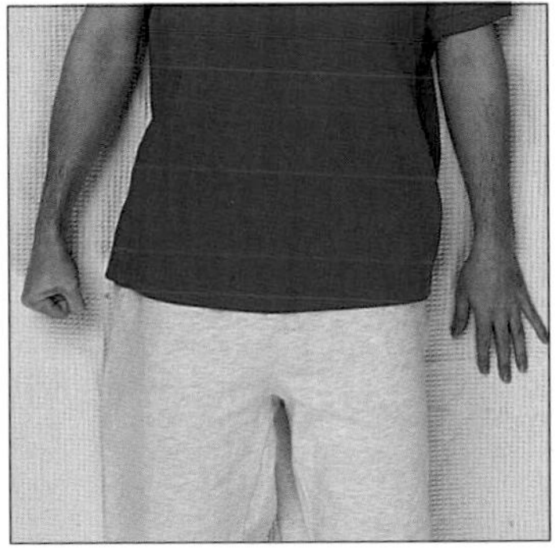

3 Tense and relax each buttock in turn, then your stomach muscles. Clench and release your right fist, then all the muscles in your arm. Repeat the process with the left arm.

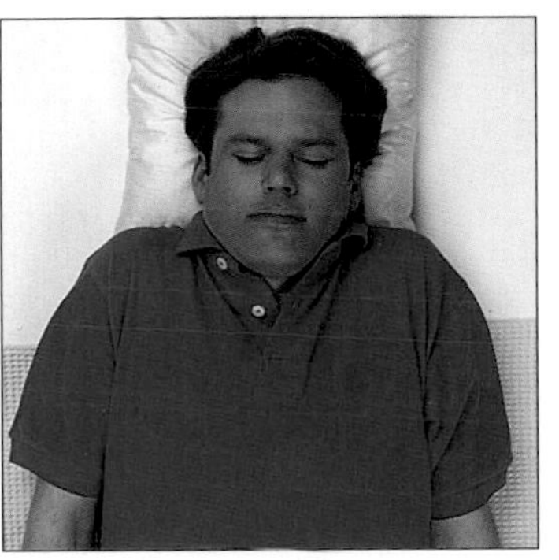

4 Lift your shoulders up to your ears. Hold for a few seconds, then lower again. Repeat 2–3 times. To free the neck, rock your head gently from side to side.

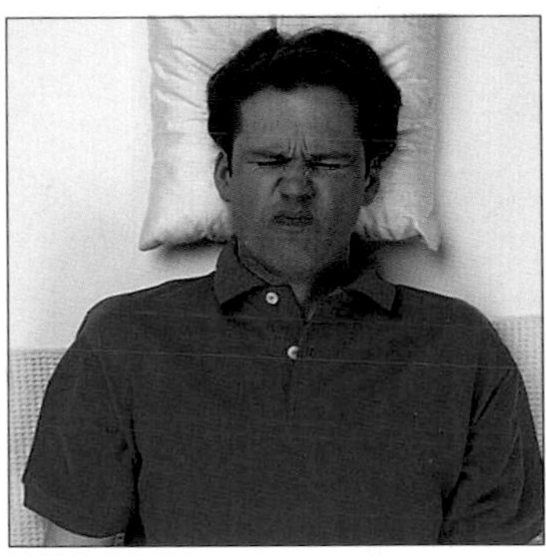

5 Yawn, then relax. Twist your mouth into a pout, and release. Frown, scrunch up your nose, then let go. Raise your eyebrows, then relax all the muscles in your face.

6 Focus on your breathing again, and tell yourself that you feel peaceful and warm. When you are ready, wriggle your toes and fingers and ease your back muscles. Gently bend your knees and roll onto one side for a while, then slowly get up.

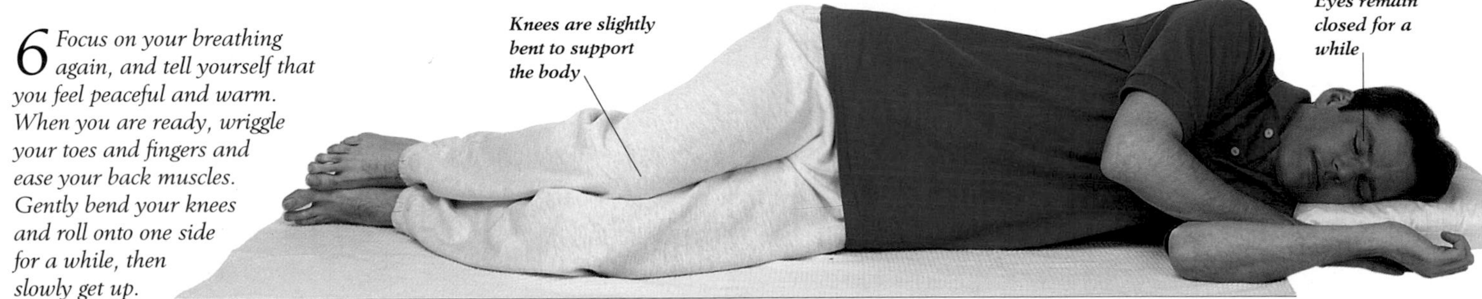

Knees are slightly bent to support the body

Eyes remain closed for a while

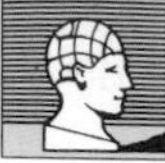

MEDITATION

RATINGS

- EVIDENCE
- MEDICAL OPINION
- PRACTITIONER
- SELF-HELP
- COMPATIBILITY

A MENTAL DISCIPLINE included in the practice of many world religions, meditation is intended to induce a state of profound relaxation, inner harmony, and increased awareness. Various techniques can be used during meditation; all involve focusing the mind on a particular object or activity, and disregarding distractions. Meditation has been shown to reverse the body's "fight-or-flight" response to stress, and while it is practiced as a means of spiritual enlightenment in Eastern societies, in the West it is widely used in a nonreligious context to treat stress-related conditions.

MAIN USES

- Stress, anxiety
- High blood pressure
- Headaches, migraines
- Fatigue, depression, insomnia
- Long-term pain
- Addictions
- Enhancing the immune system
- Personal development

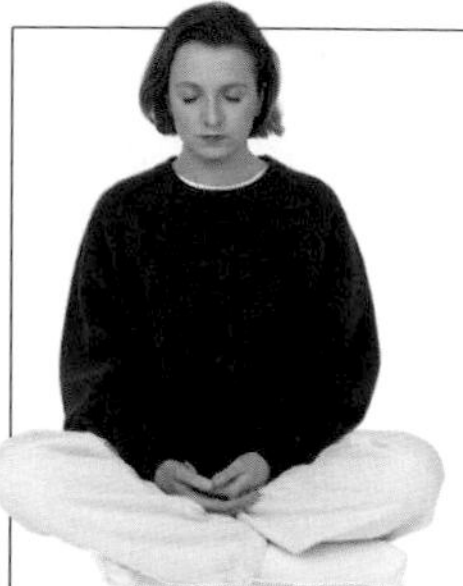

MEDITATION *is a state of heightened mental awareness and inner peace that brings mental, physical, and spiritual benefits. It is a useful self-help technique and can be practiced without adherence to any religion or philosophy.*

HISTORY

Meditative techniques are practiced in all the world's major religions, including Christianity, Judaism, Islam, Buddhism and Hinduism. In the West, meditation has traditionally taken the form of prayer and contemplation. Medieval Christian mystics, such as Hildegard of Bingen and Meister Eckhart, spoke of withdrawing to a level beyond ordinary consciousness. The Eastern Orthodox Church uses the repetitive "Jesus Prayer" as a mantra (a chant to focus the mind, formed from a single word or phrase).

In the East, meditation has long been a way of both achieving bliss and exploring consciousness itself. Indian yoga practices (see page 108) were taken to England by the Theosophists (see page 124) in the late 19th century. This was followed by the introduction of Buddhist practices, especially those of Zen Buddhism, to the US. Both were well established in Europe and the US by the 1960s, when the Indian yogi Maharishi Mahesh introduced Transcendental Meditation (TM) to the West. A form of mantra meditation based on Hindu philosophy, it attracted immense publicity, and scientific research into the therapeutic value of meditation began in the US. Dr. Herbert Benson of Harvard University defined the "relaxation response" (see page 171) after studying the physiological effects of TM meditation on practitioners, and his work encouraged the development of a nonreligious style of meditation. With the exodus of monks from Tibet, yet another form of meditation has reached the West, but TM is still one of the most popular forms of meditation.

KEY PRINCIPLES

The state of meditation can be interpreted in various ways. It may describe a condition in which the mind focuses on a thought or image, a nonjudgmental receptiveness to whatever enters the mind, a state of "relaxed awareness," or one in which the mind is "empty." All involve withdrawing from external reality and achieving deep relaxation and increased mental clarity.

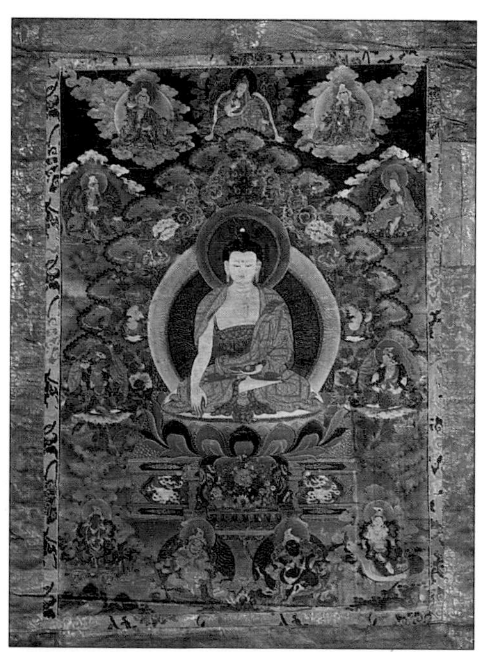

Buddha in a meditative posture, *surrounded by deities, is depicted in this Tibetan* thang-ka, *a banner for a sacred temple.*

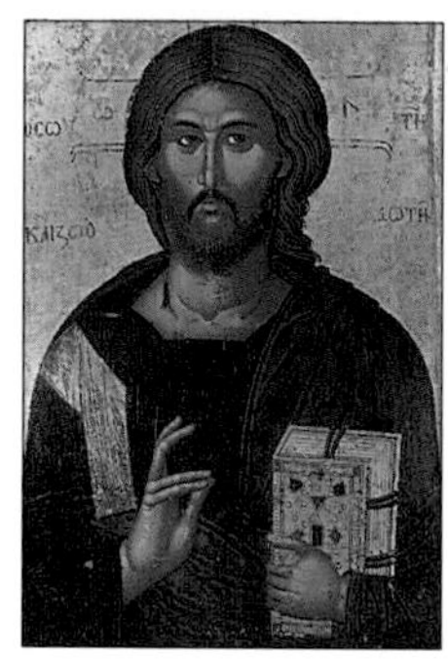

A religious depiction, *such as this 15th-century Greek icon of St. Demetrious of Thessalonik, or any image with spiritual significance for the meditator, may help the mind withdraw from and transcend everyday reality.*

Meditation has been shown to reverse the effects of stress. When under threat, the brain tells the adrenal glands to produce certain hormones in preparation for the "fight-or-flight" response. This causes blood pressure and muscle tension to increase, the heart to pound, and breathing to become fast and shallow (see page 171). Some people find that this response is provoked not only at times of real danger, but when they are faced with what they perceive as stressful situations. In meditation, the brain waves change to a distinctive alpha pattern linked with deep relaxation and mental alertness (see opposite). Regular meditators can shift into this mode at will, which allows them to deal with stress efficiently and counter conditions such as high blood pressure and muscle pain.

Various schools of meditation favor particular techniques. All, however, stress the initial need for a focus of attention to which the mind can return if distracted (see page 176). This may be the rhythm of the breathing, a mantra, a physical object, such as a religious icon, or a repetitive movement, such as t'ai chi ch'uan (see page 100).

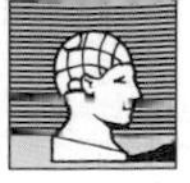

THE THEORY OF MEDITATION

The state of altered awareness and deep relaxation experienced during meditation is associated with distinctive electrical activity in the cortex, or "thinking" part of the brain. This activity can be charted as brain-wave patterns on a graph. Significant psychological and physiological benefits are linked to those patterns that occur during meditation.

THE CORTEX

The cortex is the largest part of the brain. It is where conscious thought arises and sensory perceptions are translated into actions such as speech and movement. It is also the center of imagination and dreams, and its two hemispheres are linked through the midbrain, which generates emotions. These hemispheres are each associated with different kinds of mental activity.

***The two hemispheres** consist of an outer layer rich in nerve cells, called gray matter, and inner areas rich in nerve fibers, called white matter. The "dominant" hemisphere – the left side in most people – deals with logical functions, such as rational thought, calculation, speech, and writing. The "non-dominant" hemisphere – generally the right side – is more intuitive and concerned with creativity, imagination, and emotional responses. Most of the time, the cortex is engaged with social interaction and daily tasks. Consequently, the left side has to work harder than the right side.*

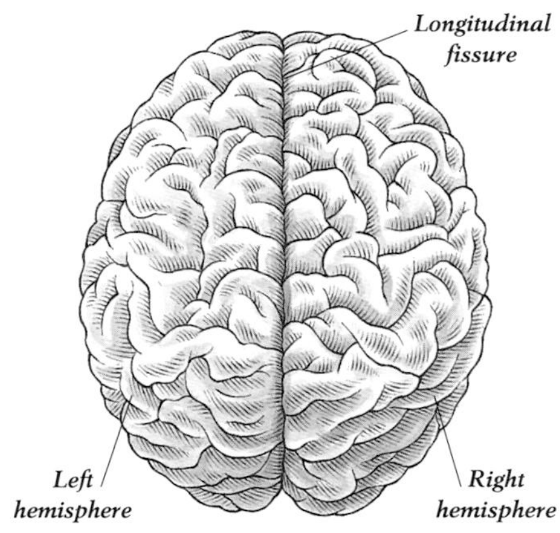

ALPHA WAVES

Normal states of consciousness – sleeping, dreaming, being awake – can be detected in the wave patterns produced by the brain. The state of meditation differs from all three. An electroencephalograph (EEG) can be used to take readings from all over the brain, through the scalp, to monitor mental states. The brain waves associated with quiet, receptive states are called alpha waves, and the EEGs reproduced below show that meditation produces alpha waves of a far higher intensity than those that occur during sleep. In alpha states, the body gradually relaxes as the parasympathetic nervous system (which reverses the fight-or-flight response) predominates.

***During meditation**, high-intensity alpha waves are produced. The hemispheres are fairly synchronized, suggesting an integration of left and right brain.*

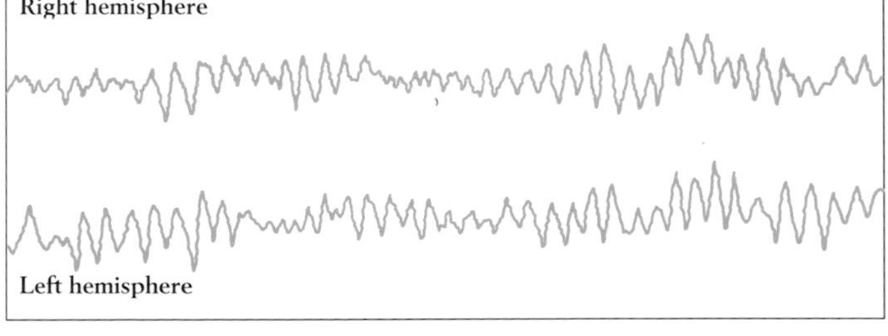

***During sleep**, alpha wave frequency in both hemispheres is of a lower intensity than during meditation, showing that the level of relaxation is less profound.*

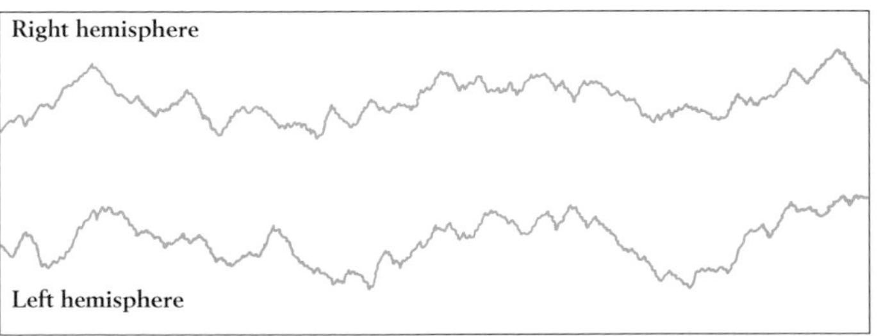

EVIDENCE & RESEARCH

Hundreds of academic papers have been written on TM alone. The American journal *Psychosomatic Medicine* published a study in 1987 comparing 2,000 meditators practicing TM with non-meditators. The TM group made fewer than half the number of doctor visits and spent 50% less time in the hospital, though skeptics point out that social factors may have had more to do with this result than meditation.

In the late 1960s, Dr. Keith Wallace of the University of California in Los Angeles found that the brain became more alert and the body more relaxed during TM. Dr. Benson's research into the relaxation response is widely documented, and his studies suggest that practitioners of advanced meditation have extraordinary physiological control.

Other systems of meditation have also been studied and while each approach has a distinctly different impact on the body and mind, patients generally report greater clarity of thought, calmness, and efficiency in managing time and energy. In the US, Dr. Dean Ornish showed in 1992 that heart disease could be reversed with a lifestyle program that included meditation (see page 243). Results of many other clinical studies include more orderly brain functioning, seen in a synchronization of brain waves between the left and right hemispheres, improved circulation in the fingers and toes, increased cerebral blood flow, and lower levels of stress hormones. Research has also shown reductions in anxiety, mild depression, insomnia, tension headaches, migraines, irritable bowel syndrome, and premenstrual syndrome.

A study reported in 1992 in the *American Journal of Psychiatry* showed that a Buddhist practice of meditation known as *Vipassana* (see page 176) could reduce anxiety, panic, and agoraphobia.

MEDICAL OPINION

A growing number of doctors believe that just as physical exercise and a healthy diet are now acknowledged to be important factors in the prevention and treatment of disease, so conventional medicine will place more emphasis on relaxation and meditation in the future. Some doctors already recommend meditation to their patients as an effective relaxation technique that can help combat stress-related illnesses.

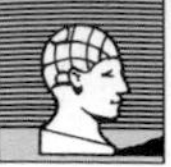

CONSULTING A PRACTITIONER

It is possible to teach yourself to meditate from books, tapes, or videos, but you will probably find it easier to consult a teacher who will show you how to achieve a meditative state, as well as supervise your progress. Sessions may take place on a one-to-one basis or in groups. Practitioners use a variety of techniques (see below); if you do not feel comfortable with one method, try another.

Whichever approach you choose, there are a few basic requirements for practicing meditation successfully: a quiet environment where you can meditate without being disturbed, a comfortable position – usually sitting so as to prevent you from becoming drowsy or falling asleep, and a focus for the mind to help it withdraw from external reality. The object of meditation is a state of "passive awareness," in which the mind is gently directed back to the focus of attention whenever it wanders, which it naturally does. Slow breathing and an awareness of the breath entering and leaving the body also help to promote deep relaxation.

Your practitioner may use language and ideas from a certain faith, such as Buddhism; it is not necessary for you to belong to this or any other faith, and techniques can be adapted to suit the individual. Many practitioners, including teachers of TM, will ask you to repeat a mantra in your head while you meditate. As the session progresses, you may start to feel sleepy, but as you continue to meditate, this will pass and you will become more alert.

You will be advised to meditate on a daily basis for around 15–20 minutes, preferably at the same time of day. First thing in the morning is an ideal time.

YOUR QUESTIONS

How long does a session last?
This depends on the method used; initially 15–20 minutes is common.

How many sessions will I need?
Again, this depends on the method used. Meditation may seem difficult at first.

Will it be uncomfortable?
Some people find it hard to sit still for long; they may prefer active meditation.

Will there be any aftereffects?
Feelings of anxiety may sometimes arise. Depression and withdrawal have been reported by long-term meditators in rare cases. The teacher should help you avoid this.

PRECAUTIONS

- Check with your doctor before starting meditation if you have a history of psychiatric problems.
- See also page 52.

MANTRA MEDITATION

A word or phrase is repeated continually, either silently or aloud. It may relate to your personal beliefs or it can simply be a positive statement.

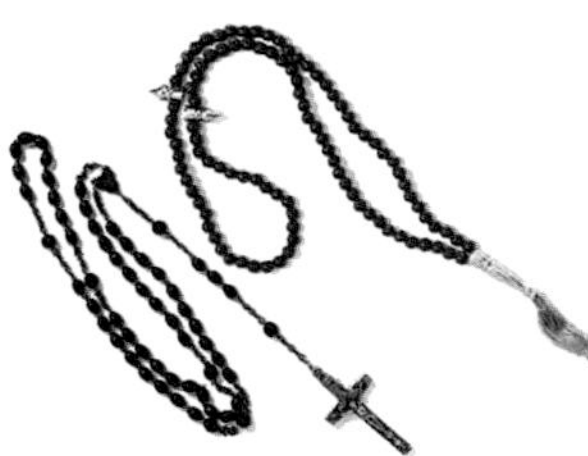

Rosaries: *Rosary beads may be used during meditation to count repetitions of a prayer.*

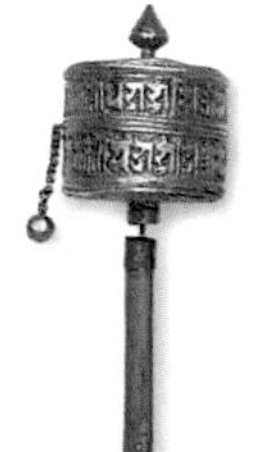

Tibetan prayer wheel: *Each rotation of the cylinder stands for one recitation of a mantra.*

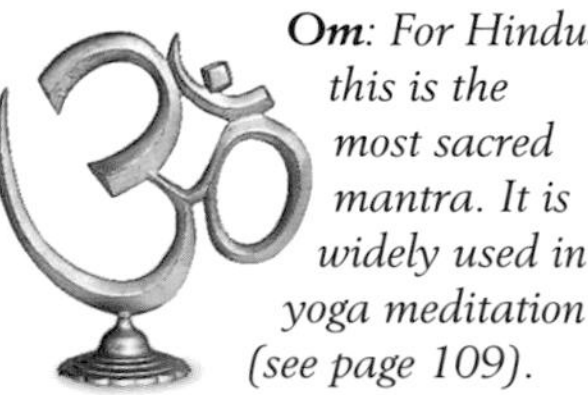

Om: *For Hindus, this is the most sacred mantra. It is widely used in yoga meditation (see page 109).*

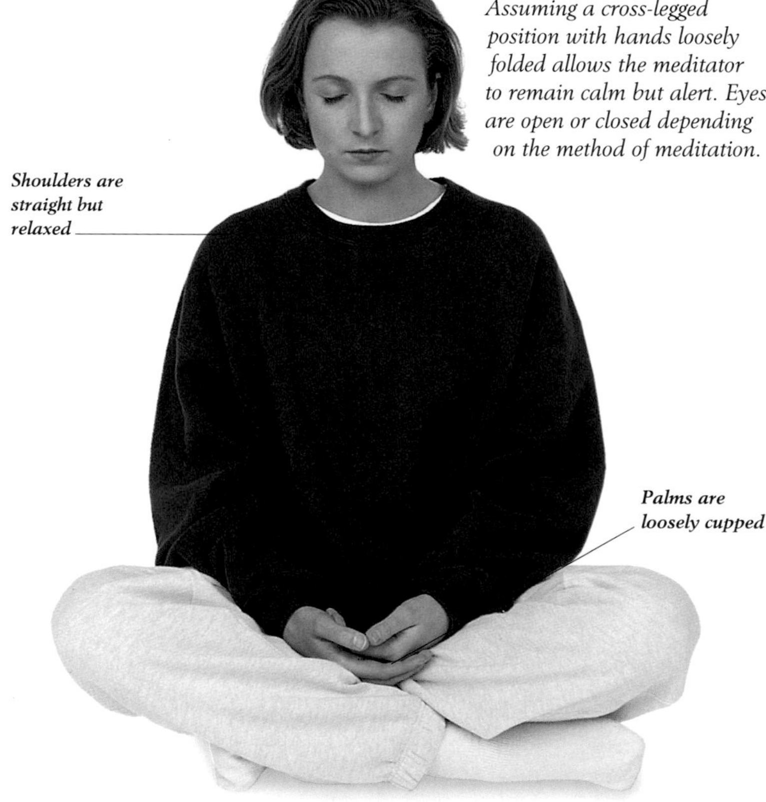

SITTING POSITION
Assuming a cross-legged position with hands loosely folded allows the meditator to remain calm but alert. Eyes are open or closed depending on the method of meditation.

Shoulders are straight but relaxed

Palms are loosely cupped

BREATH AWARENESS

The focus of attention is your breathing. You count *one*, or think of a peaceful word, with each out-breath.

VIPASSANA (MINDFULNESS)

You enter a state of "diffuse openness" – aware of, but detached from, everything you are experiencing.

ACTIVE MEDITATION

T'ai chi, walking, swimming, and other activities involving rhythmic movement can focus the mind.

OBJECT MEDITATION

An object conducive to meditation is chosen. You concentrate on it, feeling its presence and focusing on its shape, weight, texture, and other qualities.

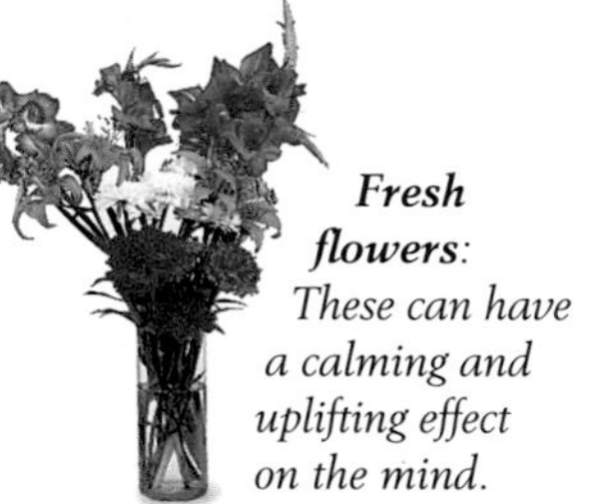

Fresh flowers: *These can have a calming and uplifting effect on the mind.*

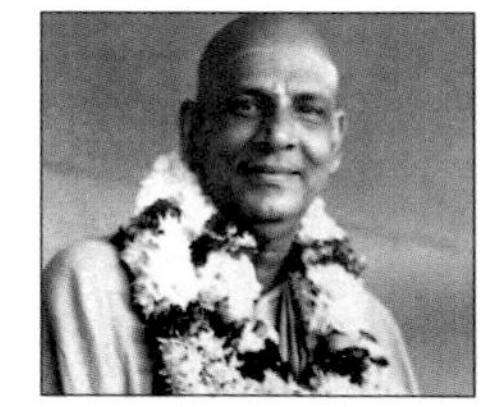

Portrait: *An image of a spiritual leader, or someone you identify with, may help you to focus.*

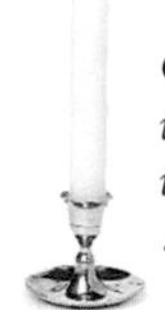

Candle: *The flame is a symbol of the inner light of pure spirituality, which is sought in meditation.*

SELF-HELP

It helps to receive instruction when you learn to meditate, but with discipline and motivation it is possible to teach yourself.

1 Find somewhere quiet and warm where you will not be interrupted as you meditate. Make sure you are wearing comfortable clothes.

2 Begin by sitting for a short time, and gradually build up to longer periods. With practice, it should be possible to sit for 15–20 minutes at least once, and preferably twice, a day, before a meal. If you must keep track of time, open your eyes occasionally to check a strategically placed clock, rather than setting an alarm that could give you a rude awakening. Eventually you will develop a sense of when to finish meditating.

3 A cross-legged pose (see opposite) is not obligatory and you may prefer to sit on an upright chair, with your back straight, and your feet firmly on the ground or a support. Rest your hands on your lap or knees. Imagine a straight line connecting your navel with the tip of your nose, or a string pulling you up from the top of your head. Close your eyes and relax.

4 Breathe slowly and rhythmically. Inhale through your nose and feel the breath move down to your abdomen. Notice which parts of your body are most tense and, as you exhale, imagine the muscles loosening.

5 Focus on the object of your meditation: the rhythm of your breathing; an image, such as a candle flame or a religious symbol; or a word or phrase repeated silently as you exhale.

6 Allow your attention to be passive. When your mind wanders, simply acknowledge what is happening, then return to the focus of meditation.

7 Try to stay as still as possible. If you develop an itch, resist the urge to scratch. Return to the focus of your meditation. The sensation will usually become less intense and disappear.

8 When you are ready, take a full minute before you open your eyes. Then take another minute to become fully aware of your surroundings. Stretch and stand up slowly. If you are interrupted, find the time later to meditate briefly again, and to enter normal consciousness slowly.

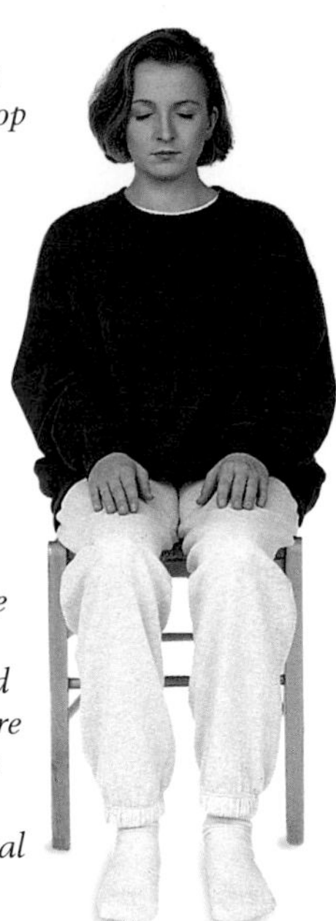

Flotation Therapy

Developed in the US during the 1970s, flotation therapy is a way of isolating body and mind from external stimuli in order to induce deep relaxation. Treatment involves lying in an enclosed and soundproofed tank of water that has sufficient salts and minerals dissolved in it to enable the body to float effortlessly. The therapy is often used to treat stress and addictions.

RATINGS	
EVIDENCE	
MEDICAL OPINION	
PRACTITIONER	
SELF-HELP	
COMPATIBILITY	

MAIN USES

- Stress, anxiety, ulcers
- High blood pressure
- Headaches, migraines
- Addictions
- Heart disease
- Back pain
- Muscle fatigue
- Enhancing the immune system

HISTORY

Flotation therapy developed from the work of Dr. John C. Lilly, an American neurophysiologist and psychoanalyst, who began research in 1954 into how the brain acted without external stimulation. He devised flotation tanks, initially known as "sensory deprivation chambers" until their therapeutic benefits in helping people achieve deep relaxation were recognized. Flotation is well established in the US and is also practiced in the UK, the rest of Europe, and Australia, often as an adjunct to meditation, hypnotherapy, or visualization (see pages 166, 174, and 178).

CONSULTING A PRACTITIONER

Most flotation tanks are installed in health clubs or "float centers," in private rooms containing the tank and a shower, which you use before and after flotation. Tanks are about 8 ft (2.5 m) long and 4 ft (1.25 m) wide, with 10 in (25 cm) of water. Most people float naked, but you may prefer to wear a bathing suit. The practitioner will give you earplugs to use. Flotation takes place in complete or semidarkness, but at any time you can switch on a light, and open the door.

During flotation, the body and mind enter a profound state of relaxation. The brain releases endorphins (see glossary), which act as natural painkillers, and you may experience mild euphoria. Your mind also becomes more receptive to suggestion and daydream. Audio speakers inside the tank may play relaxation or other therapeutic tapes. Many tanks have two-way microphones allowing you to talk to a practitioner of hypnotherapy or psychotherapy; some also have video screens. Sessions last 1–2½ hours and may be repeated as often as you like.

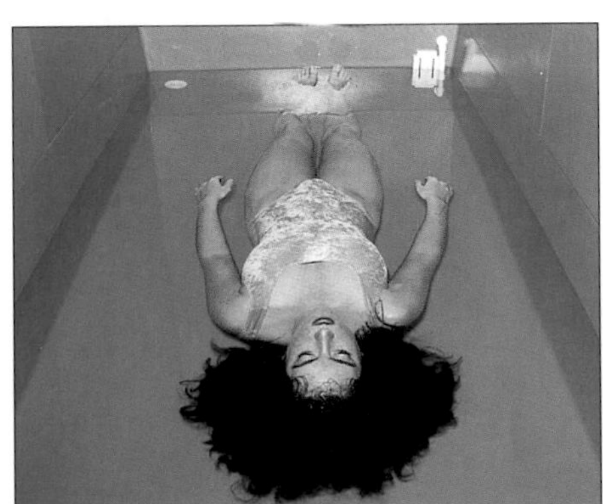

***During flotation**, external sensory stimulation, such as light or sound, is removed. The water is kept at skin temperature (93.5°F/34.2°C).*

MEDICAL OPINION

Most doctors would accept the healing potential of flotation therapy, especially since research indicates that it has the ability to reduce stress hormones in the body and affect psychological states.

PRECAUTIONS

- Make sure you have professional supervision during flotation if you are susceptible to anxiety, depression, or phobias, especially claustrophobia.
- Flotation is not suitable for those with a history of psychosis.
- See also page 52.

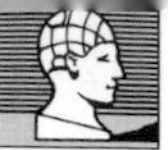

VISUALIZATION

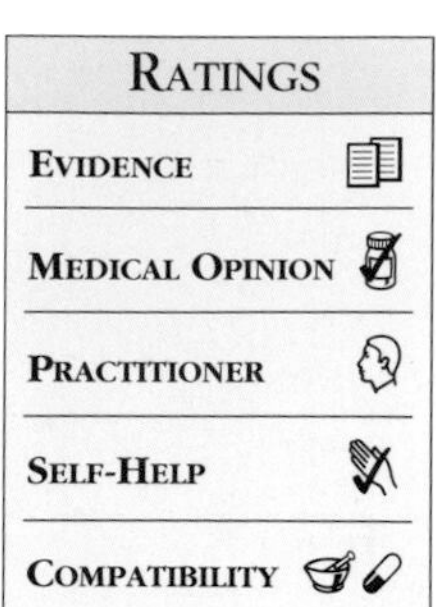

RATINGS

EVIDENCE

MEDICAL OPINION

PRACTITIONER

SELF-HELP

COMPATIBILITY

A TECHNIQUE THAT USES the imagination to help people cope with stress, fulfill their potential, and activate the body's self-healing processes, visualization was being used therapeutically by doctors and psychologists by the early 1970s. Patients are said to be able to overcome physical and emotional problems by imagining positive images and desired outcomes to specific situations, either alone or helped by a practitioner (known as "guided imagery"). Visualization forms a part of many relaxation therapies and is sometimes used as an adjunct to conventional cancer treatment.

MAIN USES

- Pain relief
- Allergies
- Heart conditions
- Anxiety, phobias
- Cancer
- Autoimmune diseases
- Stress-related conditions, including gastrointestinal & reproductive disorders
- Personal development

HISTORY

Traditional societies, especially those with shamans (see page 190), are well aware of the power of the imagination to heal or harm. Many religions also practice imagery: Tibetan Buddhists, for example, focus on the image of a deity healing symptoms.

Biofeedback researchers in the 1960s found that people used visual imagery in responding to cues from a biofeedback device (see page 169). In 1969, Dr. Carl Simonton and his wife, Stephanie Matthews-Simonton, a psychologist, carried out research into the use of visualization in cancer treatment. They encouraged patients to imagine white blood cells destroying the cancer, and claimed that, on average, these patients lived twice as long as other cancer patients. Some cancer specialists in the US, Europe, Australia, and New Zealand now include visualization as part of care programs to improve quality of life.

Psychologists worldwide have used visualization since the mid-20th century to improve motivation, for example in sports, and to change negative attitudes.

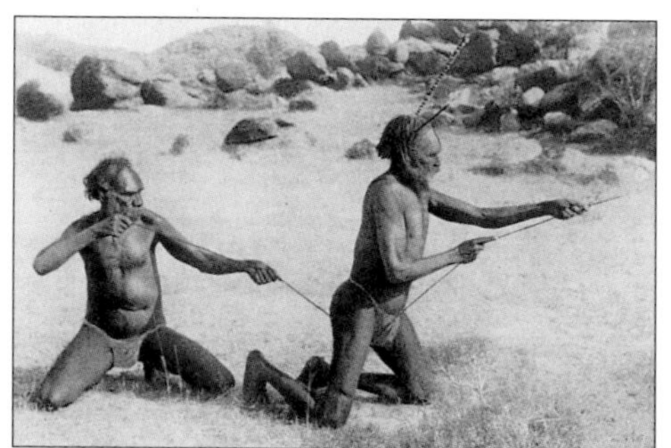

***Australian Aborigines** punish a transgressor of tribal law by ceremonially "pointing" at him to instill the image of death in his mind.*

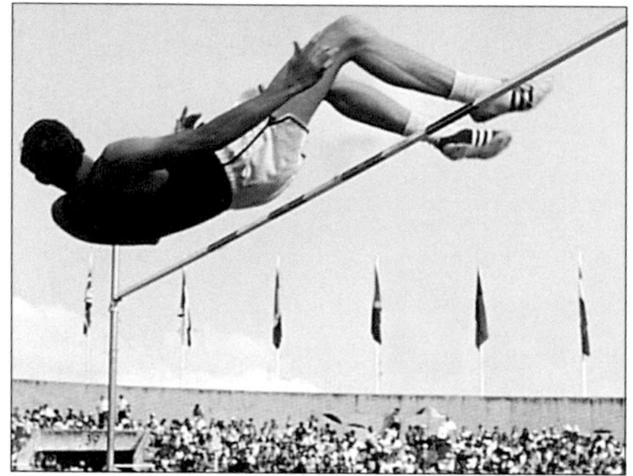

***Many athletes** use visualization in preparation for competition. Dick Fosbury, the famous high jumper, was an early exponent of the technique.*

KEY PRINCIPLES

It is unclear how visualization works, but it is said to encourage activity in the right hemisphere of the brain, which relates to creativity and emotions (see page 175). Research using positron emission tomography (PET) scans to monitor the brain during visualization exercises has shown that imagery involving sight activates the visual part of the cerebral cortex, sound imagery triggers the auditory cortex, and imagery concerning touch stimulates the sensory cortex.

A vivid image may send a message from the cerebral cortex via the lower brain to the hormonal system and the autonomic nervous system (see page 71), responsible for body functions such as heart rate and perspiration. Harnessing the power of the imagination may affect these processes and allow the body to find ways of coping with different conditions. If visualization is repeated enough, according to the theory, expectations rise and the individual begins to act as if the image were a reality. There are two common ways of using imagery, depending on the aim of treatment.

Active imagery: This works with a chosen image to control a symptom or situation, or relax the body and mind.

Receptive imagery: This helps patients gain insight into a problem by allowing images to surface that may offer clues to the emotional reasons for certain behavior.

EVIDENCE & RESEARCH

There are few scientific studies that focus solely on visualization. A number of studies since the 1960s have suggested that, when used with other stress-reducing techniques, visualization can affect physiological processes such as breathing, gastrointestinal activity, heart rate, blood pressure, sexual arousal, and the release of neurotransmitters.

A 1989 study in the Italian journal *Pediatrics* found that when mothers of premature babies listened to a relaxation and visualization audiotape, they produced 63% more milk than those who did not. In 1988, the *British Medical Journal* published a study claiming that women in the early stages of breast cancer derived greater psychological benefits from relaxation *and* visualization therapy than from relaxation alone. Studying the mind/body relationship (see page 18) may one day explain how mental imagery affects the immune system.

MEDICAL OPINION

Most doctors concede that positive thinking is a useful tool in restoring and maintaining health, and many support the inclusion of visualization techniques in treatment. Not everyone has a vivid imagination, however, and an inability to conjure up mental images of an illness being eliminated should not be seen as a sign of failure.

CONSULTING A PRACTITIONER

Visualization can be practiced on a one-to-one basis or in a group, often as part of psychotherapy or hypnotherapy (see pages 160 and 166). A practitioner may start by taking a medical history and asking what you hope to achieve from the therapy – this will affect the choice of imagery. A simple relaxation exercise, such as progressive muscle relaxation (see page 173), is practiced at the start of a session, since it is easier to learn visualization if the body is relatively free of tension.

Once you are relaxed and either lying down or sitting in a comfortable position, the practitioner will guide you through the visualization process. He will encourage you to make your chosen imagery as vivid as possible, help you to maintain your concentration, and lead you away from any thoughts that may inhibit the process. The practitioner may also ask you to repeat "positive affirmations" – phrases such as "I feel calm" or "I am in control." This helps to replace negative thoughts with positive ones.

At the end of the session, you will be asked to open your eyes and slowly become aware of your present situation.

Sessions last about 30–60 minutes, and the length of treatment will depend on your needs and your condition. You will be advised to practice daily, possibly with an audiotape or book.

PRECAUTIONS

- Do not begin to practice visualization without the guidance of a practitioner if you have a medical condition, since disturbing images may surface that could make your symptoms worse.
- See also page 52.

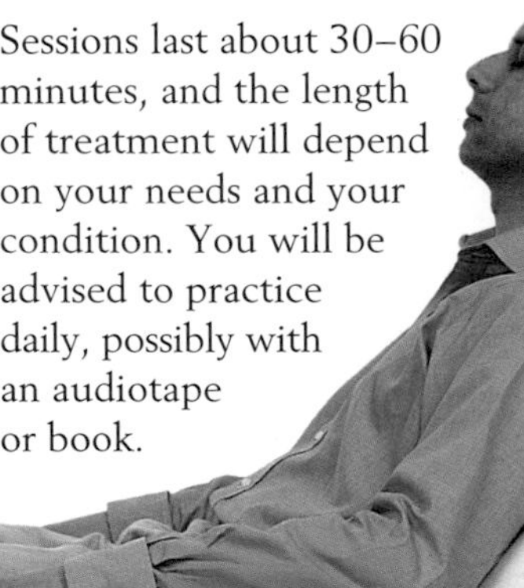

SITTING COMFORTABLY
When practicing visualization, it is essential to find a position in which the whole body can relax and the mind can "let go."

High-backed chair supports the whole body and head

SELF-HELP

Visualization is also effective as a self-help technique. Find a quiet place, lie down, or sit in a comfortable chair, and close your eyes. Breathe slowly and relax before focusing on your chosen mental image. Try to repeat the exercise 1–3 times a day.

FIGHTING ILLNESS

Create a mental picture of your illness: some people have described pain as an iron bar or a red-hot needle. Envisage any treatment you are receiving as eliminating pain and strengthening your self-healing powers. Imagine yourself healthy again.

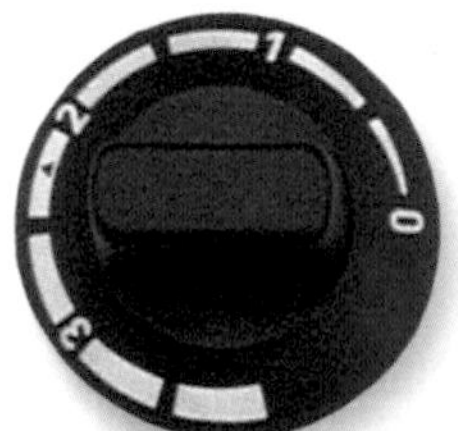

*"**Turning down**" your pain on an imaginary dial may help you to feel in control of pain and able to cope more successfully with short- or long-term illness.*

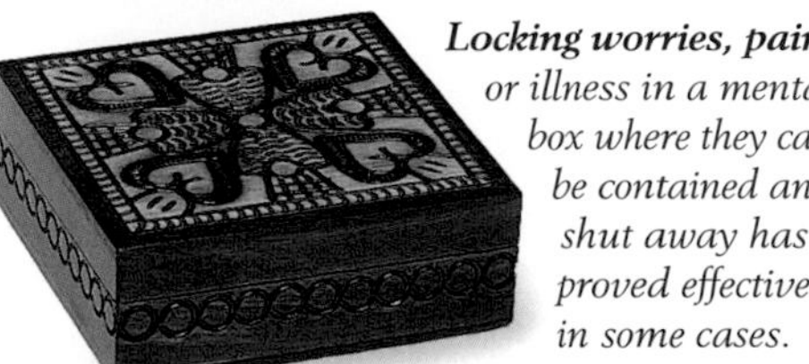

***Locking worries, pain,** or illness in a mental box where they can be contained and shut away has proved effective in some cases.*

ACHIEVING SUCCESS

Imagine a situation in which you hope to succeed. Tell yourself that you are confident and in control. If you feel that you are becoming tense at the thought of a particular difficulty, breathe slowly, relax, and detach yourself from the scene.

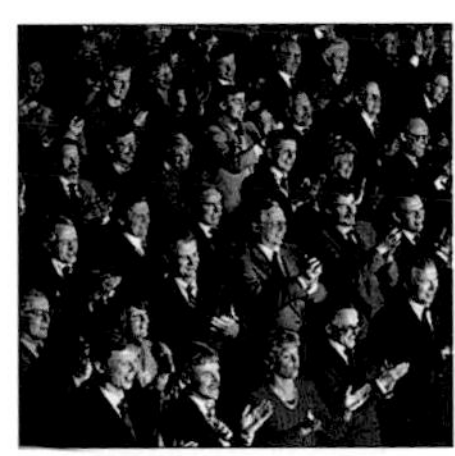

***Fear of public speaking** can be overcome by imagining yourself speaking calmly to a room of people. Hear the applause as you finish.*

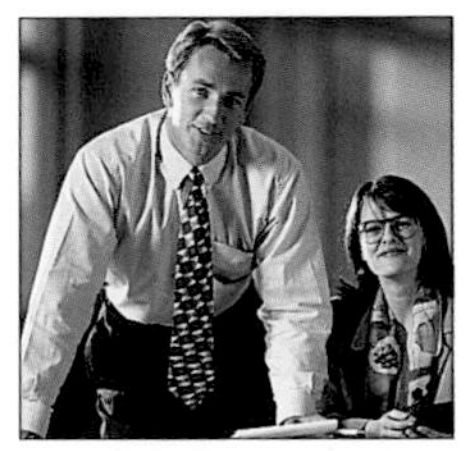

***To prepare for interviews**, visualize yourself calmly greeting the panel of interviewers and dealing confidently with their questions.*

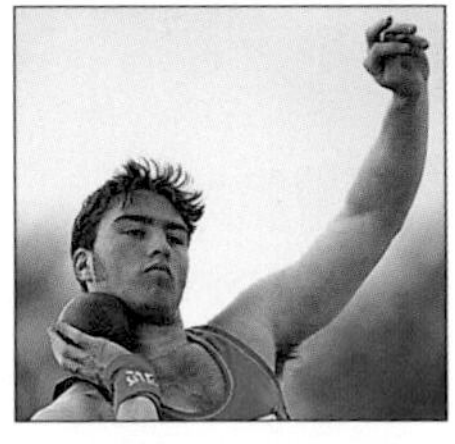

***Before a sports event**, motivation can be boosted by mentally rehearsing the precise sequence of events required for a successful performance.*

COMBATING STRESS

Visualize a calm, beautiful scene – perhaps somewhere you have been that was truly relaxing. Picture yourself there and use all your senses to make it as real as possible. Repeat to yourself phrases such as "I am relaxed and content."

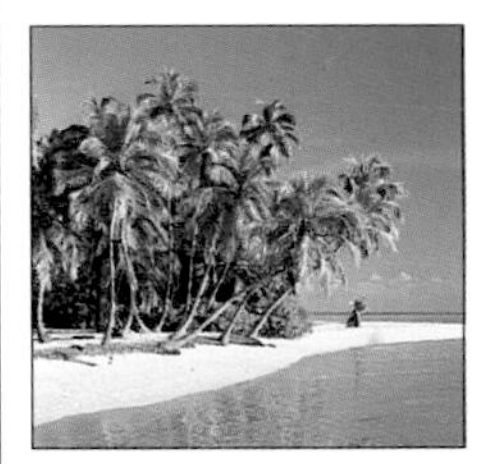

***Imagine a beach** where you can relax and unwind. Feel the warmth of the sun and the texture of the sand, hear the waves and smell the sea air.*

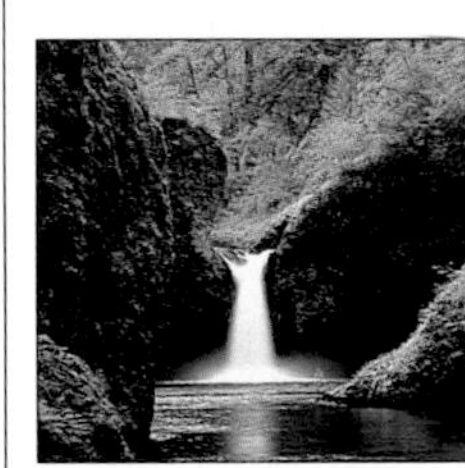

***A tropical waterfall** may help calm your mind. Listen to the sound of rushing water and mentally explore the banks of lush plants and fragrant flowers.*

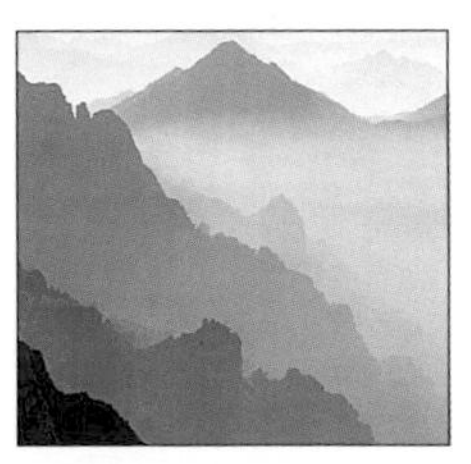

***A mountain scene** can promote a sense of harmony. Imagine the space and light around you and the sensation of filling your lungs with fresh clean air.*

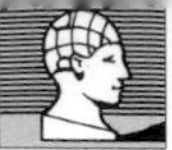

SOUND THERAPY

RATINGS	
EVIDENCE	
MEDICAL OPINION	
PRACTITIONER	
SELF-HELP	
COMPATIBILITY	

THE THERAPEUTIC POTENTIAL OF SOUND was first recognized by doctors in the late 19th century. Sound vibrates in waves at different frequencies and is said to influence both the emotions and certain physiological functions, such as heart rate and breathing. Even sounds at frequencies beyond the range of the human ear can have an impact. Practitioners use various approaches and work with the voice or with electronic or musical instruments to generate sound waves that, they claim, restore balance in the body and promote self-healing. Sound therapies are available throughout the West, and also in Japan.

MAIN USES

- Stress, anxiety
- High blood pressure
- Depression
- Autism, dyslexia, learning difficulties
- Pain relief, especially during labor
- Muscle & joint pain

HISTORY

Buddhist monks and Indian yogis have a long tradition of chanting to induce an altered physical and mental state, and the use of drumbeats to rouse soldiers before a fight is common to many cultures. Medical interest in sound first arose in 1896, when American doctors found that different types of music could stimulate blood flow and increase mental clarity.

Machines using sound waves as a form of therapy were developed in the 1950s and 1960s. The UK osteopath Dr. Peter Manners evolved cymatics therapy, which is most commonly used in the US. French ear specialists Drs. Guy Berard and Alfred Tomatis pioneered auditory integration training (AIT) and the Tomatis method respectively, both of which are attracting interest in the UK, US, and Europe. Another technique, physioacoustic methodology (PAM), was developed in Finland in the early 1990s, and is now gaining ground in Europe. Chanting is common to many cultures, and techniques such as Mongolian "overtone" chanting, introduced by practitioner Jill Purce in the UK, are gaining popularity in the West, particularly in New Age circles.

CONSULTING A PRACTITIONER

Sound travels as waves of pressure, each oscillating at its own frequency, or pitch, transmitted to the brain via the auditory nerve. In theory, auditory messages may also affect the autonomic nervous system, which regulates organs and body functions (see page 71). Some practitioners claim that, like sound waves, internal organs and cells vibrate at specific frequencies, and any disruption is symptomatic of disease. Sound therapy aims to restore disturbed inner rhythms to their natural state with the use of sound waves. Practitioners use a number of approaches.

Cymatics: A machine transmits sound waves through the skin to a specific body area. This is said to cause body cells to vibrate at an optimum, healthy resonance.

AIT and the Tomatis method: The machines aim to retrain patients who may find it hard to process certain sound frequencies, such as autistics and dyslexics, to hear and listen properly. You listen to music that emphasizes particular frequencies, forcing the brain to hear and process them afresh.

PAM: Computer-generated sound waves, played through speakers in a special chair in which you sit, are claimed to lower blood pressure and reduce muscle tension.

Chanting: You are taught to use tones in your voice to create a pure sound, said to induce a meditational state (see page 174).

Treatment usually involves weekly hour-long sessions and runs for several months. Chanting may be taught at weekend or evening workshops.

EVIDENCE & RESEARCH

Pilot studies of AIT and the Tomatis method suggest they may help treat behavioral problems. However, no convincing clinical studies validate claims for the vibration of body cells or the therapeutic effects of sound on organs and body tissues.

MEDICAL OPINION

Various body tissues absorb and reflect sound waves differently – conventional medicine makes use of this in prenatal ultrasound scans. However, most doctors are skeptical about the idea of "tuning in" to cellular vibrations to treat patients.

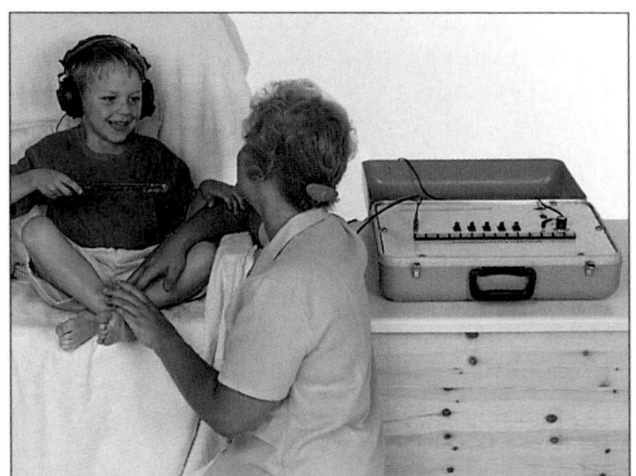

*AIT **equipment** is connected to a CD player and the patient listens to electronically filtered music that is made softer or louder to isolate difficult sound frequencies. Children with conditions such as dyslexia or autism may benefit from AIT.*

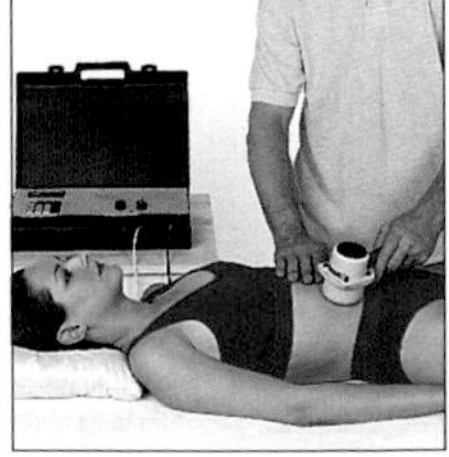

***In cymatics therapy** a machine is placed over the part of the body to be treated – here, the liver area – and set to a frequency matching that of cells in a healthy body.*

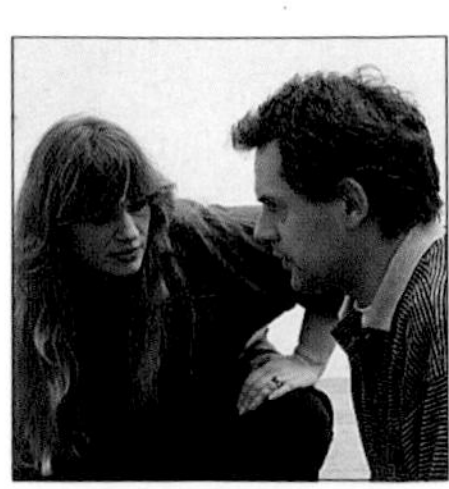

***Chanting practitioners** teach their patients to produce elongated vowel sounds that are said to resonate through the entire body and induce a state of physical and emotional well-being.*

PRECAUTIONS

- Avoid cymatics therapy if you have a pacemaker.
- See also page 52.

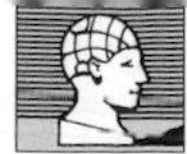

MUSIC THERAPY

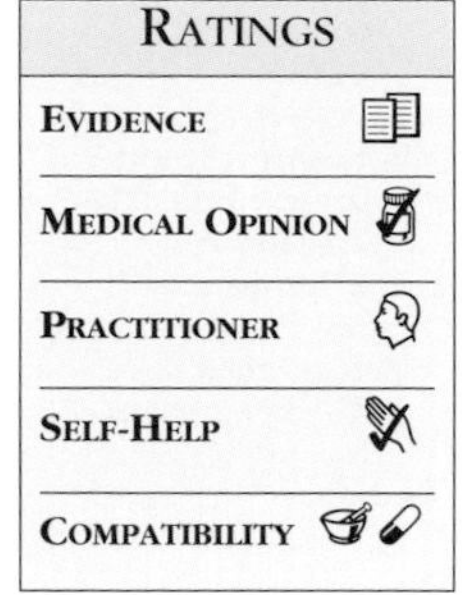

THE LINK BETWEEN MUSIC AND HEALING is an ancient one, but it is only since the 1940s that music therapy has developed in the West as a way of helping those with serious disabilities, mental illness, or psychological distress.

Making or responding to music can provide a real alternative to verbal communication, enabling the expression of emotions that may be too profound or primitive for words. Within both complementary and conventional medicine worldwide, particularly intensive care units and delivery rooms, patients are encouraged to listen to music to ease anxiety and pain, and to promote recovery.

MAIN USES

- Autism, learning difficulties
- Mental, emotional & behavioral problems
- Depression
- Stress, anxiety
- Care for the elderly
- Pain relief, especially during labor or in terminal illness

HISTORY

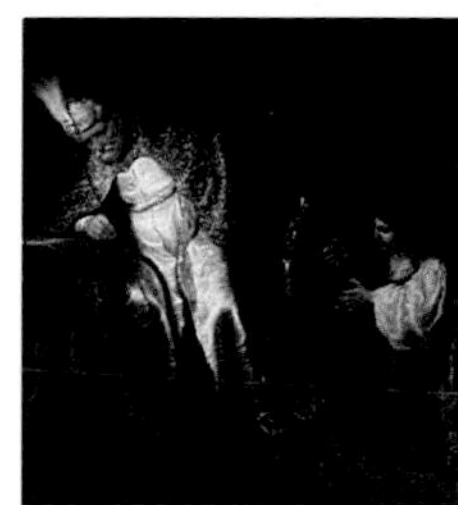

***The Old Testament** relates how David played the harp to King Saul when he was possessed by an evil spirit, and "the spirit departed from him."*

Music has long been used to stir emotions, and there are accounts of the healing power of music in the Bible and Homer's *Odyssey*. The modern practice of music therapy developed in the US at the end of World War II, in response to the psychological distress of returning war veterans. Success in their treatment led medical authorities to employ musicians in hospitals, and the National Association of Music Therapy was established in the US in 1950.

In 1958, UK concert cellist Juliette Alvin, renowned for pioneering work among children with learning difficulties, formed the British Society for Music Therapy. In 1974, American concert pianist Paul Nordoff and UK special education teacher Clive Robbins, known for their work with autistic and emotionally disturbed children, started their first training course in London. There are about 7,000 qualified music therapists in America compared with 300 in the UK and the same number in Australia.

CONSULTING A PRACTITIONER

Treatment takes place on a one-to-one or group basis, and patients range from those seeking help for emotional problems to physically or mentally disabled people. Sessions usually last an hour and the length of treatment will vary according to your condition. The aim of therapy is to help you release tension and deal with problems more effectively by expressing emotions in a nonverbal way and building a trusting relationship with the practitioner or other group members.

A session usually starts with the practitioner playing a tune or singing a song. As your confidence grows, you will be encouraged to respond, improvising on percussion instruments or with your voice. You will not be taught to play any instruments, and musical knowledge is unnecessary. Eventually, you may be able to express feelings in new ways.

For stress-related conditions and pain relief, the practitioner may ask you to select a piece of music to listen to that you find soothing. With elderly and terminally ill patients, this can stimulate memories, a therapeutic effect in itself. The rhythm of music is also said to affect physiological processes, such as heart rate or breathing, and prompt the release of endorphins, the body's own painkillers.

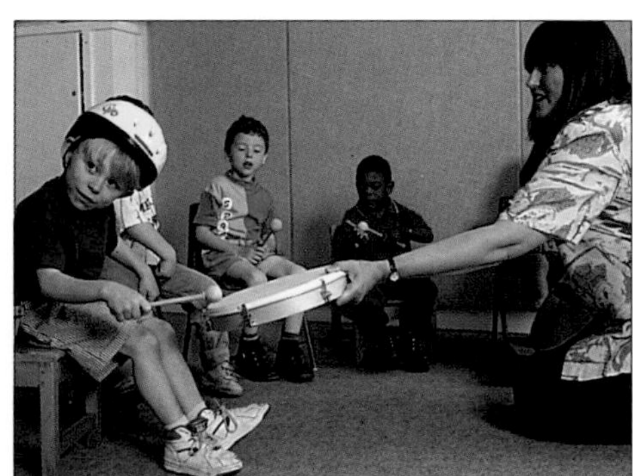

***Children with learning difficulties** – even those who are unable to speak – can be encouraged to develop communication skills by responding to music and interacting with the music therapist.*

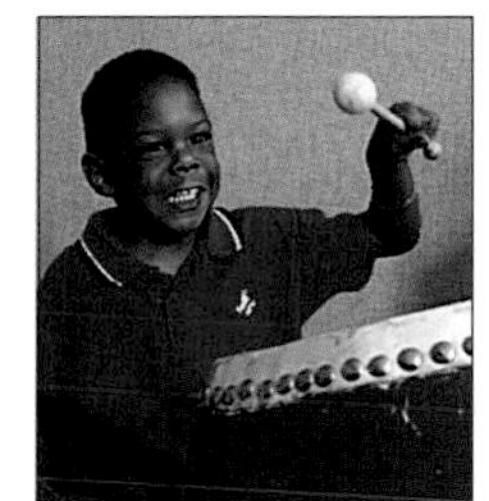

***Playing the drums** can provoke the release of exuberant emotions. Music therapy can be particularly effective with children, whose reactions to music are often spontaneous and uninhibited.*

EVIDENCE & RESEARCH

Worldwide research is taking place into the effects of music on the immune system. Studies in the US, the UK, and Germany, published in 1991, showed that patients who listened to music recovered more quickly than average and felt less anxiety and discomfort. Some studies in the 1980s and 1990s, such as those by Dr. Ralph Spintge in Germany, suggested that music with a certain rhythm may reduce stress by lowering heart rate, blood pressure, and respiration. Research in Europe, the US, and Australia in the 1980s confirmed that music therapy can benefit those with physical and mental disabilities.

MEDICAL OPINION

Doctors acknowledge that music therapy can help patients release emotions and relax, and it may have a useful part to play in the care of mentally and physically disabled people. Such patients are increasingly referred to music therapists, although most doctors are not convinced of music's ability to treat illness by affecting body systems directly.

PRECAUTIONS

- See page 52.

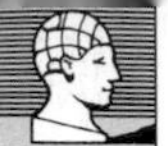

ART THERAPY

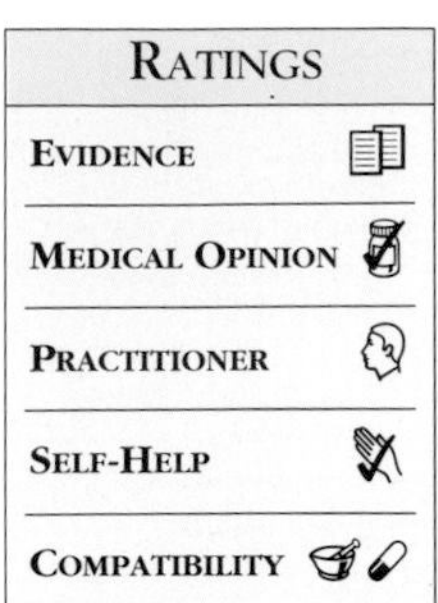

IN THE AFTERMATH OF WORLD WAR II, creative art began to be used on both sides of the Atlantic to help those who had undergone traumatic experiences deal with them and readjust to life. Spanning both conventional and complementary medicine, art therapy is now used by psychiatrists and psychotherapists worldwide as a technique in the diagnosis and treatment of mental and emotional disorders. It can also help people in emotional distress – for example, after a bereavement – providing therapeutic relief in expression through creative activities such as painting, drawing, and sculpting.

MAIN USES

- Mental & emotional disorders
- Learning difficulties
- Eating disorders
- Addictions
- Stress
- Bereavement
- Relief in Alzheimer's disease and terminal illness
- Personal development

HISTORY

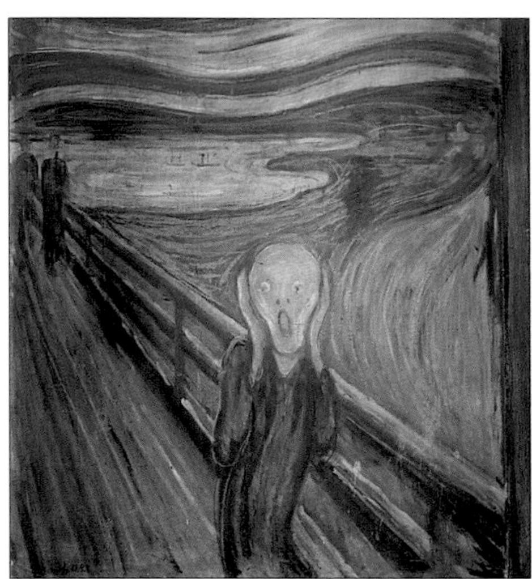

Edvard Munch's The Scream *is a well-known example of the power of art to express painful emotions that sometimes cannot be put into words.*

The expression of feelings in visual form has a long history, as ancient cave paintings attest. In the 19th century, Rudolf Steiner advocated the role of art in healing when developing anthroposophy (see page 124). In the early 20th century, Carl Jung and Sigmund Freud (see page 160) ascribed to visual images the ability to reflect a patient's subconscious state, while other psychoanalysts, such as Anna Freud and Melanie Klein, later emphasized the value of creative art in childhood development.

After World War II, art therapy was used in the rehabilitation of war veterans. Under the guidance of art therapist Margaret Naumberg, it began to be taken seriously in the US, where psychotherapy and other techniques based on Freudian theories were already well established. It is now widely practiced in the US, both for personal development and as a form of treatment for psychiatric disorders.

In the UK, art therapy developed in the 1940s, when artist Adrian Hill began to work informally with sanatorium patients. The British Association of Art Therapists was established in 1963, and there are now about 1,000 practitioners. A postgraduate Diploma of Art Therapy was recognized by the National Health Service in 1982, and art therapists were state-registered in 1997.

KEY PRINCIPLES

Patients are encouraged to express their feelings using materials such as paint, clay, crayons, and fabric, or even magazines from which they can make a collage. They are not expected to produce a "good" work of art, but simply to give two- or three-dimensional expression to threatening or confused emotions. The act of releasing such emotions in the safe confines of the practitioner's consulting room is considered

INTERPRETING ARTWORK

The images and colors *used in artwork may hold symbolic meanings, providing clues to the patient's emotional state. Art therapists believe that it is the patient – not the practitioner – who holds the key to the interpretation of his or her work. Uncovering the meaning of these works will not "solve" psychological problems, but can allow patients to understand, accept, and eventually move on from them.*

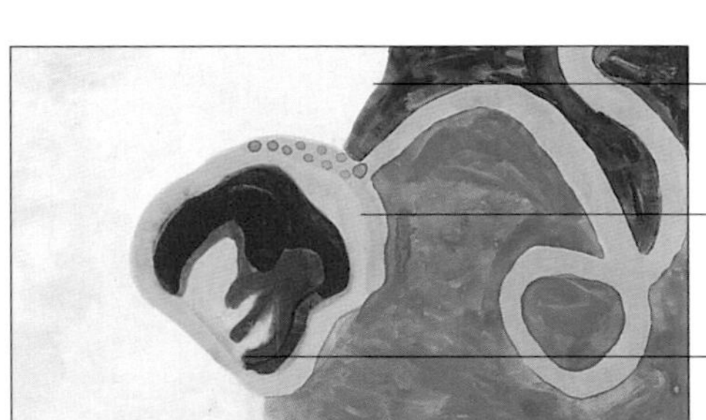

Border suggests a passage from dark to light

This image might be a tulip in bud, or a fetus and its umbilical cord

Bright colors point to rebirth and new life

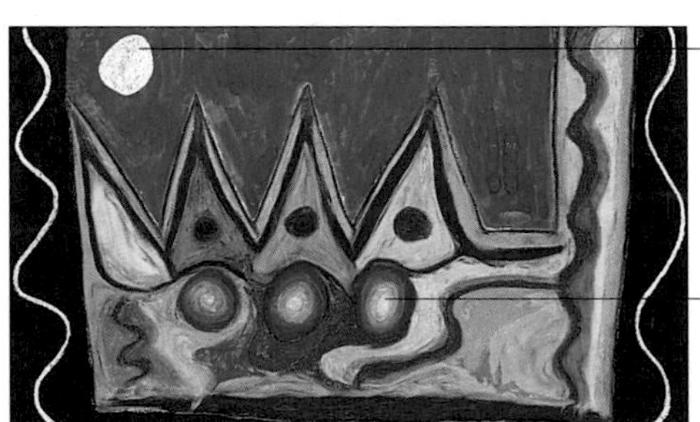

Distant moon expresses the patient's feelings about her mother

Three circles represent the patient and her siblings

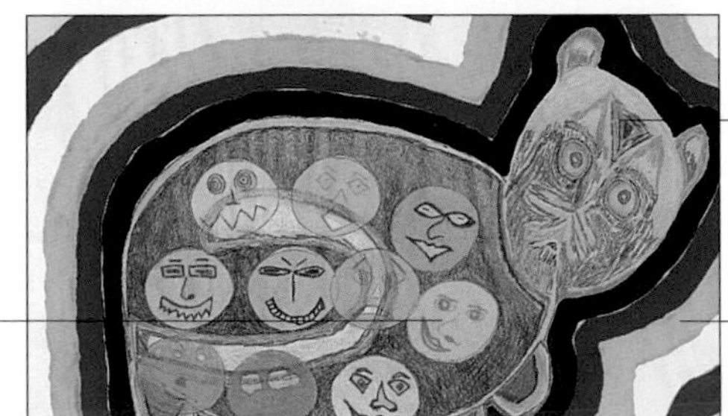

Angry face of the cat may be the key to this picture

Masks represent different roles performed by the patient

Bands of color suggest isolation from the outside world

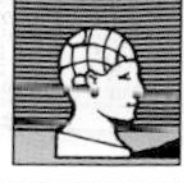

healing in itself, since the patient is able to overcome fear of self-expression and gain confidence and self-esteem. Thoughts and emotions often surface visually in a work of art long before they might appear verbally in a conventional "talk" therapy, allowing issues to be addressed at a relatively early stage. Socially unacceptable emotions, such as jealousy or rage, can also be unearthed and confronted without fear of criticism.

Many people cope with mental and emotional problems by repressing them, mistakenly believing that they are taking firm control over their lives. In the early stages of art therapy, the challenge for such patients is to relinquish control sufficiently to create a therapeutically useful image. Often, destructive impulses must be expressed before creativity and psychological insights can follow. Some patients need to make a mess, or to work carefully on an image only to destroy it, in order to achieve a breakthrough.

A further benefit of art therapy is that the work produced may contain symbols that can be interpreted by the practitioner, much as dreams may be analyzed in psychoanalysis (see page 162). Art therapy differs from psychoanalysis, however, in that it is the patient who takes the lead in interpretation, not the practitioner. Art therapists believe that the individual holds the key to the symbols he or she produces, with the practitioner playing a supporting or guiding role.

Evidence & Research

Extensive casework in North America, the UK, and Europe since the late 1980s has demonstrated the value of art therapy for a wide range of emotional and psychological disturbances, including psychotic illnesses, severe learning difficulties, eating disorders, and alcohol and drug abuse. Areas now being explored include relief from AIDS, Alzheimer's disease, and terminal illness.

Medical Opinion

Art therapy is extensively used in hospitals, prisons, and other institutions in the treatment of psychological disorders and addictions. Most psychiatrists and doctors accept its role in treating learning difficulties and exploring the profound inner conflicts that arise when a life-threatening disease is diagnosed.

Consulting a Practitioner

Before therapy begins, the practitioner assesses your condition. Many patients, especially in the UK and Australia, may have been referred by a medical doctor. If this is the case, the practitioner reviews any notes or background information resulting from your previous treatment. He asks about your emotional problems, your life situation, and your expectations from therapy. You in turn should take this opportunity to ask any questions you may have about the approach.

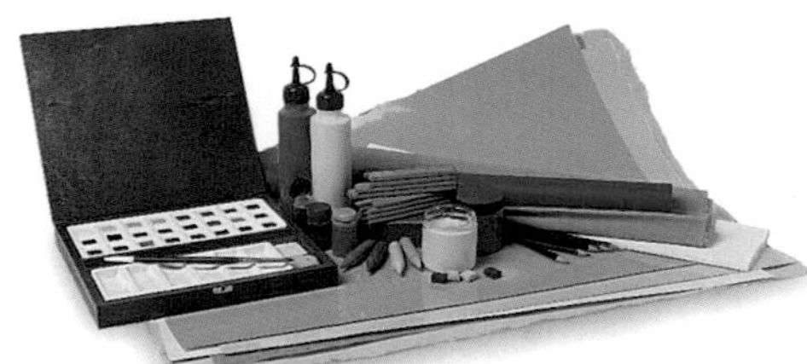

A wide range of media *will usually be offered to patients, including paints, crayons, chalk and clay. The practitioner will encourage patients to express their feelings through their artwork.*

During a session, the practitioner avoids guiding you in an intrusive manner. He may respond to what you produce with questions and comments, in order to stimulate interpretation and further development. Unexpected and disturbing images and associations may be made in the process, and the practitioner will help you explore the meanings uncovered and feelings that arise. If you are having difficulty with a particular medium, he may suggest changing to another or working with it in a different way.

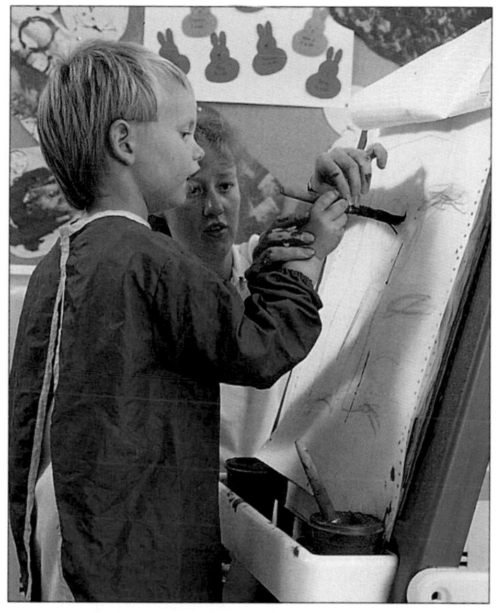

Children may find *it easier to convey emotional states through images rather than words, and art therapy may benefit those who are emotionally disturbed or who have learning difficulties.*

Adult therapy sessions usually take place once a week and are 60–90 minutes long; children's sessions may last 30 minutes. A minimum of six months' treatment is advised. Sessions may be one-to-one, or may take the form of group therapy, involving about 8–10 people. When working with a group, the practitioner might suggest theme-based exercises using dreams, relaxation, and visualization techniques (see pages 170 and 178).

Art therapy is sometimes practiced in hospitals to supplement conventional psychotherapy. Up to three quarters of practitioners work in social services, prisons, and educational institutions. Some also work in private practice.

Precautions

- See page 52.

Self-Help

Art therapy can be an ideal way to relax and allow problems to find a natural resolution. Talent or expertise is not important; the essential thing is to ignore the critical, inhibited part of yourself and let go. Choose the art media that most appeal to you. Some tips are given below.

- Begin by loosening up and allowing your intuition and spontaneity to surface. One way is to make initial sketches or paintings with your left hand if you are right-handed (or right hand if left-handed).
- Work quickly, without thinking about what you are doing. Put down the first shapes, forms, and colors that come into your head.
- If you are uncomfortable with paints or clay, make a collage with images cut from newspapers and magazines.
- When you are finished, look carefully at your work. Do any symbols, shapes, or colors hold significance? What feelings do they elicit? The meaning may not be clear, but try exploring these images in your artwork and see if they evolve.

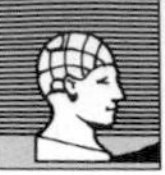

FENG SHUI

RATINGS
EVIDENCE
MEDICAL OPINION
PRACTITIONER
SELF-HELP
COMPATIBILITY

PRACTICED IN CHINA for over a thousand years, feng shui is the ancient Asian art of arranging living and working space to bring physical and spiritual benefits. Derived from the same philosophy as acupuncture and other traditional Chinese therapies, it seeks to harmonize the flow of qi *("life energy") within a room or building to enhance the health, happiness, and prosperity of those who live or work there. Feng shui has had a major impact on the development of cities such as Hong Kong and Taipei, and there is growing interest in the UK, North America, and Australasia.*

MAIN USES

- Personal development
- Stress-related problems
- Emotional problems, including poor relationships, inability to make decisions, loneliness & lack of self-confidence

HISTORY

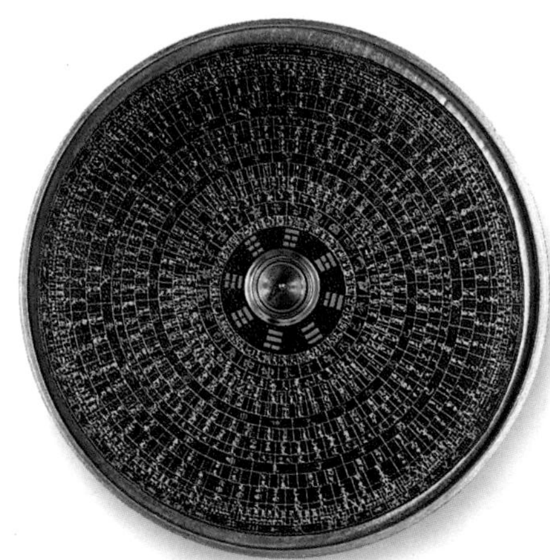

The **luo pan** ***compass*** *is a traditional feng shui tool, made individually for the practitioner, to determine "energy patterns" and other information.*

Literally translated as "wind" and "water," feng shui (pronounced "fung shoy") has its roots in the ancient Chinese belief that environmental forces shape human destiny. According to legend, a Chinese ruler, Fu Hsi, saw a tortoise emerging from the Lo River and realized that the markings on its shell symbolized universal principles. He used this pattern to devise eight configurations of energetic forces, known as trigrams (see page 90), which became the basis of the hugely influential work of divination, the *I Ching (Book of Changes)*. Considered an oracle by feng shui masters at imperial courts, it was later used throughout China as a guide to decision making.

Feng shui has survived the centuries and is taken so seriously in the Far East that Western companies based there are often obliged to acknowledge it when designing new offices. In this way, knowledge of the art is now spreading to the West.

KEY PRINCIPLES

Based on the same principles as those of Traditional Chinese Medicine (see page 140), feng shui is sometimes referred to as "space acupuncture." In the same way that an imbalance between *yin* and *yang* in the body is believed to disrupt health, disharmony in one's surroundings is said to have a negative effect on all aspects of life, from relationships to financial affairs.

Landscapes, buildings, rooms, even the tops of tables, are said to have their own flow of *qi*, or "life energy," and feng shui encourages blocked or depleted *qi* to move freely in a given area by altering the layout. To plot the flow of *qi*, an octagonal "map," known as the *ba-gua*, may be superimposed on the ground plan of a building or room (see below). If one section of the *ba-gua* is missing, or badly arranged, problems are expected in the corresponding area of the occupants' lives.

THE *BA-GUA*

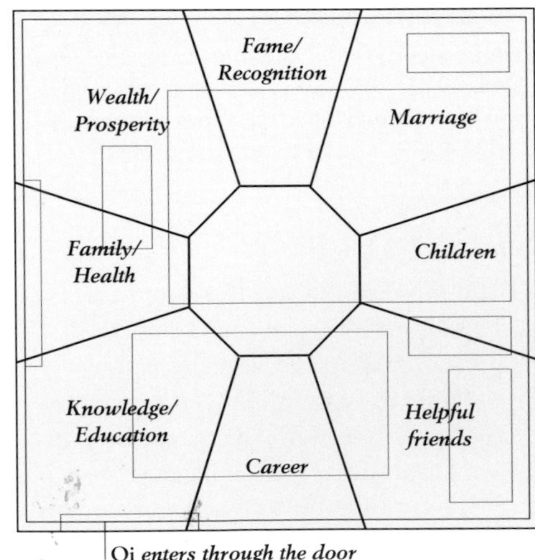

The eight "houses" *of the* ba-gua, *based on the compass points and the eight trigrams, each relate to different aspects of life. In feng shui, this mystic tool is used to plan and assess buildings and rooms.*

The Chinese concepts of the trigrams and the "five elements" – earth, fire, water, wood, and metal – are also key factors in feng shui. Depending on the school of feng shui to which the practitioner belongs, each element may be associated with a compass point, color, season, and number. The relationship between the elements is used to assess feng shui in the home or workplace and to create a state of harmony. The occupants' dates of birth are often taken into account, since these too can be categorized according to the five elements. Some practitioners also use a "map" of five symbolic animals to analyze a space.

In the West, "space clearing" techniques may be used in addition to, or instead of, feng shui. Ceremonial rituals drawn from Native American, Zulu, Maori, and Balinese cultures, involving bell-ringing, incense-burning, incantations, and crystals, are used to "cleanse" and consecrate buildings.

EVIDENCE & RESEARCH

No studies have been carried out in the West on feng shui, and research into related therapies, such as acupuncture, has failed to prove the existence of *qi*.

MEDICAL OPINION

Feng shui lies outside the boundaries of Western medical expertise and seems far removed from the conventional approach to illness and treatment. However, doctors acknowledge that social and psychological factors can affect health, and the pathological effects of discord and disorder may merit some consideration.

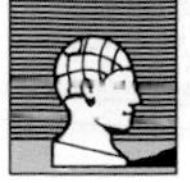

CONSULTING A PRACTITIONER

A feng shui consultation usually involves a visit to your home or workplace by a practitioner. The length of the visit depends on the size of the building, but is generally 1–2 hours. During the session, the practitioner will ask you about any areas in your life or business that you feel are in need of attention, and may also ask for the dates of birth of all the members of your household or key members of staff at your workplace.

The practitioner will make a detailed assessment of each room in the building. After the consultation, she will send you a report listing suggested changes. This may involve choosing a new color scheme, moving plants or ornaments, or avoiding certain areas altogether. For example, a washbowl in the marriage corner of your bedroom may be causing marital harmony to drain away, and the practitioner will advise that its use is discontinued. You can discuss any queries with the practitioner by telephone.

It is also possible to consult a feng shui practitioner by mail by sending her a floor plan of your home or workplace.

PRECAUTIONS

- See page 52.

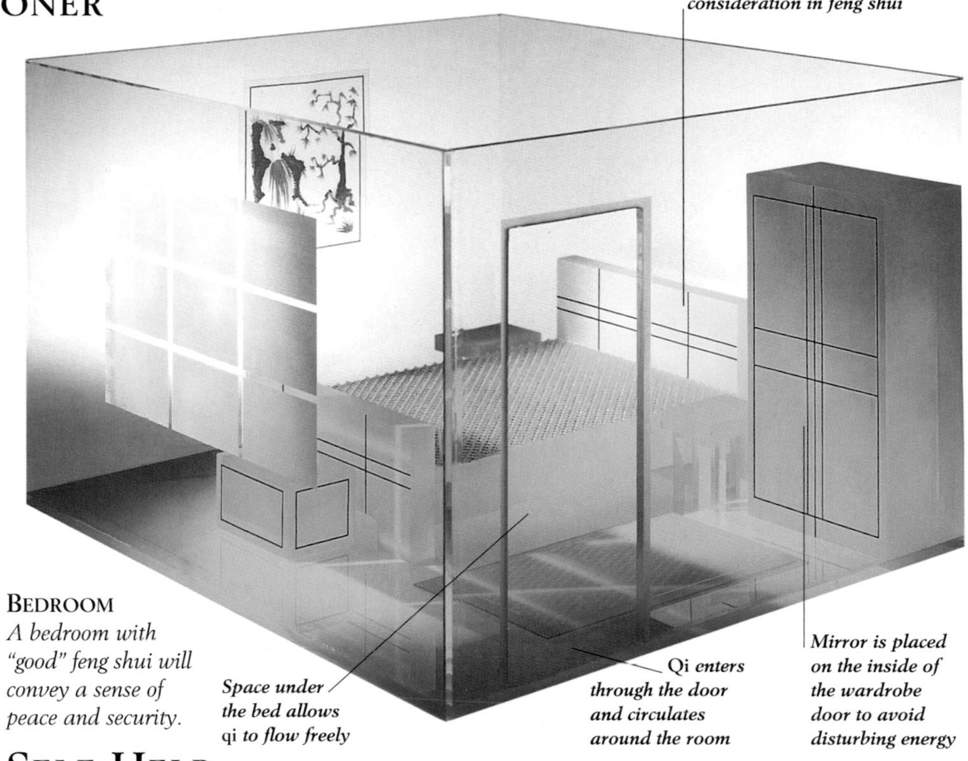

BEDROOM
A bedroom with "good" feng shui will convey a sense of peace and security.

SELF-HELP

There are various simple steps you can take to improve the feng shui of your surroundings. To enable *qi* to flow freely, remove clutter from rooms and surfaces, and make sure there is plenty of space around furniture. Check that items such as clocks are in working order, and repair broken furniture. Healthy plants attract *qi* and can counteract the electromagnetic fields surrounding computers or televisions. Avoid sharp-leaved plants, however, which are believed to "cut" *qi*. Long-stemmed flowers and images of "airy" objects, such as balloons, direct the flow of *qi* upward. Mirrors should be used with care, as they reflect *qi* and can disturb energy patterns.

Geomancy

A form of divination, geomancy is based on various theories about ways in which the environment may have a detrimental effect on health. Practitioners who believe the problems are electromagnetic refer to this as "geopathic stress," and claim to detect these harmful energies and reverse their effects.

RATINGS

- EVIDENCE
- MEDICAL OPINION
- PRACTITIONER
- SELF-HELP
- COMPATIBILITY

MAIN USES

- Anxiety, depression
- Insomnia
- Fatigue, CFS
- Headaches, migraines
- Rheumatoid arthritis

HISTORY

Societies as diverse as the Aborigines of Australia and the Chinese share a belief in the existence of invisible "energy pathways." Feng shui, a form of geomancy, is common in the Far East (see opposite). In the West, the theory of "ley lines," said to run through sites of spiritual significance, such as the prehistoric stone circle of Stonehenge in the UK, was put forward in the 1920s. Geomancy is arousing interest in countries where electromagnetic fields and pollution generated by industry cause concern.

CONSULTING A PRACTITIONER

Some practitioners relate energy fields in the environment to geological faults, underground streams, and manufactured features, such as power cables. Humans are now said to spend prolonged periods exposed to harmful fields in the home or workplace, especially in urban areas. A practitioner may use dowsing (see page 198) to detect malign energy fields, and will try to restore them to a state of harmony – for example, by moving furniture or "trapping" harmful energy with crystals.

MEDICAL OPINION

Evidence about the dangers of even relatively powerful electromagnetic fields is still highly controversial, and doctors tend to dismiss geomancy as fanciful.

PRECAUTIONS

- See page 52.

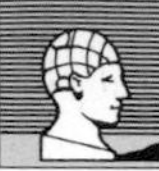

COLOR THERAPY

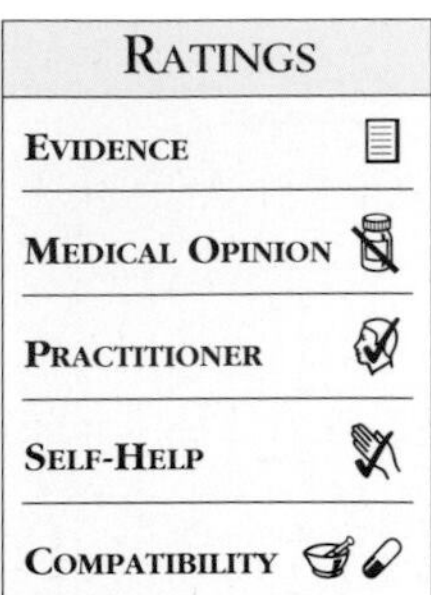

RATINGS

- EVIDENCE
- MEDICAL OPINION
- PRACTITIONER
- SELF-HELP
- COMPATIBILITY

THE IMPACT OF COLOR on mood is widely recognized. Color therapists go further, believing that different hues can treat illness and improve physical, emotional, and spiritual health. According to the theory, the vibrations of color waves can directly affect body cells and organs. Many practitioners also claim that the body emits its own "aura," or energy field, the colors of which reflect a person's state of health. Different colors are used to "heal," often in the form of colored light. The therapy has a long tradition in New Age circles in Europe, and interest is growing in the US, Australia, and Japan.

MAIN USES

- Emotional & behavioral problems
- Stress-related conditions
- Depression, insomnia
- Fatigue, CFS
- Headaches
- High blood pressure
- Arthritis
- Skin conditions
- Menstrual problems

HISTORY

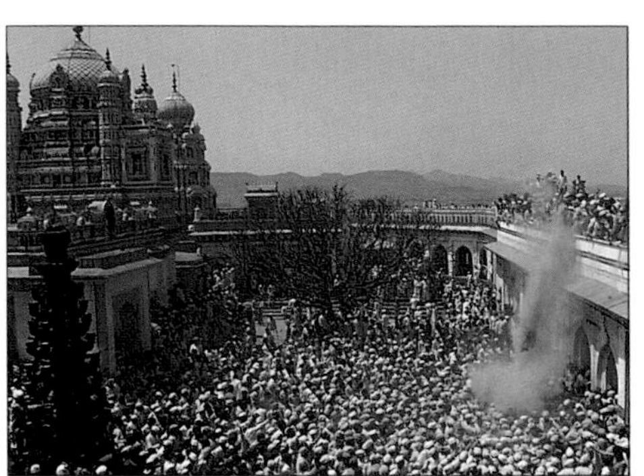

Colors have always *had symbolic overtones. In the Indian festival of* Somavati Amavasya, *yellow turmeric powder, representing the sun, is scattered.*

The earliest association of colors with symbolic meanings arose from the close relationship between prehistoric humans and nature. Green was the color of growth; blue represented the sky and heavenly peace. Cultural differences developed, however. Red, the color of blood, spelled disaster for the ancient Celts, while the Chinese associated it with the sun and considered it propitious.

In the West, healing with color remained largely a folk tradition based on superstition and the use of crystals and precious stones until the 19th century, when discoveries were made about the light spectrum and electromagnetic waves. An Indian scientist, Dinshah P. Ghadiali, was one of the first to attempt a scientific explanation of color therapy. In a book published in 1933, he claimed that colors transmitted healing vibrations, and he invented two machines for this purpose.

Modern practitioners borrow at random from folk superstition, Eastern mysticism and Western psychological research.

KEY PRINCIPLES

The sun's rays contain a whole spectrum of electromagnetic radiation that forms visible white or "full-spectrum" light. Light travels in waves, and its different wavelengths are perceived by the brain as colors. When light is passed through a prism or refracted as a rainbow, the different color waves of the spectrum can be identified (see below).

As well as having its own wavelength, each color has a certain frequency, the rate at which its wave vibrates. Practitioners of color therapy believe that cells and organs in the body also have vibrational frequencies, and they use colors to correct vibrational imbalances in the body and create a state of harmony.

Many color therapists are influenced by the *Vedic* theory of the body's *chakras*, vortexes of "life energy" into which light is believed to stream (see page 109). Each *chakra* is said to correspond to a particular part of the body and is associated with, and stimulated by, certain emotions and colors (see opposite). Practitioners use various tests to ascertain which colors are missing and which ones are required to keep the *chakras* working in harmony. Related to the *chakras* is a person's "aura," a "subtle" (nonphysical) body consisting of multicolored layers that surround an individual. Although it is invisible to most people, some practitioners claim to "see" a person's aura. They will "read" the colors of the aura to determine the patient's state of health, then visualize healing colors to counteract negative or dull colors in the aura (see page 104).

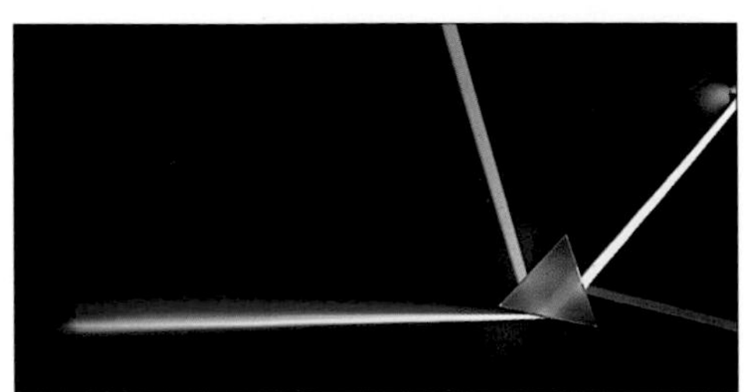

When full-spectrum light *shines into a prism, it "refracts" into the seven colors of the spectrum: red, orange, yellow, green, blue, indigo, and violet.*

EVIDENCE & RESEARCH

There is no evidence for vibrational healing through color, or for *chakras* or auras, although extensive research shows that color can affect mood. In 1984, Professor Harry Wohlfarth of the University of Edmonton, Canada, demonstrated that yellow and red are the most stimulating colors, and blue and black the most calming. Yellow was found to increase children's learning ability. Researchers in the US in 1973 found that bathing in red light for 30 minutes caused heart rate and blood pressure to rise, while blue light caused them to decrease. In the 1940s and 1950s, Swiss psychologist Dr. Max Lüscher devised tests, used in medicine and industry, to reveal subjects' states of mind and even physical illness from their response to color. In a 1948 West German study, it was found that yellow, orange, or red in the classroom increased student IQ.

MEDICAL OPINION

Doctors accept the psychological effects of color more readily than the physical. Research suggests that ultraviolet (UV) light (see page 188) can be used in treating depression, but more studies are needed on colored light. Doctors seriously question the idea of prescribing colors as medicine.

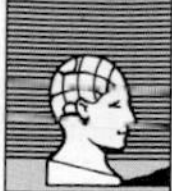

CONSULTING A PRACTITIONER

The practitioner usually begins by asking for details of your medical history and your personal color preferences. Practitioners working with the aura and *chakras* may claim simply to "see" which colors your body requires. There are two other main methods of diagnosis commonly used in color therapy.

Color reflection reading: From a range of eight colored cards, the practitioner asks you to choose three. Your physical and psychological health are assessed from your selection to provide clues as to which areas of your body are out of balance.

Color spine chart: This relates parts of the spine to different colors and body areas. Techniques vary, but the practitioner may "dowse" (see page 198) the chart for imbalances by running a finger down it to pinpoint problem areas and treatment colors, while concentrating on information you have given.

Treatment is often in the form of color illumination therapy, in which colored light is shone for a precise length of time either directly onto a specific part of your body through a quartz-tipped "crystal flashlight," or diffused around you as you sit under a light source. Different hues are selected according to their vibrational frequencies and their particular effects on internal organs. The practitioner often uses both the main color and its complementary opposite alternately in treatment. If you are being treated with violet, for example, you will usually also be exposed to yellow. This is said to ensure a healthy balance of color in the body. Sessions are usually about an hour long, and a course of treatment may last several weeks, depending on the condition.

Practitioners of other therapies, such as reflexology or acupuncture, may incorporate aspects of color therapy into their work.

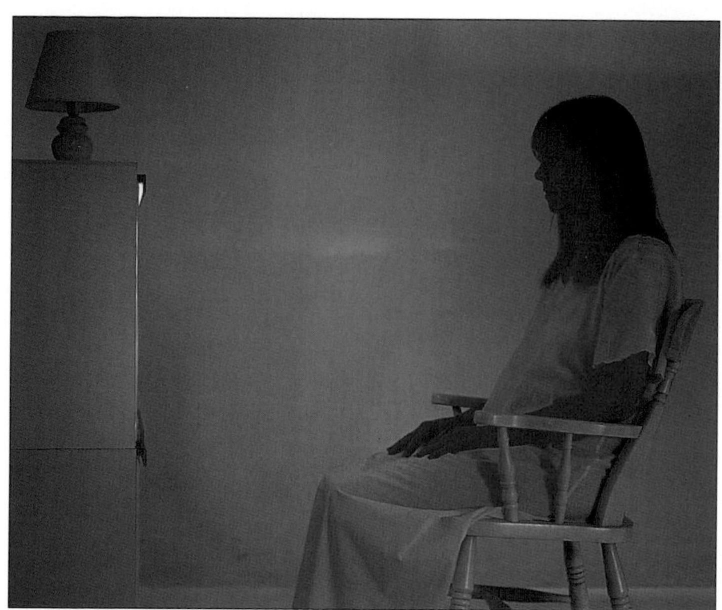

ILLUMINATION THERAPY
A computer-controlled color therapy machine directs colored light at the patient as she sits or lies in a darkened room. The main treatment color – in this case, orange – is alternated with its complementary color, blue, and each dose is precisely timed.

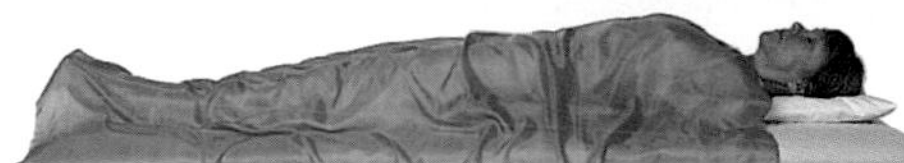

Colored silks *may be draped over the body to treat illness. For depression, a practitioner might use orange silk for 20 minutes, followed by blue – its complementary color – for 10 minutes.*

PRECAUTIONS

- See page 52.

SELF-HELP

Your practitioner may teach you how to visualize yourself bathing in a certain color or breathing it into your body. You may also be advised to include specific colors in your clothing, environment, and food, and to drink water that has been "solarized" by absorbing sunlight through stained glass of a particular color.

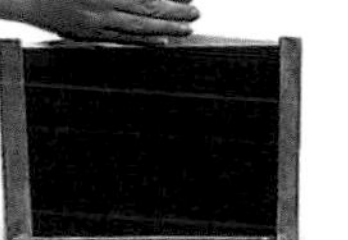

Solarized blue water *is used to treat insomnia.*

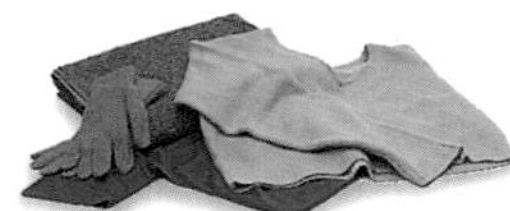

Clothing *in treatment colors may be worn.*

COLOR & THE *CHAKRAS*

COLOR	CHAKRA	PHYSICAL INFLUENCE	SPIRITUAL INFLUENCE	IN EXCESS
	Sahasrara (Color: magenta) **Situated**: Crown of the head	**Treats**: Compulsive behavior **Affects**: Pineal gland	Spiritual development, reverence, commitment, idealism	Fanaticism, domination
	Ajna (Color: violet) **Situated**: Forehead	**Treats**: Addiction **Affects**: Pituitary gland	Perception, intuition, dignity, self-respect, tolerance	Corruption, pride, arrogance
	Vishuddha (Color: blue) **Situated**: Throat	**Treats**: Insomnia, overactivity **Affects**: Thyroid gland	Creativity, inspiration, peace, relaxation, devotion, trust	Doubt, distrust, apathy, melancholy
	There is no *chakra* associated with the color turquoise	Turquoise stimulates the immune system	Independence, heightened awareness, power of articulation	Tendency to be easily influenced, immaturity
	Anahata (Color: green) **Situated**: Heart	**Treats**: Nervous tension **Affects**: Thymus gland	Freedom, balance, harmony, sympathy, love	Lethargy, lack of motivation, insecurity, jealousy
	Manipura (Color: yellow) **Situated**: Solar plexus	**Treats**: Unresolved feelings **Affects**: Pancreas	Mental energy and alertness, determination	Lack of concentration, malice, deviousness
	Swadisthana (Color: orange) **Situated**: Lower abdomen	**Treats**: Depression, low libido **Affects**: Reproductive organs	Happiness, optimism, sexual energy	Confusion, tiredness, pessimism
	Muladhara (Color: red) **Situated**: Base of coccyx	**Treats**: Inertia **Affects**: Adrenal glands	Courage, willpower, physical energy, and vitality	Domination, physical cruelty, anger, vulgarity

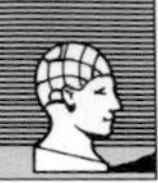

LIGHT THERAPY

RATINGS

- EVIDENCE
- MEDICAL OPINION
- PRACTITIONER
- SELF-HELP
- COMPATIBILITY

SUNLIGHT AND ARTIFICIAL LIGHT have been used for over a century to restore physical and psychological health. More recently, medical science has come to recognize the important role light plays in regulating the body's biological clock, which controls sleep, hormone production, and other functions. Light therapy is now used throughout the Western world to improve vitality and treat skin conditions such as psoriasis. It is especially associated with seasonal affective disorder (SAD), a severe manifestation of the "winter blues," thought to be caused by light deprivation in winter.

MAIN USES

- Seasonal affective disorder (SAD)
- Skin conditions
- Depression
- Insomnia
- Disturbed sleep patterns, jet lag

HISTORY

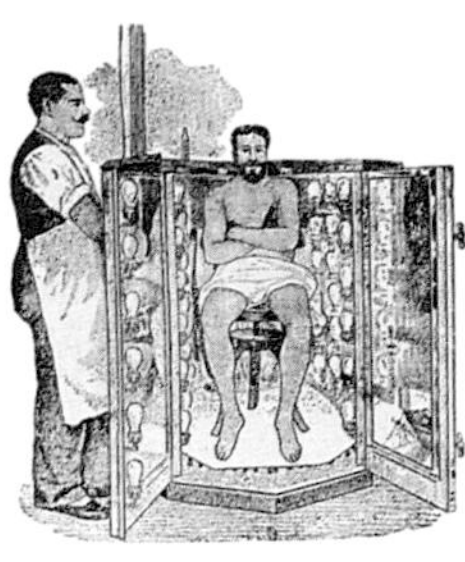

***"Incandescent electric light baths"** were used to treat many physical and mental illnesses in 19th-century European sanatoriums. Patients were also advised to get regular exercise in bright sunlight.*

The benefits of natural sunlight have been used by generations of healers, notably 19th-century naturopaths (see page 118).

Danish doctor Niels Finsen received the Nobel Prize for Medicine in 1903 for research into the ability of ultraviolet (UV) light to treat tuberculosis. About fifty years later, American photobiologist Dr. John Ott claimed that "full-spectrum" light from the sun is needed for the body to absorb key nutrients, and that pollution, windows, and eyeglasses may block vital components of the sun's rays. The discovery that reduced daylight hours can cause severe depression led to recognition of seasonal affective disorder (SAD; see page 293).

CONSULTING A PRACTITIONER

When light enters the eye, it stimulates nerve impulses to the hypothalamus, part of the brain responsible for mood, appetite, sleep, temperature, and sex drive. These nerve impulses travel to the pineal gland in the brain, which regulates hormonal balance, including the production of serotonin, a hormone linked to mood. In darkness, the gland secretes melatonin, a hormone that controls sleep patterns by causing drowsiness and is also said to affect the immune system. If the body's internal clock is disrupted by jet lag, shift work, or seasonal changes in light, physical or psychological problems may occur.

Natural daylight also stimulates the body to produce vitamin D, essential for the absorption of certain minerals, including calcium, which strengthens bones. The UV rays in daylight have an antibacterial effect, thought to help clear skin infections such as acne and psoriasis.

A practitioner places you under a fluorescent full-spectrum or bright white light for up to an hour, depending on your condition. You can also use a light box and visor at home for at least 20 minutes a day. Fluorescent full-spectrum light is the same as natural daylight, but without the toxic UV wavelengths. Bright white light (so called because the colors combine to make white) contains no UV wavelengths – some studies suggest these are not needed for an antidepressant effect.

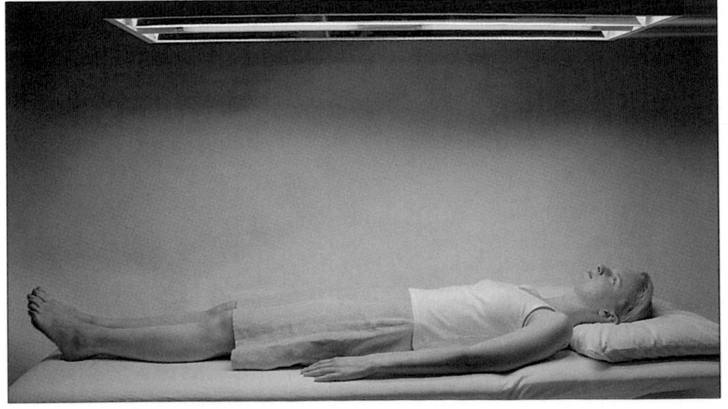

***The patient** lies with eyes open on a couch under a lamp emitting UV filtered full-spectrum or bright white light. Light is measured in a unit called the lux. At least 2,500 lux are needed to have a therapeutic effect on the body clock. Daylight averages about 5,000 lux, most offices about 500–1,000 lux.*

EVIDENCE & RESEARCH

Several studies led by Dr. Norman E. Rosenthal, notably those published in the *American Journal of Psychiatry* in the 1980s, are accepted as evidence that SAD exists and can be treated by light therapy. The studies are supported by a growing body of research. UV light is known to have antiviral, antibacterial, and antifungal properties, and has proved effective in treating psoriasis. Claims that it helps ailments such as heart disease, cancer, osteoporosis, and menstrual problems are not yet backed by research.

MEDICAL OPINION

SAD may cause depression in winter, but many doctors believe the disorder is relatively uncommon. For ailments such as psoriasis, UV light treatment is conventional practice; for others, such as cancer, its efficacy is unproved. Exposure to unfiltered UV rays must be weighed against the risk of skin cancer.

PRECAUTIONS

- Avoid overexposure to UV light, since it can cause skin cancer.
- Do not take vitamin D supplements during a course of light therapy – high doses can be toxic.
- Consult an eye specialist before a course of light therapy if you have an eye disorder.
- See also page 52.

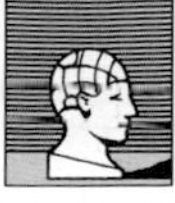

BIORHYTHMS

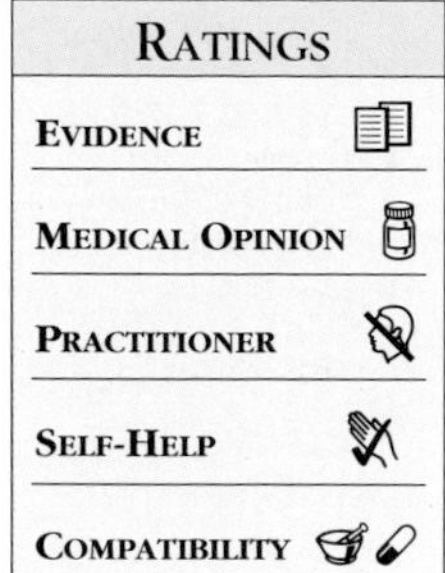

SOME DAYS WE FEEL on top of the world, our minds sharp and creative, with energy to spare. Yet at other times, for no obvious reason, we seem lethargic, irritable, or unable to concentrate. These states have been attributed to internal cycles, or "biorhythms," identified early in the 20th century, which are said to regulate physical, emotional, and intellectual functioning. Individual charts of the cycles are used to help people pinpoint days of optimum performance and take precautions at times of physical or emotional crisis. Primarily a self-help technique, biorhythms are popular worldwide, especially in Japan.

MAIN USES

- Planning vacations, surgical operations, business ventures & projects that depend on top performance & avoiding risk

HISTORY

Biorhythms were first charted in Berlin in around 1900. Dr. Wilhelm Fleiss, an eminent ear, nose, and throat specialist and associate of Sigmund Freud, analyzed medical records and concluded that a male "solar" cycle (governing physical health) and a female "lunar" cycle (controlling emotions) coexisted in everyone and accounted for most life experiences.

Dr. Fleiss's work was supported by his contemporary, the Austrian psychologist Hermann Swoboda, who noted that asthma attacks seemed to recur on a cyclical basis.

A cycle governing the intellect was first tracked in the 1920s, when an Austrian mathematician, Professor Alfred Teltscher, noted that the academic performance of his students fell into a pattern of highs and lows. Chronobiology (see right) has attracted further interest in the 1990s.

The use of biorhythm charts has become popular around the world, from the US to Russia and Japan, and mail-order charts are available through newspapers and magazines.

CONSULTING A PRACTITIONER

Specialized companies can chart your biorhythm cycles for you. Alternatively, you can work out your own chart by using biorhythm calculators or computer programs (usually obtained by mail order).

Biorhythms are calculated from your date of birth and fall into three cycles: the 23-day *physical* cycle, said to influence strength, immunity, stamina, sex drive, and coordination; the 28-day *emotional* cycle, governing mood and creativity; and the 33-day *intellectual* cycle, acting upon memory and concentration.

When charted in monthly patterns, each cycle forms a wave across a central horizontal line. Since the cycles vary in length, they coincide only occasionally.

When a cycle peaks, its force is said to be strong. The low phase of the cycle is passive and recuperative. For example, peaks in the intellectual cycle are said to be marked by increased rationality and problem-solving ability, while troughs are characterized by an increase in intuition.

"Critical," also known as "caution," days occur when the cycles cross the horizontal line. When two or three cycles intersect at this point on a given day you are said to be especially vulnerable. Although biorhythms cannot predict accidents or crises, practitioners claim they may help you avoid potentially difficult situations.

EVIDENCE & RESEARCH

Chronobiology (the study of daily rhythms in physiological processes such as hormone production, temperature, and blood pressure) arose from the discovery that these daily rhythms could influence the body's reactions to drugs and the timing of asthma and heart attacks. Evidence of long-term cycles, however, is inconclusive and ambiguous.

Professor Harold Willis, a psychologist at Southern State College in Missouri found that over half the patients who died at a local hospital in 1973 did so on their critical days, and a study in the early 1960s by the Tokyo Institute of Public Health showed that bus and taxi accidents in Japan increased on drivers' critical days. However, research published in 1979 by the British Transport and Road Research Laboratory found no significant correlation between biorhythms and accidents.

MEDICAL OPINION

The theory of biorhythms is appealing, but the evidence to back it up is very thin, and most doctors would dismiss it.

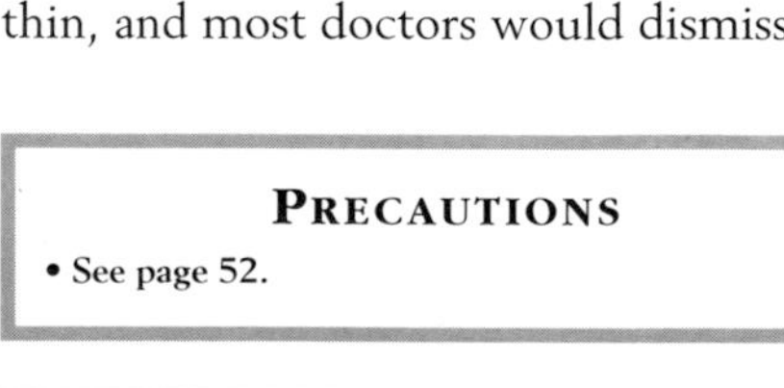

BIORHYTHM CHART

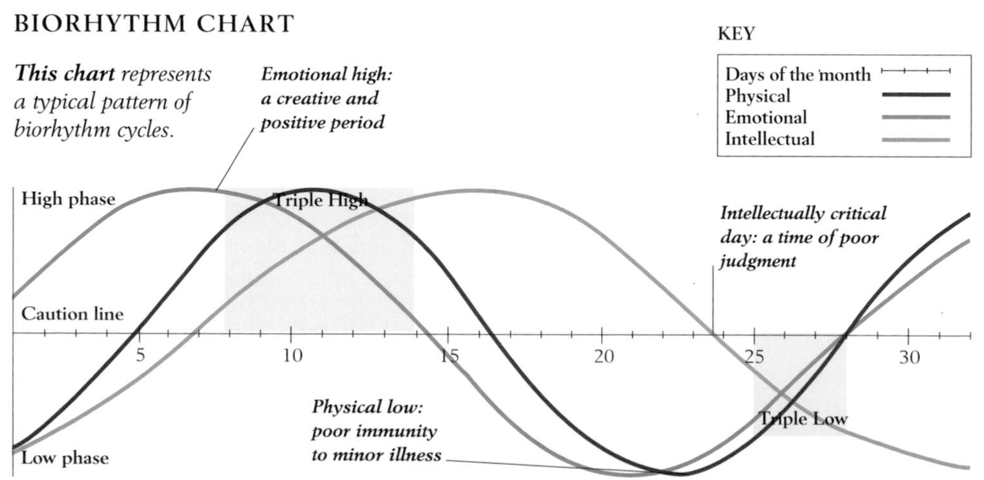

This chart *represents a typical pattern of biorhythm cycles.*

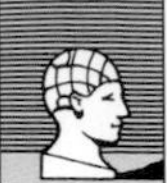

OTHER THERAPIES

SHAMANISM

The word *shaman,* from the Tungus language of Siberia, describes someone who is said to be able to "journey" to and commune with the spirit world. Shamans, variously known as witch doctors, wizards, sorcerors, medicine men, or holy men, have been revered by tribal societies from the ancient Celts to the Australian Aborigines.

Shamanism may be broadly defined as a way of healing and providing spiritual guidance that involves going into a trance. The shaman may use continuous sounds, such as drumming or shaking rattles, or hallucinogenic drugs, to enter into a state of altered consciousness in which he can determine the causes of your illness and learn how to cure it. Some practitioners claim to make contact with a spirit guide. Contemporary or neoshamanism combines traditional methods with modern therapies such as counseling and visualization (see pages 163 and 178). It first attracted interest in the US as awareness of Native American traditions grew, and then spread to the UK and Australia. A session may last from an hour to a weekend, and shamans claim to treat "conditions of the soul" that may affect emotional and physical health. Doctors tend to dismiss neoshamanism as a jumble of psychotherapy and New Age ideas.

VOICE THERAPY

German singing teacher Alfred Wolfsohn developed the basis of voice therapy in the 1920s and 1930s. When he died in 1962, Roy Hart, a South African actor and student of Wolfsohn, continued his work. The technique is most widely practiced in the UK and France.

Practitioners claim that the speed, tone, rhythm, and pitch of the voice provide vital clues to a person's mental, physical, and emotional health. Piano notes are used to help you expand the vocal and emotional range of your sounds. Emphasis is placed on exploring cries and screams as well as sighs and whispers: this is said to have a profound psychological effect and increase vocal expression. Voice therapy can help people deal with emotional barriers and vocal problems, such as stammering. Treatment may be 4–12 individual hour-long sessions, or group workshops over a week or weekend. Most doctors see voice therapy as an acceptable way to help self-expression, relaxation, and vocal flexibility.

THE SILVA METHOD

Developed in the 1960s by José Silva, a Mexican American, this technique aims to develop and control the powers of the mind through exercises that involve adjusting to different brain wavelengths or "levels." Exercises are taught at classes by registered practitioners throughout the US and UK.

Silva exercises, which are similar to those used in autogenic training (see page 168), aim to help you reach, and go beyond, the state of awareness achieved by meditation (see page 174). The exercises are designed to teach you to recognize and use different levels of consciousness. According to the Silva method, beta is associated with an everyday waking state; theta and delta are unconscious intuitive levels. "Going into alpha," Silva claimed, sharpens the mind, facilitates self-healing, and encourages extrasensory perception, telepathy, and clairvoyance. Further Silva exercises use visualization techniques (see page 178) to integrate the analytical left side of the brain with the creative right side.

Silva training involves 40 hours of seminars over two weekends. While the Silva method may enhance memory, self-confidence, and creativity, most doctors view it as essentially a self-hypnosis technique, and question its ability to promote mental ability or diagnostic skills.

PAST LIFE THERAPY

Since the 1950s, some hypnotherapists (see page 166) and psychotherapists (see page 160), mainly in the US and UK, have used regression techniques to allow patients to express what seem to be memories of earlier lives. Such regressions are often thought to be evidence of reincarnation, but some practitioners see them as the mind's way of symbolizing buried thoughts or emotions.

While regression usually takes place under hypnosis, practitioners trained in psychotherapy may work with you fully conscious, although very relaxed or in a light trance, sometimes as part of a group. You are asked about past events that may have current significance for you, and you may find yourself recalling times and places of which you have no apparent knowledge. Whatever their source, these "memories" can have a therapeutic, even cathartic, effect, and may help resolve emotional or nervous complaints, such as anxiety, phobias, and panic attacks. Sessions usually last about an hour, and treatment may continue for several months or longer.

There have been a few documented cases in which historical details recalled under hypnosis were later confirmed. However, doctors are likely to see past life therapy simply as an outlet for the imagination, and would advise against any literal interpretation of the events recalled.

AURA-SOMA

Described by its creator as "noninvasive, self-selective soul therapy," Aura-Soma is a form of color therapy (see page 186). It was developed, or "envisaged," in 1984 by Vicky Wall, a UK chiropodist who allegedly developed extrasensory powers after losing her sight. The therapy is mainly available in the UK; a small number of practitioners work in the US and Australia.

You are presented with a selection of over 90 specially prepared "balance" bottles, then asked to choose four. Each contains two colored liquids: a mixture of essential oils on a layer of springwater containing herbal extracts. The colors you choose are said to provide insights into your physical and emotional condition. The four bottles are shaken and the mixtures applied to your skin daily for as long as necessary; this supposedly allows the colors to enter the body and rebalance disturbed *chakras* (see page 109). There is no standard length of treatment or number of sessions, and the therapy is used primarily for long-standing emotional problems and stress. It is not recognized by conventional medicine.

PRECAUTIONS

- Check with your doctor before practicing any therapy that claims to alter your state of consciousness if you have a history of serious psychiatric illness.
- See also page 52.

DIAGNOSTIC TECHNIQUES

Complementary diagnostic techniques are based on one or more of three main principles: the patient's story, extrasensory perception, or examination of a specific part of the body that is said to represent the whole, as in iridology or Chinese and Ayurvedic tongue and pulse diagnosis. Dowsing and energy medicine are examples of methods that rely on processes not proved by science, professing to detect something that is not revealed by the five senses alone. Practitioners using complementary diagnostic techniques claim to find "weaknesses" or "disturbances" unidentified by conventional methods, which aim only to link recognized symptoms with named diseases that have established causes.

THE TECHNIQUES

PULSE DIAGNOSIS *page 192* ◆ TONGUE DIAGNOSIS *page 193*

HARA DIAGNOSIS *page 194* ◆ HAIR ANALYSIS *page 194*

IRIDOLOGY *page 195* ◆ APPLIED KINESIOLOGY *page 196*

TOUCH FOR HEALTH *page 197* ◆ DOWSING *page 198*

NUTRITIONAL TESTING *page 199*

ENERGY MEDICINE *page 200*

KIRLIAN PHOTOGRAPHY *page 201*

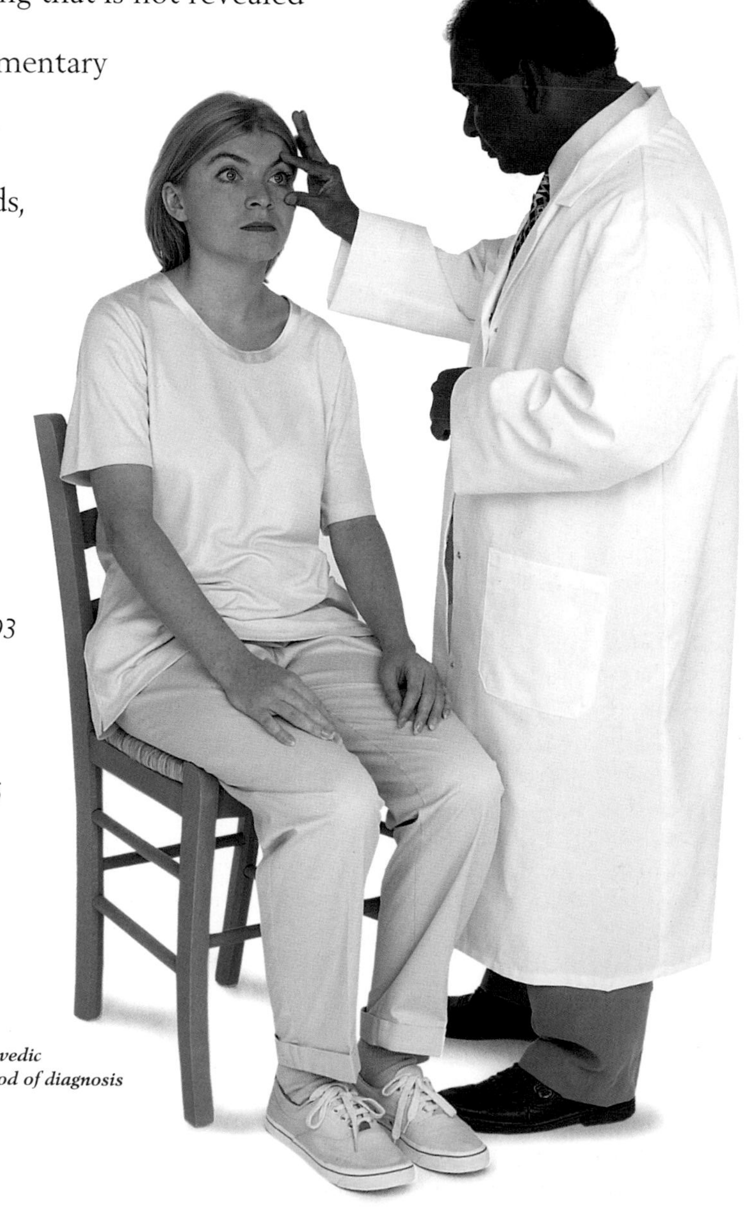

Ayurvedic method of diagnosis

PULSE DIAGNOSIS

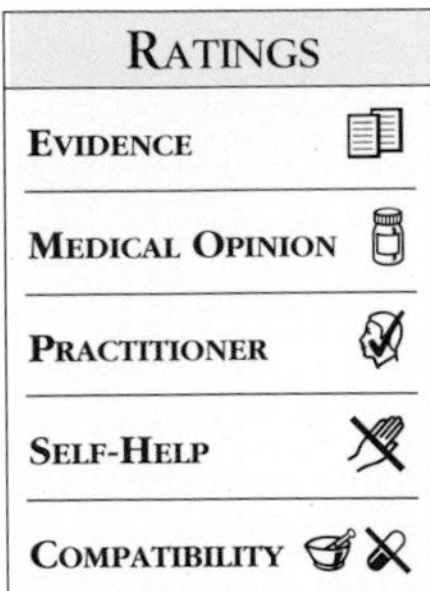

RATINGS
EVIDENCE
MEDICAL OPINION
PRACTITIONER
SELF-HELP
COMPATIBILITY

BOTH EASTERN AND WESTERN medical traditions assess health using the pulse in the radial artery of the wrist. Traditional Chinese and Ayurvedic practitioners distinguish up to nine pulses on each wrist, which are said to reflect the condition of internal organs and the flow of "life energy" throughout the body. Western practitioners use only one pulse point on the wrist to check the rate at which blood pumps from the heart. From this they may diagnose heart disorders and circulatory problems. Some complementary therapists use pulse testing to detect food allergies and intolerances.

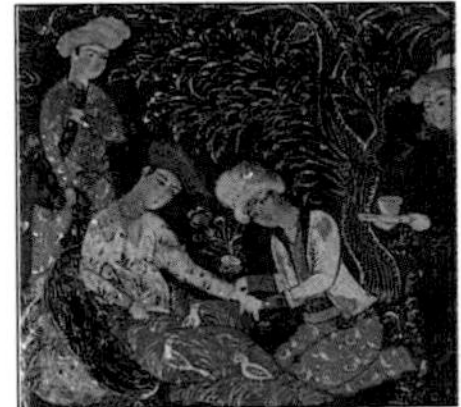

An Asian physician *tests a pulse in this illustration of 1632.*

WESTERN DIAGNOSIS

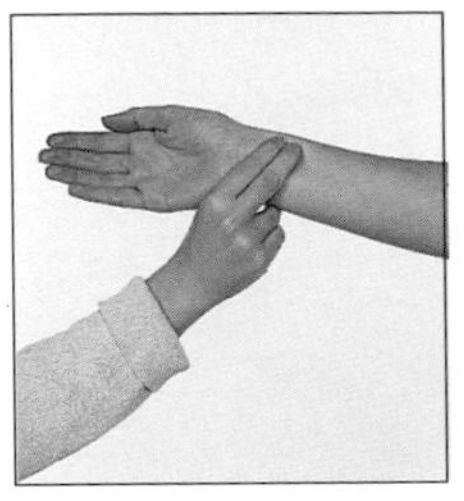

A doctor *or practitioner of Western therapies lays two fingers on the inside of the patient's wrist to test the pulse of blood. The average adult pulse is 60–80 beats per minute.*

Practitioners of Western complementary therapies often use pulse diagnosis in the same way as conventional doctors – to measure the rate at which blood pulses through the arteries after each heartbeat. The practitioner uses two fingertips to feel the pulse in the radial artery of the wrist. An abnormally fast or slow pulse may be a sign of illness. In addition to this method, two further variations are used by some practitioners:

Pulse-testing for reactions to food: Devised in the 1940s by American allergist Dr. Arthur Coca, this method claims to diagnose food allergies and intolerances. The pulse is taken before eating a suspect food, then at 10-, 20-, 40-, and 60-minute intervals afterward. An increase or decrease in the rate of 10 or more beats per minute is said to indicate an abnormal reaction.

Auriculocardiac reflex method: According to Dr. Paul Nogier, the French doctor who developed auricular acupuncture in the 1950s (see page 94), specific points on the ear relate to different parts of the body. He claimed that when a point is stimulated using a special electromagnetic indicator, types of light, or the blunt end of an acupuncture needle, a surge in the wrist pulse can occur, which indicates disharmony in the related body part.

CHINESE DIAGNOSIS

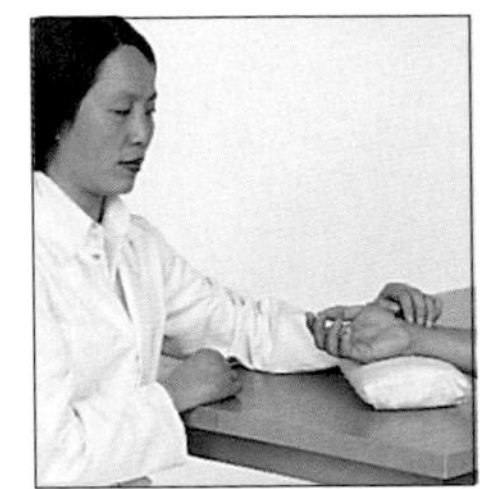

In Traditional Chinese Medicine, *the doctor assesses the flow of* qi *and the state of body organs by using three fingers to test pulse readings on each wrist.*

In Traditional Chinese Medicine (TCM), pulse-taking is an essential diagnostic technique. Three pulse points – known as *cuen*, *guan*, and *chi* – are identified on the radial artery of the wrist, using the index, middle, and ring fingers.

From the strength and rhythm of the pulses, the practitioner assesses the flow of *qi*, or "life energy," in the body, and the interaction of the forces of *yin* and *yang* (see pages 91 and 141). *Qi* is said to be carried through the body via channels linked to body organs, such as the Heart, Kidneys, Liver, Lungs, Large and Small Intestines, Spleen, and Stomach. Assessing the flow of *qi* provides information about the condition of these organs.

The practitioner will apply light, moderate, and deep pressure to the pulse points, giving nine pulse readings on each wrist. The pressure levels relate to the three qualities necessary for a healthy pulse. Under light pressure, it must be calm and regular, when it is said to have Stomach *qi*, the sign of a good constitution. Under moderate pressure, it should be even and forceful, having *shen*, or vitality. If this can still be felt when pressing firmly, the pulse has *geng*, or "root." There are 28 basic types of pulse, including "floating," "feeble," "slow," "rapid," and "slippery."

AYURVEDIC DIAGNOSIS

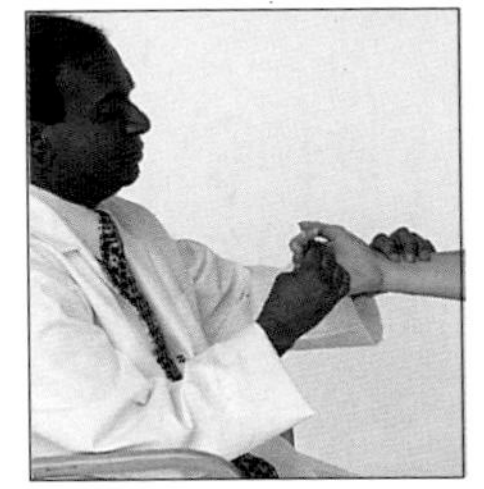

An Ayurvedic practitioner *uses the index, middle and ring fingers to locate three pulse points, which are related to the flow of* prana *in the body and the three* doshas.

Pulse diagnosis in Ayurveda is based on principles similar to those of TCM. Practitioners check three deep and three superficial pulse points on each wrist to analyze the strength, vitality, and physical state of specific organs and also of the *nadi*, channels which circulate *prana*, or "life energy," through the body (see page 109).

Each pulse point is also related to one of the *doshas*, or vital energies, believed to define every individual (see page 145). One *dosha* and one pulse tend to predominate. The pulse nearest the hand (the quick, slithery "snake pulse") is *vata*; the middle pulse (jumpy, often called "the frog") is *pitta*; and the point furthest from the hand (the slow, floating "swan pulse") is *kapha*.

MEDICAL OPINION

Pulse testing for food allergies is not seen as dependable by most doctors. There is no laboratory equipment sensitive enough to measure the pulses that practitioners of Chinese medicine and Ayurveda claim to detect, and Western doctors find it difficult to believe that such subtleties exist.

PRECAUTIONS

- See page 52.

TONGUE DIAGNOSIS

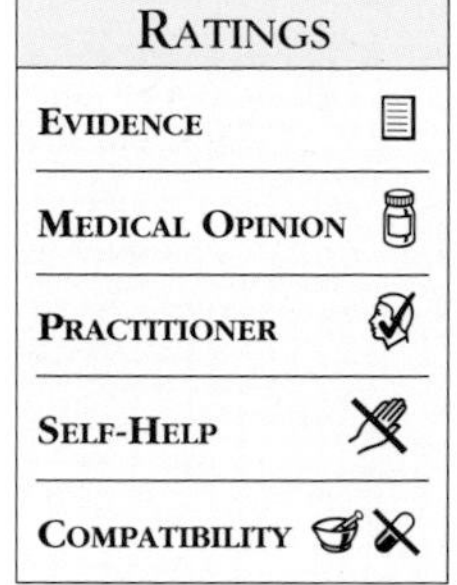

RATINGS
EVIDENCE
MEDICAL OPINION
PRACTITIONER
SELF-HELP
COMPATIBILITY

"LET ME SEE YOUR TONGUE" is a common request by doctors all over the world. The condition of the tongue is believed by all medical traditions to reflect an individual's state of health, although to an infinitely greater degree in the East. Practitioners of Traditional Chinese Medicine and Ayurveda closely observe the surface of the tongue to assess the balance of "life energy" forces in the body and the health of internal organs. Conventional doctors are also likely to examine the tongue, and may reach conclusions similar to those of their complementary counterparts, but will diagnose specific medical conditions only.

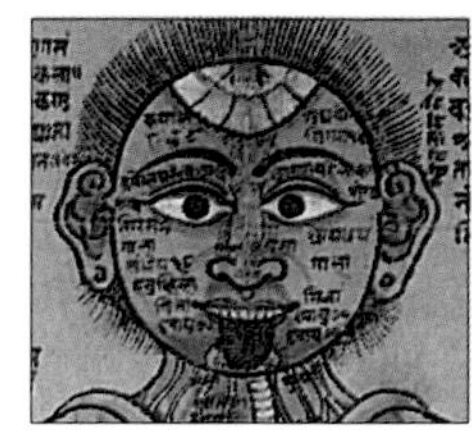

***The tongue** shown in a traditional diagnostic chart from Nepal.*

WESTERN DIAGNOSIS

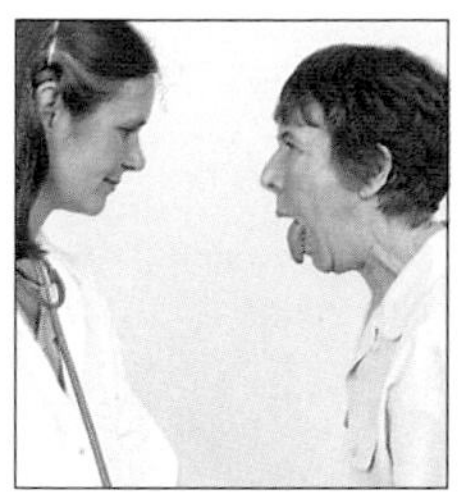

***A doctor** or Western complementary therapist assesses the patient's tongue for clues to help diagnose many conditions, including constipation and iron deficiency.*

In conventional medicine, doctors regularly examine their patients' tongues, and certain tongue conditions are associated with poor health. An inflamed tongue, for example, is a sign of severe iron deficiency. Dehydration may also be diagnosed from the appearance of the tongue, while some nervous disorders affect its movements.

In complementary medicine, the tongue may similarly be examined as an aid to diagnosis. Nutritional therapists (see page 148) claim to detect certain vitamin or mineral deficiencies in the appearance of the tongue. A smooth, sore tongue may be due to a lack of vitamin B_{12}, folic acid (a B vitamin), or iron. In some cases, it is also connected with a yeast or fungal infection. Enlarged, sore taste buds at the tip of the tongue are said to indicate a lack of vitamin B_2 or B_6, and bruising or enlargement of the veins under the tongue may be due to a deficiency of vitamin C.

The appearance of the tongue is also associated with certain conditions in homeopathy (see page 126). A red tip on the tongue, particularly if dry and cracked, is one of the key symptoms considered when prescribing *Rhus tox.*, used for rheumatism and skin conditions. A patient with chronic phlegm and a red tongue with a thick coating is likely to be given *Antim tart.*

CHINESE DIAGNOSIS

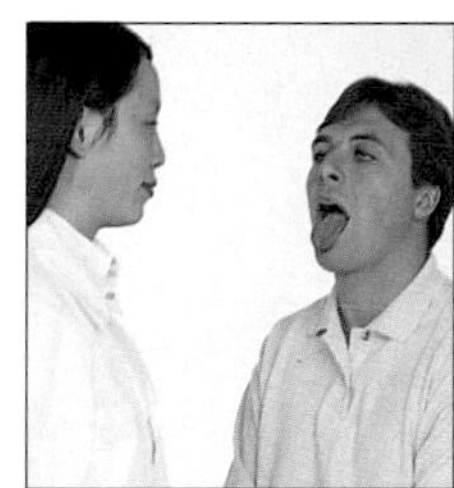

***In Traditional Chinese Medicine**, the practitioner observes the surface of the patient's tongue, noting its color, size, and coating, and which areas are moist or dry.*

According to Traditional Chinese Medicine (TCM), the tongue is linked to all the organs in the body via meridians, which act as channels for *qi*, or "life energy" (see page 91). Disharmony in the body, based on a patient's pattern of symptoms, is believed to be reflected in the tongue before manifesting as disease.

A practitioner of TCM will observe the shape, color, size, texture, and coating of the tongue. A healthy tongue should be pale red, reasonably moist, fit neatly into the mouth, and have a thin white moss (coating). A red tongue indicates "heat," or excess *qi*, and a pale tongue reflects "cold," or deficient *qi*.

The tongue is also considered when assessing the balance of *yin* and *yang* (see page 141). A puffy tongue with tooth marks on the edges is often due to fluid retention, which may be caused by *yang* deficiency. An absence of tongue moss, which Chinese doctors call a "peeled" tongue, may be the result of deficient *yin*, characterized by a lack of body fluids and secretions.

Different areas of the tongue are said to relate to different parts of the body, altering in color, shape, or texture according to internal problems. Red in the center of the tongue, for instance, could indicate "heat" in the stomach.

AYURVEDIC DIAGNOSIS

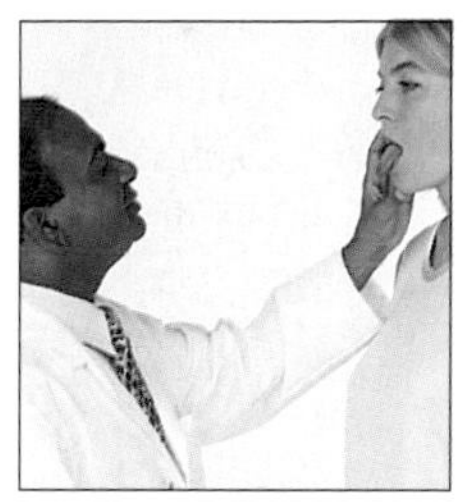

***An Ayurvedic practitioner** can assess whether the patient's three vital doshas are in harmony by examining the color, shape, and texture of the tongue.*

The tongue is analyzed by Ayurvedic practitioners in much the same way as in TCM. Abnormalities on the surface are said to indicate disturbances in the three vital energies, or *doshas* (see page 145). A whitish tongue is linked to a *kapha* disturbance, a red or yellow-green tongue suggests disrupted *pitta*, and a black or brown tongue disruptions in *vata*.

Discolorations or irregularities on different parts of the tongue are associated with disturbances in different body organs. The condition of the lungs, for example, is believed to relate to the sides of the tongue toward the front.

MEDICAL OPINION

Doctors often examine the tongue, but they consider blood tests to be a more reliable diagnostic tool. Complementary practitioners' claims to detect nutritional deficiencies from the appearance of the tongue are thus in line with conventional medicine. However, Western doctors do not accept tongue diagnosis as practiced in TCM and Ayurveda.

PRECAUTIONS

- See page 52.

HARA DIAGNOSIS

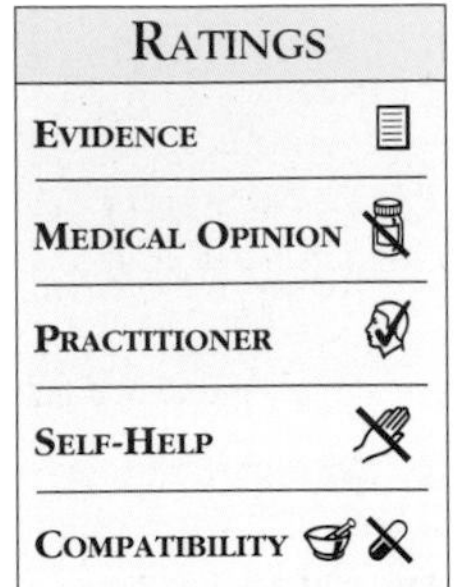

HARA IS THE JAPANESE WORD for abdomen. "Feeling" the hara *is an important diagnostic technique in Japanese medicine, and is widely used by practitioners of shiatsu massage (see page 96). It is, however, a far older practice than shiatsu – its roots lie in Traditional Chinese Medicine and in the theory of the meridians, which are channels of* ki*, or "life energy" (see page 91).* Hara *diagnosis is said to work by relating different parts of the abdomen to different internal organs and meridians. The* hara *can be interpreted and "mapped" using various systems; one of the simplest is shown below.*

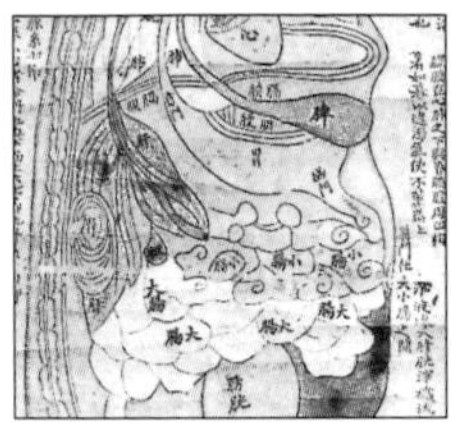

This Chinese chart *maps the internal organs for diagnosis.*

CONSULTING A PRACTITIONER

Ki is said to enter the body in the breath and to be channeled through the meridians to the organs. It is "stored" in the abdomen in an area called the *tanden*, just below the navel. In *hara* diagnosis, the patient is asked to relax and breathe deeply to allow *ki* to circulate fully. The practitioner then gently presses the *tanden* and other areas on the abdomen to assess the circulation of *ki*. Any disturbances in the flow are thought to lead to illness.

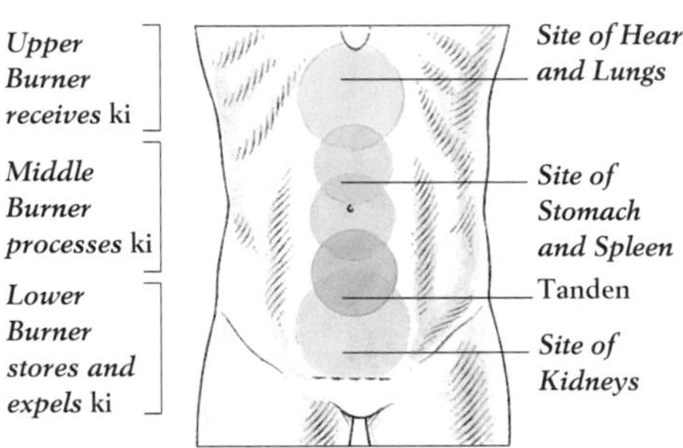

The abdomen is divided *into the three regions of the "Triple Burner," said to relate to the organs of the upper, middle, and lower body respectively.*

MEDICAL OPINION

Western doctors do not accept the theory of *ki* and internal energy channels. They are likely to view as even more far-fetched the idea that *ki* can be assessed and the condition of organs in the body diagnosed by feeling the abdomen.

PRECAUTIONS

- See shiatsu (page 97) and page 52.

HAIR ANALYSIS

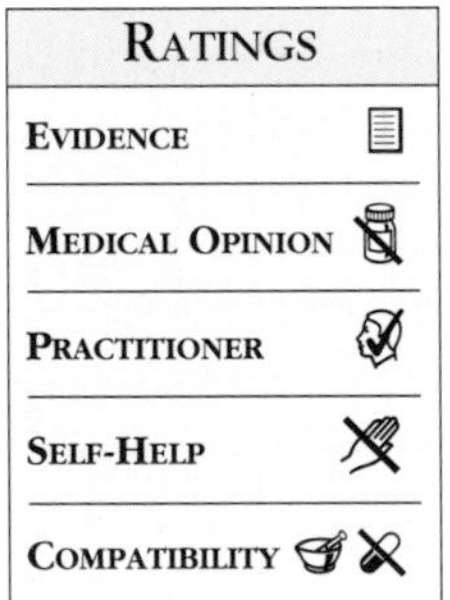

LABORATORY ANALYSIS of strands of hair has been used since the 19th century to assess levels of minerals in the body. These chemicals are absorbed from food and the environment, and many are needed for good health, but others, such as mercury and lead, are toxic if they accumulate in the body. Mineral deficiencies and toxic excesses are said to contribute to allergies, digestive problems, depression, and other ailments. Practitioners such as nutritional therapists and clinical ecologists (see pages 148 and 154), who treat patients using mineral supplements and detoxification diets, often use hair analysis.

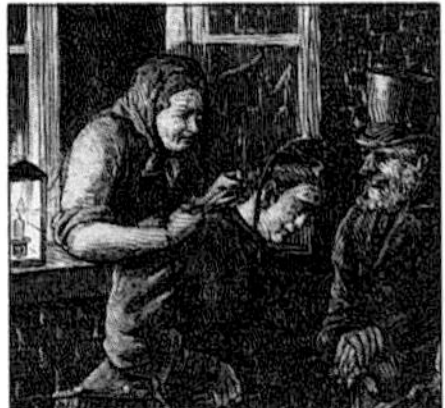

Cutting a sample *of hair in a German pharmacy in 1894.*

CONSULTING A PRACTITIONER

Hair is made of a protein known as keratin. This contains sulfur, which traps minerals from the blood supply feeding the root of the hair. Strands of hair retain minerals even after being removed from the scalp. Hair grows at a rate of about ½ in (1 cm) a month, and hair analysis works with samples taken from the 1½ in (3 cm) of hair closest to the scalp. The sample is sent to a laboratory, where it is washed and rinsed intensively, then burned and the ash analyzed. Hair analysis measures levels of essential minerals, including calcium, sodium, magnesium, phosphorus, and potassium, and toxic minerals, such as lead, arsenic, mercury, and aluminum.

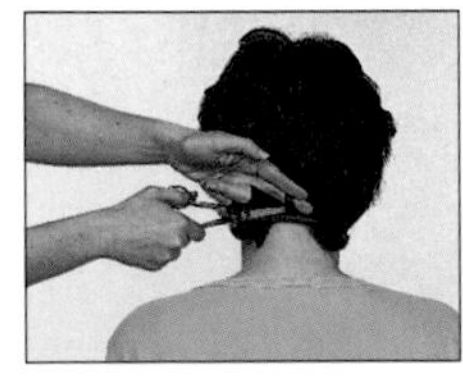

A sample *taken from the nape of the neck, near the root, contains minerals absorbed by the hair during the previous three months.*

MEDICAL OPINION

Doctors do not consider hair analysis to be a reliable test of mineral concentrations in the body. It may offer information about long-term exposure to toxic chemicals, but it is not believed to be able to reveal allergies or diagnose diseases.

PRECAUTIONS

- See page 52.

IRIDOLOGY

RATINGS

- EVIDENCE
- MEDICAL OPINION
- PRACTITIONER
- SELF-HELP
- COMPATIBILITY

PIONEERED IN HUNGARY in the 19th century, iridology uses the appearance of the eye, and in particular the iris, to assess mental and physical health. Practitioners claim to identify past and present disorders and predict future problems by studying the color, condition, and markings of a patient's iris. They claim not to diagnose an actual disease but to pinpoint weaknesses in the body so that health problems can be avoided. Iridology is sometimes used as an additional diagnostic tool by practitioners of therapies such as homeopathy and naturopathy, especially in continental Europe.

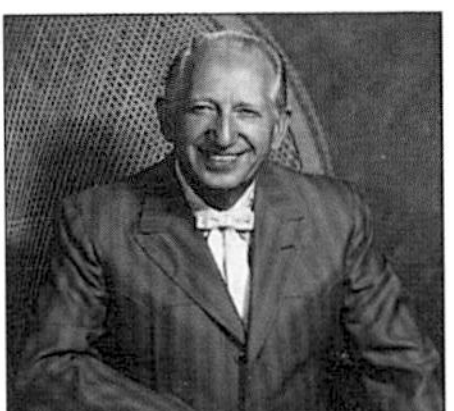

Dr. Bernard Jensen *developed the iris chart used by iridologists.*

HISTORY

Clear, shining eyes have been associated with good health since ancient times. A form of iridology may have been used by the Greek physician Hippocrates in the 5th century B.C., but only in the late 19th century was the theory of modern iridology first outlined by a Hungarian doctor, Ignatz von Peczely. As a child, von Peczely was trying to release a trapped owl when the bird broke its leg. At that moment, he noticed a dark mark appearing in the owl's iris, which turned white as the leg healed. When von Peczely became a doctor, he dedicated his career to charting patients' diseases from markings in the iris.

In 1950, a detailed map of the iris was constructed by American doctor Bernard Jensen. It is this diagnostic tool that is used by iridologists today (see below).

EXAMINING THE EYE

The practitioner may use a camera with a special lens and sidelighting to produce a photographic slide of each iris. The slides are later projected onto a large screen for detailed analysis.

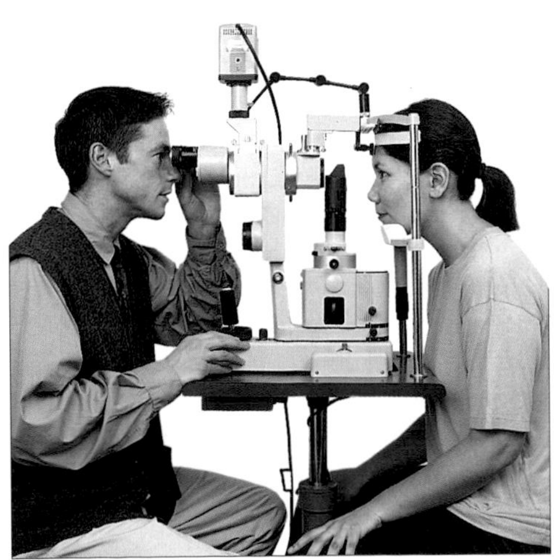

CONSULTING A PRACTITIONER

An iris includes thousands of nerve endings, and iridologists claim that it is therefore linked to every body organ and tissue. Neuro-optic reflexes in the iris are said to react to disorders in the body, marking or discoloring the related part of the iris.

The first consultation lasts about an hour. Some iridologists use a camera to make slides of your irises (see below), but other practitioners may simply examine your eyes with an ophthalmoscope or even a flashlight and magnifying glass.

The fibers radiating from the pupil are closely examined, as is the condition of the iris. White marks, for example, are said to indicate inflammation in the organ related to that part of the iris; a dark rim around the iris reveals the presence of "toxins." Eye color is believed to be linked to constitution: those with blue eyes are said to be prone to complaints such as arthritis, brown eyes to a slow metabolic rate, and mixed irises to a weak digestion. The practitioner will treat any conditions identified using the therapy with which he works, or will refer you to a specialist.

EVIDENCE & RESEARCH

Clinical trials have so far indicated that iridology fails to diagnose disease even when it is present. These trials include a UK study of iridology photographs reported in *Complementary Therapies in Medicine* in 1996; a 1988 study in the *British Medical Journal*, using gallbladder disease as the test; and a 1979 study of patients with kidney disease in the *Journal of the American Medical Association.*

MEDICAL OPINION

Most doctors see iridology as a misleading diagnostic technique. They caution that patients may be unnecessarily distressed by inaccurate and alarmist diagnoses.

PRECAUTIONS

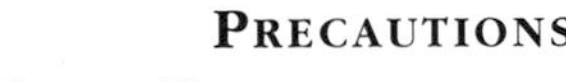

- See page 52.

MAP OF THE IRISES

Each iris is divided into sections corresponding to different parts of the body and body systems.

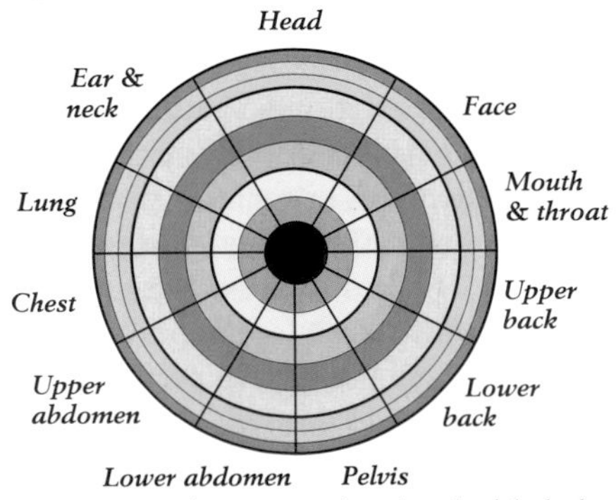

Right iris *is said to represent the right side of the body*

KEY

- Skin
- Muscle
- Arteries
- Veins
- Lymph
- Intestines
- Skeleton
- Stomach

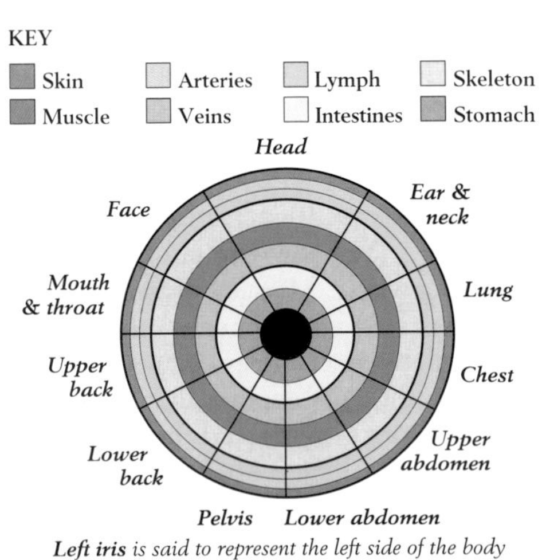

Left iris *is said to represent the left side of the body*

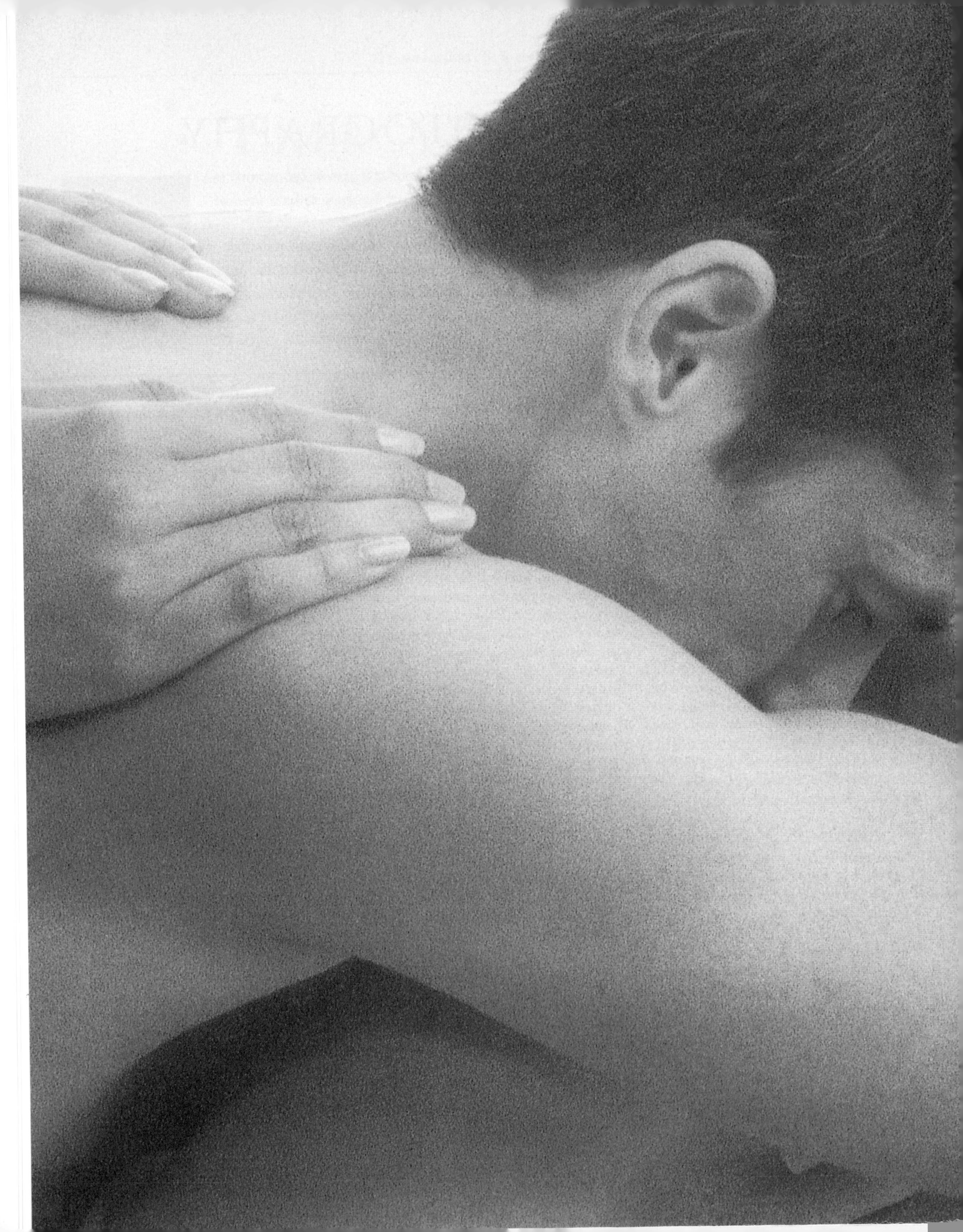

Treating Ailments

4

Both complementary and conventional medicine have their place in health care. For life-threatening conditions, modern surgery and powerful drugs are essential, but complementary therapies can play a supporting role, helping body and mind develop greater resilience. For other health problems, however, such as long-term and recurring disorders, where mainstream medicine can run out of solutions, nonconventional therapies may come into their own and can be extraordinarily effective. But how do you choose from the wide range of therapies available and determine which is most likely to benefit you?

This section helps you make an informed choice by highlighting the best complementary treatment options for over 200 health problems, from headaches and colds to heart disease and cancer. There is a clear explanation of the causes, symptoms, and conventional treatment for each condition, together with expert advice on prevention and self-help. The key complementary therapies for every ailment are summarized, with information on what each therapy involves, why it is thought to be beneficial, and details of any research that supports claims of its effectiveness.

HOW TO USE THIS SECTION

THE FOLLOWING PAGES offer a guide to choosing complementary therapies for over 200 health problems, ranging from colds and acne to cancer and heart disease. Each condition is summarized and its conventional treatment described, followed by an outline of the approach taken by the most commonly used complementary therapies. Where possible, information is based on research and clinical experience. To discover which type of therapy most appeals, see the questionnaire on pages 50–51. See pages 318–23 for advice on finding a practitioner and a list of useful addresses.

SAFETY ISSUES

Before embarking on any treatment, it is important to read the precautions below and the red light symptoms (see right), in addition to the relevant therapy entry (see pages 48–190) and the guidelines for choosing a practitioner (see page 318).

PRECAUTIONS

- Do not attempt to diagnose a health problem yourself. Always consult your doctor.
- Consult a doctor immediately if you have any of the red light symptoms.
- Check with a doctor if there is no improvement within 2–3 weeks (48 hours in children under five) or if symptoms get worse.
- Do not stop taking any prescribed medication without first consulting your doctor.
- Tell your complementary practitioner about any prescribed medication you are taking, and any other complementary treatments you are receiving.
- Tell your doctor about any complementary treatments or remedies you are taking.
- Always check with a doctor before embarking on any complementary treatment if you have any medical condition or symptoms of illness.
- Do not embark on vigorous exercise without first consulting a doctor if you have any serious medical condition, such as back pain, high blood pressure, or heart disease, or if you are pregnant.
- People with persistent mental illness may be disturbed by hypnosis, visualization, and meditation.
- Advise your practitioner if you have any sexually transmitted disease.
- Do not begin a course of complementary therapy without first consulting your doctor if you are pregnant, or trying to conceive.
- Do not take or use any herbal or aromatherapy products during the first three months of pregnancy or if breastfeeding unless supervised by an experienced practitioner.
- Consult your doctor before allowing babies or infants to receive complementary treatments, as some, such as enemas and certain herbal remedies, are unsuitable for small children.
- Children under 12 should follow complementary treatments only with professional supervision and a doctor's consent.
- Children under 12 should not fast.
- Do not take supplements of iron or vitamin A without first consulting your doctor. Do not exceed the recommended dosage of other supplements.
- Do not take high doses of nutritional supplements without professional supervision.
- Do not embark on fasts lasting longer than two days without professional supervision.

RED LIGHT SYMPTOMS

Consult a doctor *immediately* for:

- Chest pain or shortness of breath; if there is acute pain in the chest, arms, jaw, or throat, call an ambulance
- Unexplained dizziness
- Persistent hoarseness, cough, sore throat
- Difficulty in swallowing
- Persistent abdominal pain or indigestion
- Coughing up blood
- Persistent weight loss or fatigue
- A mole changing shape, size, or color, or itching or bleeding
- Change in bowel or bladder habits
- Passing blood in the stool
- Vaginal bleeding between periods, after sex or after menopause, or unusual vaginal discharge
- Thickening or lump in a breast; discharge or bleeding from a nipple; change in shape or size of a breast
- Swelling or lump in a testicle; change in shape or size of a testicle; total and persistent failure to get an erection
- Severe headaches; persistent one-sided headaches; vision disturbance
- A sore that does not heal, or swellings
- Frequent and persistent back pain
- Unexplained leg pain and swelling

THERAPY RATINGS

Each therapy is assessed according to three categories using the following ratings symbols:

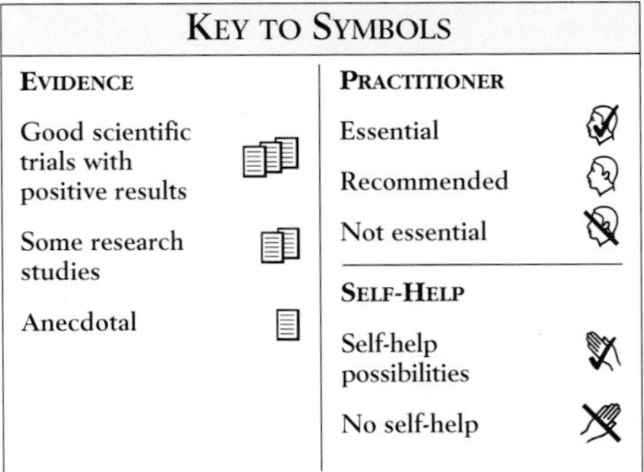

EVIDENCE

***Good scientific trials with positive results**: There is a credible base of research evidence for the efficacy of this therapy.*

***Some research studies**: There are some published studies, but no well-designed clinical trials, and little conclusive evidence.*

***Anecdotal**: Evidence of efficacy is purely via oral tradition or word-of-mouth; any research has been inconclusive or in some cases negative.*

PRACTITIONER

***Essential**: This therapy should not, or cannot, be attempted without guidance from a qualified practitioner.*

***Recommended**: While supervision may not be essential, it is definitely to be recommended initially or if you have a serious condition.*

***Not essential**: It is perfectly possible to learn about this therapy from books, videos, or tapes; while supervision may help, it is not necessary.*

SELF-HELP

***Self-help possibilities**: It is possible to practice this therapy on yourself, either self-taught or on the advice of a practitioner.*

***No self-help**: Do not try any treatment without the supervision of a practitioner.*

TYPICAL AILMENTS PAGES

Below are sample pages that show the typical coverage of an ailment. Annotations explain how the pages are organized and how information is presented.

ORGANIZED BY BODY SYSTEM
The ailments are grouped according to the body system they affect.

Key to symbols *explains clearly what each symbol means*

At-a-glance symbols *assess the efficacy, practitioner involvement, and self-help options for each treatment*

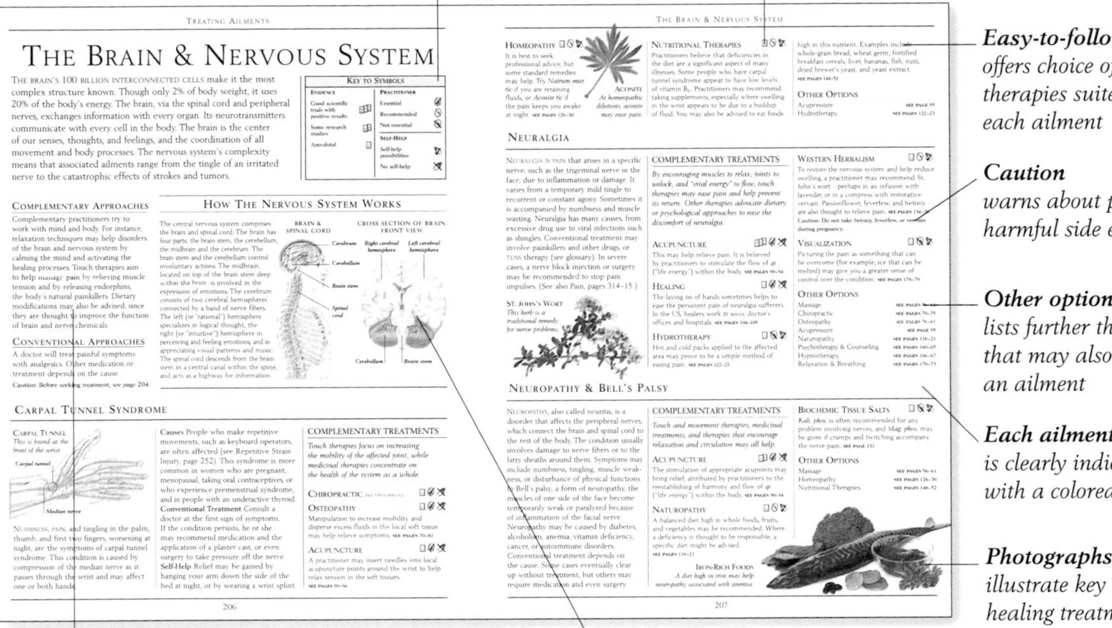

Easy-to-follow text *offers choice of key therapies suited to each ailment*

Caution *warns about possible harmful side effects*

Other options *lists further therapies that may also benefit an ailment*

Each ailment entry *is clearly indicated with a colored band*

Photographs *illustrate key healing treatments*

Complementary and conventional approaches *are summarized for easy comparison*

Cross sections *and detailed diagrams illustrate how the body systems work*

FEATURE PAGES
Ten two-page features focus in detail on the best treatment options for particularly common ailments, such as headaches.

Causes & symptoms *summarizes medical thinking on why the ailment occurs*

Prevention *gives self-help ideas for avoiding the condition or easing it*

Touch & movement approaches *work on the body at a structural level, improving the function of the spine, for example*

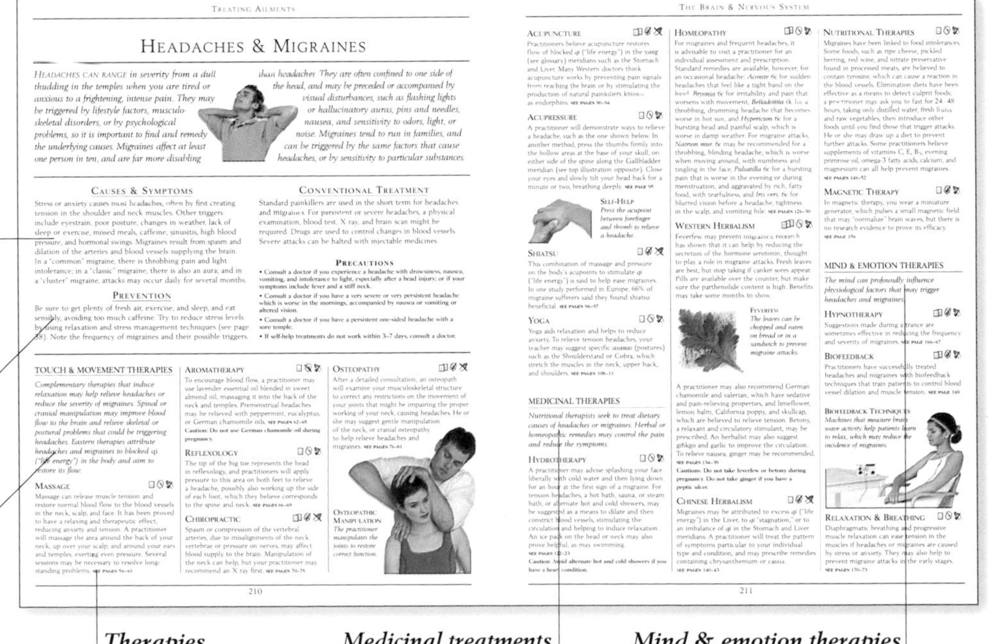

Therapies *are listed in the order in which they appear in the book*

Medicinal treatments, *usually herbal remedies or dietary approaches, aim to redress imbalances*

Mind & emotion therapies *have a direct impact on body functions by restoring a sense of self-control and calm*

AILMENT GROUPS

- THE BRAIN & NERVOUS SYSTEM *(see pages 206–13)*
- SKIN *(see pages 214–19)*
- EYES *(see pages 220–21)*
- EARS *(see pages 222–23)*
- THE RESPIRATORY SYSTEM *(see pages 224–27)*
- MOUTH & THROAT *(see pages 228–29)*
- DIGESTION *(see pages 230–39)*
- THE URINARY SYSTEM *(see pages 240–41)*
- HEART & CIRCULATION *(see pages 242–49)*
- MUSCLES, BONES & JOINTS *(see pages 250–61)*
- HORMONES *(see pages 262–63)*
- WOMEN'S HEALTH *(see pages 264–75)*
- MEN'S HEALTH *(see pages 276–77)*
- CHILDREN'S HEALTH *(see pages 278–85)*
- MIND & EMOTIONS *(see pages 286–97)*
- ALLERGIES *(see pages 298–303)*
- CANCER *(see pages 304–307)*
- THE IMMUNE SYSTEM *(see pages 308–13)*
- PAIN *(see pages 314–15)*
- FIRST AID *(see pages 316–17)*

THE BRAIN & NERVOUS SYSTEM

THE BRAIN'S 100 BILLION INTERCONNECTED CELLS make it the most complex structure known. Though only 2% of body weight, it uses 20% of the body's energy. The brain, via the spinal cord and peripheral nerves, exchanges information with every organ. Its neurotransmitters communicate with every cell in the body. The brain is the center of our senses, thoughts, and feelings, and the coordination of all movement and body processes. The nervous system's complexity means that associated ailments range from the tingle of an irritated nerve to the catastrophic effects of strokes and tumors.

KEY TO SYMBOLS

EVIDENCE
- Good scientific trials with positive results
- Some research studies
- Anecdotal

PRACTITIONER
- Essential
- Recommended
- Not essential

SELF-HELP
- Self-help possibilities
- No self-help

COMPLEMENTARY APPROACHES

Complementary practitioners try to work with mind and body. For instance, relaxation techniques may help disorders of the brain and nervous system by calming the mind and activating the healing processes. Touch therapies aim to help manage pain by relieving muscle tension and by releasing endorphins, the body's natural painkillers. Dietary modifications may also be advised, since they are thought to improve the function of brain and nerve chemicals.

CONVENTIONAL APPROACHES

A doctor will treat painful symptoms with analgesics. Other medication or treatment depends on the cause.

Caution: Before seeking treatment, see page 204.

HOW THE NERVOUS SYSTEM WORKS

The central nervous system comprises the brain and spinal cord. The brain has four parts: the brain stem, the cerebellum, the midbrain and the cerebrum. The brain stem and the cerebellum control involuntary actions. The midbrain, located on top of the brain stem deep within the brain, is involved in the expression of emotions. The cerebrum consists of two cerebral hemispheres connected by a band of nerve fibers. The left (or "rational") hemisphere specializes in logical thought, the right (or "intuitive") hemisphere in perceiving and feeling emotions, and in appreciating visual patterns and music. The spinal cord descends from the brain stem in a central canal within the spine, and acts as a highway for information.

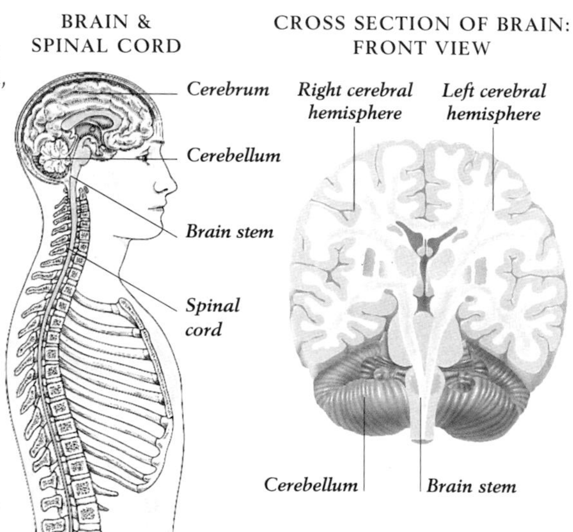

CARPAL TUNNEL SYNDROME

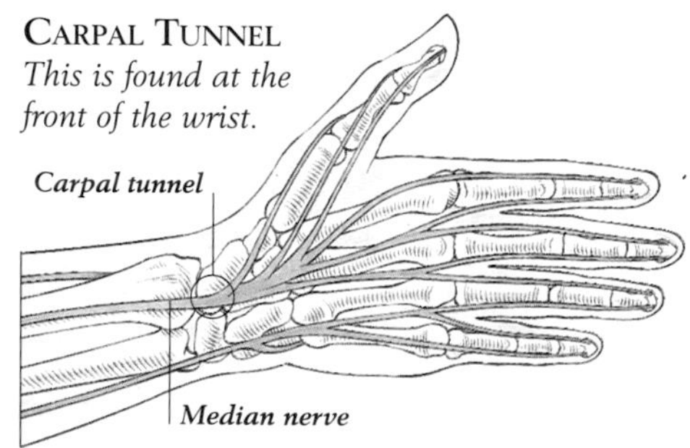

CARPAL TUNNEL
This is found at the front of the wrist.

NUMBNESS, PAIN, and tingling in the palm, thumb, and first two fingers, worsening at night, are the symptoms of carpal tunnel syndrome. This condition is caused by compression of the median nerve as it passes through the wrist and may affect one or both hands.

Causes People who make repetitive movements, such as keyboard operators, are often affected (see Repetitive Strain Injury, page 252). This syndrome is more common in women who are pregnant, menopausal, taking oral contraceptives, or who experience premenstrual syndrome, and in people with an underactive thyroid.
Conventional Treatment Consult a doctor at the first sign of symptoms. If the condition persists, he or she may recommend medication and the application of a plaster cast, or even surgery to take pressure off the nerve.
Self-Help Relief may be gained by hanging your arm down the side of the bed at night, or by wearing a wrist splint.

COMPLEMENTARY TREATMENTS

Touch therapies focus on increasing the mobility of the affected joint, while medicinal therapies concentrate on the health of the system as a whole.

CHIROPRACTIC (SEE OSTEOPATHY)

OSTEOPATHY

Manipulation to increase mobility and disperse excess fluids in the local soft tissue may help relieve symptoms. SEE PAGES 70–81

ACUPUNCTURE

A practitioner may insert needles into local acupuncture points around the wrist to help relax tension in the soft tissues.
SEE PAGES 90–94

HOMEOPATHY

It is best to seek professional advice, but some standard remedies may help. Try *Natrum mur.* *6c* if you are retaining fluids, or *Aconite 6c* if the pain keeps you awake at night. SEE PAGES 126–30

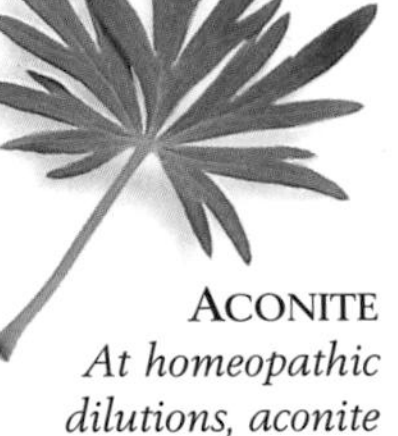

ACONITE
At homeopathic dilutions, aconite may ease pain.

NUTRITIONAL THERAPIES

Practitioners believe that deficiencies in the diet are a significant aspect of many illnesses. Some people who have carpal tunnel syndrome appear to have low levels of vitamin B_6. Practitioners may recommend taking supplements, especially where swelling in the wrist appears to be due to a buildup of fluid. You may also be advised to eat foods high in this nutrient. Examples include whole-grain bread, wheat germ, fortified breakfast cereals, liver, bananas, fish, nuts, dried brewer's yeast, and yeast extract.
SEE PAGES 148–52

OTHER OPTIONS

Acupressure SEE PAGE 95
Hydrotherapy SEE PAGES 122–23

NEURALGIA

NEURALGIA IS PAIN that arises in a specific nerve, such as the trigeminal nerve in the face, due to inflammation or damage. It varies from a temporary mild tingle to recurrent or constant agony. Sometimes it is accompanied by numbness and muscle wasting. Neuralgia has many causes, from excessive drug use to viral infections such as shingles. Conventional treatment may involve painkillers and other drugs, or TENS therapy (see glossary). In severe cases, a nerve block injection or surgery may be recommended to stop pain impulses. (See also Pain, pages 314–15.)

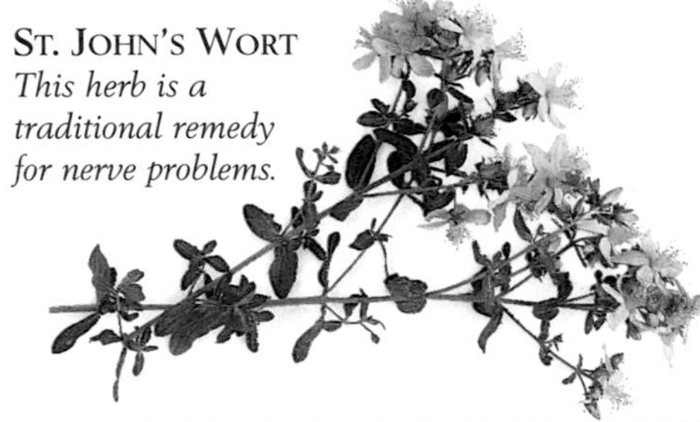

ST. JOHN'S WORT
This herb is a traditional remedy for nerve problems.

COMPLEMENTARY TREATMENTS

By encouraging muscles to relax, joints to unlock, and "vital energy" to flow, touch therapies may ease pain and help prevent its return. Other therapies advocate dietary or psychological approaches to ease the discomfort of neuralgia.

ACUPUNCTURE

This may help relieve pain. It is believed by practitioners to stimulate the flow of *qi* ("life energy") within the body. SEE PAGES 90–94

HEALING

The laying on of hands sometimes helps to ease the persistent pain of neuralgia sufferers. In the US, healers work in some doctor's offices and hospitals. SEE PAGES 104–105

HYDROTHERAPY

Hot and cold packs applied to the affected area may prove to be a simple method of easing pain. SEE PAGES 122–23

WESTERN HERBALISM

To restore the nervous system and help reduce swelling, a practitioner may recommend St. John's wort – perhaps in an infusion with lavender, or in a compress with restorative vervain. Passionflower, feverfew, and betony are also thought to relieve pain. SEE PAGES 134–39
Caution: Do not take betony, feverfew, or vervain during pregnancy.

VISUALIZATION

Picturing the pain as something that can be overcome (for example, ice that can be melted) may give you a greater sense of control over the condition. SEE PAGES 178–79

OTHER OPTIONS

Massage SEE PAGES 56–61
Chiropractic SEE PAGES 70–75
Osteopathy SEE PAGES 76–81
Acupressure SEE PAGE 95
Naturopathy SEE PAGES 118–21
Psychotherapy & Counseling SEE PAGES 160–65
Hypnotherapy SEE PAGES 166–67
Relaxation & Breathing SEE PAGES 170–73

NEUROPATHY & BELL'S PALSY

NEUROPATHY, also called neuritis, is a disorder that affects the peripheral nerves, which connect the brain and spinal cord to the rest of the body. The condition usually involves damage to nerve fibers or to the fatty sheaths around them. Symptoms may include numbness, tingling, muscle weakness, or disturbance of physical functions. In Bell's palsy, a form of neuropathy, the muscles of one side of the face become temporarily weak or paralyzed because of inflammation of the facial nerve. Neuropathy may be caused by diabetes, alcoholism, anemia, vitamin deficiency, cancer, or autoimmune disorders. Conventional treatment depends on the cause. Some cases eventually clear up without treatment, but others may require medication and even surgery.

COMPLEMENTARY TREATMENTS

Touch and movement therapies, medicinal treatments, and therapies that encourage relaxation and circulation may all help.

ACUPUNCTURE

The stimulation of appropriate acupoints may bring relief, attributed by practitioners to the reestablishing of harmony and flow of *qi* ("life energy") within the body. SEE PAGES 90–94

NATUROPATHY

A balanced diet high in whole foods, fruits, and vegetables may be recommended. Where a deficiency is thought to be responsible, a specific diet might be advised.
SEE PAGES 118–21

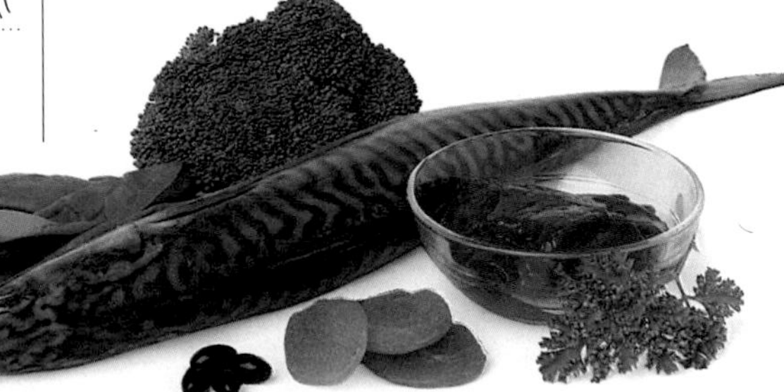

IRON-RICH FOODS
A diet high in iron may help neuropathy associated with anemia.

BIOCHEMIC TISSUE SALTS

Kali. phos. is often recommended for any problem involving nerves, and *Mag. phos.* may be given if cramps and twitching accompany the nerve pain. SEE PAGE 131

OTHER OPTIONS

Massage SEE PAGES 56–61
Homeopathy SEE PAGES 126–30
Nutritional Therapies SEE PAGES 148–52

Dizziness

Dizziness usually results from a brief drop in the amount of blood flowing to the brain, due to getting up too quickly. Other possible causes include fatigue, stress, hyperventilation (rapid breathing), heat, anemia, or low blood sugar. If you feel dizzy, lie down or sit with your head between your knees and breathe slowly and evenly. Tell your doctor about frequent or prolonged attacks of dizziness; they may be a symptom of a cardiovascular, hormonal, or nerve disorder, or a psychiatric condition.

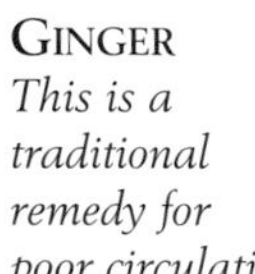

Ginger
This is a traditional remedy for poor circulation.

Complementary Treatments

To relieve dizziness, some practitioners work on tension in the body's musculoskeletal structure. Others aim to improve "energy" flow or redress nutritional deficiencies.

Chiropractic (see Osteopathy)

Osteopathy

Dizziness is sometimes a sign that tension around the joints of the upper neck is affecting the nerves and blood vessels to the head. To alleviate the tension, practitioners may manipulate the neck and the spine. SEE PAGES 70–81

Acupressure

A practitioner will demonstrate techniques that may help relieve dizziness, such as massaging points found on the arch of the foot, behind the earlobe, and between the nose and upper lip. SEE PAGE 95

Western Herbalism

Ginkgo may be helpful when dizziness is due to insufficient blood flow to the brain. Ginger may relieve dizziness that is associated with morning sickness. SEE PAGES 134–39

Caution: Do not take ginger if you have a peptic ulcer.

Chinese Herbalism

Dizziness may be ascribed to "Liver heat," "Kidney deficiency," or after illness, to "wind invasion," and may be treated with mulberry and ginger, among other herbs. SEE PAGES 140–43

Nutritional Therapies

If you have low blood sugar levels, a nutritionist may suggest frequent, small, high-protein meals. Iron-rich diets may be recommended for anemia. Vitamins B_2 and B_3 may be prescribed to prevent fatigue. SEE PAGES 148–52

Other Options

Acupuncture SEE PAGES 90–94
Naturopathy SEE PAGES 118–21

Vertigo

Vertigo is the sensation that you or your surroundings are spinning. Arising from a disturbance in the inner ear, acoustic nerve, brain stem, or eyes, vertigo may be caused by something as trivial as a carnival ride disrupting balance, or as serious as a tumor affecting the brain or inner ear. Stomach disorders, infections, stress, migraines, epilepsy, or heart disease can also cause vertigo. A doctor may advise drugs to reduce the sensation and to treat any underlying infection.

Complementary Treatments

Vertigo may sometimes be helped by dietary modifications, herbal infusions, and rubs.

Naturopathy

According to naturopaths, vertigo may respond to reducing caffeine, sugary and fried foods, salt, nicotine, and alcohol. SEE PAGES 118–21

Western Herbalism

To ease the effects of an attack, practitioners may advise an infusion of a circulatory stimulant, such as betony or fresh ginger, or of a relaxant, such as lemon balm. SEE PAGES 134–39

Cautions: Do not take betony during pregnancy. Do not take ginger if you have a peptic ulcer.

Ayurveda

After asking you about your diet and lifestyle, a practitioner may advise a blend of sesame oil, camphor, cardamom, and cinnamon applied to the head to stimulate the senses. SEE PAGES 144–47

Other Options

Acupuncture SEE PAGES 90–94
Acupressure SEE PAGE 95

Dyslexia

As much as 10% of the population is thought to have some degree of dyslexia, in which letters are misperceived and written incorrectly. For a minority of sufferers, dyslexia also brings emotional and behavioral problems. A recent theory holds that impaired communication between the brain hemispheres may play a role. It is best to treat dyslexia early. If your child shows signs – low literacy skills, clumsiness, or poor memory – you should consult an educational psychologist, who will perform tests. The child may be entitled to special educational help.

Complementary Treatments

Therapies may help by improving coordination, concentration, and confidence.

CranioSacral Therapy

Gentle adjustments to the cranium and spine may correct any misalignments contributing to the problem. SEE PAGE 81

Anthroposophical Medicine

Eurythmy, a movement therapy in which sounds are represented through gesture, may help harmonize communication between the hemispheres of the brain. SEE PAGES 124–25

Relaxation & Breathing

Knowing how and when to relax can help reduce some of the stress and frustration dyslexia may bring. A practitioner will guide you through a series of breathing exercises designed to release tension. SEE PAGES 170–73

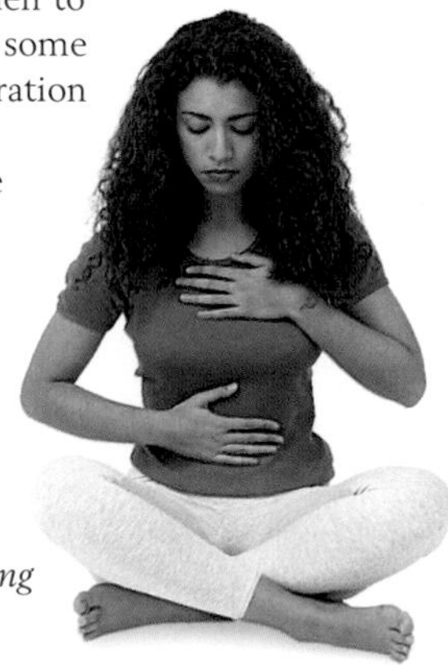

Breathing Exercise
Diaphragmatic breathing encourages relaxation.

MEMORY IMPAIRMENT

AS PEOPLE GROW OLDER they tend to become more forgetful. But memory problems can occur at any age, due to depression, stress, anxiety, lack of sleep, or lack of mental stimulation. Allergies, glandular disorders, fungal infections, and nutritional imbalances have also been blamed. Sometimes traumatic events are "forgotten" in order to cope, and brain injury or stroke can cause irreversible memory loss. Loss of short-term memory may herald Alzheimer's disease (see below). Consult a doctor if memory loss is accompanied by confusion, inability to concentrate, and changes in behavior.

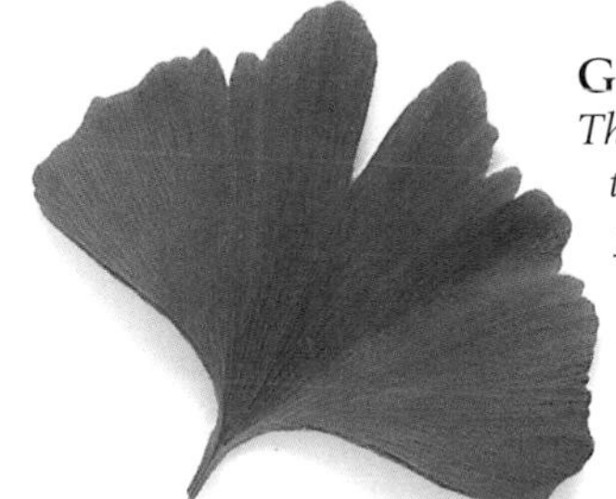

GINKGO
This herb is widely taken in Europe for poor memory and dementia.

COMPLEMENTARY TREATMENTS

Gentle exercise can increase circulation to the brain, perhaps enhancing brain power. It may also be possible to increase brain activity with the help of supplements, medicinal remedies, or changes in diet. Focusing the mind through activities like meditation may also improve the memory.

QIGONG

This therapy combines breathing techniques with physical movement, which encourages "energy" flow and stimulates the brain and its powers of concentration. SEE PAGE 99

HOMEOPATHY

Standard remedies include *Sulfur 6c* for difficulty in remembering words and names, and *Calcarea 6c* for poor concentration. SEE PAGES 126–30

FLOWER ESSENCES

Rosemary, comfrey, broom, yew, forget-me-not, and the Himalayan teakwood flower are said to be helpful. SEE PAGE 132

WESTERN HERBALISM

A practitioner may prescribe ginkgo. Research has shown that this herb increases the blood supply to the brain, accelerates nerve impulse transmission, and offsets damage from free radicals (see glossary). SEE PAGES 134–39

NUTRITIONAL THERAPIES

A practitioner may recommend that you take lecithin, a substance that is thought to boost acetylcholine, a neurotransmitter involved in memory. Some therapists also attribute memory loss to food allergies, food intolerances, and anemia, and may recommend dietary changes or nutritional supplements. SEE PAGES 148–52

RELAXATION & BREATHING

By learning methods of relaxing the body and mind, you may bring about an improvement in memory. SEE PAGES 170–73

OTHER OPTIONS

T'ai Chi Ch'uan SEE PAGES 100–101
Yoga SEE PAGES 108–11
Meditation SEE PAGES 174–77
Visualization SEE PAGES 178–79

SENILE DEMENTIA & ALZHEIMER'S DISEASE

MARKED BY MEMORY LOSS, confusion, emotional swings, and mental deterioration, senile dementia is thought to affect 10% of those aged over 65 and 20% of those over 75. Impaired circulation of blood to the brain causes some of the cases, but about 50% are attributable to Alzheimer's disease, a disorder in which brain cells progressively degenerate. Alzheimer's is diagnosed from behavioral symptoms and sometimes from a brain scan. There may be a genetic cause and some believe that susceptibility to environmental toxic substances such as aluminum and mercury may play a role, because abnormally high levels of these chemicals have been found in the brain cells of some patients.

Conventional Treatment Dementia resulting from malnutrition or drug abuse can be reversed in some cases. There is currently no cure for Alzheimer's disease but conventional treatment aims to sustain the patient's quality of life to the greatest extent possible. In later stages, sedatives and other drugs may be prescribed to control symptoms.

COMPLEMENTARY TREATMENTS

Various therapies may bring psychological relief, but the patient has to be a willing participant in whichever therapy is chosen.

AROMATHERAPY

Aromas often trigger memories and so may benefit patients. Evidence suggests that the oils of German chamomile and rose are calming, while lemon and peppermint are stimulating. SEE PAGES 62–65

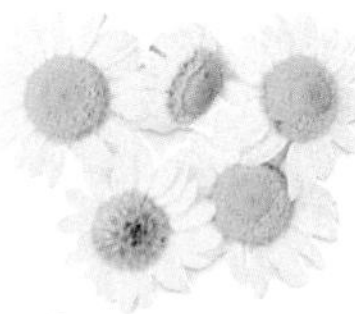

GERMAN CHAMOMILE
The essential oil of these flowers has a calming effect.

T'AI CHI CH'UAN

Millions of elderly Chinese people regularly practice t'ai chi, a meditative series of movements. They believe that this gentle exercise helps to maintain mental agility. SEE PAGES 100–101

WESTERN HERBALISM

To treat memory loss, an herbalist may recommend ginkgo, widely thought to boost blood flow to the brain. In German studies in 1991 and 1994, ginkgo was shown to improve the memory and social function of patients with early Alzheimer's disease. SEE PAGES 134–39

CHINESE HERBALISM

A practitioner may recommend ginseng and Chinese angelica *(dang gui)*, both stimulants, to increase vitality. SEE PAGES 140–43

NUTRITIONAL THERAPIES

Practitioners link Alzheimer's disease with deficiencies of a wide range of vitamins, minerals, and enzymes, and will recommend supplements such as folic acid and vitamin B complex. SEE PAGES 148–52

CLINICAL ECOLOGY

A practitioner may suggest replacing amalgam dental fillings, which contain mercury, and avoiding environmental toxins. SEE PAGES 154–55

CHELATION THERAPY

While little supporting evidence exists, this therapy is said to increase the brain's blood supply and to remove heavy metals implicated in Alzheimer's disease. SEE PAGE 157

HEADACHES & MIGRAINES

HEADACHES CAN RANGE in severity from a dull thudding in the temples when you are tired or anxious to a frightening, intense pain. They may be triggered by lifestyle factors, musculoskeletal disorders, or by psychological problems, so it is important to find and remedy the underlying causes. Migraines affect at least one person in ten, and are far more disabling than headaches. They are often confined to one side of the head, and may be preceded or accompanied by visual disturbances, such as flashing lights or hallucinatory auras, pins and needles, nausea, and sensitivity to odors, light, or noise. Migraines tend to run in families, and can be triggered by the same factors that cause headaches, or by sensitivity to particular substances.

CAUSES & SYMPTOMS

Stress or anxiety causes most headaches, often by first creating tension in the shoulder and neck muscles. Other triggers include eyestrain, poor posture, changes in weather, lack of sleep or exercise, missed meals, caffeine, sinusitis, high blood pressure, and hormonal swings. Migraines result from spasm and dilation of the arteries and blood vessels supplying the brain. In a "common" migraine, there is throbbing pain and light intolerance; in a "classic" migraine, there is also an aura; and in a "cluster" migraine, attacks may occur daily for several months.

PREVENTION

Be sure to get plenty of fresh air, exercise, and sleep, and eat sensibly, avoiding too much caffeine. Try to reduce stress levels by using relaxation and stress management techniques (see page 38). Note the frequency of migraines and their possible triggers.

CONVENTIONAL TREATMENT

Standard painkillers are used in the short term for headaches and migraines. For persistent or severe headaches, a physical examination, blood test, X ray, and brain scan might be required. Drugs are used to control changes in blood vessels. Severe attacks can be halted with injectable medicines.

PRECAUTIONS

- **Consult a doctor if you experience a headache with drowsiness, nausea, vomiting, and intolerance to light, especially after a head injury; or if your symptoms include fever and a stiff neck.**
- **Consult a doctor if you have a very severe or very persistent headache which is worse in the mornings, accompanied by nausea or vomiting or altered vision.**
- **Consult a doctor if you have a persistent one-sided headache with a sore temple.**
- **If self-help treatments do not work within 3–7 days, consult a doctor.**

TOUCH & MOVEMENT THERAPIES

Complementary therapies that induce relaxation may help relieve headaches or reduce the severity of migraines. Spinal or cranial manipulation may improve blood flow to the brain and relieve skeletal or postural problems that could be triggering headaches. Eastern therapies attribute headaches and migraines to blocked qi *("life energy") in the body and aim to restore its flow.*

MASSAGE

Massage can release muscle tension and restore normal blood flow to the blood vessels in the neck, scalp, and face. It has been proved to have a relaxing and therapeutic effect, reducing anxiety and tension. A practitioner will massage the area around the back of your neck, up over your scalp, and around your ears and temples, exerting even pressure. Several sessions may be necessary to resolve long-standing problems. SEE PAGES 56–61

AROMATHERAPY

To encourage blood flow, a practitioner may use lavender essential oil blended in sweet almond oil, massaging it into the back of the neck and temples. Premenstrual headaches may be relieved with peppermint, eucalyptus, or German chamomile oils. SEE PAGES 62–65

Caution: Do not use German chamomile oil during pregnancy.

REFLEXOLOGY

The tip of the big toe represents the head in reflexology, and practitioners will apply pressure to this area on both feet to relieve a headache, possibly also working up the side of each foot, which they believe corresponds to the spine and neck. SEE PAGES 66–69

CHIROPRACTIC

Spasm or compression of the vertebral arteries, due to misalignments of the neck vertebrae or pressure on nerves, may affect blood supply to the brain. Manipulation of the neck can help, but your practitioner may recommend an X ray first. SEE PAGES 70–75

OSTEOPATHY

After a detailed consultation, an osteopath will examine your musculoskeletal structure to correct any restrictions on the movement of your joints that might be impairing the proper working of your neck, causing headaches. He or she may suggest gentle manipulation of the neck, or cranial osteopathy to help relieve headaches and migraines. SEE PAGES 76–81

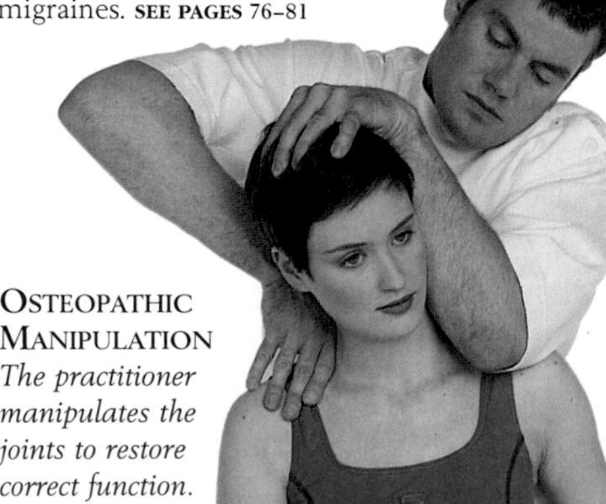

OSTEOPATHIC MANIPULATION *The practitioner manipulates the joints to restore correct function.*

ACUPUNCTURE

Practitioners believe acupuncture restores flow of blocked *qi* ("life energy") in the *yang* (see glossary) meridians such as the Stomach and Liver. Many Western doctors think acupuncture works by preventing pain signals from reaching the brain or by stimulating the production of natural painkillers known as endorphins. SEE PAGES 90–94

ACUPRESSURE
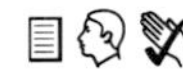

A practitioner will demonstrate ways to relieve a headache, such as the one shown below. In another method, press the thumbs firmly into the hollow areas at the base of your skull, on either side of the spine along the Gallbladder meridian (see top illustration opposite). Close your eyes and slowly tilt your head back for a minute or two, breathing deeply. SEE PAGE 95

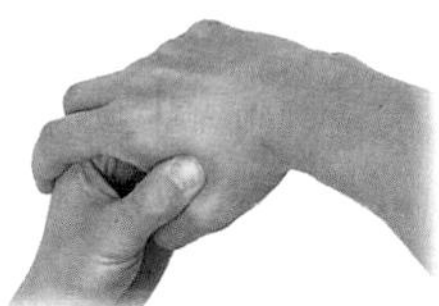

SELF-HELP
Press the acupoint between forefinger and thumb to relieve a headache.

SHIATSU
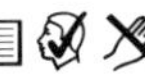

This combination of massage and pressure on the body's acupoints to stimulate *qi* ("life energy") is said to help ease migraines. In one study performed in Europe, 66% of migraine sufferers said they found shiatsu beneficial. SEE PAGES 96–97

YOGA
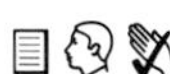

Yoga aids relaxation and helps to reduce anxiety. To relieve tension headaches, your teacher may suggest specific *asanas* (postures) such as the Shoulderstand or Cobra, which stretch the muscles in the neck, upper back, and shoulders. SEE PAGES 108–11

MEDICINAL THERAPIES

Nutritional therapists seek to treat dietary causes of headaches or migraines. Herbal or homeopathic remedies may control the pain and reduce the symptoms.

HYDROTHERAPY
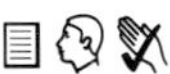

A practitioner may advise splashing your face liberally with cold water and then lying down for an hour at the first sign of a migraine. For tension headaches, a hot bath, sauna, or steam bath, or alternate hot and cold showers, may be suggested as a means to dilate and then constrict blood vessels, stimulating the circulation and helping to induce relaxation. An ice pack on the head or neck may also prove helpful, as may swimming.
SEE PAGES 122–23

Caution: Avoid alternate hot and cold showers if you have a heart condition.

HOMEOPATHY

For migraines and frequent headaches, it is advisable to visit a practitioner for an individual assessment and prescription. Standard remedies are available, however, for an occasional headache: *Aconite 6c* for sudden headaches that feel like a tight band on the head, *Bryonia 6c* for irritability and pain that worsens with movement, *Belladonna 6c* for a throbbing, drumming headache that becomes worse in hot sun, and *Hypericum 6c* for a bursting head and painful scalp, which is worse in damp weather. For migraine attacks, *Natrum mur. 6c* may be recommended for a throbbing, blinding headache, which is worse when moving around, with numbness and tingling in the face, *Pulsatilla 6c* for a bursting pain that is worse in the evening or during menstruation, and aggravated by rich, fatty food, with tearfulness, and *Iris vers. 6c* for blurred vision before a headache, tightness in the scalp, and vomiting bile. SEE PAGES 126–30

WESTERN HERBALISM

Feverfew may prevent migraines; research has shown that it can help by reducing the secretion of the hormone serotonin, thought to play a role in migraine attacks. Fresh leaves are best, but stop taking if canker sores appear. Pills are available over the counter, but make sure the parthenolide content is high. Benefits may take some months to show.

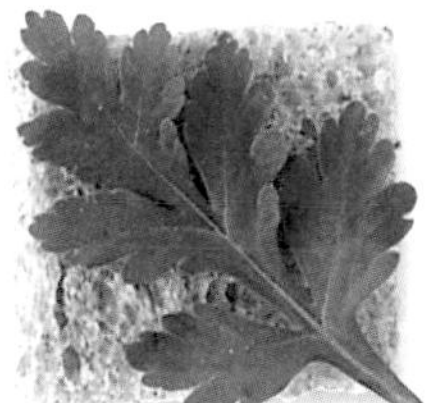

FEVERFEW
The leaves can be chopped and eaten on bread or in a sandwich to prevent migraine attacks.

A practitioner may also recommend German chamomile and valerian, which have sedative and pain-relieving properties, and limeflower, lemon balm, California poppy, and skullcap, which are believed to relieve tension. Betony, a relaxant and circulatory stimulant, may be prescribed. An herbalist may also suggest ginkgo and garlic to improve the circulation. To relieve nausea, ginger may be recommended.
SEE PAGES 134–39

Cautions: Do not take feverfew or betony during pregnancy. Do not take ginger if you have a peptic ulcer.

CHINESE HERBALISM
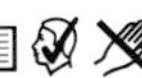

Migraines may be attributed to excess *qi* ("life energy") in the Liver, to *qi* "stagnation," or to an imbalance of *qi* in the Stomach and Liver meridians. A practitioner will treat the pattern of symptoms particular to your individual type and condition, and may prescribe remedies containing chrysanthemum or cassia.
SEE PAGES 140–43

NUTRITIONAL THERAPIES

Migraines have been linked to food intolerances. Some foods, such as ripe cheese, pickled herring, red wine, and nitrate preservative found in processed meats, are believed to contain tyrosine, which can cause a reaction in the blood vessels. Elimination diets have been effective as a means to detect culprit foods; a practitioner may ask you to fast for 24–48 hours, taking only distilled water, fresh fruits, and raw vegetables, then introduce other foods until you find those that trigger attacks. He or she may draw up a diet to prevent further attacks. Some practitioners believe supplements of vitamins C, E, B_3, evening primrose oil, omega-3 fatty acids, calcium, and magnesium can all help prevent migraines.
SEE PAGES 148–52

MAGNETIC THERAPY

In magnetic therapy, you wear a miniature generator, which pulses a small magnetic field that may "normalize" brain waves, but there is no research evidence to prove its efficacy.
SEE PAGE 156

MIND & EMOTION THERAPIES

The mind can profoundly influence physiological factors that may trigger headaches and migraines.

HYPNOTHERAPY
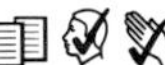

Suggestions made during a trance are sometimes effective in reducing the frequency and severity of migraines. SEE PAGE 166–67

BIOFEEDBACK
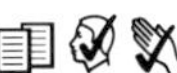

Practitioners have successfully treated headaches and migraines with biofeedback techniques that train patients to control blood vessel dilation and muscle tension. SEE PAGE 169

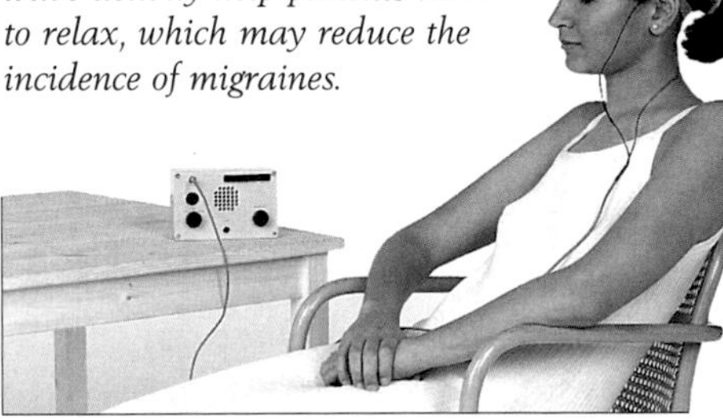

BIOFEEDBACK TECHNIQUES
Machines that measure brain wave activity help patients learn to relax, which may reduce the incidence of migraines.

RELAXATION & BREATHING

Diaphragmatic breathing and progressive muscle relaxation can ease tension in the muscles if headaches or migraines are caused by stress or anxiety. They may also help to prevent migraine attacks in the early stages.
SEE PAGES 170–73

ACNE

AFFECTING SEVEN OUT OF TEN young people, and occasionally persisting into adulthood, acne is caused by the blockage and infection of the oil-producing sebaceous glands adjacent to hair follicles in the skin. A plug of sebum, the skin's natural oil, forms in the follicle and eventually darkens to become a blackhead. If the sebum becomes infected, a pus-filled pimple forms.

Causes A tendency toward acne may be hereditary. Hormones play a part; for example, the production of the hormone testosterone, particularly in puberty, may stimulate an overproduction of sebum, leading to blocked follicles. While conventional medicine holds that diet and stress play no role, some doctors believe that high-fat junk food and anxiety may aggravate the condition.

Conventional Treatment If standard skin preparations or prescription antibiotic lotions do not work, doctors may advise a preparation containing tretinoin, a derivative of vitamin A. Oral contraceptives may be recommended. For scarring, removal of the top layer of skin by dermabrasion or laser may be suggested.

Self-Help It is important to keep affected areas clean by washing twice daily with a medicated cleanser and hot water. Never squeeze spots, since this may leave scars.

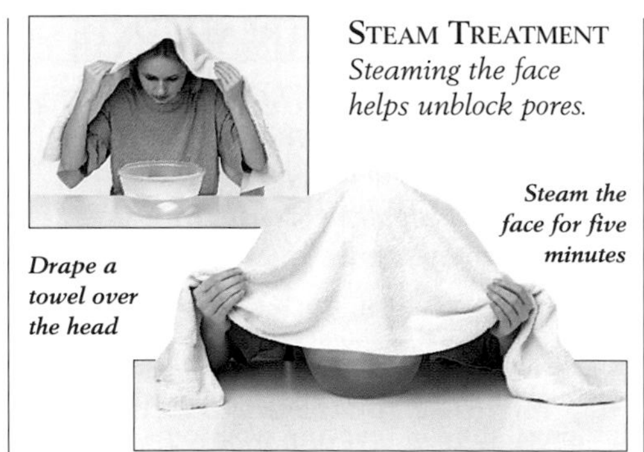

STEAM TREATMENT
Steaming the face helps unblock pores.

COMPLEMENTARY TREATMENTS

There are two main approaches to acne: treating the outbreaks directly with cleansing facials and the application of healing substances, and improving skin health through diet.

AROMATHERAPY

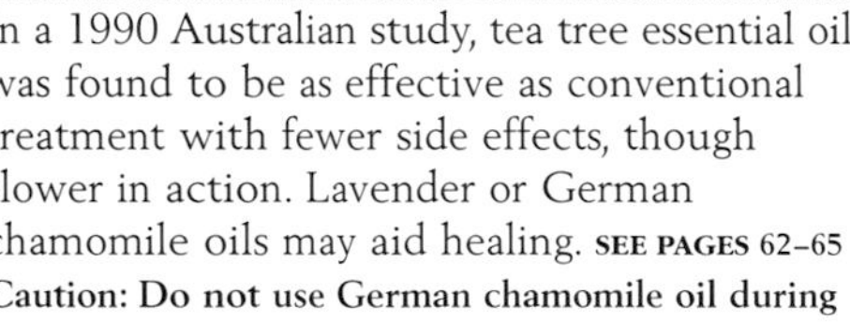

In a 1990 Australian study, tea tree essential oil was found to be as effective as conventional treatment with fewer side effects, though slower in action. Lavender or German chamomile oils may aid healing. SEE PAGES 62–65

Caution: Do not use German chamomile oil during pregnancy.

NATUROPATHY

Practitioners believe that acne indicates a hormonal or digestive disturbance or a problem with elimination. You might be advised to eat plenty of fresh fruits and vegetables, and to avoid dairy products. Regular short fasts and a raw-foods diet may also be suggested to help eliminate waste products. SEE PAGES 118–21

HYDROTHERAPY

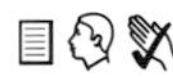

Facial steam baths can help open pores and remove blocked sebum. A practitioner may suggest you take hot Epsom salts baths to cleanse the system. Thalassotherapy (seawater jets and baths) is popular in Europe to cleanse and tone the skin. SEE PAGES 122–23

Caution: Avoid Epsom salts baths if elderly or frail.

WESTERN HERBALISM

Practitioners believe that acne results from an overload of toxins in the body or a hormonal imbalance. You may be advised to take cleansing herbs such as dandelion root or nettle, perhaps combined with immunity-enhancing echinacea. Wild yam might be prescribed for its ability to help regulate hormone production. Facial steam baths incorporating various herbs may be advised to cleanse the pores, followed by applications of witch hazel or herbal infusions. Propolis, an antibiotic substance made by bees, can be effective in the form of a cream dabbed on spots. SEE PAGES 134–39

Caution: Do not take wild yam during pregnancy.

OTHER OPTIONS

Homeopathy — SEE PAGES 126–30
Chinese Herbalism — SEE PAGES 140–43
Ayurveda — SEE PAGES 144–47
Nutritional Therapies — SEE PAGES 148–52
Relaxation & Breathing — SEE PAGES 170–73
Light Therapy — SEE PAGE 188

HIVES

ALSO KNOWN AS URTICARIA, this condition affects as many as 20% of the population at some point in their lives. It is an intensely itchy rash, with inflamed red, or red-and-white, weals on the skin. It usually lasts for several hours, and no longer than a day. The cause is not always known, but hives commonly result from an allergic reaction (see Allergies, page 298). Triggers may include substances in food, particularly the proteins found in meat, fish, and shellfish; certain drugs; plants; heat or cold; and insect bites. Stress can also provoke hives. It is important to identify and avoid the allergens. A doctor may advise calamine lotion to ease itching, but oral antihistamines bring the swiftest relief.

COMPLEMENTARY TREATMENTS

Homeopathic preparations, essential oils, or other preparations may soothe the itching, and most therapists will also undertake a thorough inquiry to determine and treat the underlying cause.

NATUROPATHY

To discover the source of the reaction, a practitioner may suggest an exclusion diet, removing common triggers such as shellfish, strawberries, tomatoes, chocolate, eggs, meat, wheat, nuts, and milk. SEE PAGES 118–21

HYDROTHERAPY

To relieve itching, a practitioner may suggest adding sodium bicarbonate or oatmeal to a warm bath. Vinegar can help the condition by normalizing the skin's pH level. SEE PAGES 122–23

HOMEOPATHY

Among the remedies that may help is *Urtica 6c*, derived from nettle. It is said to be especially appropriate for intense itching triggered by shellfish and plants, including nettles themselves. SEE PAGES 126–30

NETTLE
Homeopaths use nettle to treat hives.

OTHER OPTIONS

Western Herbalism — SEE PAGES 134–39
Chinese Herbalism — SEE PAGES 140–43
Nutritional Therapies — SEE PAGES 148–52
Clinical Ecology — SEE PAGES 154–55

COLD SORES, GENITAL HERPES & SHINGLES

RELATED HERPES VIRUSES are responsible for these three conditions, characterized by painful blisters on the skin or mucous membranes. When the blisters appear around the lips, they are commonly known as cold sores. Herpes blisters may also erupt on the genitals, in the eyes, or, rarely, in the brain. Shingles takes the form of a painful, itchy rash that usually develops along the path of a nerve supplying the skin, most commonly around the ribs or lower trunk, or on the upper face, neck, or limbs. Red spots turn into very painful, yellow blisters, which take several weeks to subside. Residual nerve pain may linger for months or even years after the blisters have healed.

Causes Cold sores and genital herpes blisters are caused by exposure to the herpes simplex virus, and are contagious on contact. Once in the body, the virus remains for life, generally dormant. Eruptions may be activated by illness, lowered immunity, overexposure to sunlight, poor diet, and other factors. Shingles is caused by the related varicella-zoster virus, which also causes chicken pox (see page 283); most adults with shingles also had chicken pox as children. The virus remains inactive for years, reemerging as shingles when immunity is low or during periods of stress.

Conventional Treatment Cold sores and genital herpes can be treated with an antiviral ointment. Severe cases may require an oral antiviral drug, such as acyclovir, which has been shown to reduce the severity and frequency of attacks. A doctor will refer herpes simplex infections of the eye to an eye specialist. The severity of a shingles attack and the possibility of lingering pain can also be reduced with the drug acyclovir. Local anesthetics, atropine ointments, and oral painkillers can help relieve the pain of blisters. TENS therapy (see glossary) may block long-term nerve pain which sometimes persists for many years and can resist treatment.

TOUCH & MOVEMENT THERAPIES

To speed healing and ease post-shingles nerve pain, touch therapies such as aromatherapy and acupuncture may be useful.

AROMATHERAPY

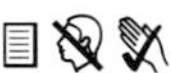

To speed healing of cold sores, a practitioner may suggest gently massaging the affected area with well-diluted soothing essential oils, such as geranium and lavender, and antiseptic oils such as tea tree or eucalyptus. SEE PAGES 62–65

Caution: Do not use oils on a shingles rash.

ACUPUNCTURE

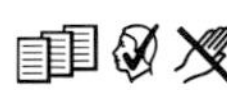

This can be an effective form of long-term pain relief. Western scientists believe that acupuncture may work by blocking the pain pathways to the brain and releasing natural painkillers known as endorphins. Your practitioner will treat acupoints that correspond to the location of the outbreak. SEE PAGES 90–94

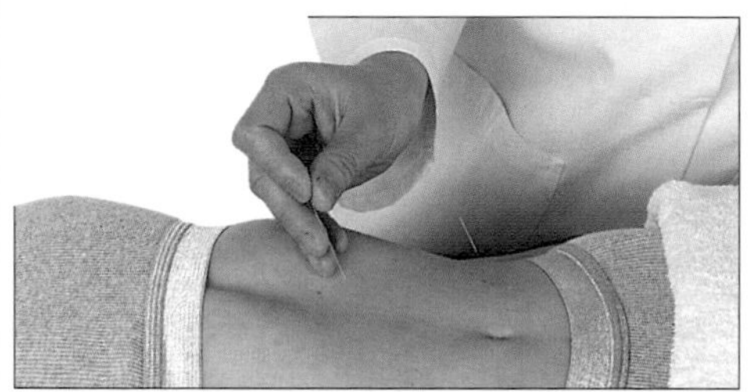

PAIN RELIEF
To relieve pain, an acupuncturist inserts a fine needle into the acupoint.

MEDICINAL THERAPIES

Medicinal therapies seek to to ease pain and boost the immune system to prevent attacks from recurring.

NATUROPATHY

Practitioners will aim to strengthen your immune system to fight infection and may advise you to avoid carbohydrates, coffee, alcohol, and tobacco, which are believed to depress immunity. Garlic, known to support the immune system, may help.
SEE PAGES 118–21

HYDROTHERAPY

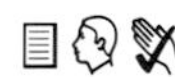

A practitioner might suggest you treat shingles rashes with ice packs and cold compresses.
SEE PAGES 122–23

HOMEOPATHY

Standard remedies associated with herpes include *Rhus tox.*, *Mezereum*, and *Natrum mur.*, depending on the characteristics of the illness.
SEE PAGES 126–30

WESTERN HERBALISM

In an article published in the British journal *Nature* in 1979, Italian researchers reported that glycyrrhizic acid, one of the constituents of licorice, deactivated cells infected with the herpes simplex virus. Swabbing the area with a cream containing this substance may help. In another study, capsaicin extracted from chilies was found to relieve nerve pain in 80% of post-shingles patients.
SEE PAGES 134–39

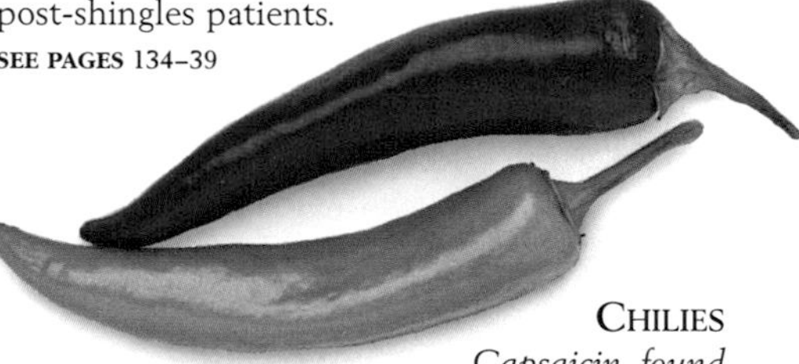

CHILIES
Capsaicin, found in chilies, relieves pain.

NUTRITIONAL THERAPIES

The amino acid lysine, found in kidney beans, potatoes, eggs, chicken, fish, and meat, is thought to inhibit the herpes simplex virus. Your practitioner may suggest you eat these foods, while avoiding foods such as peanuts, chocolate, and seeds, which contain the amino acid arginine, on which the virus seems to thrive. Antioxidants (see glossary), such as vitamins C and E, may help prevent attacks.
SEE PAGES 148–52

OTHER OPTION

Chinese Herbalism SEE PAGES 140–43

MIND & EMOTION THERAPIES

Herpes outbreaks have been linked to high levels of stress. Therapies that focus on relaxing the mind and body may counteract this, help to control recurrences of the condition, and reduce persistent pain.

RELAXATION & BREATHING

A practitioner will guide you through exercises designed to help you learn to relax and to gain a level of mastery over stressful situations. SEE PAGES 170–73

VISUALIZATION

Picturing calm, soothing scenes can help you to relax, releasing physical and emotional tension. A practitioner will teach you to imagine the pain as something that is diminishing, such as a lump of melting ice.
SEE PAGES 178–79

OTHER OPTIONS

Autogenic Training SEE PAGE 168
Meditation SEE PAGES 174–77

ECZEMA & DERMATITIS

ECZEMA IS A COMMON REACTION of the skin to a wide range of irritants and allergies (see also Allergies, page 298). Symptoms include reddening, itching, blistering, and oozing. In severe cases, the skin thickens into scabs. The term "dermatitis" means inflammation of the skin and it is often used interchangeably with eczema.

Causes *Atopic eczema*, the most common form, occurs especially in children and may run in the family. It is often associated with hay fever and asthma. *Contact eczema*, also known as contact dermatitis, is a localized and temporary allergic response to an irritant. *Seborrheic eczema* tends to occur when there is an overproduction of the skin's natural oils.

Conventional Treatment Doctors may prescribe steroid hydrocortisone creams to relieve inflammation, and antihistamines and antibiotics to control itching and infection. Moisturizing creams and soap substitutes are recommended for dry skin. Seborrheic eczema may respond to antifungal medication. Avoiding known allergens, especially house dust and detergents, may be suggested.

Caution: Test remedies on healthy skin before applying to eczema patches.

COMPLEMENTARY TREATMENTS

Treating the skin, strengthening the digestion and elimination processes, and helping the patient cope with stress may all help.

AROMATHERAPY

Diluted essential oils of lavender, bergamot, and geranium may help relieve itching and inflammation. Lavender oil in a bath may be suggested to lower stress. SEE PAGES 62–65

Caution: Only a qualified aromatherapist should treat eczema.

LAVENDER OIL
A relaxant, lavender oil may also relieve itching.

NATUROPATHY

Eczema is believed to be a sign of poor digestion and elimination, so fasting and special diets may be advised. Tests to identify allergies may also be undertaken; some of these techniques are not substantiated by research. SEE PAGES 118–21

CHINESE HERBALISM 

Research at London's Great Ormond Street Hospital for Children found a formula of Chinese herbs very effective in treating atopic eczema in children. A practitioner may prescribe remedies including Chinese wormwood, Chinese gentian, peony root, and rehmannia. SEE PAGES 140–43

Caution: Do not take peony root during pregnancy.

NUTRITIONAL THERAPIES 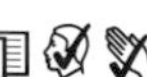

A practitioner may suggest evening primrose oil supplements. Several studies, including two published in *The Lancet* in 1981 and 1982, found that this substance relieved the symptoms of atopic eczema. SEE PAGES 148–52

CLINICAL ECOLOGY 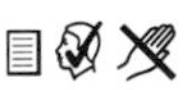

Environmental chemicals and pollutants are said to cause eczema. Various tests will be performed to find the culprits. SEE PAGES 154–55

PSYCHOTHERAPY & COUNSELING 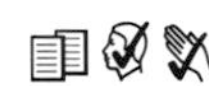

A German study found that psychotherapy could lessen the severity of eczema and reduce patients' need for cortisone treatment, possibly by reducing stress-related physiological changes that trigger itchiness. SEE PAGES 160–65

HYPNOTHERAPY 

This therapy may be effective in controlling itching and has proved particularly useful in childhood atopic eczema. SEE PAGES 166–67

OTHER OPTIONS

Homeopathy	SEE PAGES 126–30
Western Herbalism	SEE PAGES 134–39
Autogenic Training	SEE PAGE 168

PSORIASIS

THERE IS NO KNOWN CAUSE or cure for psoriasis, in which the epidermis produces new cells too fast, resulting in raised, rough, and reddened areas of skin covered with silvery gray scales. Psoriasis is hereditary in 50% of cases, and a child with one infected parent has a 25% chance of getting it. A metabolic disorder may be responsible. Psoriasis may improve with exposure to ultraviolet light or with application of coal tar and dithranol lotions and shampoos. A doctor will advise a healthy diet, moderate alcohol intake, and stress management.

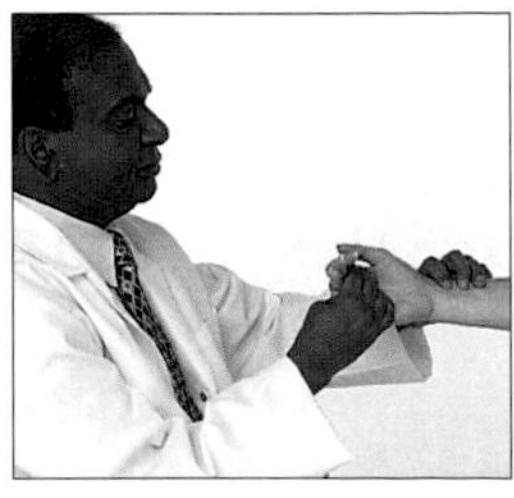

AYURVEDIC PULSE TESTING
A practitioner will use this and other tests to assess your doshic constitution, and will treat accordingly.

COMPLEMENTARY TREATMENTS

In addition to attempting to relieve the discomfort of psoriasis, practitioners will try to find the trigger factors. Many complementary therapists believe that a buildup of waste products in the body is responsible.

NATUROPATHY 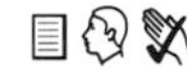

Practitioners will suggest diets to clear waste products from the body and to boost the immune system. Some practitioners link psoriasis with an overgrowth of bacteria in the bowel and may suggest a high-fiber diet and probiotics (see glossary) to counter this. SEE PAGES 118–21

HYDROTHERAPY

To stimulate the circulation and eliminate waste products, your practitioner may recommend hot baths with Epsom salts. SEE PAGES 122–23

Caution: Avoid Epsom salts baths if elderly or frail.

AYURVEDA 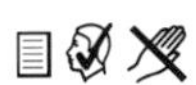

Practitioners believe that psoriasis is caused by blood impurities, possibly associated with emotional factors. Herbal remedies include *Guggulu tiktaka ghrita* (gum resin with five bitter herbs) to cleanse the bowels, promote digestion, stimulate the liver, and purify the blood. SEE PAGES 144–47

LIGHT THERAPY 

Exposure to sunlight, especially ultraviolet rays, alleviates psoriasis. SEE PAGE 188

Caution: Overexposure to ultraviolet radiation can be harmful.

OTHER OPTIONS

Acupuncture	SEE PAGES 90–94
Acupressure	SEE PAGE 95
Western Herbalism	SEE PAGES 134–39
Chinese Herbalism	SEE PAGES 140–43
Clinical Ecology	SEE PAGES 154–55
Psychotherapy & Counseling	SEE PAGES 160–65
Hypnotherapy	SEE PAGES 166–67
Visualization	SEE PAGES 178–79

DANDRUFF

FINE WHITE SCALES flaking from the scalp is a common problem at all ages, although dandruff tends to be at its worst in adolescence. In babies, the condition is known as cradle cap. A form of seborrheic eczema (see opposite), dandruff may respond to medicated shampoos. In severe cases, a doctor may prescribe lotions containing corticosteroid or antifungal medication.

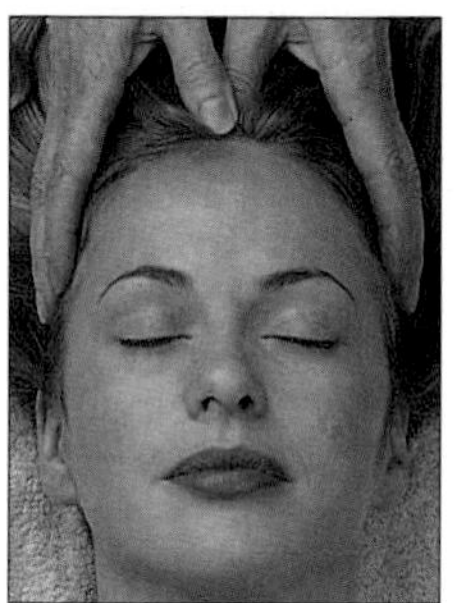

SCALP MASSAGE *Gentle massage improves blood flow, alleviating dandruff.*

COMPLEMENTARY TREATMENTS

Enhancing the circulation to the scalp may help to reduce dandruff, as may medicinal therapies, which help by improving the elimination process.

MASSAGE

Therapists believe that stimulating the circulation in the scalp may reduce a dandruff problem. They will demonstrate techniques that you can do by yourself. SEE PAGES 56–61

AROMATHERAPY

Certain essential oils, such as cedarwood, rosemary, and tea tree, may help to control dandruff if diluted in a carrier oil, applied to the scalp and left on overnight.
SEE PAGES 62–65

NATUROPATHY

Practitioners believe that dandruff indicates toxic overload and poor digestion, and will treat accordingly. Some naturopaths say that dandruff may result from overconsumption of citrus fruits. Practitioners may recommend vitamin E in the form of a cream or lotion to rub onto the scalp.
SEE PAGES 118–21

HOMEOPATHY

Some standard remedies that may help are *Arsenicum 6c* for a dry, itchy scalp, *Sepia 6c* if your scalp is moist and greasy, and *Sulfur 6c* for thick dandruff that is itchy at night.
SEE PAGES 126–30

OTHER OPTIONS

Western Herbalism SEE PAGES 134–39
Nutritional Therapies SEE PAGES 148–52

CHAPPED SKIN

COLD, WET, AND WINDY weather can result in the skin on the hands and face becoming rough, sore, and cracked. Skin also loses elasticity and cracks if it is exposed to cold after immersion in hot, soapy water. Applying moisturizing creams, wearing gloves and protective clothing, drying skin before exposure to cold, and using a humidifier in a centrally heated atmosphere will all help, as may exercise, which stimulates circulation in the skin.

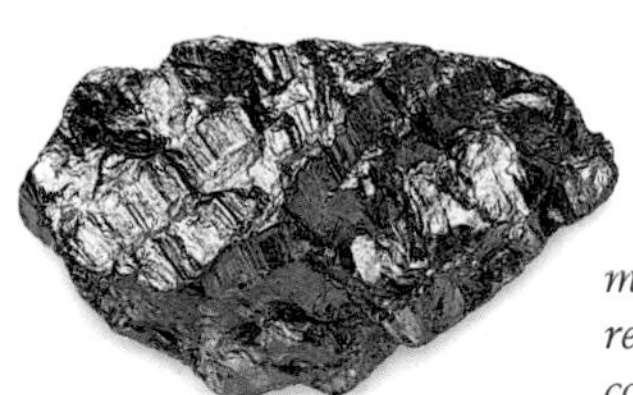

GRAPHITE *This form of carbon is ground into a powder to make a homeopathic remedy for skin conditions.*

COMPLEMENTARY TREATMENTS

Since ancient times, soothing oils and other natural remedies have been applied to irritated skin. More recently, diet has been implicated in skin disorders. Therapists may seek to rectify imbalances by suggesting changes in eating habits.

AROMATHERAPY 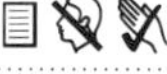

If your face is affected, a steam bath with geranium essential oil may be advised.
SEE PAGES 62–65

NATUROPATHY

Naturopaths believe that persistent chapped skin may respond to supplements of essential fatty acids, vitamins E and B complex, kelp, and bioflavonoids. Vitamin D and vitamin E oil rubbed into the skin may also be recommended.
SEE PAGES 118–21

HYDROTHERAPY 

Hot and cold compresses applied to the affected area can help to stimulate the circulation. SEE PAGES 122–23

HOMEOPATHY

For persistent chapped skin, a practitioner may suggest *Petroleum 6c* for deep cracks and a watery discharge, *Graphites 6c* for chapping with a yellow crust, and *Natrum mur. 6c* for lips that have become cracked due to sea air.
SEE PAGES 126–30

WESTERN HERBALISM

Calendula ointment or cream may be recommended to soothe discomfort and heal the irritated tissues. SEE PAGES 134–39

NAIL PROBLEMS

COMMON NAIL PROBLEMS include splitting, poor growth, nail bed infections caused by fungi or bacteria, irritation due to biting or injury, and ingrown toenails. Nail problems may indicate more general health disorders, and a doctor will try to treat the underlying problem, which may be a nutritional deficiency or a medical condition. Surgery may be necessary for ingrown toenails.

COMPLEMENTARY TREATMENTS

Dietary improvements and healing plant substances may improve the health of nails.

AROMATHERAPY 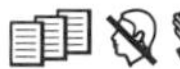

You may be advised to apply tea tree oil, which has antibacterial properties. SEE PAGES 62–65

AYURVEDA

Nail diagnosis is an important element of Ayurvedic medicine. Practitioners may recommend applying aloe vera and turmeric for fungal infections, and neem oil for infections of the nail and cuticle. SEE PAGES 144–47

NUTRITIONAL THERAPIES 

Supplements and foods rich in zinc and B_6 may be suggested. SEE PAGES 148–52

OTHER OPTION

Western Herbalism SEE PAGES 134–39

EYES

WHEN LIGHT ENTERS THE EYE, it stimulates electrical and chemical changes in the retina, a tissue lining the back of the eye. Nerve fibers transmit messages from the retina to the visual cortex of the brain, which interprets the information as images. It is important to have regular eye tests to detect visual problems, such as nearsightedness, and to make sure that the eyes are healthy. The most common eye problems are infections of the mucous lining and the degenerative effects of aging. Complementary treatments can soothe sore eyes and redress any nutritional problems that may contribute to visual impairment.

KEY TO SYMBOLS

EVIDENCE	PRACTITIONER
Good scientific trials with positive results	Essential
Some research studies	Recommended
Anecdotal	Not essential
	SELF-HELP
	Self-help possibilities
	No self-help

COMPLEMENTARY APPROACHES

Complementary therapists attribute eye problems to poor nutrition, muscle strain, pollution, the side effects of drugs, and failure to exercise the eye muscles. Traditional Chinese Medicine associates the eyes with the Liver. Practitioners will attempt to nourish and strengthen that organ with herbal remedies and, in certain cases, dietary adjustments.

CONVENTIONAL APPROACHES

Practitioners usually treat serious eye problems, such as glaucoma, with medication or surgery.

Cautions: Consult a doctor immediately if you have any visual impairment or eye pain. Before seeking treatment, see page 204.

HOW THE EYE WORKS

The eye is surrounded by a protective outer coat, the sclera, which is transparent at the front (the cornea) to allow light to enter. The cornea focuses light through the pupil onto the lens, which in turn focuses the light onto the retina at the back of the eye. The amount of light entering the eye is regulated by the contraction and dilation of muscles in the iris (the colored part of the eye). From the retina, messages are transmitted through the optic nerve to the brain for interpretation.
The conjunctiva, a mucous membrane covering the white of the eye and lining the eyelids, protects the eye, bathing it in a protective film of tears that ensures clear vision and prevents drying and infection. To maintain its shape, the eyeball is filled with a watery liquid.

CROSS SECTION OF THE EYE

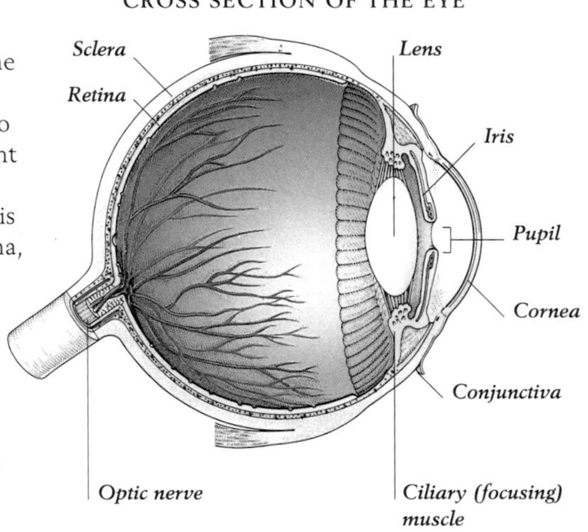

CATARACTS

A CATARACT ARISES when ordinarily transparent proteins in the lens cloud over, resulting in hazy vision. Cataracts most commonly occur as part of the aging process, but they may also stem from eye disease, injury, steroid use, metabolic or congenital disorders, poisoning, or radiation. A cataract cannot be reversed. It is usually removed in a simple operation and replaced with an artificial lens.

BATES EXERCISES
Focusing on one pencil and then on the other is said to enhance vision.

COMPLEMENTARY TREATMENTS

Gentle eye exercises, herbal remedies, and improved nutrition may all help cataracts.

ACUPRESSURE

A therapist may direct you to massage the Stomach meridian acupoint found on the bone below the pupil of the eye. SEE PAGE 95

THE BATES METHOD

According to the Bates method, bad habits, such as staring, make many eye problems, including cataracts, worse. A practitioner will assess your eyesight and prescribe exercises to "reeducate" the eyes. SEE PAGE 114

CHINESE HERBALISM

In Traditional Chinese Medicine, eye problems are associated with "deficiency of Liver *yin*" (see glossary). A practitioner may suggest dietary changes and lycium berries, thought to promote good eyesight. SEE PAGES 140–43

NUTRITIONAL THERAPIES

Practitioners believe that antioxidants (see glossary) such as vitamin C, vitamin E, and beta-carotene can help prevent free radicals (see glossary) from damaging the protein of the lens. In a UK study, people with the most beta-carotene in their diet had 39% fewer cataracts than those with the least, and those who took vitamin C supplements for more than ten years were 45% less likely to have cataracts.
SEE PAGES 148–52

OTHER OPTIONS

Acupuncture SEE PAGES 90–94
Homeopathy SEE PAGES 126–30
Ayurveda SEE PAGES 144–47

CONJUNCTIVITIS & STIES

ALSO KNOWN AS "PINK EYE," conjunctivitis is an inflammation of the eye's protective mucous membrane. It is marked by swelling, redness, watering, discharge, a feeling of grittiness and itchiness, and sometimes by sensitivity to light. It may be a symptom of an allergy such as hay fever, or be caused by environmental irritants or a virus. Conventionally, antibiotic ointment or drops are prescribed for an infection, and antihistamine or steroid drops for an allergy. Sties are small pus-filled abscesses that form at the roots of eyelashes. They generally clear up of their own accord, but, if recurrent, a doctor will prescribe antibiotic ointment.

Caution: Consult a doctor if conjunctivitis lasts longer than 48 hours, if there is a thick discharge, if vision is affected, or if light hurts the eyes.

COMPLEMENTARY TREATMENTS

Practitioners of Traditional Chinese Medicine try to improve Liver health. Western therapies see infections as a sign that the immune system is overloaded.

NATUROPATHY

Eating raw foods or fasting may be suggested to eliminate waste products, followed by a healthy whole-grain diet rich in fruits and vegetables. To speed healing of a sty, a naturopath may suggest that you wrap absorbent cotton around a wooden spoon, dip it in very hot water and hold it adjacent to (not on) the stye to encourage it to discharge pus. SEE PAGES 118–21

HOMEOPATHY

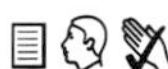

These standard remedies treat eye problems: *Euphrasia 6c* for eyes that water continuously, *Pulsatilla 6c* for itching eyes and a yellow discharge, and *Staphysagria 6c* for sties that develop a head of pus. SEE PAGES 126–30

WESTERN HERBALISM

A practitioner may suggest applying warm compresses of eyebright, burdock, or calendula frequently to the eye, and taking garlic, echinacea, or other herbs to boost your immune system. SEE PAGES 134–39

CHINESE HERBALISM

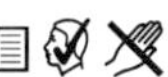

A practitioner may ascribe conjunctivitis to "wind heat" in the Liver meridian and advise an eyebath of boiled bamboo leaves, violets, and chrysanthemum flowers to soothe symptoms. SEE PAGES 140–43

OTHER OPTIONS

Nutritional Therapies SEE PAGES 148–52
Clinical Ecology SEE PAGES 154–55

GLAUCOMA

IN GLAUCOMA, pressure in the eye damages retinal and optic nerves, in severe cases leading to blindness. The pressure is caused by a buildup of fluid within the eyeball and blockage of drainage channels. This can occur suddenly, but in "open-angle" glaucoma, the buildup is so gradual that deteriorating vision may not be noticed. Aging and hereditary abnormalities are the most frequent causes of glaucoma. Conventional medical treatment is essential and drugs and surgery can relieve pressure.

Cautions: Consult a doctor immediately if you experience pain or visual disturbance. Those over 40 with a family history of glaucoma should have eye tests every 2 years.

COMPLEMENTARY TREATMENTS

Practitioners attempt to reduce the buildup of pressure in the eyes in order to minimize nerve damage in the retina.

CRANIAL OSTEOPATHY

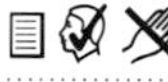

Gentle manipulation of the cranium is said to boost blood circulation and improve fluid dispersal within the head. It may help to relieve buildup of fluid in the eyes. SEE PAGE 81

THE BATES METHOD

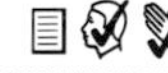

Practitioners claim that visual exercises may help relax the eyes, countering the visual deterioration that accompanies glaucoma. SEE PAGE 114

CHINESE HERBALISM

Practitioners may suggest dietary changes to decrease pressure in the eyes and herbal remedies such as lycium and rehmannia, both thought to support the Liver. SEE PAGES 140–43

NUTRITIONAL THERAPIES

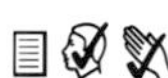

Antioxidants (see glossary), such as vitamin C and bioflavonoids, may be advised. Vitamin C is thought to boost levels of collagen (a protein involved in tissue building), while bioflavonoids work with vitamin C to strengthen the capillaries of the eye. SEE PAGES 148–52

OTHER OPTIONS

Naturopathy SEE PAGES 118–21
Homeopathy SEE PAGES 126–30
Western Herbalism SEE PAGES 134–39

MACULAR DEGENERATION

IN MACULAR DEGENERATION, blood vessels behind the central area of the retina (the macula) constrict, reducing blood flow. Vision deteriorates as a result, and the ability to read and do fine work is lost. Aging is the main cause, but high blood pressure, atherosclerosis, smoking, nutritional deficiencies, and other factors have also been implicated. If caught early, macular degeneration may be arrested with laser surgery.

COMPLEMENTARY TREATMENTS

Practitioners aim to stimulate blood flow and strengthen the eyes with appropriate remedies and supplements.

NUTRITIONAL THERAPIES

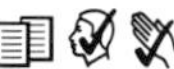

Antioxidants (see glossary) are thought to delay the aging process that can lead to degeneration of the retina. Vitamin A as beta-carotene (found in parsley, spinach, carrots, and other vegetables and fruits) is considered particularly important to strengthen the layer of lutein and zeaxanthin in the retina, which filters out damaging short-wave light rays. Zinc supplements may be recommended to stimulate eye enzymes. SEE PAGES 148–52

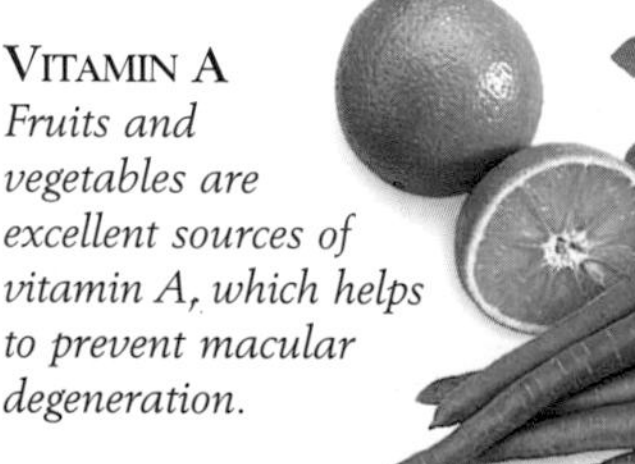

VITAMIN A *Fruits and vegetables are excellent sources of vitamin A, which helps to prevent macular degeneration.*

EARS

THE EARS ARE RESPONSIBLE for both hearing and balance. The outer and middle ears convey sound to the inner ear, which turns the sound waves into nerve impulses and transmits them to the brain via the auditory nerve. Semicircular canals in the inner ear control balance. The eustachian tube, running from the middle ear to the back of the throat, admits air and keeps pressure from building up in the middle ear. Unfortunately it can also admit viruses and bacteria that cause inflammation. Other ear disorders include temporary or permanent loss of hearing and malfunction of the balance mechanism.

KEY TO SYMBOLS

EVIDENCE	PRACTITIONER
Good scientific trials with positive results	Essential
Some research studies	Recommended
Anecdotal	Not essential
	SELF-HELP
	Self-help possibilities
	No self-help

COMPLEMENTARY APPROACHES

Persistent ear infections are generally seen by complementary practitioners as an accumulation of mucus, to be treated with diet and herbs. Traditional Chinese Medicine relates the ears to the Kidney; hearing problems may therefore indicate a Kidney disharmony, or a lack of Kidney *jing* (essence), that worsens with age.

CONVENTIONAL APPROACHES

Antibiotic or anti-inflammatory drops are prescribed for skin problems affecting the outer ear. Middle-ear infections are treated with antibiotics, and some doctors give decongestants to help dry out the middle ear. Balance problems are treated with sedative drugs.

Caution: Before seeking treatment, see page 204.

THE FUNCTIONS OF THE EAR

The main function of the external ear (the pinna or auricle) and the external canal is protection. Wax collects here on fine hairs and helps stop infection from entering the delicate middle ear. At the threshold to the middle ear is the tympanic membrane or eardrum. Airwaves striking the eardrum trigger movements in three tiny bones (ossicles) in the middle ear, which affect fluid in the inner ear and send signals via the auditory nerve to the brain, where they are perceived as sounds. The eustachian tube, which keeps air pressure on both sides of the eardrum equal, runs from the middle ear to the upper part of the throat behind the nose.

The ears are also organs of balance. The three semicircular canals of the inner ear are filled with fluid, and contain hair cells that are able to monitor the smallest changes in acceleration and movement. This information is relayed by nerve fibers to the brain, allowing the body to adjust by making further changes necessary to maintain balance.

CROSS SECTION OF THE EAR

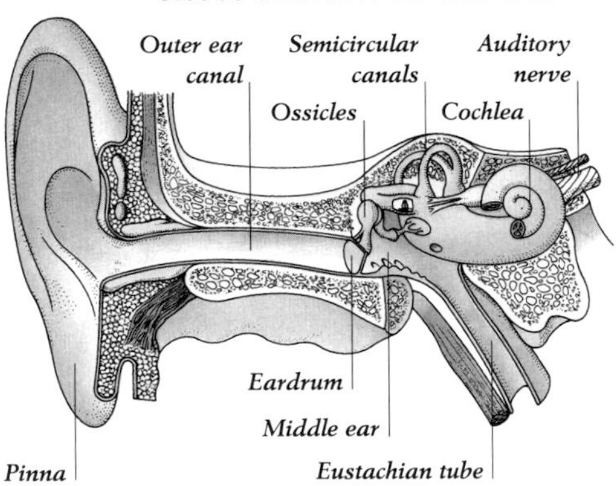

TINNITUS

PEOPLE AFFECTED by tinnitus hear a continuous ringing, hissing, or buzzing, but the sound has no external source. Many people worry that tinnitus might indicate a serious illness or that it will get louder, but these fears are unjustified. Excess ear wax, a blocked or impaired eustachian tube, and damage to the inner ear's cochlea are often to blame. Tinnitus has also been linked with use of certain drugs, such as aspirin, chloroquine, and quinine, and with persistent loud noise, smoking, and shock. There is no cure for tinnitus, but a masker, which fits into the ear like a hearing aid, may be used to suppress the noise with other sounds.

COMPLEMENTARY TREATMENTS

Mind therapies aim to focus attention away from the sound. Acupuncture and osteopathy seek to restore the body's natural balance.

ACUPUNCTURE

In Traditional Chinese Medicine, tinnitus is seen as evidence of "disharmony." A low-pitched noise suggests Kidney disharmony, while a high-pitched noise suggests Liver disharmony. The practitioner will insert various needles along the appropriate meridians. SEE PAGES 90–94

ACUPUNCTURE *A practitioner checks for evidence of disharmony.*

WESTERN HERBALISM

Ginkgo may be recommended to improve blood circulation to the inner ear. SEE PAGES 134–39

RELAXATION & BREATHING

A therapist will teach techniques to ease tension and induce a sense of calm, which may help to lower awareness of the noise. SEE PAGES 170–73

OTHER OPTIONS

Cranial Osteopathy SEE PAGE 81
Psychotherapy & Counseling SEE PAGES 160–65
Biofeedback SEE PAGE 169

EAR INFECTIONS & EARACHE

AN INFECTION of the outer ear may be caused by swimming or poking an object into the ear canal. An infection of the middle ear usually follows an infection in the nose or throat, when viruses and bacteria gain access via the eustachian tube. An acute middle ear infection brings intense, throbbing pain, fever, and, in severe cases, if the infection bursts the eardrum, a yellow-green discharge of pus. A chronic infection causes intermittent discomfort and discharge. Earache does not result only from an ear infection; other common causes may include problems with the teeth or jaw, phlegmy congestion, a buildup of wax, and boils or neuralgia affecting the outer ear.

Conventional Treatment Painkillers are usually recommended for short-term relief. Symptoms that continue for longer than a few days indicate an underlying infection, which a doctor will probably treat with antibiotics.

Cautions: Consult a doctor promptly if there is loss of hearing, dizziness, or discharge. Do not push objects into the ear, since there is a risk of perforating the eardrum.

COMPLEMENTARY TREATMENTS

Most acute earaches settle spontaneously within 48 hours. Soothing herbal medicines, dietary advice, and gentle touch and movement therapies can all help and, for those with recurring or chronic earache, might also improve resistance to infection.

CRANIAL OSTEOPATHY

Manipulation of the bones of the skull is said to help drain a buildup of fluid from the ear. SEE PAGE 81

ACUPRESSURE

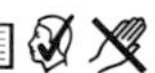

A practitioner may suggest two ways to relieve earache that is not due to an infection: pressing firmly with three fingers on the area in front of the ear, and pressing gently in the hollows behind the earlobes with the middle fingers. SEE PAGE 95

NATUROPATHY

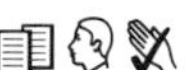

Holding a warmed pack against the ear may help to ease pain. A naturopath may also advise testing for intolerances to milk, wheat, or other foods. Food intolerances are thought to cause swelling that blocks the eustachian tube, encouraging a buildup of fluid in the middle ear. SEE PAGES 118–21

HOMEOPATHY

Standard remedies that may help acute ear infections include *Aconite 6c* for pain brought on by cold, and *Belladonna 6c* for throbbing pain with fever (especially in children) and sensitivity to touch. SEE PAGES 126–30

BIOCHEMIC TISSUE SALTS

Ferrum phos. may be advised to help relieve pain, congestion, and fever. SEE PAGE 131

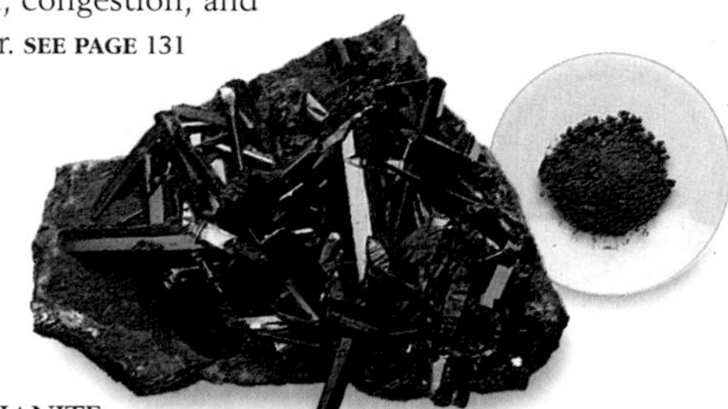

VIVIANITE
This mineral is the source of the biochemic tissue salt remedy Ferrum phos., *for ear infections.*

WESTERN HERBALISM

Herbs such as German chamomile, echinacea, and skullcap soothe pain and fight infection. St. John's wort is an excellent antiseptic and a practitioner may recommend placing a few drops of the extract in the ear and plugging it with a cotton ball. SEE PAGES 134–39

DEAFNESS

THERE ARE TWO forms of deafness: conductive deafness and nerve deafness.

Causes Conductive deafness occurs when the transmission of sound waves to the inner ear is prevented by an abnormality in the external or middle ear. Causes include inflammation, otosclerosis (hardening causing lack of mobility between the bones in the middle ear), foreign objects, and wax. Nerve deafness occurs if there is an abnormality in the auditory nerve. Causes of this form of deafness include viral infections, exposure to loud noise, the aging process, and some metabolic disorders.

Conventional Treatment Syringing to remove wax, and operations on the eardrum and middle ear, can help in some cases of conductive deafness. Hearing aids are the usual treatment for nerve deafness, while cochlear implants (electrical implants in the inner ear) can sometimes help the profoundly deaf.

COMPLEMENTARY TREATMENTS

Boosting the local circulation and improving the diet may reduce deafness. Acupuncture aims to improve the flow of qi *("life energy").*

CRANIAL OSTEOPATHY

Cranial osteopathy is said to be effective in treating deafness caused by middle ear problems. SEE PAGE 81

ACUPUNCTURE

For deafness caused by phlegm or accompanied by tinnitus a practitioner may use needles to stimulate the Kidney and Bladder meridians. SEE PAGES 90–94

NUTRITIONAL THERAPIES

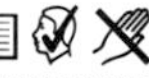

Vitamin D may help otosclerosis. According to nutritional therapists, vitamin A is required for the cochlea to function efficiently. Since vitamin E improves uptake of vitamin A you may be advised to take the two supplements together. This combination is considered to be a particularly effective treatment for age-related deafness. Ginger and ginkgo are also thought to help alleviate deafness by improving blood circulation in the ear. SEE PAGES 148–52

AYURVEDA

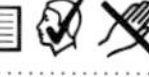

An Ayurvedic practitioner may use albad oil, supplements, and herbs such as black pepper and ashwanganda to treat hearing loss by boosting the circulation of blood in the ear. SEE PAGES 144–47

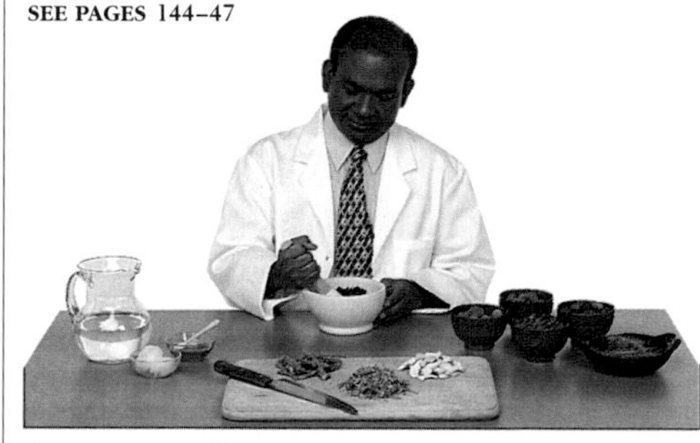

AYURVEDIC REMEDIES
As many as 20 different plants and minerals may be ground up to form a remedy.

OTHER OPTIONS

Naturopathy SEE PAGES 118–21
Homeopathy SEE PAGES 126–30
Western Herbalism SEE PAGES 134–39

THE RESPIRATORY SYSTEM

THE RESPIRATORY SYSTEM enables oxygen from the air to be taken into the bloodstream to provide the energy the body needs to function. As we breathe in, air is filtered by the nose, then travels down the windpipe (trachea) and bronchial tubes to the lungs, into millions of tiny sacs. Oxygen passes through the thin sac walls into the blood, in exchange for carbon dioxide, a waste product, which is breathed out. Mucus may collect in little-used parts of the lungs, encouraging bacteria to grow. In urban areas the air is often laden with chemicals from industry and traffic, placing a strain on the respiratory mucous membranes' defenses.

KEY TO SYMBOLS	
EVIDENCE	**PRACTITIONER**
Good scientific trials with positive results	Essential
Some research studies	Recommended
Anecdotal	Not essential
	SELF-HELP
	Self-help possibilities
	No self-help

COMPLEMENTARY APPROACHES

Treatment aims to reduce the intake of pollutants and allergens, and lessen their effects on the lungs. Building up the immune system helps the body resist attack by microorganisms inhaled through the nose and mouth.

CONVENTIONAL APPROACHES

Infections of the respiratory tract are often triggered by viruses. Irritation of the mucous membranes may constrict the airways, making breathing difficult. Decongestants, antihistamines, and bronchodilators may be prescribed. Any secondary bacterial infections (those that occur after viral infections) are treated using antibiotics.

Caution: Before seeking treatment, see page 204.

HOW AIR ENTERS THE LUNGS

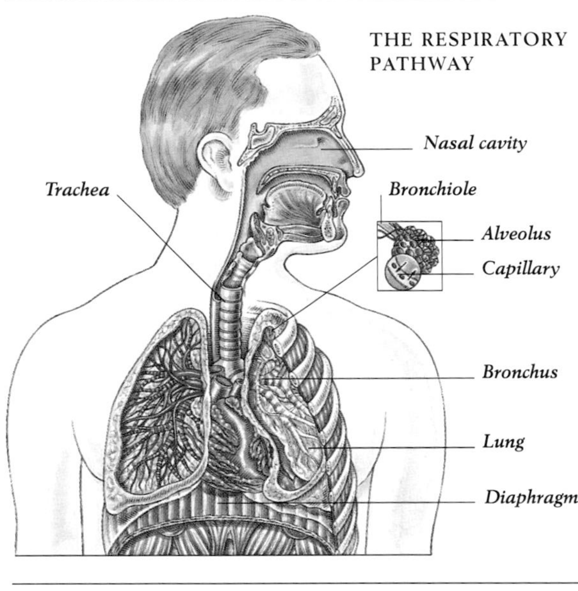

Air inhaled via the nose or mouth enters the windpipe (trachea) in the throat. The trachea divides into two tubes (bronchi) that enter the lungs – spongy, elastic air-filled organs on either side of the heart. Within each lung, the bronchi branch into smaller and smaller tubes. The very smallest tubes (bronchioles) carry air into tiny sacs (alveoli) which are surrounded by microscopically fine blood vessels (capillaries), whose walls are so thin that oxygen from the air easily diffuses through them and into the red blood corpuscles, where it is carried in hemoglobin to body tissues. The respiratory tract is lined with mucous membranes.

PHLEGM

PHLEGM IS THE OVERPRODUCTION of mucus in the respiratory tract. It gives rise to sneezing, a runny nose, blocked sinuses, and loss of smell and taste. Inflammation of the mucous membranes is the usual cause, often triggered by cold and flu viruses, other infections, allergies, or a stuffy environment. Most cases of phlegm clear quickly but, if persistent, a doctor may prescribe decongestants. Antibiotics may be given if phlegm results from a bacterial infection, and antihistamines if it is caused by an allergy.

Self-Help Measures include avoiding possible allergens, such as pollen and house dust, keeping rooms well ventilated, and reducing intake of dairy foods and sugar.

COMPLEMENTARY TREATMENTS

Touch and movement techniques such as aromatherapy, as well as medicinal therapies, are used to relieve the symptoms of congestion and boost the immune system.

AROMATHERAPY

To relieve congestion, a practitioner may recommend adding a few drops of essential oils, such as eucalyptus, lemon, or cedarwood, to a bath. SEE PAGES 62–65

NATUROPATHY

Eliminating dairy foods may reduce mucus. A therapist may advise fasting with plenty of water and fruit juice to expel toxins, followed by a raw-foods diet and zinc supplements. SEE PAGES 118–21

HYDROTHERAPY

A hydrotherapist may recommend taking long, hot showers, saunas, and steam baths to relieve symptoms. Mustard baths and sitz baths may also help. SEE PAGES 122–23

WESTERN HERBALISM

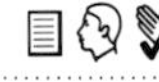

A practitioner will prescribe herbs to loosen mucus, such as hyssop. If phlegm persists, an astringent herb such as nettle may be suggested. Garlic and echinacea may also be recommended to fight infection. SEE PAGES 134–39

OTHER OPTIONS

Acupuncture SEE PAGES 90–94
Acupressure SEE PAGE 95
Homeopathy SEE PAGES 126–30
Nutritional Therapies SEE PAGES 148–52

SINUSITIS

THE SINUSES ARE CAVITIES in the facial bones. Lined with mucous membranes, they surround the nose and are joined to the nasal cavity. Infection, inflammation, and excess mucus can block the sinuses. Severe pain can result in the forehead, upper jaw, and cheekbones. Symptoms often improve after a few days, but conventionally, antihistamines and decongestants may be advised. To treat infection, antibiotics may be prescribed. Sometimes surgery or flushing the sinuses are necessary to clear a long-term blockage.

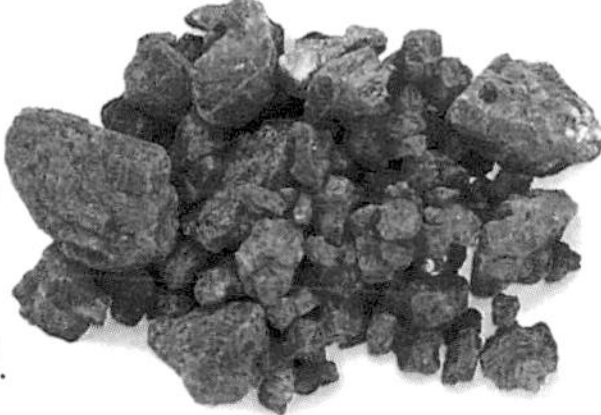

POTASSIUM DICHROMATE *The homeopathic remedy* Kali bich. *is made from this mineral.*

COMPLEMENTARY TREATMENTS

Therapies focus on fighting any underlying infection, reducing mucus production, and clearing blocked sinuses.

AROMATHERAPY

To help fight infection and clear blocked passages, a practitioner may recommend a steam inhalation with eucalyptus, tea tree, or lavender essential oil. Massaging the face and throat with a mixture of well-diluted essential oils may also help. SEE PAGES 62–65

Caution: Use steam inhalations with care if you have asthma.

ACUPRESSURE

A practitioner may recommend pressing firmly at the base of the nose on either side of the nostrils. This stimulates acupoints on the Large Intestine meridian and is considered to help sinusitis. SEE PAGE 95

HOMEOPATHY

The following standard remedies may help: *Kali bich. 6c* for pressure on the bridge of the nose and thick stringy discharge, and *Sticta pulmonaria 6c* for chronic sinusitis with no discharge. SEE PAGES 126–30

CHINESE HERBALISM

Traditional Chinese Medicine regards sinusitis as a sign of "wind and heat invasion," and of deficient *qi* ("life energy") in the Lung. A practitioner may recommend herbal remedies such as Minor Blue Dragon Formula, Pueraria "N" Formula, and Asarum Formula.

Caution: Minor Blue Dragon Formula contains ephedra, which can overstimulate the heart. SEE PAGES 140–43

OTHER OPTIONS

Acupuncture SEE PAGES 90–94
Naturopathy SEE PAGES 118–21
Western Herbalism SEE PAGES 134–39

COMMON COLD

ANY ONE OF MORE THAN 200 viruses can cause a common cold. Infection leads to inflammation of the membranes that line the nose, sinuses, and throat, resulting in a blocked or runny nose, sneezing, sore throats, coughs, mild fever, and headaches. **Cause** The virus is contracted by breathing in tiny droplets coughed or sneezed into the air by an infected person. Infection is most likely when the immune system is weakened by poor diet, overwork, or stress. In an otherwise healthy person, a cold will usually run its course in about a week. A doctor may recommend pain-relieving drugs, such as aspirin, acetaminophen, and ibuprofen, to help alleviate symptoms.

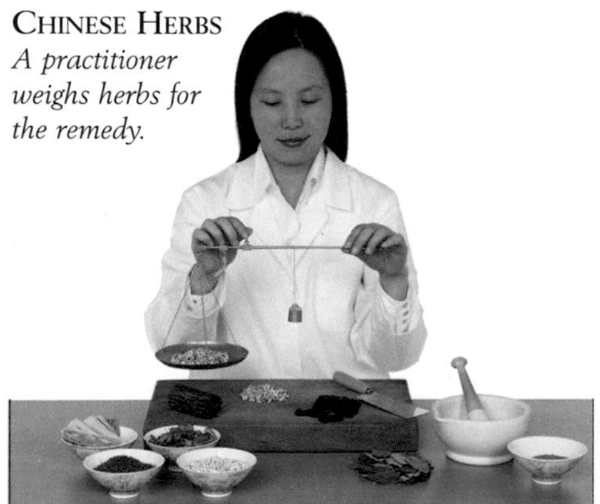

CHINESE HERBS *A practitioner weighs herbs for the remedy.*

COMPLEMENTARY TREATMENTS

Since there is no cure for a cold, treatment will usually focus on relieving symptoms and on building up the immune system to resist any further infection.

AROMATHERAPY

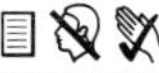

To help ward off colds, a practitioner may advise steam inhalations with essential oils of eucalyptus, lavender, and tea tree, which are all believed to have antiviral properties. To ease congestion and coughs, steam inhalation of peppermint oil may be advised. Massage with the same essential oils diluted in a carrier oil may also help. SEE PAGES 62–65

Caution: Use steam inhalations with care if you have asthma.

NATUROPATHY

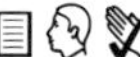

Naturopaths believe that having more than two colds a year indicates that the immune system is under strain. A practitioner will recommend adopting a healthy diet that includes fresh fruits, vegetables, and whole grains, and drinking plenty of liquids to keep the respiratory tract moist, which will help repel the cold virus. For a sore throat, a soothing gargle made with hot water, honey, lemon juice, and garlic may be advised to help fight infection. Steam inhalations and mustard foot baths, which stimulate the circulation, may also help. SEE PAGES 118–21

Caution: Use steam inhalations with care if you have asthma.

WESTERN HERBALISM

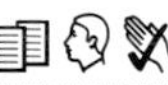

A 1994 review of German trials determined that echinacea could help boost the immune system. An herbalist may recommend this and other herbs to relieve aches and pains, reduce fever, and clear mucus. Boneset is used to shorten the duration of a cold. A red sage gargle or garlic, either raw or in capsules, may be suggested to help fight infection. Expectorant herbs are used to ease coughs (see also page 226). SEE PAGES 134–39

Cautions: Do not take medicinal doses of sage during pregnancy. Boneset in high doses can be toxic.

CHINESE HERBALISM

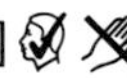

Practitioners may prescribe astragalus root. In Chinese studies, astragalus appeared to reduce the incidence of colds and shorten their duration by stimulating production of proteins that prevent viral infection. SEE PAGES 140–43

Caution: Do not take astragalus if you have a skin disorder.

NUTRITIONAL THERAPIES

High doses of vitamin C may be recommended. Several, but not all, studies suggest that this can shorten the duration of a cold and reduce its severity. In a series of clinical trials since 1984, zinc gluconate has been tested as a means to shorten the duration of colds, with some positive results. SEE PAGES 148–52

OTHER OPTIONS

Acupressure SEE PAGE 95
Homeopathy SEE PAGES 126–30

BRONCHITIS & COUGHS

BRONCHITIS IS A CONDITION in which the mucous lining of the bronchial tubes becomes inflamed. It may be "acute" or "chronic." In acute bronchitis, infection by a virus or bacteria produces thick, yellow-green phlegm that collects in the tubes, causing fever, a painful cough, raw throat, shortness of breath, and wheezing. Symptoms usually last about a week, but the cough may take longer to clear. Chronic bronchitis tends to affect smokers and the elderly. The mucous membrane becomes permanently thickened, clogging the tubes and causing a persistent cough and breathlessness.

Causes Acute bronchitis usually begins with a cold or flu and is exacerbated by a cold or damp environment, or by breathing polluted air. Chronic bronchitis arises from repeated attacks of acute bronchitis and is linked to long-term irritation by dust, smoke, and other environmental pollutants.

Conventional Treatment Acute bronchitis is generally treated with bed rest and drugs, such as aspirin or acetaminophen, for pain and fever. If it is due to a bacterial infection, antibiotics will be prescribed. Expectorants may help to loosen phlegm. Those with chronic bronchitis will be advised to stop smoking, lose weight if appropriate, and have a flu vaccination every winter. In addition, bronchodilator drugs (to widen the airways) and oxygen inhalers are often prescribed.

Self-Help Stop smoking and lose any excess weight. Avoid polluted air and use a humidifier to keep the air moist.

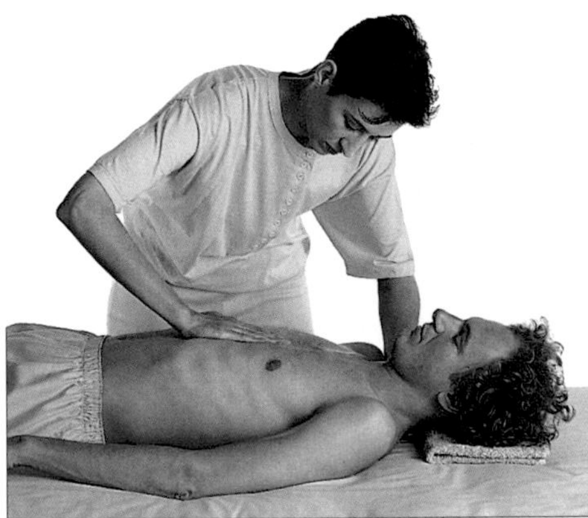

MASSAGE
Tapping and massaging the chest helps to dislodge phlegm and improve breathing.

TOUCH & MOVEMENT THERAPIES

Therapies work on unblocking the airways to improve breathing and alleviate symptoms.

MASSAGE 

For patients with chronic bronchitis, a practitioner may suggest a physical therapy massage, which involves tapping the back and chest to help dislodge phlegm and improve breathing. SEE PAGES 56–61

AROMATHERAPY 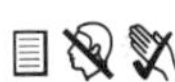

A practitioner may recommend an inhalation using tea tree, which is antiseptic, eucalyptus, for its expectorant properties, thyme, both antiseptic and expectorant, and lavender, which helps relax muscles and aids breathing.
SEE PAGES 62–65

Caution: Use steam inhalations with care if you have asthma.

CHIROPRACTIC (SEE OSTEOPATHY) 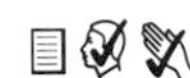

OSTEOPATHY

If airways are obstructed by chronic bronchitis, the muscles of the neck, shoulders, chest, and back become tense. Soft-tissue techniques may help breathing capacity.
SEE PAGES 70–81

MEDICINAL THERAPIES

Medicinal therapies, such as naturopathy and herbalism, aim to boost the body's responses to infection.

NATUROPATHY 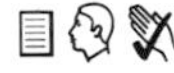

A practitioner will attempt to stimulate the immune system to fight infection and reduce mucus production. Fasting for 1–2 days and then a raw-foods or fruit diet may be suggested. You may be asked to cut out dairy products, sugar, and other kinds of refined carbohydrates. Hot spicy foods may be recommended to open the air passages. Practitioners also recommend a hot-water bottle or mustard poultice on the chest to bring warmth to the area. Postural drainage (lying on a bed with the top half of the body hanging over the side) might loosen and expel phlegm. SEE PAGES 118–21

Caution: Restricted diets may lead to malnutrition.

HYDROTHERAPY 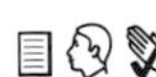

Steam inhalations, steam baths, or saunas may be advised to ease bronchial congestion. Hot and cold compresses may also be helpful.
SEE PAGES 122–23

Caution: Use steam inhalations with care if you have asthma.

WESTERN HERBALISM 

Rather than suppressing a cough, an herbalist will prescribe expectorants – many of which are believed to have antibacterial and antiviral properties – to encourage coughing and expel phlegm. Expectorant herbs include elecampane and thyme. Echinacea, garlic, and goldenseal may be suggested to fight infection, along with warming herbs such as ginger.
SEE PAGES 134–39

Cautions: Do not take goldenseal during pregnancy or if you have high blood pressure. Do not take ginger if you have a peptic ulcer.

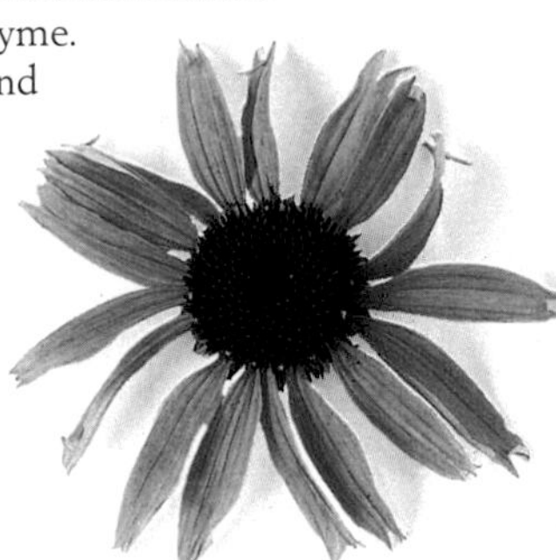

ECHINACEA
This herb appears to stimulate the body's defenses.

CHINESE HERBALISM 

Acute bronchitis is associated with "external wind," "cold," or "heat" and practitioners may recommend herbs such as fritillary, plantain, and balloon flower. Chronic bronchitis is considered to be due to a deficiency of *qi* ("life energy") in the Spleen or Lung. Classic remedies include Platycodon and Fritillaria Formula for a cough with sticky phlegm "heat" and deficiencies of Lung *yin* (see glossary) and Lung *qi*.
SEE PAGES 140–43

Caution: Take fritillary or Fritillaria Formula only under professional supervision.

OTHER OPTIONS

Homeopathy	SEE PAGES 126–30
Biochemic Tissue Salts	SEE PAGE 131
Ayurveda	SEE PAGES 144–47
Nutritional Therapies	SEE PAGES 148–52

MIND & EMOTION THERAPIES

Learning to relax not only relieves stress, it improves breathing. Both are especially important for those with chronic bronchitis.

RELAXATION & BREATHING 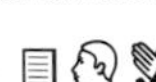

Most people use only half the lungs' potential capacity in breathing. Your therapist may demonstrate diaphragmatic breathing to help you use your chest and lungs more efficiently. This can also have the effect of calming the body and mind, and help to give you a sense of self-control if you have chronic bronchitis.
SEE PAGES 170–73

INFLUENZA

AN INFECTION of the respiratory tract, influenza (flu) is caused by one of a group of viruses. It produces symptoms similar to those of a common cold but worse: high temperature, sweating and shivering, muscle aches, fatigue and feelings of heaviness, a dry sore throat, painful breathing, and headaches. Occasionally the digestive system is also affected. Influenza usually lasts about a week, but it may persist if a secondary bacterial infection develops. Fighting the infection puts the body under stress, and a bout of flu may leave sufferers tired and depressed for weeks afterward.

Conventional Treatment Drugs such as aspirin and acetaminophen help to relieve pain, and decongestants and antihistamines may reduce mucus. Annual immunization can give up to 70% protection and is recommended for the elderly, those with bronchitis, asthma, or emphysema, and others with weak immune systems.

COMPLEMENTARY TREATMENTS

Therapies such as aromatherapy, naturopathy, and Chinese herbalism aim to boost the body's ability to cope with infection.

NATUROPATHY

Practitioners may suggest fasting for 48 hours to eliminate toxins and stimulate the immune system, and will advise plenty of fluids and rest. Hot baths and compresses help ease aching muscles. Fever is considered a sign that the body is healing itself, and naturopaths say it should not be suppressed in adults unless it gets dangerously high (104°F/40°C). SEE PAGES 118–21

HOMEOPATHY

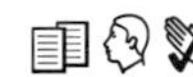

The following remedies may be suggested: *Gelsemium 6c* for feelings of fatigue, heaviness, and chills up and down the spine, *Rhus tox. 6c* if the patient is restless with stiff, painful muscles, and *Bryonia 6c* for thirst, headaches, and a painful cough. In a French study reported in 1989, the remedy *Oscillococcinum* was significantly more effective in relieving symptoms than a placebo. SEE PAGES 126–30

WESTERN HERBALISM

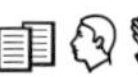

In a study in Israel in 1995, black elderberry was shown to be effective against flu. SEE PAGES 134–39

CHINESE HERBALISM

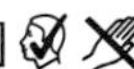

Flu may be linked with "wind cold," "damp," and "wind heat." Moxibustion may be advised, and remedies may include cinnamon. SEE PAGES 140–43

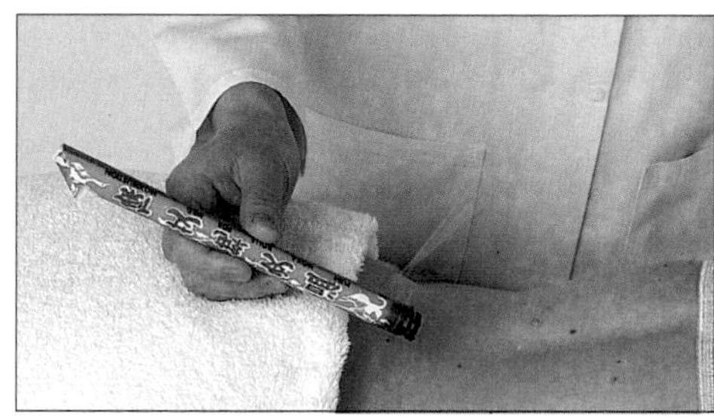

MOXIBUSTION
The herb moxa is lit and held over the acupoint to generate heat and improve the flow of qi ("life energy").

OTHER OPTION

Aromatherapy SEE PAGES 62–65

PNEUMONIA

PNEUMONIA IS AN INFECTION of one or both lungs, spreading from the bronchial airways. It causes fever, breathlessness, chest pains, chills, and a cough that produces green-yellow mucus, which is sometimes bloodstained. The infection generally follows a cold or influenza attack and is caused by a virus or bacteria. Pneumonia can be life-threatening in the very young, very old, and those whose immune systems are compromised by illness, drugs, or alcohol. Conventionally, antibiotics are usually prescribed for bacterial pneumonia, and for viral pneumonia if a secondary infection is suspected. Severe infections require hospital treatment, and physiotherapy is sometimes recommended to drain mucus from the chest.

Cautions: Call a doctor if you suspect pneumonia. Consult a doctor before undergoing any complementary treatment.

COMPLEMENTARY TREATMENTS

Massage and steam treatments help to loosen phlegm. Naturopaths and nutritional therapists aim to build up the body's innate healing ability to overcome the infection.

CHIROPRACTIC (SEE OSTEOPATHY)

OSTEOPATHY

Soft-tissue techniques may help to expel mucus and support the body's self-healing abilities. SEE PAGES 70–81

NATUROPATHY

Naturopaths may suggest a whole-foods diet, with plenty of fruit and vegetable juices and garlic to strengthen the immune system. Postural drainage (lying on a bed with the top half of the body hanging over the side) might expel phlegm. SEE PAGES 118–21

WHOLE-FOODS DIET
A healthy diet should include fresh fruits and vegetables.

HYDROTHERAPY

Steam inhalation with eucalyptus essential oil may loosen phlegm. A therapist may suggest applying a hot-water bottle to the chest and back for 30 minutes daily to ease congestion. SEE PAGES 122–23

Caution: Use steam inhalations with care if you have asthma.

WESTERN HERBALISM

A practitioner will treat pneumonia with remedies containing expectorant herbs, such as lobelia, and herbs to fight infection, such as echinacea and garlic. SEE PAGES 134–39

Caution: Take lobelia only under professional supervision.

NUTRITIONAL THERAPIES

Unconfirmed and possibly unreliable US studies early this century showed that large doses of vitamin C taken soon after infection could help defeat pneumonia by boosting the immune system. Recommended dosage is 500 mg every two hours until improvement, but this may cause nausea and other side effects. Beta-carotene, flavonoids, zinc, and thymus extract may also be suggested. SEE PAGES 148–52

OTHER OPTION

Homeopathy SEE PAGES 126–30

MOUTH & THROAT

SPEECH, TASTE, AND THE START of the digestion process are centered in the mouth. The teeth chew and grind food, breaking it up so that it can be mixed with saliva and softened for swallowing. The tongue, covered in nerve endings that respond to different tastes, helps push food toward the esophagus and down to the stomach. In the throat, the larynx uses breath to produce sounds that are shaped by the tongue, teeth, and palate to make speech. The most common mouth disorders are infections, ulcers, and dental problems. General health is reflected in the condition of the tongue and the mucous membranes of the mouth.

KEY TO SYMBOLS

EVIDENCE	PRACTITIONER
Good scientific trials with positive results	Essential
Some research studies	Recommended
Anecdotal	Not essential
	SELF-HELP
	Self-help possibilities
	No self-help

COMPLEMENTARY APPROACHES

Maintaining the health of gums and teeth is necessary for good digestive function. Traditional Chinese Medicine, Ayurveda, and all other traditional medical systems believe that the state of general health, and especially that of digestion and elimination, can be determined by examining the surface of the tongue.

CONVENTIONAL APPROACHES

Regular dental checkups are important to prevent tooth decay and gum infection. Painkillers, antibiotics, and sometimes surgery may be advised if tonsils or sinuses become infected.

Caution: Before seeking treatment, see page 204.

HOW THE MOUTH & THROAT WORK

The roof of the mouth consists of the hard palate at the front and the soft palate at the back, which stops food from entering the nose during swallowing. The tongue is the largest structure in the mouth. Consisting mainly of muscle, its surface is covered with tastebuds. The tongue is involved in speech and in chewing and swallowing food. Set into the jaws are the teeth, which grind and chop food into particles that the digestive enzymes can break down. The pharynx is a channel both for air and for food. Most of the time, air flows down the pharynx through the larynx (voice box) into the lungs. During swallowing, however, a flap of cartilage called the epiglottis blocks the entrance to the larynx, so that food or drink can pass safely into the esophagus.

STRUCTURE OF THE MOUTH & THROAT

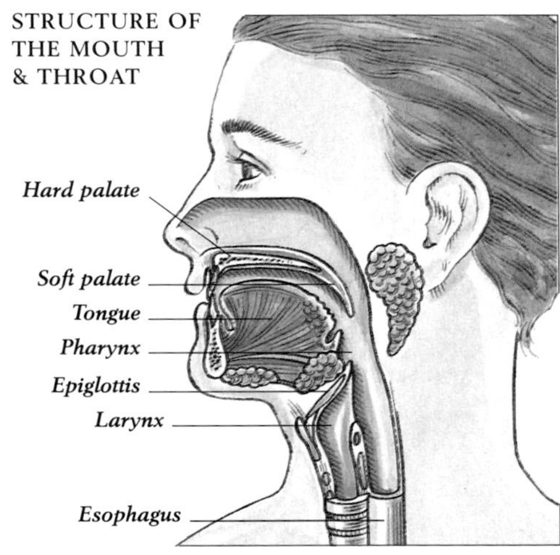

SORE THROAT & TONSILLITIS

MOST SORE THROATS are caused by a viral infection, but bacteria may also be the cause. Symptoms usually last only a few days, but could be the first signs of other problems, such as tonsillitis, an infection of the tonsils. These are two almond-shaped glands at the back of the throat that are part of the body's defense system. Inflammation causes flulike symptoms, pain on swallowing, and hoarseness. Those prone to sore throats or tonsillitis should strengthen the immune system with plenty of vitamin C, garlic, and a whole-grain diet rich in fruits and vegetables. Reducing stress levels may also be of benefit. Conventionally, painkillers, antiseptic lozenges, and gargles can help soothe a sore throat, and a doctor may prescribe antibiotics for a bacterial infection.

COMPLEMENTARY TREATMENTS

Most complementary treatments will be designed to reduce inflammation and strengthen the body's natural defenses.

AROMATHERAPY

To ease discomfort, practitioners may suggest a gargle of geranium or tea tree essential oil well diluted in water, or a gentle neck massage with diluted eucalyptus oil. SEE PAGES 62–65

NATUROPATHY

A naturopath may recommend a short fast to eliminate toxins, and garlic to ease symptoms and fight infection. Plenty of fruit juice rich in vitamin C may also be advised to soothe irritated membranes. SEE PAGES 118–21

FRUIT & GARLIC
Citrus fruits, rich in vitamin C, and garlic are valuable remedies for sore throats.

HYDROTHERAPY

Dry air can exacerbate a sore throat, so your practitioner may recommend using a humidifier. A cold abdominal pack and throat compress may aid circulation and stimulate the immune system. SEE PAGES 122–23

WESTERN HERBALISM

A practitioner will recommend gargling, perhaps with an infusion of an antiseptic herb such as calendula or sage, as soon as symptoms develop. Echinacea may be suggested to help fight infection. SEE PAGES 134–39

OTHER OPTIONS

Homeopathy SEE PAGES 126–30
Biochemic Tissue Salts SEE PAGE 131

CANKER SORES

CANKER SORES (APHTHOUS ULCERS) are small white or gray spots with inflamed edges that form on the inside of the cheek, or on the gums, lips, or tongue. Causes include nutritional deficiencies, food allergies, viral infection, injury, stress, and exhaustion. Doctors may advise antiseptic or painkilling lozenges and mouthwashes to relieve symptoms. Hydrocortisone pellets, pastes, or antibiotics may be prescribed if canker sores persist.

COMPLEMENTARY TREATMENTS

Therapies aim to redress any nutritional deficiencies and relieve symptoms.

NATUROPATHY

Practitioners may attribute recurring canker sores to a food intolerance, and a restriction diet may be suggested to detect culprit foods. Vitamin B deficiency may also be suspected, and foods rich in this vitamin, such as whole grains, milk, and potatoes, may be advised. **SEE PAGES 118–21**

WESTERN HERBALISM

An herbalist may suggest a mouthwash with myrrh, which has antimicrobial properties, or purple sage, to aid healing. Echinacea may be given to combat infection. **SEE PAGES 134–39**

Caution: Do not use myrrh during pregnancy.

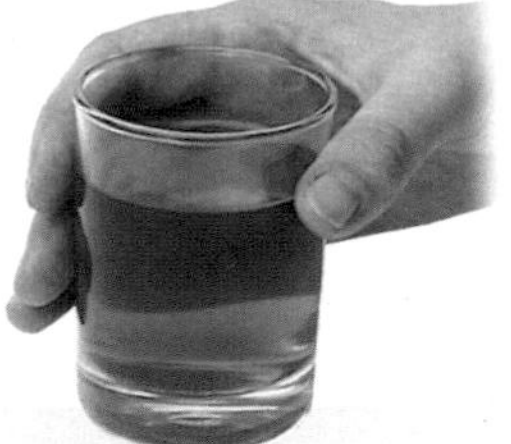

MYRRH GARGLE
A myrrh rinse can help to heal canker sores caused by bacterial infection.

LARYNGITIS

INFLAMMATION OF THE LARYNX (voice box) causes hoarseness, sometimes leading to loss of voice and a dry, rasping cough. A bacterial or viral infection is usually responsible; voice strain, heavy smoking or drinking, or stress may also be the cause. Painkillers, gargles, and medicated lozenges may ease symptoms; antibiotics can fight a bacterial infection.

Caution: See a doctor if hoarseness persists.

COMPLEMENTARY TREATMENTS

Both Western and Chinese herbalism may be effective in treating symptoms. They aim to enhance the body's healing processes.

WESTERN HERBALISM

Practitioners may advise echinacea to help resist infection and white horehound to ease a dry cough. A calendula gargle may also alleviate symptoms. **SEE PAGES 134–39**

CHINESE HERBALISM

Laryngitis is believed to be linked with toxins and "heat in the Lung." Herbs to cleanse and balance the system may include honeysuckle and peppermint. **SEE PAGES 140–43**

Caution: Do not give peppermint to children under 5.

OTHER OPTIONS

Aromatherapy	SEE PAGES 62–65
Naturopathy	SEE PAGES 118–21
Homeopathy	SEE PAGES 126–30

TOOTHACHES

THE MOST COMMON cause of a toothache is erosion of tooth enamel, exposing the dentine and the pulp at the center of the tooth to bacterial infection. In severe cases, the infection spreads to the bone to form a pus-filled abscess. Painkillers may bring relief until a dental appointment can be arranged. Antibiotics are usually prescribed for an abscess.

COMPLEMENTARY TREATMENTS

Touch and movement therapies, especially aromatherapy and acupuncture, can bring temporary relief from a toothache.

AROMATHERAPY

As an emergency measure, it is traditional to dab the affected tooth with clove essential oil. **SEE PAGES 62–65**

ACUPRESSURE

The acupoint to relieve a toothache is found on the back of the hand, between the thumb and index finger. **SEE PAGE 95**

OTHER OPTIONS

Acupuncture	SEE PAGES 90–94
Hydrotherapy	SEE PAGES 122–23
Homeopathy	SEE PAGES 126–30
Western Herbalism	SEE PAGES 134–39

GINGIVITIS & HALITOSIS

INFLAMED, BLEEDING GUMS (gingivitis) are usually a sign of infection, often due to tooth decay or dental plaque. Doctors may prescribe antibiotics in severe cases. Bad breath (halitosis) may be caused by gingivitis or digestive problems.

ORAL HYGIENE
Regular brushing helps prevent gum disease.

COMPLEMENTARY TREATMENTS

Therapies aim to improve elimination and maintain healthy teeth and gums.

NATUROPATHY

Juices high in beta-carotene, such as carrot or cantaloupe, may help restore healthy gums. Naturopaths believe that bad breath is a symptom of poor elimination of waste from the body, and may recommend a high-fiber diet with plenty of raw vegetables and water to improve digestion. Charcoal tablets are thought to help by absorbing waste products from the bowel. **SEE PAGES 118–21**

AYURVEDA

A practitioner may recommend drinking diluted lemon juice and massaging the gums with coconut oil, goldenseal, or myrrh to counter infection and speed healing. Dabbing bleeding gums with cutch may also be suggested. **SEE PAGES 144–47**

Cautions: Do not use myrrh or goldenseal during pregnancy, or goldenseal if you have high blood pressure.

OTHER OPTIONS

Homeopathy	SEE PAGES 126–30
Western Herbalism	SEE PAGES 134–39

DIGESTION

DIGESTION IS THE PROCESS that breaks down food into a form that can be absorbed into the bloodstream, so that the body can use it for energy and to build and repair tissues. Digestion begins in the mouth, with the action of saliva on food, but most of it takes place in the stomach and the small intestine. Practitioners agree that a healthy digestive system is a crucial factor in maintaining general physical and emotional well-being. Digestive-system disorders are result of a number of causes, including a poor diet, emotional disturbances, inherited problems, allergies, and infections.

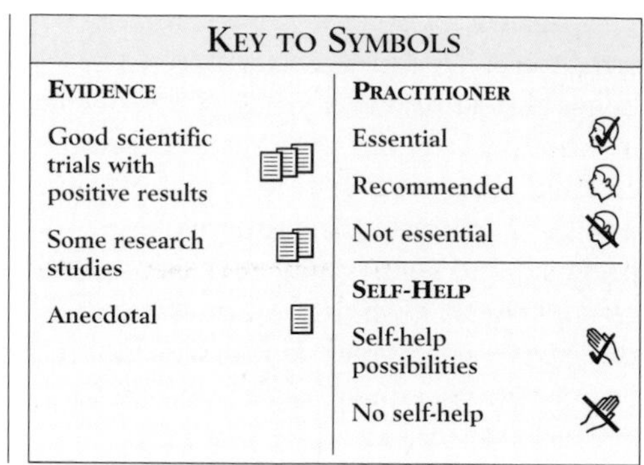

KEY TO SYMBOLS

EVIDENCE	PRACTITIONER
Good scientific trials with positive results	Essential
Some research studies	Recommended
Anecdotal	Not essential
	SELF-HELP
	Self-help possibilities
	No self-help

COMPLEMENTARY APPROACHES

Complementary treatments for almost *any* disease will pay attention to diet and the state of the gut, usually by improving the elimination of waste products, supporting the liver, and cleansing the colon. Therapies also seek to restore natural levels of the gut's beneficial bacteria, and identify and eliminate foods that irritate the digestive tract.

CONVENTIONAL APPROACHES

Drugs and surgery can be lifesaving treatments for some gut problems. They are less effective for stress-related digestive disorders.

Caution: Before seeking treatment, see page 204.

HOW FOOD IS DIGESTED

Digestion starts in the mouth, where saliva moistens food to make it easier to chew, and enzymes begin breaking down carbohydrates. Once chewed, food passes down the esophagus to the stomach, and is further broken down by acids and enzymes before passing into the small intestine. Here, digestive juices from the pancreas, liver, and gallbladder (bile) attack the now semisolid food, breaking it down into fats, proteins, and carbohydrates for absorption into the blood. The liver assists in the digestion of fats and helps to eliminate fat-soluble toxins from the body. Undigested matter passes into the colon to be excreted.

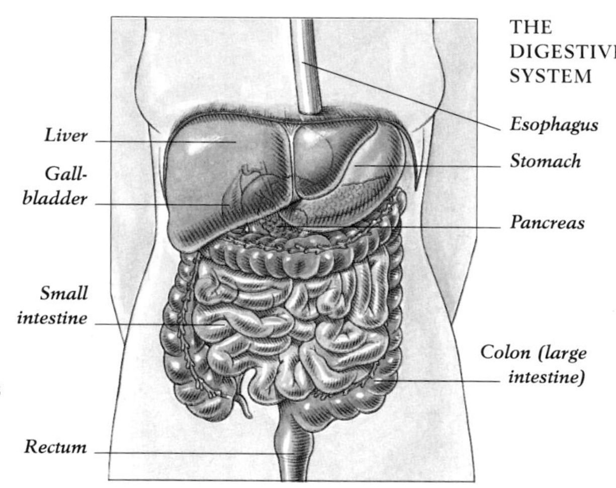

THE DIGESTIVE SYSTEM

GASTROENTERITIS

GASTROENTERITIS IS AN INFLAMMATION of the lining of the stomach and intestines, usually caused by bacteria from contaminated food, a virus, or an allergy or intolerance to a particular food. Symptoms can last from six to 36 hours, and include nausea, vomiting, diarrhea, stomach cramps, and mild fever. A doctor will advise you to take only liquids until the attack passes. A salt and glucose rehydration solution helps if vomiting and diarrhea are severe. When symptoms ease, eating small amounts of bananas, white rice, apples, and dry toast (the "BRAT" diet) helps, followed by a gradual return to a normal diet.

Caution: Consult a doctor if diarrhea continues for more than three days (24 hours for a baby) or if there is mucus or blood in the stools.

COMPLEMENTARY TREATMENTS

Soothing, healing remedies help to restore an irritated digestive tract.

NATUROPATHY

Like conventional doctors, practitioners will recommend fasting, taking only liquids, and perhaps a rehydration solution, until the worst is over. "Live" yogurt or supplements of acidophilus powder may be suggested to help restore beneficial intestinal bacteria.

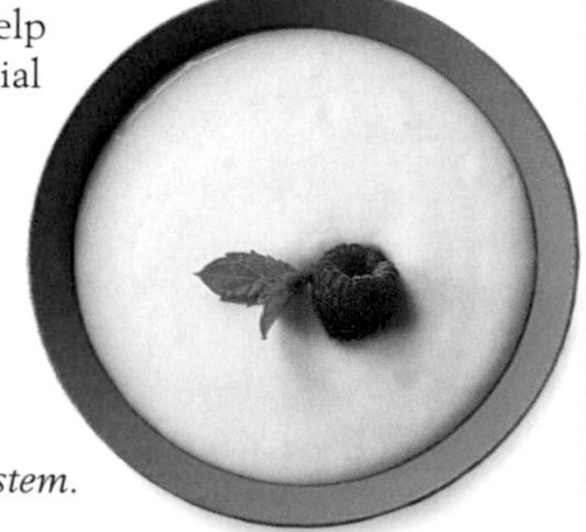

YOGURT
The bacteria in "live" yogurt benefit the digestive system.

You may be advised to avoid other dairy foods for a while, since an intolerance to lactose (the sugar found in milk and milk products) is more likely when the digestive tract is inflamed, and can lead to irritable bowel syndrome. SEE PAGES 118–21

WESTERN HERBALISM

A practitioner may suggest an infusion or tincture of meadowsweet or cinnamon to soothe the gut, reduce acidity, and ease nausea. Other recommended herbs include ginger, peppermint, or German chamomile to ease cramps and thyme or fennel to clear infection. Arrowroot mixed with a little water can soothe the bowel.

SEE PAGES 134–39

Cautions: Do not take medicinal doses of cinnamon or fennel during pregnancy, or ginger if you have a peptic ulcer. Do not take meadowsweet if you are allergic to aspirin.

NAUSEA & VOMITING

NAUSEA AND VOMITING are common symptoms. Vomiting rids the body of harmful ingested substances. It also occurs in reaction to toxins produced by illnesses or drugs. Causes range from food poisoning and the hormonal changes of early pregnancy to shock, migraines, nervous tension, and head injury, or disturbances in the inner ear and central nervous system. For vomiting caused by food poisoning, a doctor will suggest avoiding solid food for 24 hours, and in some instances may recommend a salt and glucose rehydration solution. Drugs that suppress the vomiting reflex may be prescribed in severe cases, and standard medication is available for preventing motion sickness.

Cautions: Call a doctor if vomiting recurs or if an attack lasts for more than 12 hours, particularly in children, or if it is associated with abdominal pain, high fever, drowsiness, headaches, or aversion to light. Do not use medication for nausea and vomiting in the first three months of pregnancy.

COMPLEMENTARY TREATMENTS

Therapies such as acupressure and herbalism may prove especially effective in settling the digestive system.

ACUPRESSURE

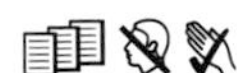

In Traditional Chinese Medicine, nausea and vomiting are considered to be symptoms of "ascending Stomach *qi* ('life energy')." In UK clinical studies reported between 1990 and 1996, stimulation of the acupoint "Pericardium 6" was shown to relieve nausea and vomiting after an anesthetic, during chemotherapy, and in morning and motion sickness. This point is located on the inner arm (see left); a practitioner will show you how to press it, or you can use special elasticized wristbands. SEE PAGE 95

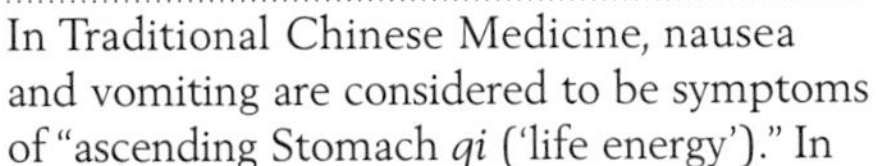

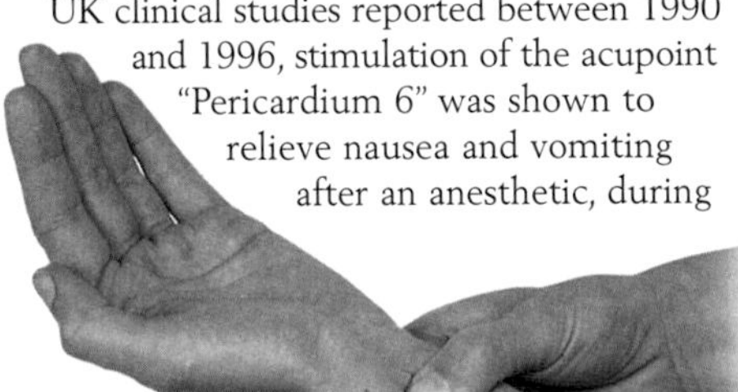

SELF-HELP
Pressing this acupoint on the inner arm may relieve nausea associated with pregnancy, chemotherapy, or anesthetics.

WESTERN HERBALISM

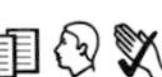

A practitioner may suggest sipping an infusion of ginger, since studies show that this herb can be even more effective than antinausea drugs in bringing relief. Peppermint, fennel, and German chamomile teas may also be recommended. If nausea is caused by an infection or food poisoning, a practitioner may advise taking garlic or diluted lemon juice.
SEE PAGES 134–39

Cautions: Do not take medicinal doses of fennel during pregnancy. Do not take ginger if you have a peptic ulcer. Do not give peppermint to children under five.

HYPNOTHERAPY

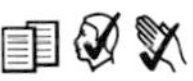

Undertaken in advance, hypnotherapy has been shown to help avert vomiting in morning sickness and after chemotherapy.
SEE PAGES 166–67

PEPTIC ULCERS & GASTRITIS

"PEPTIC ULCER" IS THE TERM commonly applied to ulcers of the stomach (gastric ulcers) and to ulcers of the duodenum (duodenal ulcers). They are breaks in the lining of the digestive tract and cause pain, burping, bloating, vomiting, weight loss, and, in severe cases, internal bleeding with tarry stool. Gastritis – inflammation of the stomach lining – produces symptoms similar to those of a peptic ulcer. The bacterium *Helicobacter pylori* is thought to play a role in both conditions; other causes include poor diet and stress.

Conventional Treatment Drugs known as H_2 blockers reduce acid production, allowing the ulcer to heal. Antibiotics to kill bacteria, and antacids to neutralize the acid, may also be prescribed. Surgery is now rare unless the ulcer has perforated the stomach wall, causing peritonitis. Ulcer-healing drugs will also be given for gastritis. Those prone to ulcers or gastritis should avoid large meals, spicy food, aspirin, caffeine, tobacco, and alcohol, which can irritate the stomach.

Caution: Consult a doctor if you notice blood in the stools, or if you are passing black, tarry stool.

COMPLEMENTARY TREATMENTS

Some therapies focus on reducing acidity. Other techniques, such as acupuncture and relaxation, can be used to relieve stress.

ACUPUNCTURE

Stimulating points on the appropriate meridians may be useful in treating peptic ulcers. This is said to induce relaxation and reduce the secretion of stomach acids.
SEE PAGES 90–94

NATUROPATHY

Practitioners recommend small, frequent meals so as not to overload the stomach. A diet rich in fiber, thought to promote the secretion of mucus, which protects the walls of the digestive tract, may be advised. A juice drink made from raw cabbage leaves is a traditional remedy for peptic ulcers.
SEE PAGES 118–21

WESTERN HERBALISM

Studies show that specially prepared licorice tablets are effective in treating peptic ulcers (licorice appears to increase the mucus that lines the digestive tract). An herbalist may also suggest remedies such as slippery elm to soothe ulcerated tissues and reduce acidity. Relaxants and tonics that may help relieve stress include lemon balm and skullcap. SEE PAGES 134–39

Caution: Do not take licorice during pregnancy, or if you have high blood pressure or anemia.

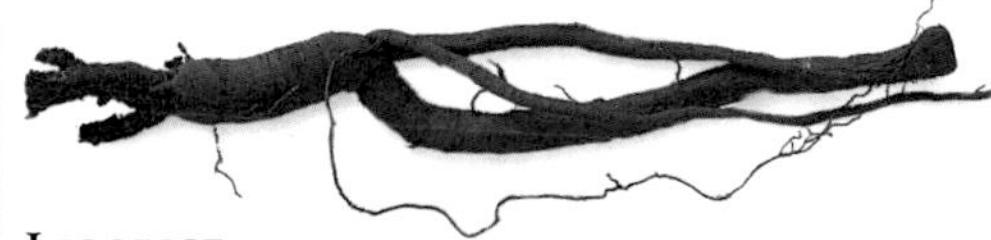

LICORICE
This powerful, soothing herb has proved as effective in healing ulcers as some conventional treatments.

NUTRITIONAL THERAPIES

Certain foods may encourage excess stomach acid production by irritating the stomach lining, and practitioners will suggest an exclusion diet to identify the foods responsible. The following supplements may also be given: vitamin A (to prevent and treat ulceration), vitamin C (deficiencies have been linked with bleeding ulcers), vitamin E (to protect membranes), and zinc (to inhibit chemicals that weaken the stomach lining). SEE PAGES 148–52

RELAXATION & BREATHING

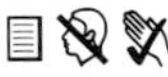

A practitioner will demonstrate techniques that may reduce acid production and help you cope with stressful situations. SEE PAGES 170–73

OTHER OPTION

Hypnotherapy SEE PAGES 166–67

INDIGESTION, ACID INDIGESTION & HEARTBURN

INDIGESTION IS A BLANKET TERM for any discomfort in the upper abdomen, usually felt after eating. It is also known as dyspepsia and acid indigestion. Symptoms include heartburn (a burning acidic sensation in the chest), burping, hiccups, nausea, and gas. Persistent indigestion may be a symptom of a peptic ulcer or of liver, gallbladder, or pancreatic disease.

Causes Too much rich, spicy, or fatty food, excess alcohol, eating too quickly, swallowing air, and eating unripe fruit can all lead to increased production of gastric acid, which irritates the stomach lining. In some cases, the acid may flow back (reflux) into the esophagus. Pregnant women and people who are overweight are more susceptible to reflux because their internal organs are pressing on the digestive tract. Stress and emotions such as anxiety and fear can also affect normal digestive secretions.

Conventional Treatment Drugs known as H_2 blockers are often prescribed to reduce acid in the stomach. Antacids may give temporary relief.

Self-Help Eat small meals at regular intervals, without rushing, and follow a fiber-rich diet to help prevent indigestion. Avoiding tobacco, alcohol, spicy or acidic foods, strong coffee, and carbonated drinks may also help.

Caution: Consult a doctor if symptoms last more than a few days, or if you are over 40 and suddenly experience indigestion.

COMPLEMENTARY TREATMENTS

All practitioners investigate the underlying cause and treat accordingly. Herbalists will also suggest remedies that prevent indigestion and treat symptoms.

CHIROPRACTIC (SEE OSTEOPATHY)

OSTEOPATHY

Manipulation of the lower thoracic area of the spine, where nerve and blood supplies to the digestive organs arise, may relieve symptoms in some people. SEE PAGES 76–81

ACUPUNCTURE

In Traditional Chinese Medicine, the digestion and assimilation process is known as "Spleen." To relieve digestive problems, a practitioner will work on the Stomach, Large Intestine, and Spleen meridians to remove any blockage of *qi* ("life energy"), which is thought to cause indigestion. SEE PAGES 90–94

NATUROPATHY

Naturopaths believe too little hydrochloric acid (one of the gastric juices) can cause indigestion, as well as contribute to most other digestive disorders, and may suggest a course of betaine hydrochloride capsules. Some claim indigestion indicates a food intolerance or allergy, and will advise an exclusion diet to identify the offending foods. "Live" yogurt, containing beneficial bacteria, may help if dysbiosis (an imbalance of microorganisms in the gut) is involved. You will also be advised to follow a whole-foods diet excluding sugar and other highly refined carbohydrates, which stimulate the secretion of gastric acid but provide no fiber or protein to neutralize it. See also Food Intolerances, page 303. SEE PAGES 118–21

WESTERN HERBALISM

Slippery elm tablets may be advised to protect the stomach lining. Dandelion and burdock taken before eating are said to enhance digestion. Goldenseal increases the flow of gastric juices, and peppermint and fennel are calming. SEE PAGES 134–39

Cautions: Do not take medicinal doses of fennel or goldenseal during pregnancy, or take goldenseal if you have high blood pressure. Do not give peppermint to children under five.

NUTRITIONAL THERAPIES

The Hay diet, in which carbohydrates and proteins are eaten separately because they are thought to require different conditions for digestion, may be advised. Vitamin C, zinc, and beta-carotene may be also be suggested. SEE PAGES 148–52

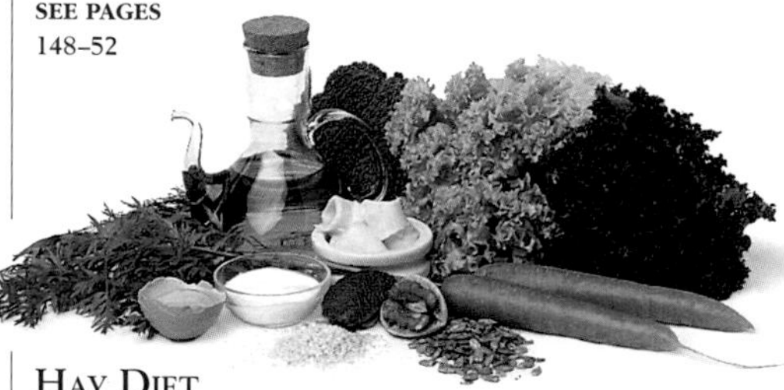

HAY DIET
Fruits and vegetables are "neutral" foods that can be eaten with either proteins or carbohydrates.

RELAXATION & BREATHING

A practitioner will demonstrate exercises to ease the mind and reduce tension and other physiological signs of stress. SEE PAGES 170–73

OTHER OPTIONS

Reflexology SEE PAGES 66–69
Acupressure SEE PAGE 95
Homeopathy SEE PAGES 126–30
Chinese Herbalism SEE PAGES 140–43

APPETITE DISTURBANCE

APPETITE IS INFLUENCED by the smell, appearance, and taste of food, as well as by general well-being and the emotions. We tend to lose our appetite during an acute illness such as flu, or because of a digestive disorder. Zinc deficiency, other nutritional factors and certain drugs can also cause loss of appetite, and it is often an early symptom of depression. Increased appetite is common in people with an overactive thyroid, and in those with low blood sugar levels; it may also be a response to emotional stress.

Caution: Consult a doctor if appetite disturbance is persistent.

COMPLEMENTARY TREATMENTS

Therapies that address physiological and emotional well-being can help to restore normal appetite.

NUTRITIONAL THERAPIES

Lack of zinc is said to reduce the senses of smell and taste, important in stimulating the appetite, and practitioners may recommend zinc-rich foods such as oysters, poultry, or eggs. Potassium deficiency, found mostly in the elderly and those taking diuretics, also affects appetite. Foods rich in potassium include broccoli, yeast extract, and bananas. SEE PAGES 148–52

PSYCHOTHERAPY & COUNSELING

If appetite is disturbed because of emotional disorders, a course of psychotherapy or counseling may help. SEE PAGES 160–65

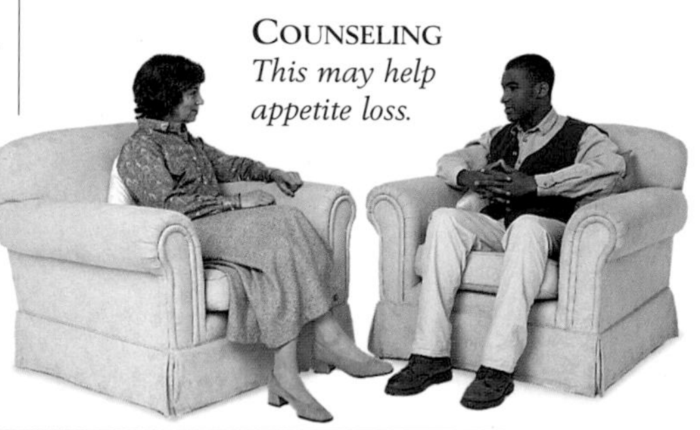

COUNSELING
This may help appetite loss.

HEPATITIS

HEPATITIS IS AN INFLAMMATION of the liver cells. It may be acute (healing eventually), or chronic (leading to ongoing liver problems). Symptoms of acute hepatitis include jaundice (yellowing of the skin), fatigue, fever, nausea, vomiting, loss of appetite, pain in the abdomen, and liver tenderness. In chronic hepatitis, symptoms may be no more than a general feeling of being unwell.
Causes Acute hepatitis is usually caused by one of several viruses. Hepatitis A (infectious hepatitis) is carried in food or water contaminated by infected feces. Hepatitis B and C are spread through blood or body fluids, by transfusion, sharing needles to inject drugs, tattooing, or sexual intercourse. Chronic hepatitis sometimes follows acute hepatitis or may develop over a long period, perhaps as a result of heavy drinking. It can destroy the liver, causing cirrhosis.
Conventional Treatment Acute hepatitis is treated with bed rest, plenty of fluids, and a diet with no meat, fats, or alcohol. Steroids may be given to reduce liver swelling. Chronic hepatitis generally resists treatment, although steroid, cytotoxic, or antiviral drugs may be used, or a liver transplant performed.

COMPLEMENTARY TREATMENTS

Careful monitoring of the diet, and certain nutritional supplements may aid recovery from acute hepatitis. The chronic form of the disease is difficult to treat, and expert professional help is essential.

NATUROPATHY

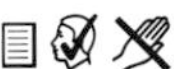

A high-fiber diet is said to increase elimination of bile acids and toxins from the liver. A naturopath may advise a high-protein, vegetarian whole-foods diet with plenty of fluids (especially vegetable juices), together with dietary supplements. Some practitioners recommend vitamins E and B_{12} and folic acid to shorten recovery time. SEE PAGES 118–21

WESTERN HERBALISM

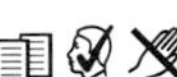

Practitioners will usually approach all cases of hepatitis with gentle liver remedies. Dandelion is a traditional detoxifying remedy and a rich source of vitamins, minerals, and beta-carotene, thought to enhance the flow of bile (a digestive juice). Studies show that milk thistle contains silymarin, a potent constituent that inhibits liver damage and increases liver cell regeneration. The active ingredient in globe artichokes, a favorite folk remedy, is cynarin, which has been shown to have a significant effect in protecting the liver and helping it to regenerate, as well as in stimulating digestive secretions. Licorice and catechin, an extract from the herb pale catechu, are also considered to be effective remedies. SEE PAGES 134–39
Cautions: Do not take licorice during pregnancy or if you are anemic or have high blood pressure. Take pale catechu only under professional supervision.

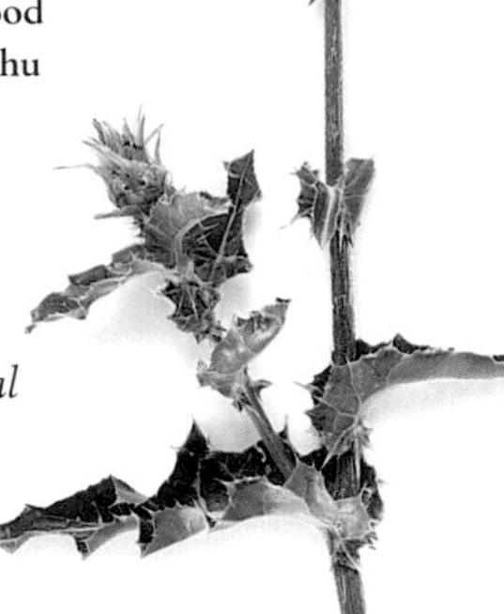

MILK THISTLE
Scientific research supports the traditional use of milk thistle for protecting the liver.

ORTHOMOLECULAR THERAPY

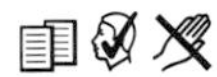

According to some studies, large doses of vitamin C (4,000–10,000 mg by mouth or injection) may alleviate viral hepatitis. Practitioners may recommend supplements of 1,000–5,000 mg a day, or as much as can be tolerated without causing diarrhea. Vitamin B_{12} supplements may also be suggested.
SEE PAGE 153

OTHER OPTIONS

Hydrotherapy SEE PAGES 122–23
Homeopathy SEE PAGES 126–30
Chinese Herbalism SEE PAGES 140–43
Ayurveda SEE PAGES 144–47
Nutritional Therapies SEE PAGES 148–52

GALLSTONES

GALLSTONES ARE PEBBLELIKE lumps in the gallbladder, where bile is stored. A thick, bitter liquid, bile contains waste products from the liver, cholesterol, and salts that help break down fats. Gallstones, which consist of cholesterol, bile pigments, and calcium salts, form when the composition of bile changes. They can cause intense abdominal pain, with bloating, gas, and nausea. If a stone blocks the gallbladder, there will be pain, inflammation and possibly jaundice (yellowing of the skin), and serious infection of the liver. Gallstones tend to occur in those who are obese, pregnant, diabetic, or taking oral contraceptives. Conventionally, drugs may dissolve small stones; others can be broken up by ultrasound. Surgery may be necessary to remove the stones or, in severe cases, the gallbladder.

COMPLEMENTARY TREATMENTS

Practitioners will use dietary regimes and herbal remedies to encourage the body to expel gallstones, while at the same time supporting the digestive system.

NATUROPATHY

Naturopaths see gallstones as a problem caused by poor digestion, absorption, and elimination, which overloads the liver. A practitioner will offer dietary advice and herbal remedies to flush out gallstones. A juice fast followed by a low-fat diet high in soluble fiber may be recommended, along with plenty of water. Olive oil and other unsaturated oils are said to help stimulate the gallbladder to cleanse itself. SEE PAGES 118–21

OLIVE OIL
Regular intake of olive oil may help prevent gallstones.

WESTERN HERBALISM

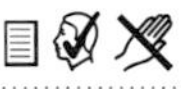

Herbal remedies known as chologogues may be prescribed to improve bile flow and dissolve gallstones. These include balmony, a Native North American remedy, globe artichoke, rosemary, sage, boldo, and dandelion.
SEE PAGES 134–39
Caution: Do not take boldo or medicinal doses of sage during pregnancy.

CHINESE HERBALISM

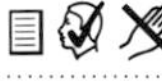

Gallstones are associated with "Gallbladder damp heat" for which Li Dan Formula is a popular patent Chinese herbal remedy.
SEE PAGES 140–43

OTHER OPTION

Nutritional Therapies SEE PAGES 148–52

CROHN'S DISEASE

CHRONIC INFLAMMATION of the digestive tract, particularly the lower small intestine, is known as Crohn's disease, one of two forms of inflammatory bowel disease (see also Ulcerative Colitis, below). Crohn's disease is becoming more common in the West, and occurs most often in people aged between 15 and 35. It can cause pain, bloating, fever, fatigue, and weight loss, and vitamin and mineral deficiencies. In the worst cases, the intestine becomes blocked by scars. The joints, skin, and eyes may also become inflamed.

Causes Crohn's disease may be an autoimmune response in which the body attacks its own tissue following infection, or it may be a reaction to stress or unknown environmental factors. It has also been linked with the measles vaccination, food intolerances, and diet. There may also be a genetic factor, as the disease appears to run in families.

Conventional Treatment Antibiotics and corticosteroids are usually prescribed to fight infection and ease inflammation. In severe cases, the damaged tissue may have to be removed surgically.

COMPLEMENTARY TREATMENTS

Naturopaths consider inflammation of the bowel to be caused by poor digestion, absorption, and elimination, and use diet and supplements to rectify this. Therapies such as herbalism aim to relieve inflammation.

NATUROPATHY

Treatment will focus on cleansing the bowel and resting and supporting the liver. An initial juice fast may be recommended, gradually progressing to a diet high in soluble fiber (found in fresh and dried fruits and leafy green vegetables). Supplements of vitamins, minerals, and digestive enzymes may be given. You may also be advised to eat "live" yogurt to rectify any disturbance of the gut's beneficial bacteria. There is evidence from Addenbrooke's Hospital, Cambridge, UK, that over 50% of sufferers of Crohn's disease may benefit from medically supervised exclusion diets, which seek to identify potential food intolerances. Dairy products and wheat are the most common offenders, and as a first step, a practitioner may suggest a diet excluding such foods. A bacterium present in milk even after pasteurization is especially suspect, so milk in particular may be excluded. SEE PAGES 118–21

WESTERN HERBALISM

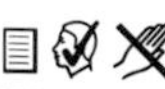

Robert's Formula is a traditional herbal preparation for tackling symptoms of inflammatory bowel disease. A modified version contains marshmallow and slippery elm to soothe and protect tissues, wild indigo for gastrointestinal infection, echinacea and goldenseal to inhibit bacteria, pokeroot to heal ulceration, and comfrey to ease inflammation.
SEE PAGES 134–39

Caution: Take wild indigo, goldenseal, pokeroot, and comfrey only under professional supervision.

RELAXATION & BREATHING

Techniques to induce relaxation are beneficial for all body functions.
SEE PAGES 170–73

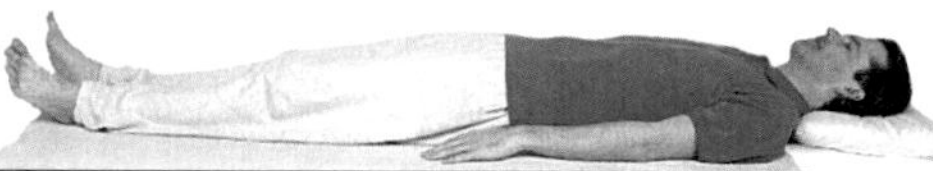

STRESS MANAGEMENT
Relaxation techniques can help you deal with stress, which may be a cause of Crohn's disease.

OTHER OPTIONS

Yoga SEE PAGES 108–11
Nutritional Therapies SEE PAGES 148–52
Autogenic Training SEE PAGE 168

ULCERATIVE COLITIS

ONE OF TWO FORMS of inflammatory bowel disease (see also Crohn's Disease, above), ulcerative colitis mainly affects people between the ages of 20 and 25. It causes inflammation of the colon and rectum, leading to ulceration of the gut lining. Symptoms include abdominal pain, diarrhea, blood and mucus in the feces, nausea, and fever. Complications include anemia from blood loss and toxins from the gut entering the bloodstream. The condition may lead to cancer of the bowel.

Cause The cause is unknown, although like Crohn's disease this may be an autoimmune disorder. It is most common in the developed world, suggesting links with a low-fiber diet, and appears to be exacerbated by stress. A doctor will give dietary advice, along with steroids to reduce inflammation. Intravenous feeding or fasting may be recommended to rest the colon. Surgery to remove the affected part of the colon is a last resort.

COMPLEMENTARY TREATMENTS

All therapies focus on easing symptoms. Acupuncture aims to restore the balance of qi ("life energy") in the body. Treatments listed for Crohn's disease may also help.

ACUPUNCTURE

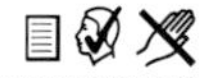

A practitioner will concentrate on stimulating acupoints on the Gallbladder meridian, either with needles or moxibustion, to correct any disturbance in the flow of *qi*.
SEE PAGES 90–94

ACUPRESSURE

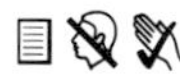

A practitioner may demonstrate several ways to relieve symptoms, such as applying deep pressure to acupoints on the Stomach and Spleen meridians. SEE PAGE 95

NATUROPATHY

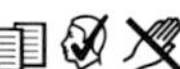

See Crohn's Disease, above. Exclusion diets, however, are less helpful. SEE PAGES 118–21

WESTERN HERBALISM

See Crohn's Disease, above. SEE PAGES 134–39

CHINESE HERBALISM

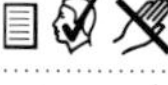

Chinese herbalists believe poisoned Blood and excess "damp" may give rise to inflammatory bowel disease. Remedies may include dandelion and astragalus to detoxify and balance the system. SEE PAGES 140–43

Caution: Do not take astragalus if you have a skin disorder.

DANDELION
An effective cleansing herb, dandelion may be used to "purify" the blood.

NUTRITIONAL THERAPIES

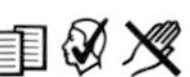

Omega-3 fatty acids (found in oily fish and fish-oil supplements) have been found to ease symptoms. Practitioners may also recommend beta-carotene (a source of vitamin A) and vitamin E. Inflammatory bowel diseases lead to a heavy loss of essential nutrients, so supervised supplementation may be needed.
SEE PAGES 148–52

CELIAC DISEASE

IN THIS DISEASE, a protein (gluten) in rye, wheat, and other cereal grains damages the lining of the small intestine so that it fails to absorb nutrients. Celiac disease usually appears in early childhood, but can affect adults. Symptoms include bulky stools, diarrhea, failure to gain weight, a bloated stomach, and fatigue. Adults may experience depression, infertility, skin complaints, canker sores, and constipation. While often hereditary, the disease may also develop after a bout of gastroenteritis. Once diagnosed, a lifelong gluten-free diet must be followed, and vitamin supplements may be advised. There may be a connection between celiac disease and bottlefeeding, and some doctors also recommend restricting cow's milk.

COMPLEMENTARY TREATMENTS

Most people are diagnosed with celiac disease in childhood. A less severe form of wheat intolerance may develop in others later in life, especially in the relatives of people who have celiac disease. Naturopaths and nutritional therapists will offer dietary guidance and suggest means of supporting the digestive system.

NATUROPATHY

A practitioner will help you change to a gluten-free diet, excluding all grains except brown rice, millet, and corn. You may also be advised to restrict your intake of cow's milk. Papain, a protein-digesting enzyme in papaya, is said to help deactivate wheat gluten, and eating plenty of fresh papaya or taking papain supplements may be suggested, along with vitamins and minerals to compensate for nutrient loss. SEE PAGES 118–21

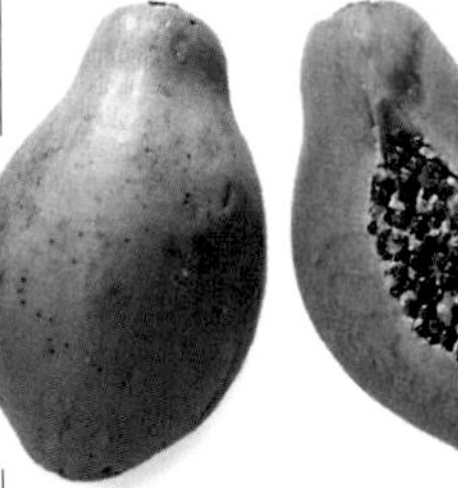

PAPAYA
Fresh papaya is said to improve the digestion of protein.

NUTRITIONAL THERAPIES

A wide range of essential nutrients is likely to be poorly absorbed in people who have celiac disease. A practitioner will supervise the supplementation of vitamins, minerals, and other substances in order to avoid deficiencies and to improve overall health.
SEE PAGES 148–52

CANDIDIASIS

CANDIDA ALBICANS is a yeastlike microorganism that occurs naturally in the mouth, gut, and vagina, and on the skin. It is normally kept under control by "friendly" bacteria, but if the immune system has been weakened by infection, stress, or nutritional deficiencies, or if the protective bacteria have been destroyed by antibiotics, it can multiply rapidly, causing infection. This condition is known as candidiasis (also called thrush, when in the mouth, or yeast infection, when in the vagina, see page 273).

Complementary practitioners believe that overgrowth of the microorganism is a widespread problem, responsible for symptoms ranging from chronic fatigue and irritability to aching muscles and joints, irregular periods, diarrhea, and constipation. They suspect the yeast causes fermentation in the small intestine and damages the mucous lining, allowing waste products to leak into the bloodstream. See also Food Intolerances, page 303.

Conventional Treatment Doctors believe candidiasis in the gut is a problem only for people whose immune systems are impaired – those people with AIDS, for example, or anyone taking steroids or hormonal drugs such as oral contraceptives. Doctors rarely treat candidiasis in the gut.

COMPLEMENTARY TREATMENTS

Candida albicans *overgrowth in the intestine is a common diagnosis made by complementary practitioners, who will attempt to deal with the infection with diet, herbs, and nutritional supplements.*

NATUROPATHY

A practitioner will advise you to exclude all forms of yeast from your diet, as well as all foods containing yeast, mold, or fungi, and starches and refined sugar, on which yeast feeds. Many naturopaths will recommend "live" yogurt, containing *Lactobacillus acidophilus*, or supplements of acidophilus powder to restore the natural balance of microorganisms in the digestive tract. Some practitioners may suggest avoiding other milk products and limiting intake of high-sugar fruits. Nutritional supplements to build up the immune system are often considered helpful.
SEE PAGES 118–21

Caution: Restricted diets may lead to malnutrition.

WESTERN HERBALISM

Remedies to control the growth of *Candida albicans* will be prescribed. Berberine, an antimicrobial alkaloid that is said to prevent the overgrowth of yeast and stimulate the immune system, is found in barberry. Pau d'arco, a South American tree, contains lapachol, believed to have an anticandida effect. SEE PAGES 134–39

Caution: Take barberry only under professional supervision.

AYURVEDA

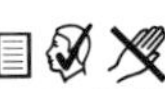

Candidiasis is said to be caused by *ama* (toxins) associated with poorly digested food. Your practitioner will try to improve digestion and strengthen natural defenses with herbs. *Panchakarma*, a detoxification process, may be suggested.
SEE PAGES 144–47

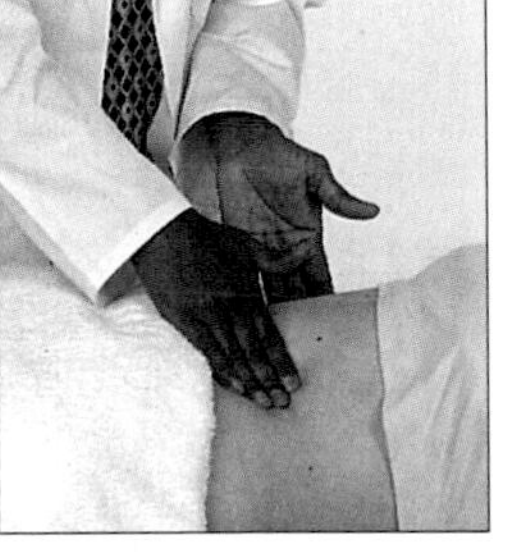

DIAGNOSIS
A practitioner will feel the abdomen to detect any disturbance in the body's "vital energies."

NUTRITIONAL THERAPIES

Practitioners may recommend "live" yogurt or acidophilus powder, which contain beneficial bacteria, to help fight the infection. Natural antifungals – garlic, aloe-vera juice, and caprylic acid, an extract of coconut – may also be advised. Nutritional supplements to restore the immune system include vitamin B complex, beta-carotene (vitamin A), vitamin C, vitamin E, and other antioxidants, as well as zinc, selenium, magnesium, essential fatty acids, and folic acid. SEE PAGES 148–52

Caution: Do not take aloe vera during pregnancy, if you are breastfeeding, or if you have hemorrhoids or kidney disease.

OTHER OPTIONS

Aromatherapy SEE PAGES 62–65
Colonic Hydrotherapy SEE PAGE 157

IRRITABLE BOWEL SYNDROME

KNOWN IN THE PAST as spastic colon and mucous colitis, irritable bowel syndrome (IBS) is one of the most common gastrointestinal complaints. It is believed to affect one person in ten, particularly women aged between 20 and 45. Peristalsis, the wavelike action of the gut that propels feces toward the rectum, becomes irregular, causing erratic bowel movements with constipation, diarrhea, and abdominal pain. IBS occurs for no apparent reason, since there is no inflammation, infection, or malignancy involved, and it can come and go for long periods at a time. Symptoms generally respond to treatment, although they can be distressing and in severe cases may be difficult to control.

CAUSES & SYMPTOMS

In IBS, the muscular wall of the colon pushes its contents toward the rectum either too quickly, resulting in diarrhea, or too slowly, causing constipation. Overactivity or spasm causes cramps. Other symptoms include a swollen abdomen, slimy mucus in the feces, and a feeling of incomplete evacuation. Exact causes of IBS are unknown, but stress appears to trigger and aggravate symptoms, and a diet low in fiber is often blamed. IBS sometimes begins after an infection of the intestines or a course of antibiotics.

PREVENTION

Eat a high-fiber diet. Make mealtimes as relaxed as you can, eat slowly, and always chew food thoroughly. Practice stress management techniques (see page 38) and get plenty of exercise: as well as reducing stress, it is good for all muscles, especially those of the abdomen and the lower back.

CONVENTIONAL TREATMENT

Although the diagnosis is usually clear, it is important to rule out other more serious complaints. A doctor will make a full examination. A colonoscopy (a procedure in which a tube is inserted through the rectum to view the bowel) or barium enema (X ray of the intestines) may be carried out. In unusual cases, bowel contractions may be measured, and the stool examined. There is no conventional cure for IBS, but symptoms can be relieved. Treatment may include a high-fiber diet or bulking agents to soften stool, and drugs to control diarrhea or muscular spasm. Counseling may also be recommended.

PRECAUTIONS

- **Consult a doctor if you are over 40 and your bowel habits have recently changed.**
- **Check with a doctor if there is blood in the stool.**
- **If you are over 60 and have IBS symptoms for the first time, see a doctor.**

TOUCH & MOVEMENT THERAPIES

Techniques such as massage and reflexology and systems of movement such as qigong and yoga can release tension and induce a sense of well-being. Acupuncture aims to balance the energy forces in the body. All may help to restore regular bowel action.

MASSAGE

Massage can promote a general feeling of well-being by releasing both muscular and emotional tension. As well as massaging you, a practitioner may demonstrate gentle self-help techniques for massaging the bowel area, with the aim of regulating bowel function.
SEE PAGES 56–61

REFLEXOLOGY

Reflexology is believed not only to aid relaxation, but to stimulate the body to heal itself. Practitioners claim that massaging the appropriate reflex points on the feet can improve digestion, helping to relieve symptoms.
SEE PAGES 66–69

FOOT MASSAGE
Applying pressure to certain points on the feet is said to stimulate the digestive system.

ACUPUNCTURE

A practitioner will treat you according to your individual symptoms, aiming to restore balance in the autonomic nervous system (see glossary). Meridians that may be worked on include the Spleen for bloating, the Stomach for diarrhea, gas, and cramps, and the Large Intestine for constipation. **SEE PAGES 90–94**

QIGONG

A teacher will demonstrate exercises to help you relax and improve the flow of *qi* ("life energy") around the body. This is believed to encourage all body systems, including the digestive tract, to function more effectively.
SEE PAGE 99

YOGA

A yoga therapy teacher will show you positions that stimulate digestion and the elimination of waste products. Gentle yoga exercises can also relax the body and calm the mind, helping you to deal with stress, which often seems to trigger symptoms of IBS.
SEE PAGES 108–11

MEDICINAL THERAPIES

Naturopaths and nutritional therapists will investigate dietary factors, which appear to play a part in at least 50% of cases of IBS. Herbal and homeopathic remedies may help to control symptoms.

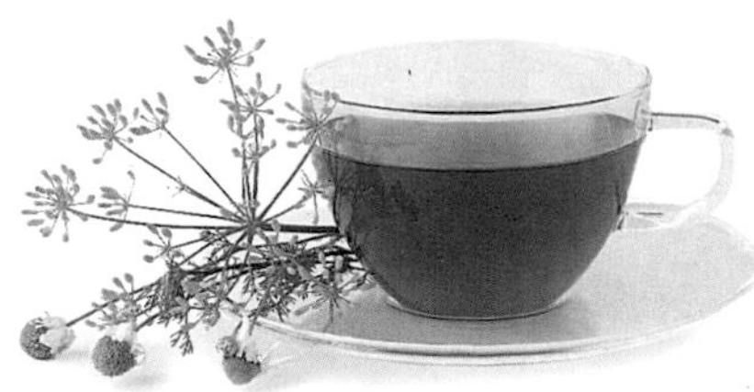

HERBAL TEA
Infusions of calming herbs, such as German chamomile and fennel, soothe the digestive tract.

NATUROPATHY 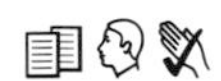

Practitioners attribute IBS to a number of factors, including food intolerance (see page 303), overgrowth of the yeast *Candida albicans* in the gut (see Candidiasis, page 235), and disturbance of the beneficial bacteria that protect the gut from toxin-producing organisms. If diarrhea is not a problem, dietary fiber and at least 2 qts (2 liters) of water a day may be recommended to help feces progress through the bowel. Water-soluble fiber (found in leafy vegetables, fruits, and oat bran) is easier to digest than insoluble fiber (found in wheat bran, beans, and lentils), which may irritate the gut and produce gas.

Stress and medication can destroy beneficial bacteria in the intestine. Since roughly half the mass of stool is made up of microorganisms, the destruction is likely to affect bowel health. Practitioners will aim to redress the balance with yogurt or supplements containing "friendly" bacteria such as *Lactobacillus acidophilus, Lactobacillus bulgaricus,* and *Bifidobacillus.*

Some practitioners claim that two-thirds of IBS sufferers have an intolerance to at least one food, so exclusion diets may be suggested to identify the substances involved. Wheat and dairy products are common culprits; citrus fruits, tea, coffee, and alcohol may also be implicated. Food combining (see the Hay diet, page 152) may be helpful in some cases. SEE PAGES 118–21

HOMEOPATHY 

A homeopath will assess your constitutional type and prescribe accordingly. The following standard remedies may also help: *Argent. nit. 6c* for constipation alternating with diarrhea, *Cantharis 6c* for burning pains in the abdomen, *Nux vomica 6c* for gas and spasms with an ineffectual urge to move the bowels, *Colchicum 6c* for watery stool, cramps, and nausea, and *Arsen. alb. 6c* for profuse diarrhea with colic and anxiety. SEE PAGES 126–30

WESTERN HERBALISM 

Peppermint is traditionally used to relieve intestinal spasm and trapped gas. Several studies have found that peppermint oil capsules, specially coated so that the oil is not released until the capsules reach the colon, work well in reducing contractions of the intestinal muscle. A practitioner may also suggest peppermint tea. Ginger, too, has long been used to relieve gastrointestinal distress. Other herbal antispasmodics said to relieve intestinal cramps, expel wind, tone the stomach, and ease pain include German chamomile, fennel, valerian, rosemary, and lemon balm. A practitioner may suggest a tea made with a combination of wild yam, goldenseal, German chamomile, peppermint, agrimony, and marshmallow to soothe the bowel, with hops and extra German chamomile if stress is a factor. SEE PAGES 134–39

Cautions: Do not take wild yam, medicinal doses of fennel, or goldenseal during pregnancy, or goldenseal if you have high blood pressure. Do not take ginger if you have a peptic ulcer. Do not take hops if you have clinical depression.

CHINESE HERBALISM 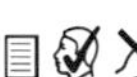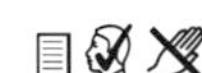

In Traditional Chinese Medicine, the symptoms of IBS are thought to be associated with a "weakness of the Kidney and Spleen," "excess dampness in the Intestine," or "stagnation of *qi* ('life energy') in the Liver." A practitioner may prescribe remedies that include dandelion with magnolia bark to ease bloating, Chinese rhubarb, and Chinese angelica (*dang gui*) to prevent constipation, and poria for diarrhea. SEE PAGES 140–43

Cautions: Do not take Chinese rhubarb or Chinese angelica during pregnancy. Do not take Chinese rhubarb if prone to gout or kidney stones.

OTHER OPTIONS

Nutritional Therapies SEE PAGES 148–52
Colonic Hydrotherapy SEE PAGE 157

MIND & EMOTION THERAPIES

Psychological factors clearly play an important part in the incidence of IBS. It may be that the body responds to continual stress or anxiety, even of a low level, in a way that interferes with the digestive process, affecting the muscle action of the bowel. Studies have shown that stress management techniques can be highly effective in treating the disorder.

PSYCHOTHERAPY & COUNSELING 

Most people with IBS who consult a practitioner report concurrent mental and emotional problems such as anxiety, hostility, depression, and disturbed sleep. People with IBS do seem to experience more stress than most, and stress naturally provokes contractions of the colon. Psychological therapies may help to change ways of thinking and behaving. SEE PAGES 160–65

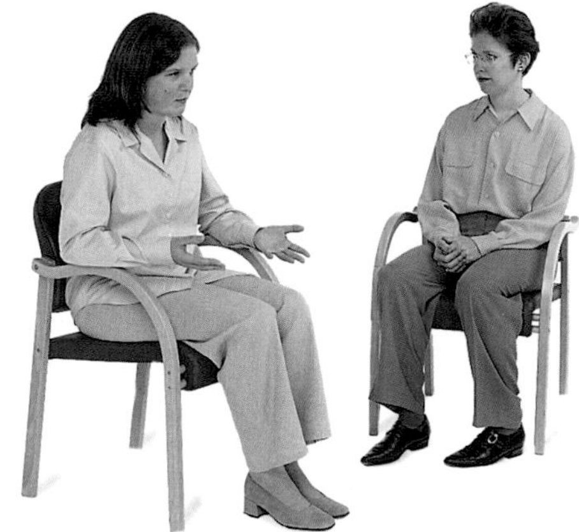

COUNSELING
A counselor will help you to change the way you respond to stress, which often contributes to IBS.

HYPNOTHERAPY 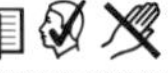

In a UK study reported in *The Lancet* in 1989, hypnotherapy proved successful in relieving symptoms of IBS when medical treatment had failed. A practitioner will aim to induce a state of deep relaxation and a feeling of abdominal warmth, which appear to be highly effective in relieving symptoms. SEE PAGES 166–67

AUTOGENIC TRAINING 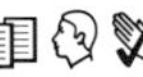

A form of meditation, autogenic training is particularly useful for stress-related conditions such as IBS. A practitioner will teach you a series of mental exercises that enable you to relax the mind and body at will. SEE PAGE 168

BIOFEEDBACK 

Biofeedback works on the principle that you can learn to control physiological functions with the use of electronic monitors. Various forms of biofeedback have been shown to be effective in treating IBS, especially when combined with other behavioral and psychological therapies. SEE PAGE 169

RELAXATION & BREATHING 

Techniques to enhance breathing, induce relaxation, and release muscle tension may help you to manage stress and relieve anxiety. A study reported in the Swiss journal *Digestion* in 1991 reported fewer and less severe attacks in two-thirds of patients with IBS after a stress management program that included relaxation exercises. SEE PAGES 170–73

OTHER OPTION

Meditation SEE PAGES 174–77

GAS

A BUILDUP OF GAS in the digestive tract can cause abdominal pain and bloating. It is relieved by burping or expulsion through the anus. It is often caused by nervous swallowing of air, or gulping food and drink too quickly, but can also be caused by poor digestion or inappropriate diet. Gas may also be a symptom of digestive disorders such as constipation, irritable bowel syndrome, ulcers, or diverticular disease. Conventionally, a doctor will advise taking charcoal tablets to absorb gas, chewing food well, and avoiding gas-producing foods such as legumes. Any underlying condition should be investigated and treated.

COMPLEMENTARY TREATMENTS

Massage and medicinal therapies aim to restore balance to the digestive system and relieve discomfort.

AROMATHERAPY

A practitioner may massage the abdomen in a clockwise direction with cinnamon, ginger, or clove essential oil to ease gas. SEE PAGES 62–65

NATUROPATHY

Naturopaths may suspect food intolerance or candidiasis as a possible cause. An exclusion diet may be suggested. SEE PAGES 118–21

CHINESE HERBALISM

Gas is attributed to "stagnant Stomach *qi* ('life energy')" or "damp heat," and remedies containing orange peel and magnolia bark may be offered. Standard Chinese medicines for dealing with stagnation of Stomach *qi* include Curing Formula (Healthy Quiet Pills) and Bupleurum and Cinnamon Formula.
SEE PAGES 140–43

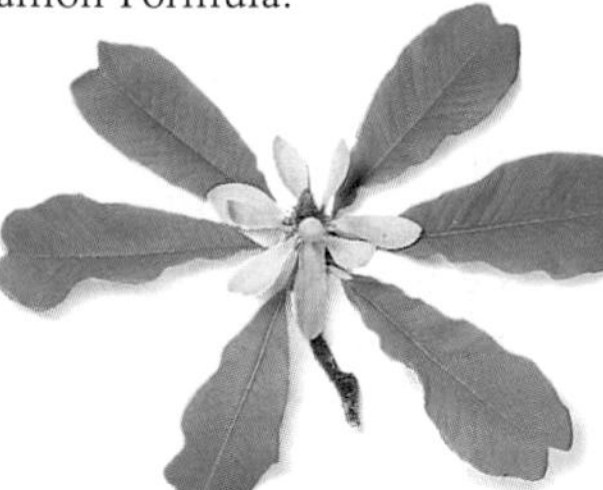

MAGNOLIA
Called hou po *in China, magnolia may be used to relieve bloating.*

OTHER OPTIONS

Yoga	SEE PAGES 108–11
Western Herbalism	SEE PAGES 134–39
Nutritional Therapies	SEE PAGES 148–52
Relaxation & Breathing	SEE PAGES 170–73

DIARRHEA

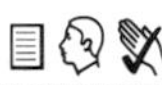

DIARRHEA – RUNNY, WATERY stool and explosive bowel movements – has many causes. Sudden bouts may be due to gastroenteritis, dysentery, or a food allergy. Prolonged or repeated bouts may be due to Crohn's disease or ulcerative colitis, irritable bowel syndrome, or more rarely, bowel cancer. Excess vitamin C or magnesium can cause diarrhea, as can stress or anxiety. A short attack is not serious, but loss of fluid and body salts may lead to dehydration, which can be life-threatening.

Caution: Consult a doctor if diarrhea lasts longer than three days (24 hours in a baby or elderly person), or if there is mucus or blood in the stools.

COMPLEMENTARY TREATMENTS

A short bout of diarrhea is sometimes considered part of a cleansing reaction, but repeated attacks suggest other problems, which naturopaths will attempt to redress. Mind and emotion therapies aim to reduce stress, whatever the diagnosed cause.

NATUROPATHY

Naturopaths regard persistent diarrhea as one of the most common symptoms of food allergy or intolerance and will suggest tests and an elimination diet. In the absence of a diagnosable medical condition, advice on rectifying poor digestion, pancreatic dysfunction, or underactivity of digestive enzymes will also be given. SEE PAGES 118–21

RELAXATION & BREATHING

Strong emotions, such as anxiety, may be interpreted by the body as an emergency situation. In an involuntary response, food may be pushed too quickly through the intestines, resulting in sudden diarrhea. A practitioner will teach you breathing techniques and relaxation exercises which, if practiced regularly, may help to reduce stress hormone levels and restore the smooth working of the digestive system. SEE PAGES 170–73

OTHER OPTIONS

Homeopathy	SEE PAGES 126–30
Western Herbalism	SEE PAGES 134–39
Chinese Herbalism	SEE PAGES 140–43
Nutritional Therapies	SEE PAGES 148–52
Meditation	SEE PAGES 174–77

HEMORRHOIDS

HEMORRHOIDS (OR PILES) are swollen, protruding veins inside the anus. They tend to produce a blood-tinged mucous discharge and bleed when the bowels are opened. If very large, they may descend with the bowel movement and become inflamed and painful. Chronic constipation is the usual cause, and a low-fiber diet, circulatory disorders, and lack of exercise may all contribute. Conventional treatment includes advice on diet and exercise, and suppositories and creams to ease discomfort and reduce inflammation. Surgery may be necessary for severe cases.

COMPLEMENTARY TREATMENTS

Practitioners treat and prevent flare-ups with diet and herbal remedies. Hydrotherapy may be especially effective in relieving discomfort.

NATUROPATHY

Diets to cleanse and stimulate the system will be advised. To soothe inflammation, you may be given a combination of zinc oxide, vitamin E, and aloe vera gel or olive oil. SEE PAGES 118–21

HYDROTHERAPY

A practitioner may suggest applying cold compresses. A warm sitz bath may also help.
SEE PAGES 122–23

HOMEOPATHY

While practitioners advocate treatment on the basis of constitutional assessment, a standard remedy for hemorrhoids is *Hamamelis 6c*.
SEE PAGES 126–30

WESTERN HERBALISM

Witch hazel or the aptly named pilewort may reduce pain and swelling. Papaya juice applied externally is said to be helpful. SEE PAGES 134–39

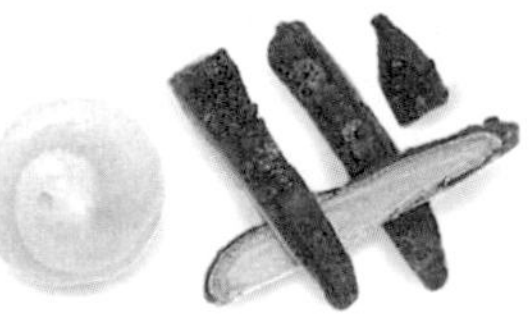

WITCH HAZEL
The astringent properties of witch hazel help to restore distended veins.

CONSTIPATION

CONSTIPATION IS THE INFREQUENT and difficult passing of small, hard stool, which can cause hemorrhoids, anal fissures, and other painful problems.

Causes Usually due to lack of fiber in the diet, constipation may also be the result of dehydration, a bowel blockage, lack of exercise, aging (when muscle tone may be lost), habitual laxative use, a thyroid problem, or pregnancy (when hormones can affect bowel routine). Constipation can be a symptom of irritable bowel syndrome, liver or gallbladder dysfunction, and diverticulosis. The onset of constipation after middle age may be an early sign of bowel cancer.

Conventional Treatment A doctor will advise you to get regular exercise and include more fiber and fluids in your diet. Mild laxatives may be prescribed. Chronic constipation may be investigated with a rectal examination and a barium enema (bowel X ray) or colonoscopy (an internal examination using a fiber-optic tube) to see if there is an abnormality.

Caution: Consult a doctor if constipation lasts longer than two weeks.

COMPLEMENTARY TREATMENTS

Touch and movement techniques can help to restore normal bowel action. Medicinal therapies, such as naturopathy and Ayurveda, aim to stimulate the whole digestive system using diet and exercise.

MASSAGE 

To relieve constipation quickly, a therapist may demonstrate a technique in which you massage the abdomen carefully in small circles. SEE PAGES 56–61

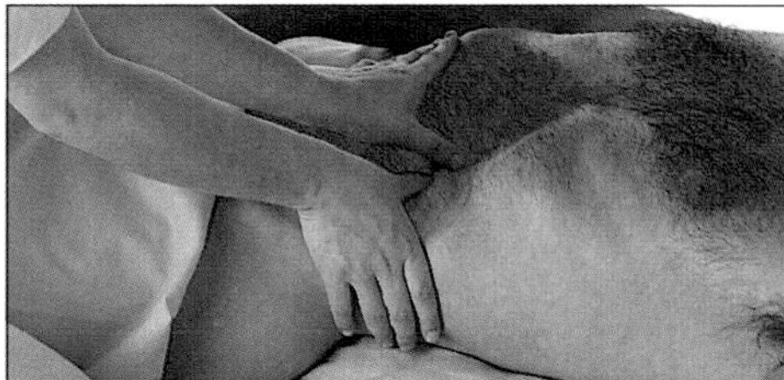

TOUCH THERAPY
Massaging the abdomen stimulates the bowel, and may give relief from constipation.

ACUPUNCTURE 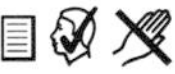

A practitioner will try to restore the natural contractions of the colon, possibly by stimulating acupoints along the Large Intestine and Liver meridians. SEE PAGES 90–94

ACUPRESSURE 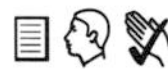

A practitioner may suggest lying on your back and gently pressing the fingertips at a point three finger widths below the navel. SEE PAGE 95

NATUROPATHY

Naturopaths pay serious attention to elimination because the bowel is seen as a potential source of toxins. "Fiber, fluid, and exercise" is their main therapeutic approach to constipation. Not all fiber is thought to be effective: psyllium husks, oat bran, and corn bran are less irritating than wheat bran. If a laxative is needed, linseed, senna, or cascara may be advised, although the last two can eventually make the colon more sluggish, and should be taken for only a few weeks. SEE PAGES 118–21

AYURVEDA 

Ayurvedic practitioners link well-being with a healthy gastrointestinal tract. Triphala powder is often advised as a laxative. A diet including plenty of fruits, leafy green vegetables, bran, and whole-wheat flour will also be effective. Practitioners may also recommend yoga techniques and exercise. SEE PAGES 144–47

OTHER OPTIONS

Homeopathy SEE PAGES 126–30
Western Herbalism SEE PAGES 134–39
Nutritional Therapies SEE PAGES 148–52

DIVERTICULAR DISEASE

THE PRESENCE OF DIVERTICULA, small fingerlike pouches that protrude from the lining of the large intestine, is known as diverticulosis. The pouches tend to occur with age and, in the West, are common in people over 70. There may be no symptoms, but some people complain of pain, bloating, constipation, or diarrhea. The condition known as diverticulitis occurs when the pouches are clogged with feces and become infected and inflamed, causing pain in the lower abdomen, diarrhea, and fever.

Causes Diverticula are caused by a buildup of pressure and weakness in the muscular wall, usually resulting from a low-fiber diet and an excess of refined foods. Constipation, stress, and poor abdominal muscle tone may also contribute.

Conventional Treatment A doctor will advise bed rest, plenty of fluids but no solid food, antibiotics to clear infection, and antispasmodic drugs to relieve pain.

COMPLEMENTARY TREATMENTS

Dietary changes may be advised for constipation. Herbalists offer calming, anti-inflammatory remedies to soothe irritation and ease pain.

NATUROPATHY 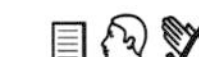

Practitioners claim that switching to a high-fiber diet clears up diverticular disease in 90% of cases, but the change must be gradual, usually taking 6–8 weeks. They often recommend a juice and water fast until painful symptoms subside, followed by the careful addition of semisolid food, such as mashed banana and puréed steamed carrots. Finally they recommend adding high-fiber foods such as brown rice to help soften motions and prevent constipation. You will be advised to avoid fibrous fruits and vegetables with seeds that may lodge in the diverticula and cause inflammation; bran can also be an irritant. Dietary supplements may be recommended to fight infection, restore the immune system, and heal inflamed tissues. SEE PAGES 118–21

HYDROTHERAPY 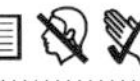

Practitioners consider that the alternate use of hot and cold water eases inflammation, and may advise hot and cold sitz baths and hot moist compresses to bring relief. SEE PAGES 122–23

Caution: Avoid cold, or alternate hot and cold, showers or baths if you have a heart condition.

WESTERN HERBALISM 

Practitioners may suggest garlic to help fight infection, and herbs to calm the gut and check inflammation. Slippery elm, which protects and soothes the mucous lining of the bowel, is thought to be particularly useful. German chamomile, marshmallow, and peppermint number among the herbs that may be given for their anti-inflammatory properties. SEE PAGES 134–39

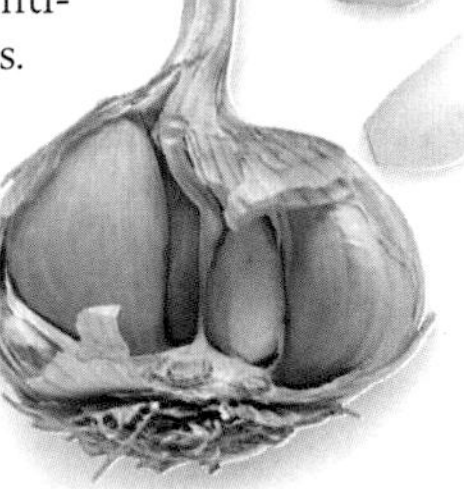

GARLIC
The oil in garlic cloves has powerful antibiotic and antiseptic properties.

THE URINARY SYSTEM

EVERY DAY THE KIDNEYS filter 37 gallons (140 liters) of fluid, removing excess water, salts, and waste products, and returning all but 1–2 pints (0.5–1 liter) of it back into circulation. Besides filtering waste, the kidneys also help to regulate blood pressure and reclaim essential substances, such as minerals. The waste fluid, urine, is excreted on average three to four times daily. In men, the urethra is five times longer than in women. As a result, men experience problems with urinary control and infection less frequently than women. Kidney stones, by contrast, are several times more common in men.

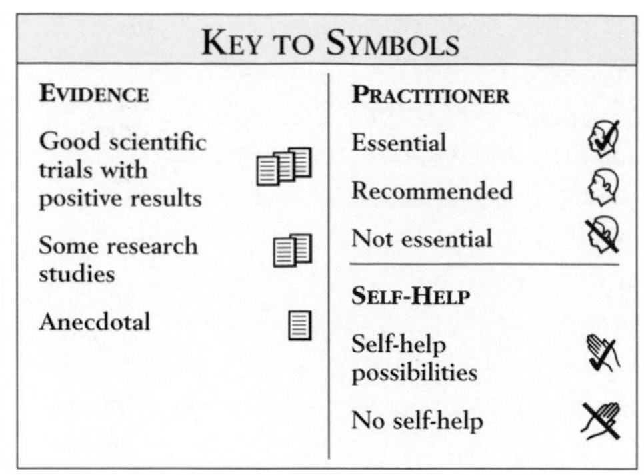

COMPLEMENTARY APPROACHES

The kidneys are seen as the key to the elimination of toxins. The strength of the kidneys is thought to indicate an individual's constitutional ability to resist disease. Many traditional remedies act by increasing the rate of urine production. In Traditional Chinese Medicine, the kidney is said to store *jing*, the essence of life.

CONVENTIONAL APPROACHES

Many drugs act on the kidneys to influence blood pressure and also the balance of body fluids and chemicals. Persistent low-grade renal infection is now seen as a major cause of kidney damage and failure, so any childhood infections should be carefully monitored.

Caution: Before seeking treatment, see page 204.

HOW THE URINARY TRACT WORKS

Filtered fluid (urine) passes from the kidneys down two tubes (ureters) into the bladder. The bladder is a muscular bag that expands as urine collects. As bladder pressure builds up, the nervous system sends a message of discomfort to the brain. In response, the brain will relay a message to the bladder muscles, the sphincter muscle governing the exit of the bladder, and the pelvic-floor muscles. In normal circumstances, the message is consciously inhibited until a convenient place for urination is found. Once it is, the bladder muscles are allowed to contract and the sphincter and pelvic-floor muscles to relax, so that urine flows out of the body through the urethra, removing waste products and excess fluid.

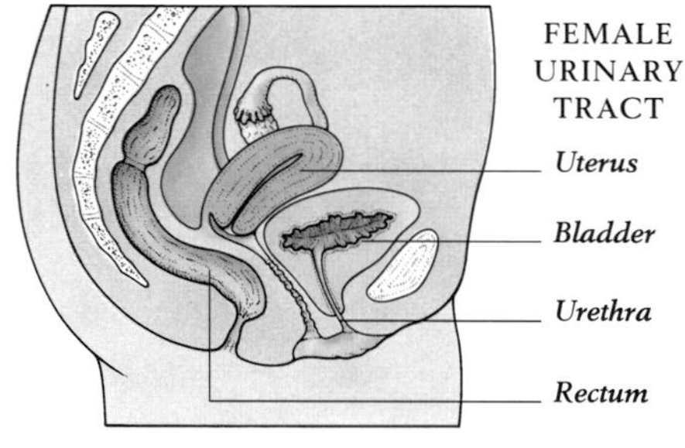

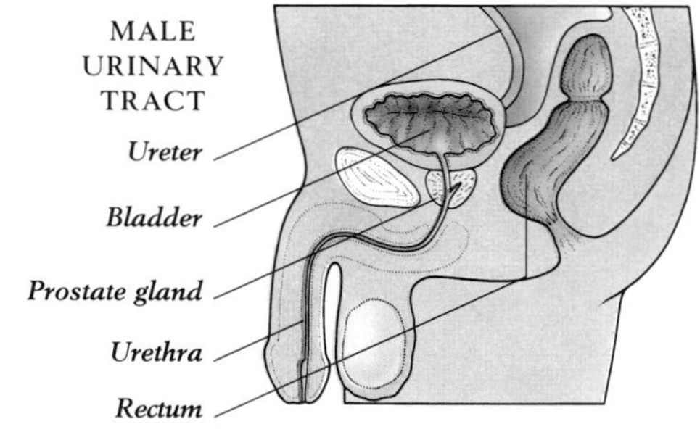

NONSPECIFIC URETHRITIS

MEN MAKE UP 75% of those with nonspecific urethritis (NSU), an inflammation of the urethra signaled by soreness in the penis, especially after urination, discharge, and sometimes pain. Women may have no symptoms other than heavier-than-usual vaginal discharge. The condition is generally caused by chlamydial infection and is treated with antibiotics.

Caution: Consult a doctor if you suspect NSU.

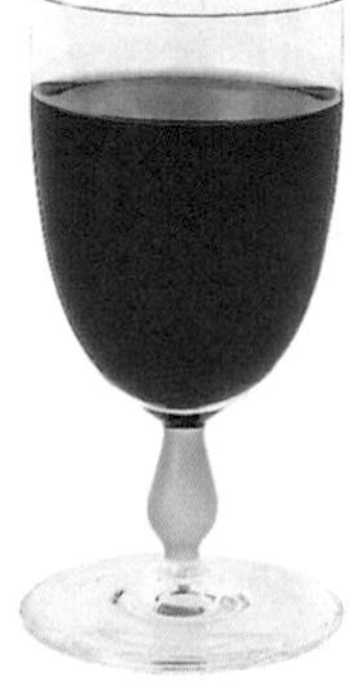

CRANBERRY JUICE
Studies suggest that cranberry juice helps NSU.

COMPLEMENTARY TREATMENTS

For conditions such as NSU that tend to recur, complementary therapies may offer valuable help in boosting immunity.

NATUROPATHY

A naturopath might advise a short fast followed by a vegetable and whole-grain diet to stimulate the body's healing mechanisms and enhance immunity. Other recommendations may include adequate sleep, plenty of fluids, foods rich in vitamin A, and "live" yogurt to restore gut bacteria if you are taking antibiotics. Foods with a diuretic effect, such as asparagus and celery, have long been used to treat NSU. Cranberry juice, also diuretic, may prevent bacteria from sticking to the walls of the urinary tract. SEE PAGES 118–21

WESTERN HERBALISM

Herbs such as celery seed, buchu, or bearberry may be recommended for their properties as urinary antiseptics. SEE PAGES 134–39

CHINESE HERBALISM

Urethritis is linked with "damp heat" in the Bladder and Kidney. Dianthus Formula is often given to clear this. SEE PAGES 140–43

NUTRITIONAL THERAPIES

Vitamin B_1 is believed to reduce irritation, zinc and the antioxidant (see glossary) vitamins A and E to boost immunity, and baking soda to alkalize the urinary tract. SEE PAGES 148–52

OTHER OPTIONS

Homeopathy SEE PAGES 126–30
Orthomolecular Therapy SEE PAGE 153

URINARY INCONTINENCE

THE INVOLUNTARY RELEASE of urine can range from slight leaking to total loss of bladder control. In *stress incontinence,* coughing or other sudden movements cause weakened muscles to allow the escape of a small amount of urine. In *urge incontinence,* an overwhelming need to urinate precedes complete emptying of the bladder. Urge incontinence is often due to a bladder infection (see page 273). *Overflow incontinence* occurs when some form of blockage, usually an enlarged prostate gland, impedes normal elimination (see page 277).

Conventional Treatment Incontinence pads and appliances may lessen the nuisance, and simple exercises can be practiced to help strengthen the pelvic-floor muscles responsible for regulating urine flow. Medical treatment depends on the type and the cause of the condition. Drugs may be given for an infection, or to help loss of control caused by nervous-system impairment. Incontinence linked to menopause may improve with hormone replacement therapy. In severe cases, catheterization may be necessary.

COMPLEMENTARY TREATMENTS

Therapists will attempt to stop incontinence by isolating and eliminating causes and by suggesting remedies thought to strengthen the urinary system.

NATUROPATHY

A practitioner will address factors such as obesity that can aggravate incontinence. Caffeine has a diuretic property that increases urine output. Artificial sweeteners, carbonated drinks, and tomato-based foods, which can irritate the bladder, may be discouraged.
SEE PAGES 118–21

HOMEOPATHY

The following standard remedies may help: *Causticum 6c* for involuntary urination after coughing, sneezing, laughing, or enforced retention, or *Pulsatilla 6c* for involuntary urination when lying down or getting feet wet. SEE PAGES 126–30

WESTERN HERBALISM

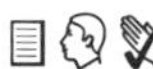

An herbalist may prescribe cypress oil to reduce fluid production, or horsetail, which is thought to act as a "tonic" for the urinary tract. SEE PAGES 134–39

Cautions: Do not take horsetail for longer than six weeks. Do not use cypress oil during pregnancy.

CHINESE HERBALISM

Practitioners link incontinence to Kidney *yang* (see glossary) deficiency with "internal cold," and may prescribe Rehmannia Eight Plus Formula. Ginkgo seeds are a traditional kidney and bladder tonic, and are advised for incontinence and frequent urination.
SEE PAGES 140–43

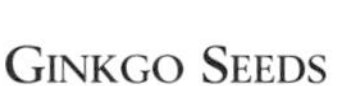

GINKGO SEEDS
Chinese herbalists commonly prescribe ginkgo seeds to tone the urinary system.

BIOFEEDBACK

Sensors can help people identify and strengthen the muscles that are needed for bladder control. The US Department of Health and Human Services analyzed 22 studies and came to the conclusion that muscular reeducation through biofeedback training had a 54–95% success range. SEE PAGE 169

OTHER OPTIONS

Acupuncture SEE PAGES 90–94
Acupressure SEE PAGE 95

KIDNEY STONES

MINERALS IN THE URINE can crystallize into stones in the kidney and bladder, sometimes causing agonizing pain or even kidney failure. Causal factors include kidney infection, metabolic and nutritional problems (e.g., gout), and inadequate fluid intake. Doctors may suggest ultrasound to fragment large stones into smaller, passable pieces, but some require surgical removal.

Caution: See a doctor if stones are suspected.

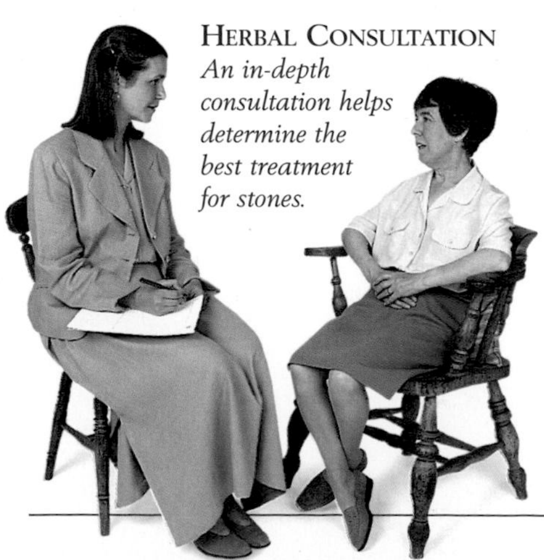

HERBAL CONSULTATION
An in-depth consultation helps determine the best treatment for stones.

COMPLEMENTARY TREATMENTS

Dietary changes, supplements, and herbal remedies may help in preventing the recurrence of stones. Some substances are also said to break down existing stones.

NATUROPATHY

A practitioner will seek to reduce sugar and salt in the diet, which are implicated in the formation of kidney stones. She will also recommend increasing fluid intake to 2–3 qts (2–3 liters) daily and eating more green vegetables: the magnesium content encourages the absorption of calcium, and the fiber hastens the elimination of waste. Many stones are made of calcium oxalate. It may therefore be important to reduce the intake of oxalate, a substance found in a number of foods, including beets, rhubarb, spinach, strawberries, and chocolate. Asparagus may be recommended; it contains asparagine, which is said to break up oxalate crystals. Cranberry juice helps to reduce urinary calcium levels in some people.
SEE PAGES 118–21

WESTERN HERBALISM

Treatment concentrates on diluting the urine with diuretic herbs. These include stone root and gravel root, parsley piert, dandelion, cleavers, and horsetail. Marshmallow and couch grass may have a soothing effect on an inflamed urinary passage. Visnaga, a traditional Egyptian herb for kidney stones, relaxes the muscles of the ureter, possibly helping stones to pass. SEE PAGES 134–39

Caution: Take visnaga only under professional supervision. Do not take horsetail for longer than six weeks.

NUTRITIONAL THERAPIES

Advice will depend on the chemical makeup of the stones. Kidney stones frequently consist of calcium and oxalate. To prevent crystallization of these elements, you may be given vitamin B_6, magnesium, and vitamin K. To lower calcium excretion, the amino acid lysine may be given, as may vitamin A, certain enzymes, and citrate, a salt that binds with calcium. SEE PAGES 148–52

OTHER OPTIONS

Homeopathy SEE PAGES 126–30
Chinese Herbalism SEE PAGES 140–43

HEART & CIRCULATION

A MIRACLE OF MOTION, the heart is a hollow muscle about the size of a clenched fist that circulates blood around the body, supplying the tissues with oxygen and nutrients. Circulatory, or cardiovascular, disorders tend to fall into two categories: problems with the heart's pumping power and rhythm; and disruption of blood flow through narrowed or blocked arteries. Conventional doctors now agree with complementary therapists that diet and lifestyle changes are essential in treating heart problems. The difference in the two approaches now lies in the extent to which it is thought possible to avoid drugs and surgery.

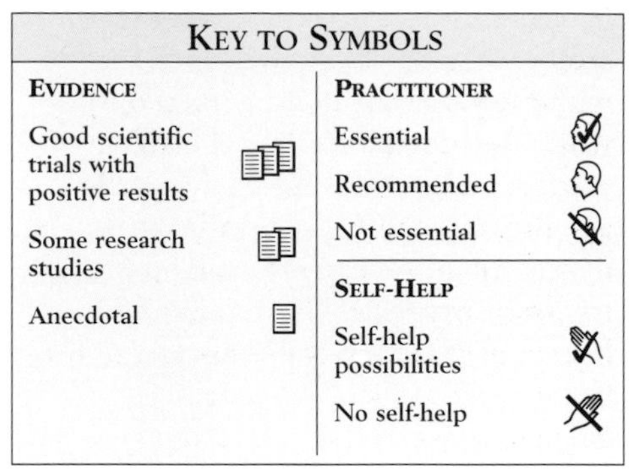

COMPLEMENTARY APPROACHES

Dietary measures and lifestyle changes, such as getting more exercise and giving up smoking, are the major planks of complementary medicine's approach to the treatment of heart disease. Proper functioning of the heart, according to complementary practitioners, also depends on the health and harmonious workings of other organs, such as the liver and kidneys.

CONVENTIONAL APPROACHES

Conventional medicine will advocate dietary and lifestyle changes to lower blood pressure and reduce levels of fats in the blood. Drugs may also be used to achieve this as well as to stabilize heart rhythm and improve blood flow. Surgery may be advised if blood vessels or heart muscle is badly damaged.

Caution: Before seeking treatment, see page 204.

HOW THE HEART PUMPS BLOOD

The heart pumps blood around the body in a network of arteries (see right, red) and veins (blue). These are linked by tiny capillaries, whose thin walls allow oxygen and nutrients to pass from the blood to the cells, and waste products such as carbon dioxide to pass back. The heart has distinct halves, each with two chambers (an atrium and a ventricle). Deoxygenated blood flows into the right side via two major veins, the superior and inferior vena cava, and is pumped via the pulmonary artery to the lungs. Oxygenated blood returns to the left side of the heart and is pumped to the body via the aorta (the largest artery). The heart has its own circulation system, fed by the coronary arteries.

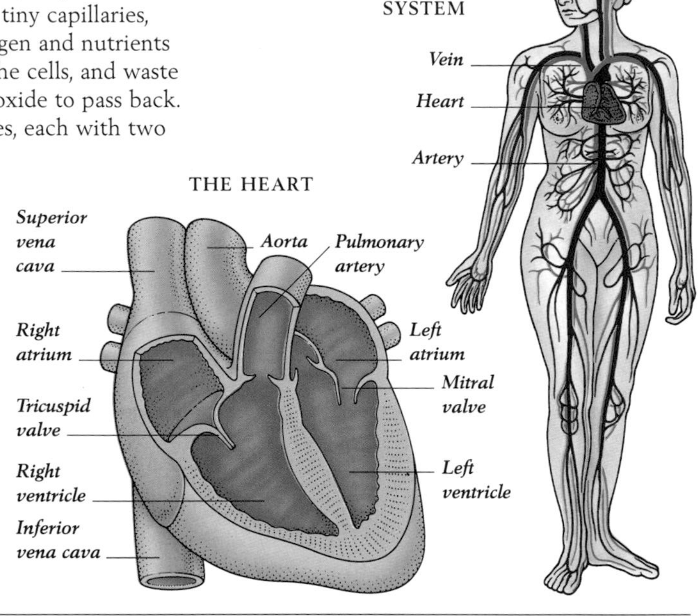

ANGINA PECTORIS

ANGINA PECTORIS MEANS "throttling the chest," a graphic description of the cramp-like pain it causes. It is a sign that too little oxygen is reaching the heart because the arteries have become narrowed. Conventionally, nitrate drugs may be given to improve blood supply to the heart, and other types of medication to reduce blood pressure. A graduated exercise program can help strengthen the heart. Angioplasty (a balloon inserted into the artery to reopen it) or coronary artery bypass surgery may be necessary as a last resort.

COMPLEMENTARY TREATMENTS

Eastern therapies may be beneficial in offsetting angina attacks. Studies show that Western herbalism can improve the health of the heart and circulation.

ACUPUNCTURE

Scandinavian studies between 1986 and 1992 showed that acupuncture can increase the heart's working capacity, reducing anginal pain and the need for medication. Sham acupuncture (on false meridians) was, however, sometimes seen to be just as effective. SEE PAGES 90–94

WESTERN HERBALISM

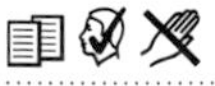

You may be prescribed hawthorn to relax and strengthen the heart. German studies show that the bioflavonoids found in hawthorn dilate the coronary arteries, improving the supply of blood and oxygen to the heart, and reducing the symptoms of angina. SEE PAGES 134–39
Caution: Take hawthorn only under professional supervision.

OTHER OPTIONS

T'ai Chi Ch'uan SEE PAGES 100–101
Yoga SEE PAGES 108–11
Naturopathy SEE PAGES 118–21

ATHEROSCLEROSIS & CORONARY ARTERY DISEASE

IN ATHEROSCLEROSIS, THE INSIDES of the artery walls gradually become clogged with fatty plaque deposits (atheroma), which restrict the flow of blood. If the coronary arteries, which supply the heart, are affected, the heart muscle is deprived of oxygen and nutrients, making it unable to pump properly. This condition is known as coronary artery disease and, if unchecked, eventually leads to angina, or even a heart attack.

Causes Atherosclerosis begins with damage to the artery walls, caused by wear and tear, viral infections, or chemical agents. This is made worse by smoking, stress, and high blood pressure. White blood cells cling to the damaged artery walls and attract droplets of fat, particularly cholesterol, which gradually build up into plaque deposits. These impede blood flow or, at worst, completely block the artery.

Conventional Treatment A doctor may prescribe drugs to improve blood flow, lower cholesterol levels, and reduce the burden on the heart. Surgical options include a coronary artery bypass, or if that is impossible because all the arteries that serve the heart are furred up, an angioplasty to widen the narrowed arteries.

Self-Help The following measures can help ward off atherosclerosis.

- Eat a low-fat diet. The Cretan Mediterranean diet, based on vegetables, fruits, fish, garlic, and olive oil with 1–2 glasses of red wine a day, may help.
- Give up smoking and learn to manage stress, both of which raise blood pressure, and do aerobic exercise at least three times a week to improve the strength and efficiency of the heart.
- Take half an aspirin twice a week, especially if you have already had a heart attack. Aspirin reduces the stickiness of the blood platelets, making them less likely to clump together and form a clot.
- Women might consider hormone replacement therapy after menopause, particularly if there is a family history of coronary heart disease. Tests have shown that HRT may reduce the risk of a heart attack by as much as 44%.

TOUCH & MOVEMENT THERAPIES

Massage therapies and the gentle exercises practiced in Traditional Chinese Medicine are known to relieve stress and induce relaxation, reducing strain on the heart.

AROMATHERAPY

A relaxing aromatherapy massage reduces stress and stimulates the circulation. According to some practitioners, a massage with essential oils of lavender, peppermint, marjoram, and rose may help to strengthen heart action. SEE PAGES 62–65

Cautions: If you have a heart condition, consult an experienced practitioner. Do not use marjoram oil during pregnancy.

PEPPERMINT
The stimulating properties of its oil may aid circulation.

T'AI CHI CH'UAN

Practitioners believe that the movement and breathing exercises of t'ai chi encourage an even flow of *qi* ("life energy") around the body. Western cardiologists have advised heart patients to take up t'ai chi as a gentle form of exercise that does not strain the heart. SEE PAGES 100–101

OTHER OPTIONS

Massage SEE PAGES 56–61
Yoga SEE PAGES 108–11

MEDICINAL THERAPIES

Therapies such as naturopathy and nutritional therapies aim to improve dietary habits and redress nutritional deficiencies.

NATUROPATHY

Improving the diet and lifestyle of people with coronary artery disease has shown promising results. In the US, Dr. Dean Ornish has devised a program to reverse heart disease without surgery or drugs. It consists of a high-fiber diet, in which only 10% of calories come from fats, exercise three times a week, group therapy, and stress management techniques. In one study, 82% of Dr. Ornish's patients experienced improved arterial blood flow and a reduction in chest pain, while symptoms grew worse in 53% of the control group. SEE PAGES 118–21

NUTRITIONAL THERAPIES

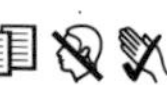

As well as advocating a healthy low-fat diet based on whole grains, a practitioner will also recommend foods that protect the heart: antioxidant (see glossary) fruits and vegetables, and oily fish such as mackerel, which contain omega-3 essential fatty acids. Food supplements may also be suggested: vitamin B to reduce levels of homocysteine, a substance that damages artery walls, carnitine, niacin, calcium, chromium, and lecithin to reduce cholesterol, magnesium to dilate the arteries, and pantethine to reduce fat levels in the blood. In 1996, a UK study found that vitamin E supplements could reduce the risk of heart attack in patients with atherosclerosis by 77%. SEE PAGES 148–52

Caution: Take supplements for heart conditions only with professional advice.

MIND & EMOTION THERAPIES

Those with a mistrustful, hostile attitude to life are especially susceptible to coronary heart disease. Meditation and other therapies aim to reduce negative feelings.

MEDITATION

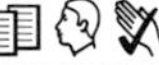

During periods of persistent stress, the body produces excess stress hormones and fats. These raise levels of cholesterol in the blood, a risk factor in coronary artery disease. A practitioner will show you how to attain a state of "relaxed awareness," which helps to reduce the stress response. SEE PAGES 174–77

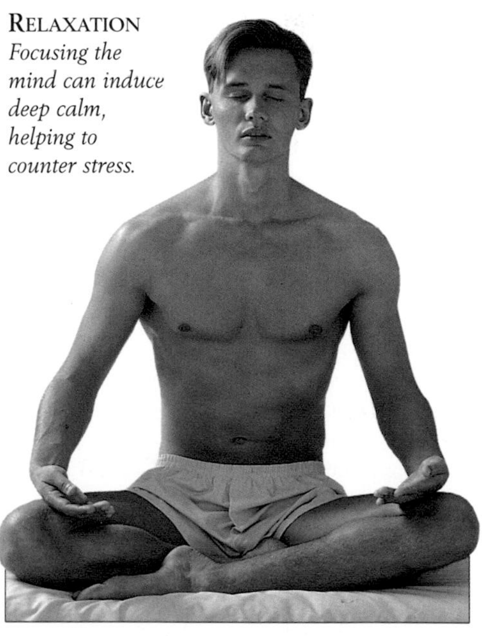

RELAXATION
Focusing the mind can induce deep calm, helping to counter stress.

OTHER OPTION

Biofeedback SEE PAGE 169

HIGH BLOOD PRESSURE

BLOOD PRESSURE CONSTANTLY fluctuates. It is low early in the morning, for example, and rises during any kind of physical exertion or in response to stress. Sometimes, however, blood pressure becomes permanently high, even during periods of rest, indicating that the heart is having to work harder to pump blood around the body because the arteries have become constricted. High blood pressure, or hypertension, eventually damages the blood vessels, leading to stroke, coronary artery disease, heart failure, and many other ailments. Complementary therapies aim to lower blood pressure by natural means, which in some cases may reduce or eliminate the need for conventional drugs.

CAUSES & SYMPTOMS

Symptoms occur only if blood pressure is very high, and may include dizziness, headaches, fatigue, ringing in the ears, visual disturbance, breathlessness, and insomnia. No specific cause has been identified for the majority of cases, but lifestyle seems to play an important role: people in remote areas of the world show virtually no evidence of hypertension, but if they move to developed countries their blood pressure rises dramatically.

PREVENTION

Although population studies show that most people with high blood pressure are aged between 50 and 60, it is not an inevitable part of the aging process. To avoid high blood pressure, adopt a healthy lifestyle: give up smoking, lose excess weight, exercise regularly, reduce stress, eat a low-fat diet, and reduce intake of alcohol, salt, and caffeine (see pages 23–48).

CONVENTIONAL TREATMENT

Hypertension rarely causes symptoms, so it is advisable to have your blood pressure checked at least once a year starting at the age of 40; once detected, the condition is usually controllable. Changes in lifestyle and diet may be enough to lower mildly high blood pressure; if it does not respond, antihypertensive drugs will be prescribed, which may include diuretics, beta-blockers, vasodilators (see glossary), and drugs that act on the nervous system. Although it is highly effective, drug treatment will probably be for life and can cause side effects.

PRECAUTIONS

- **Do not discontinue any prescribed medication or treatment without consulting your doctor.**
- **Consult your doctor before taking dietary supplements or herbal remedies, since some may be incompatible with conventional medication.**
- **Consult your doctor before starting an exercise program.**

TOUCH & MOVEMENT THERAPIES

Stress triggers the release of the hormone epinephrine, which causes the smaller arteries to tense up, increasing blood pressure. Both Eastern and Western therapies focus on techniques that are aimed at promoting relaxation and reducing stress.

MASSAGE

Slow, stroking massage helps release muscle tension and may be effective, even in those who find it difficult to unwind. Several studies have proved that massage can lower blood pressure temporarily, although it cannot control it permanently. SEE PAGES 56–61

AROMATHERAPY

A practitioner may massage you with essential oils of lavender, geranium, sandalwood, rose, or clary sage, all of which have sedative qualities. SEE PAGES 62–65

Caution: Do not use clary sage oil during pregnancy.

ACUPUNCTURE

Practitioners may stimulate acupoints to calm excess Liver *yang* (see glossary), tone the Kidney, and disperse "phlegm damp disharmonies" associated with high blood pressure. SEE PAGES 90–94

QIGONG

Practitioners believe that qigong, which combines gentle exercise with meditation, using simple flowing postures, improves the balance and flow of *qi* ("life energy") in the body. It is considered that this helps lower blood pressure and calms hostile feelings. SEE PAGE 99

CALMING POSTURES
The gentle controlled movements of qigong help to promote inner calm.

T'AI CHI CH'UAN

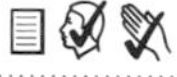

This more dynamic form of qigong can help you cope with stress, keep your blood pressure under control, and provide benefits of exercise without straining the heart. SEE PAGES 100–101

YOGA

A practitioner will teach you appropriate *asanas* (postures) and breathing techniques. Yoga is a powerful way of reducing stress because it combines breathing, relaxation, and meditation techniques, and stretching exercises. A trial reported in *The Lancet* in 1973 found that a combination of yoga, meditation, and biofeedback allowed 25% of patients with high blood pressure to give up their medication, and 35% to reduce it. However, more recent research has not confirmed these findings. SEE PAGES 108–11

Caution: Do not attempt Headstands.

OTHER OPTIONS

Chiropractic — SEE PAGES 70–75
Osteopathy — SEE PAGES 76–81
The Alexander Technique — SEE PAGES 86–87

MEDICINAL THERAPIES

Medicinal practitioners aim to reduce the need for conventional medication either by helping to improve diet or by recommending remedies that will have a beneficial effect on blood vessels and tissues.

NATUROPATHY

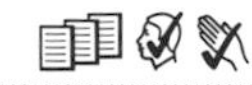

There is a strong link between high blood pressure and diet, and your practitioner will suggest improvements. A well-balanced diet should contain plenty of whole grains, fruits, and vegetables, and low-fat dairy products. These are rich in potassium, complex carbohydrates, polyunsaturated fat, fiber, calcium, magnesium, vitamin C, and beta-carotene – all claimed in varying degrees to lower blood pressure. Practitioners also believe that high-fiber foods, especially oat bran and psyllium seeds, can treat and prevent high blood pressure. Garlic and onion also seem to have the ability to bring down blood pressure. Results are mixed, but a UK study reported that subjects with mildly raised high blood pressure who ate garlic regularly had a drop in diastolic blood pressure (see glossary) from 102 to 89 after three months. In addition, studies have shown that vegetarians tend to have lower blood pressure and a lower incidence of cardiovascular disease than people who eat meat. SEE PAGES 118–21

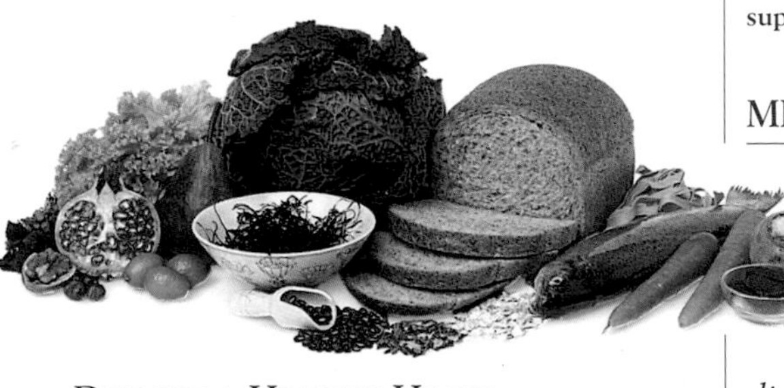

DIET FOR A HEALTHY HEART
A diet that is rich in complex carbohydrates, oily fish, and fruits and vegetables is recommended to prevent and treat high blood pressure.

HOMEOPATHY

A homeopath will make an individual assessment in order to choose the remedy most suited to your constitution. *Baryta carb.* *6c*, *Adrenalin 6c*, *Eel serum 6c*, and *Baryta mur.* *6c* are typical specific remedies for high blood pressure. In one research study, a few individuals showed strongly positive responses to *Baryta carb. 6c.*, although results from other studies have been mixed. SEE PAGES 126–30

WESTERN HERBALISM

After a detailed consultation, a practitioner will prescribe remedies on an individual basis, possibly containing herbs such as hawthorn, lime flower, buckwheat, and yarrow, to help dilate constricted blood vessels and so lower the pressure in the arteries. Diuretics such as dandelion or parsley may also be given to support the kidneys, and you may be recommended herbs to help you relax, such as German chamomile, lemon balm, lavender, and rosemary. SEE PAGES 134–39

Cautions: Do not take yarrow or medicinal doses of parsley during pregnancy. Take hawthorn only under professional supervision.

CHINESE HERBALISM

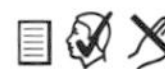

In Traditional Chinese Medicine, high blood pressure is associated with several common "disharmonies," including "rising Liver *yang* (see glossary)," "Kidney *yin* deficiency," and "phlegm damp." Your practitioner will assess your condition and prescribe a formula, possibly including the herbs *tian ma* and *gou teng* to calm Liver *yang*, rehmannia to restore Kidney *yin*, and *chen pi* and *fu ling* to dispel "phlegm damp." SEE PAGES 140–43

NUTRITIONAL THERAPIES

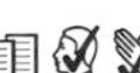

A nutritional therapist will assess your diet and lifestyle and suggest modifications and nutritional supplements. Calcium-rich foods are often recommended; there seems to be a link between low calcium intake and hypertension. Supplements commonly recommended include omega-3 fatty acids, magnesium, potassium, vitamin C, and a substance called coenzyme Q10. SEE PAGES 148–52

Caution: Do not take potassium or magnesium supplements without professional supervision.

MIND & EMOTION THERAPIES

Various mind and emotion therapies help lower high blood pressure by encouraging relaxation. Being able to relax at will is the best possible way of reducing stress, and has a direct effect on blood pressure.

PSYCHOTHERAPY & COUNSELING

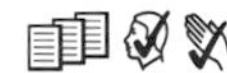

Practitioners try to help people recognize and change those attitudes and aspects of behavior that are associated with stressful situations. Cognitive behavioral therapy is particularly useful for those with "hostile" tendencies (impatient, cynical people who tend to be mistrusting and easily angered, and who are especially likely to develop other health problems if they have high blood pressure). SEE PAGE 160–65

HYPNOTHERAPY

A practitioner will train you to relax under hypnosis. It is thought that the memory of the hypnotically induced state of relaxation may enable you to reenter it when necessary, helping you to cope more effectively with stressful situations or psychological conflicts. SEE PAGES 166–67

AUTOGENIC TRAINING

Your therapist will teach you mental exercises designed to help you recognize stressful situations and induce relaxation. SEE PAGE 168

BIOFEEDBACK

Biofeedback makes use of devices that monitor physiological responses, for example heartbeat and brain wave patterns. It can help you to recognize when you are relaxed so that you can recreate the feeling at will. Studies have shown that biofeedback techniques may help people with mildly raised blood pressure. SEE PAGE 169

RELAXATION & BREATHING

Under stress, breathing becomes rapid and shallow. Learning how to breathe slowly and evenly (diaphragmatic breathing) counters this effect and promotes deep muscle relaxation. Scientific studies by Professor Benson of the Harvard Medical School have shown that, during the "relaxation response," both blood pressure and metabolic rate are lowered and the heartbeat is temporarily slowed. SEE PAGES 170–73

MEDITATION

Techniques that calm and focus the mind can help generate deep alpha brain waves, which are associated with relaxation. SEE PAGES 174–77

VISUALIZATION

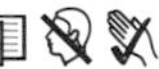

A practitioner can show you how to reduce stress by teaching you to picture soothing and reassuring scenes, which may calm the mind, relieve muscle tension, and induce relaxation. SEE PAGES 178–79

SOOTHING SCENES
Exercises that encourage people to picture positive outcomes to certain events help them to feel calm and in control, and so cope with stress.

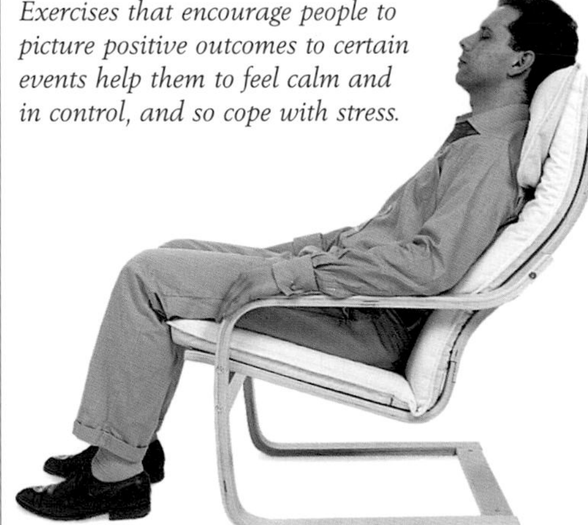

MUSIC THERAPY

Studies have shown that music can have a temporary beneficial effect on blood pressure. Listening to a piece of music or taking part in a music session may release tension and help you to relax. SEE PAGE 181

LOW BLOOD PRESSURE

WHEN BLOOD PRESSURE DROPS, the arteries do not always constrict rapidly enough in response. This means that the supply of blood to the brain is decreased, which can result in dizziness and fainting. The causes of low blood pressure, or hypotension, include ill health, pregnancy, diabetes, lack of food, heat exhaustion, antidepressant drugs, or an excessive dose of a drug prescribed for high blood pressure. Some research suggests that people with persistently low blood pressure may experience depression, fatigue, and lethargy more frequently than those with normal blood pressure. Conventional treatment depends on the underlying cause.

COMPLEMENTARY TREATMENTS

Naturopathy improves health and hydrotherapy boosts the circulation.

NATUROPATHY

Your practitioner will suggest a balanced diet based on whole grains, and plenty of exercise in fresh, unpolluted air to restore well-being and proper sleep patterns. SEE PAGES 118–21

HYDROTHERAPY

Practitioners believe cold showers and baths help blood vessels to contract, then dilate, to restore the normal pumping of blood and oxygen to the upper body. SEE PAGES 122–23

Caution: Avoid cold, or alternating hot and cold, showers or baths if you have a heart condition.

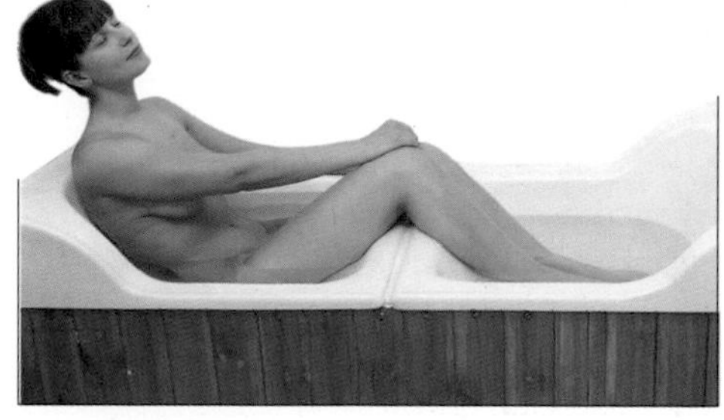

SITZ BATH
Circulation is stimulated by a sitz bath that involves sitting in cold water with your feet in hot water and then changing over.

OTHER OPTIONS

Western Herbalism SEE PAGES 134–39
Nutritional Therapies SEE PAGES 148–52

HEART VALVE DISEASE

THE HEART VALVES prevent blood from running backward when the heart muscle contracts. If they become inflamed or leaky they cannot do their job properly. Severe valve disease can cause irregular heartbeat, heart attack, heart failure, or angina. Valve problems may require surgery.

Caution: Consult a doctor before undertaking any complementary treatments.

COMPLEMENTARY TREATMENTS

If the heart is damaged it is important to avoid stressing it further. Relaxation techniques are an essential part of healing.

NUTRITIONAL THERAPIES

Practitioners suggest a balanced diet low in saturated fat. They may advise supplements of carnitine to lower cholesterol, panthetine to reduce blood fat levels, and coenzyme Q10, a substance essential for energy production. SEE PAGES 148–52

RELAXATION & BREATHING

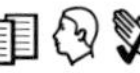

A practitioner may show you diaphragmatic breathing techniques, which encourage even, calm breathing, and progressive relaxation sequences to help release tension and promote sleep. SEE PAGES 170–73

HEART FAILURE

SOMETIMES THE PUMPING ACTION of the heart becomes inefficient, a condition known as heart failure. If the right side is affected, blood returning from all parts of the body to the heart is held back, forcing fluid into the tissues, and causing fatigue, weakness, and palpitations. If failure is on the left side, blood has difficulty returning to the heart from the lungs. These become congested, resulting in breathlessness and coughing, especially on lying down. Causes of heart failure include anemia, high blood pressure, other heart problems and lung disease. Conventionally, diuretics and a drug called digoxin may be prescribed to reduce fluid buildup and strengthen the heartbeat. Further treatment depends on the cause.

Cautions: Avoid excessive exercise and fluid intake and temperature extremes. Consult a doctor before undertaking any complementary treatments.

COMPLEMENTARY TREATMENTS

Aromatherapy and dietary improvements aim to relieve the symptoms of heart failure. In addition, traditional herbal remedies may help steady the heartbeat.

MASSAGE

"Manual lymph drainage" massage is a gentle stroking technique that stimulates the lymphatic system. This is thought to remove waste products more effectively and may help reduce fluid retention. SEE PAGES 56–61

Caution: If you have a heart condition, consult an experienced practitioner.

NATUROPATHY

A practitioner will assess your lifestyle and suggest changes. If fluid retention is a problem, you may be advised to avoid salt, which encourages this condition, and to cut down on sweet foods, which require a lot of water to be metabolized. Tea and coffee should also be avoided. SEE PAGES 118–21

WESTERN HERBALISM

A practitioner may treat heart failure with foxglove, the source of the conventional drug digoxin. Hawthorn and lily of the valley are other traditional remedies used for heart failure. SEE PAGES 134–39

Caution: Take foxglove, hawthorn, and lily of the valley only under professional supervision.

FOXGLOVE
Foxglove contains cardiac glycosides, which help the heart to pump more evenly and slowly.

OTHER OPTION

Chinese Herbalism SEE PAGES 140–43

HEART ATTACK

A HEART ATTACK, or myocardial infarction, can be fatal and is the most serious consequence of coronary artery disease (see page 243). An attack occurs when part of the heart muscle dies because its blood supply is cut off due to narrowing or a blood clot in one of the coronary arteries. Symptoms include intense pain in the chest, spreading to the left arm, throat, or jaw and lasting up to an hour. Sweating, breathlessness, pallor, or collapse may also occur. However, sometimes in older people a heart attack may cause little or no pain.
Conventional Treatment Heart attack patients are often admitted to coronary or intensive care units for round-the-clock monitoring and care. A doctor will prescribe morphine to relieve pain, and medication to correct heartbeat disturbances, and to treat heart failure and shock. Rehabilitation focuses on improving the diet and lifestyle, with regular exercise being an important feature. Taking half an aspirin twice a week improves blood flow, helping to ward off another attack.

Cautions: Call an ambulance immediately if you suspect a heart attack. Consult a doctor before undergoing any complementary treatment in convalescence after a heart attack.

COMPLEMENTARY TREATMENTS

Several types of treatment can help those recuperating from a heart attack. Gentle movement therapies can lower stress levels without straining the heart, and mind therapies teach stress management techniques. A naturopath or nutritional therapist may recommend dietary changes and food supplements.

T'AI CHI CH'UAN 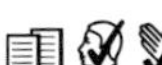

These ancient Chinese exercises concentrate on movements to develop inner calm and encourage relaxation. A 1996 UK study revealed that when patients recovering from a heart attack practiced t'ai chi, their blood pressure was lowered. SEE PAGES 100–101

NATUROPATHY 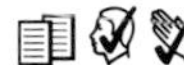

A practitioner will look at your overall diet and lifestyle and suggest changes such as getting gentle exercise in the fresh air at least three times a week, cutting out saturated fat, and eating more antioxidant (see glossary) fruits and vegetables. Certain foods such as oily fish, chili, garlic, and ginger help protect the heart and may be particularly recommended. SEE PAGES 118–21

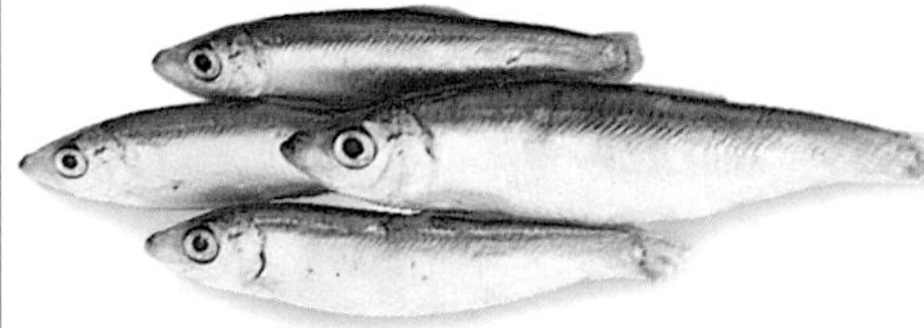

OILY FISH
Fish such as whitebait contain omega-3 essential fatty acids, which help protect the heart.

NUTRITIONAL THERAPIES 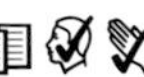

Practitioners consider that magnesium and potassium deficiency may cause spasms of the coronary arteries and induce a heart attack. They may prescribe supplements to strengthen heart muscle contraction. Although it is not scientifically proven, some practitioners believe milk is linked to heart problems because it affects the absorption of magnesium into the bloodstream. They may therefore recommend that you exclude milk and milk products from your diet. SEE PAGES 148–52
Caution: Do not take potassium or magnesium supplements without professional supervision.

RELAXATION & BREATHING 

Proper breathing is a key step toward relaxation. A practitioner will teach techniques that, if practiced regularly, will help reduce stress and encourage a calm outlook on life. SEE PAGES 170–73

OTHER OPTIONS

Qigong SEE PAGE 99
Western Herbalism SEE PAGES 134–39
Visualization SEE PAGES 178–79

PALPITATIONS

PALPITATIONS are the sensation experienced when the heart seems to beat irregularly or more forcibly than usual. There may be fluttering and a feeling of weakness or of missing a beat. This may be alarming but it is usually harmless. Emotions, including anxiety, shock and anger, are common causes. Other triggers include indigestion, vigorous exercise, hyperventilation (rapid breathing), smoking, drinking too much alcohol, coffee or tea, medication, an overactive thyroid, or coronary artery disease. Treatment may include anti-arrhythmic drugs to regulate the heart, or beta-blockers (see glossary). If the trigger is psychological, relaxation techniques or a course of psychotherapy may be advised.

Caution: Consult a doctor if palpitations persist, recur, or are accompanied by dizziness, chest pains, breathlessness, or nausea.

COMPLEMENTARY TREATMENTS

Palpitations often have emotional triggers, so therapies that induce relaxation may prevent their recurrence. Dietary and herbal remedies aim to treat physical causes.

MASSAGE 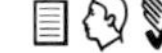

Regular massage may aid relaxation, lowering raised blood pressure and reducing stress levels. SEE PAGES 56–61

ACUPRESSURE 

A practitioner may show you how to press the Pericardium and Heart meridian acupoints on the wrist, which are considered to have a calming effect. SEE PAGE 95

NATUROPATHY 

A naturopath will aim to improve your general health. Some believe palpitations may be due to food intolerances, and will recommend that you follow an exclusion diet to pinpoint suspect foods. SEE PAGES 118–21

CHINESE HERBALISM 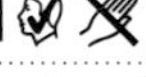

Palpitations are associated with "deficiencies of Heart blood," and a practitioner will prescribe nourishing herbs. SEE PAGES 140–43

AUTOGENIC TRAINING 

If palpitations have a psychological trigger, such as anxiety, a practitioner may be able to show you techniques to control them. These involve exercises that enable you to switch off the body's alarm system at will, inducing relaxation. SEE PAGE 168

RELAXATION & BREATHING 

A practitioner may show you progressive muscle relaxation and yoga breathing exercises (*pranayama*), which are considered helpful for palpitations. SEE PAGES 170–73

OTHER OPTIONS

Yoga SEE PAGES 108–11
Homeopathy SEE PAGES 126–30
Western Herbalism SEE PAGES 134–39
Biofeedback SEE PAGE 169

ANEMIA

IN ANEMIA, levels of hemoglobin, the substance that binds with oxygen and carries it around the body in the blood, are reduced. Symptoms include dizziness, fainting, pallor, fatigue, irritability, recurrent infections, poor concentration, heart palpitations, shortness of breath, vision problems, sore tongue, and loss of appetite. **Causes** Anemia is most commonly caused by a deficiency of iron, an essential component of hemoglobin. Too little dietary iron, blood loss from accidents, heavy menstruation, or surgery, or a hemorrhoid or peptic ulcer can all result in iron-deficiency anemia. Other types of anemia include *megaloblastic anemia* and *pernicious anemia*, which both involve a deficiency of folate or vitamin B_{12}, and *sickle cell anemia* and *thalassemia*, which are inherited disorders. Conventionally, blood-sample monitoring along with dietary advice and iron or vitamin B_{12} supplements are the usual treatments.

Caution: Take supplements only under professional supervision.

COMPLEMENTARY TREATMENTS

Therapies aim to increase intake of iron and improve its absorption into the blood.

WESTERN HERBALISM

To remedy iron deficiencies, a practitioner may suggest adding iron-rich herbs, such as parsley, dandelion, and watercress, to salads and soups. Infusions of raspberry, burdock, and nettle may also be prescribed. SEE PAGES 134–39

Caution: Do not take medicinal doses of raspberry in early pregnancy.

RASPBERRY
Both leaves and fruit are astringent, helping to reduce bleeding.

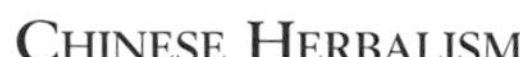

CHINESE HERBALISM

As well as a diet of iron-rich foods, a practitioner is likely to prescribe herbal remedies to help the process of iron absorption. Malabsorption may be attributed to a failure of the Spleen to process *qi* ("life energy"), and you may be asked to take "Return Spleen" tablets. The Tang Kuei Four Formula may be suggested for Blood deficiency, along with a *qi* tonic, such as ginseng. SEE PAGES 140–43

Caution: Do not take ginseng during pregnancy or if you have high blood pressure.

AYURVEDA

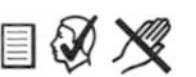

In Ayurveda, anemia is thought to be due to an imbalance of *pitta*, one of the three "vital energies." Purging is the usual treatment, and *punarnava mandura*, a mild laxative rich in iron, is often given. Sour and fried foods that might impair liver function are prohibited, and iron-rich green vegetables and sesame seeds are recommended. SEE PAGES 144–47

NUTRITIONAL THERAPIES

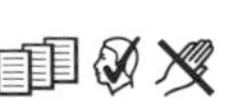

Practitioners treat anemia with dietary advice and supplements of iron, folic acid, or vitamin B_{12}. You may be advised to eat foods with a high iron content and to take supplements of vitamin C and zinc, which aid the absorption of iron. SEE PAGES 148–52

OTHER OPTIONS

Naturopathy SEE PAGES 118–21
Homeopathy SEE PAGES 126–130
Biochemic Tissue Salts SEE PAGE 131

VARICOSE VEINS

VARICOSE VEINS are blue swollen veins that show just beneath the surface of the skin, generally in the legs. They may appear in one leg only, but usually affect both, and are four times more common in women than in men. They may be accompanied by swollen ankles, fatigue, eczema, and by ulceration of the skin covering the affected veins. Varicose veins occur when the valves in the veins become weak, stopping blood from flowing back toward the heart efficiently, causing it to stagnate. Factors that contribute include heredity, aging, obesity, pregnancy, constipation, long periods of time standing, menopause, and a sedentary lifestyle. Conventional treatment includes advice such as getting exercise, wearing support stockings, and resting with the feet above chest level to help blood flow back to the heart. In severe cases, the veins are injected with chemicals that cause them to collapse, or they are stripped out through incisions in the leg.

Caution: Varicose veins can bleed profusely if injured.

COMPLEMENTARY TREATMENTS

Therapies aim to improve the circulation and the tone of the vein walls, and to address possible causes, such as constipation.

AROMATHERAPY

A practitioner will choose essential oils that may have a tonic action on the circulation. Cypress, which is astringent and diuretic, is often used. SEE PAGES 62–65

Caution: Do not use cypress essential oil in the first three months of pregnancy.

YOGA

Postures such as the Headstand, or the Inverted Corpse, lying on the back with the legs at 45 degrees against a wall, may ease varicose veins. SEE PAGES 108–11

Caution: Do not attempt Headstands in pregnancy or if you have high blood pressure.

HEADSTAND
This may be recommended to reduce blood pressure in the legs.

NATUROPATHY

Dietary advice focuses on avoiding constipation and improving the elasticity of the walls of the veins. Citrus fruits, apricots, cherries, and bilberries, which contain bioflavonoids (see glossary), may be recommended to strengthen the blood vessels. SEE PAGES 118–21

HYDROTHERAPY

Alternate hot and cold baths, showers, or compresses may be recommended to improve the circulation. SEE PAGES 122–23

Caution: Avoid alternating hot and cold baths or showers if you have a heart condition.

WESTERN HERBALISM

A practitioner may recommend witch hazel or calendula lotion to tone the walls of the veins and relieve discomfort. Studies indicate that gotu kola extract taken orally may enhance connective tissue structure and improve blood flow. Aescin, found in horse chestnut, has an anti-inflammatory effect. It also reduces fluid retention and tones vein walls. Butcher's broom is anti-inflammatory and improves the elasticity of the veins. SEE PAGES 134–39

Caution: Do not take butcher's broom if you have high blood pressure.

PHLEBITIS

PHLEBITIS IS AN INFLAMMATION of a surface leg vein, which may be accompanied by clotting (thrombophlebitis). Phlebitis can result from injury, infection, or irritation of the vein wall and is often associated with pregnancy and varicose veins. Conventional treatment includes pain relief, dressings, anti-inflammatory drugs, and antibiotics, as well as advice on keeping the leg raised. If the condition is due to a blood clot, anticoagulants will be prescribed.

Caution: Consult a doctor if you think you may have phlebitis; blood clots can be dangerous.

COMPLEMENTARY TREATMENTS

External treatments are said to improve vein-wall elasticity, and dietary advice aims to prevent the blood from clotting too easily.

HOMEOPATHY

A practitioner will prescribe remedies according to your constitutional type that will raise resistance and increase the natural reabsorption of blood clots. *Arnica 6c* may be recommended for phlebitis that follows an injury, *Lachesis 6c* if the skin has a purplish tinge, and *Pulsatilla 6c* if the pain is worse in heat. SEE PAGES 126–30

WESTERN HERBALISM

You may be asked to apply compresses and lotions made with arnica, hawthorn, or calendula to the affected area. Horse chestnut extract (aescin), butcher's broom, witch hazel, and other herbs are reported to have a beneficial effect on the veins (see Varicose Veins, page 248). SEE PAGES 134–39

NUTRITIONAL THERAPIES

A practitioner may recommend bromelain, a digestive enzyme found in pineapple, since there is evidence suggesting that it may help to break up blood clots.
SEE PAGES 148–52

FROSTBITE

SOME PEOPLE are particularly susceptible to frostbite: the itchy, reddish-blue swellings on fingers and toes that appear in cold weather. They are caused by the superficial blood vessels in the skin constricting excessively, due to poor circulation. Poor diet, insufficient warm clothing, and lack of exercise are also factors. Keeping warm and boosting the circulation by getting exercise will help prevent frostbite, and creams and tablets are available to help treat them. Doctors may prescribe medication to diabetics, the elderly, or those with arthritis in the hands or feet, to help boost the circulation.

COMPLEMENTARY TREATMENTS

Therapies that improve the circulation can help counter the condition.

MASSAGE

Regular massage may boost circulation in the skin and help prevent frostbite. SEE PAGES 56–61

ACUPRESSURE

To ease discomfort, a practitioner may show you how to press the Pericardium meridian acupoint on the wrist. SEE PAGE 95

NATUROPATHY

A balanced whole-foods diet will be suggested, together with garlic and ginger. SEE PAGES 118–21
Caution: Do not take ginger if you have a peptic ulcer.

HYDROTHERAPY

Alternate hot and cold hand or foot baths stimulate the circulation. Warm and cold compresses between the shoulder blades may be advised to improve circulation to the peripheries.
SEE PAGES 122–23

FOOTBATH
Soaking frostbite in hot, followed by cold, water stimulates blood flow.

NUTRITIONAL THERAPIES

Supplements of vitamin E, vitamin C, bioflavonoids, and rutin may be recommended.
SEE PAGES 148–52

RAYNAUD'S DISEASE & RAYNAUD'S PHENOMENON

IN THESE CONDITIONS, the blood vessels serving the fingers and toes become hypersensitive to cold and contract so that blood circulation is restricted. The affected areas grow very cold, turn white and numb, then blue, and become red and painful when warmed. If there is no known cause, the condition is called Raynaud's disease, but if it is the result of an underlying disorder, which can include high blood pressure, arteriosclerosis, diabetes, or neuralgia, it is known as Raynaud's phenomenon. Battery-powered heated socks and gloves are available to help sufferers keep warm; medical treatment includes drugs to relax and open the blood vessels.

COMPLEMENTARY TREATMENTS

Manipulative treatments, dietary regimes, and mind therapies can help improve the circulation to the hands and feet.

CHIROPRACTIC

(SEE OSTEOPATHY)

OSTEOPATHY

Manipulating the neck and spine may improve peripheral circulation. SEE PAGES 70–81

SPINAL MANIPULATION
Easing distortions of the vertebrae may improve blood circulation.

NATUROPATHY

A practitioner may suggest foods high in vitamin E, such as wheat germ and nuts, and magnesium-rich foods, such as soybeans, to help dilate the blood vessels. Hydrotherapy (see pages 122–23) may also help to boost the circulation. SEE PAGES 118–21

BIOFEEDBACK

Practitioners believe that you can learn to control skin temperature. They will teach you to focus mentally on warming the fingers and toes with the help of temperature sensors. In studies, symptoms were reduced by two thirds in some people. SEE PAGE 169

OTHER OPTIONS

Western Herbalism SEE PAGES 134–139
Autogenic Training SEE PAGE 168

MUSCLES, BONES & JOINTS

MUSCLES, BONES, AND JOINTS, and the soft tissues around the joints, make up the musculoskeletal system, which protects the internal organs and gives us mobility. There are more than 200 bones in the skeleton. The place where two bones meet is called a joint. It may either be fixed, as in the skull, or mobile, as in the elbow. Muscles are tissues that contract and enable the body to move, some being under our control, others not. Disorders of the musculoskeletal system are one of the major causes of health problems today, responsible for widespread disability and accounting for a quarter of all visits to the doctor.

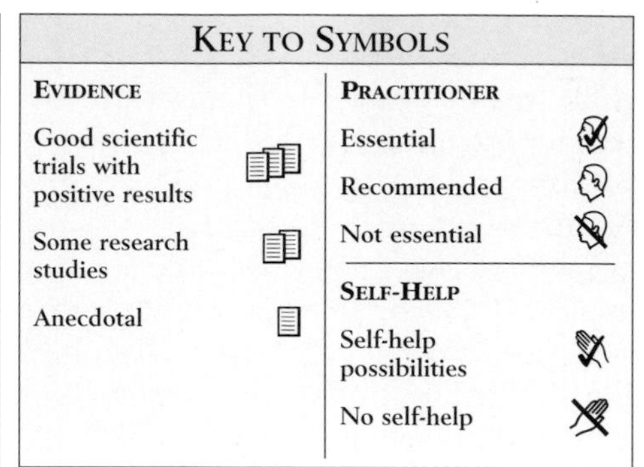

COMPLEMENTARY APPROACHES

Osteopaths, chiropractors, and other complementary therapists believe that poor function in one area of the body affects the entire system. "Trigger points," for example, are taut bands of muscle felt as hard, twitchy nodules, which can be caused by tension in other areas of the body, especially around the spine. Significantly, these points are very often situated along acupoint meridians (see page 91). A practitioner will work on trigger points as well as on the area that is causing the problem.

CONVENTIONAL APPROACHES

Inflammation and pain in joints and muscles is often treated with aspirinlike anti-inflammatory drugs. Physical therapy is also important. Joint replacement (especially the hip) can be highly effective.
Caution: Before seeking treatment, see page 204.

HOW THE MUSCULOSKELETAL SYSTEM WORKS

The spinal column comprises 33 girdle-shaped vertebrae, which protect the spinal cord. Many therapists believe that a stiff or misaligned spinal column adversely affects other body elements, even internal organs. Mobile joints, such as the knuckles, move within a sheath of fibrous tissue. The membrane lining this sheath produces a lubricating fluid. The sheath terminates in ligaments, tough bands of tissue that fuse into the bones and link them. Muscles are attached to the skeleton and to other muscles by tendons, strong flexible cords or sheets of fibers.

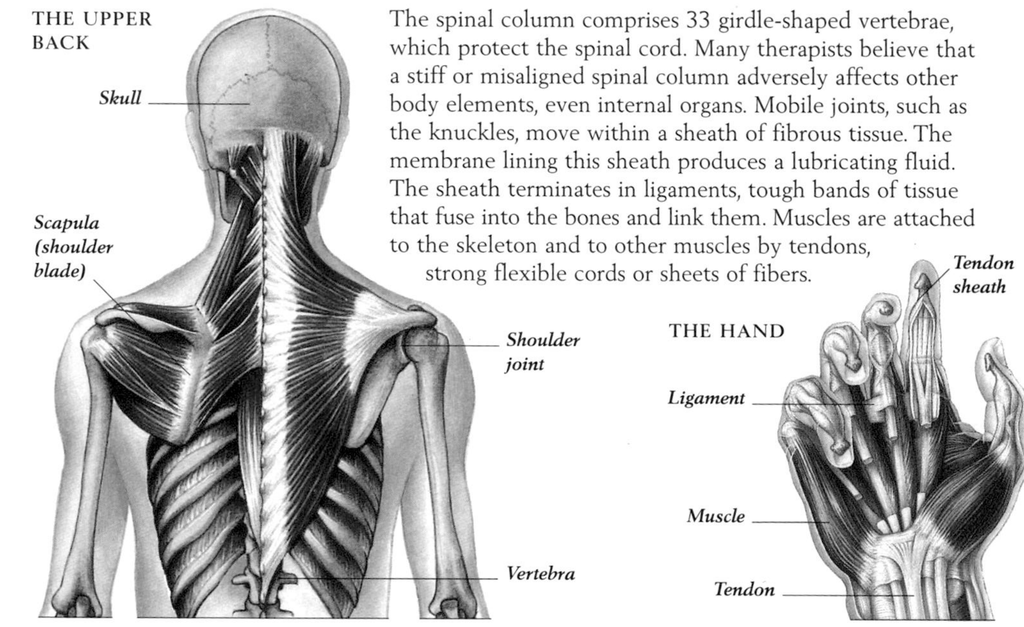

CRAMPS

PAINFUL, INVOLUNTARY MUSCLE SPASMS are a common complaint, particularly in children, the elderly, and pregnant women. Cramps can be triggered by exercise, repetitive action, or extended immobility in an awkward position. Rubbing and stretching the muscle usually brings relief. Another cause of cramps, salt loss through sweating, is easily prevented and treated with a drink of saltwater. Poor circulation in the legs may cause night cramps. A doctor might advise treating night cramps with drugs containing quinine or calcium.

COMPLEMENTARY TREATMENTS

Most touch and movement therapies are suitable for relieving and preventing muscle tension. Medicinal therapists tend to regard diet and deficiencies as significant factors, and will treat according to the cause.

MASSAGE

Massage stimulates the circulation and encourages the elimination of lactic acid. This substance, a waste product of intensive muscular exertion, accumulates in the tissue and causes muscle spasms. Your practitioner will show you how to knead, stroke, and stretch the affected area. SEE PAGES 56–61

WESTERN HERBALISM

Cramp bark has had long use as a muscle relaxant. A practitioner may advise a rubbing lotion made with this herb. SEE PAGES 134–39

NUTRITIONAL THERAPIES

Zinc or magnesium supplements may help people suffering from cramps. According to clinical observations in the US in the 1970s, vitamin E supplements may also bring relief. SEE PAGES 148–52

OTHER OPTIONS

Acupressure SEE PAGE 95
Yoga SEE PAGES 108–11
Homeopathy SEE PAGES 126–30

Muscle Pain

Muscle pain varies dramatically in terms of severity, site, and cause. Certain kinds are easily treated with over-the-counter painkillers, but other kinds may last for years, having no identifiable cause. Additional information may be found in Pain (see pages 314–15), Backache (see pages 254–55), and Sports Injuries (see page 261).

Types of Pain When muscle fibers are torn, internal bruising occurs, which results in pain and possible swelling. Such injuries are common in sporting activities. In any situation where the muscle is stretched beyond its capacity, it may respond by becoming tense and irritable, and may even develop an intensely tender "trigger point," which may radiate pain to other areas. This is called *myofascial pain*. Myofascial pain from trigger points is not generalized, but affects particular muscles and may contribute to other soft-tissue problems, including repetitive strain injury (see page 252) and frozen shoulder (see page 253).

Generalized muscle pain and stiffness, occurring without an evident cause but with a characteristic pattern of tender spots, is known as *fibromyalgia syndrome* (FMS), formerly called *fibrositis*. Often affecting the neck and back, it frequently occurs with other conditions, such as chronic fatigue syndrome, menstrual complaints, and irritable bowel syndrome. Tension, poor posture, and sleep disturbance may all be contributing factors.

Conventional Treatment Muscle pain from injury generally responds to painkillers and anti-inflammatory drugs, but myofascial pain and FMS may prove resistant. Small doses of antidepressants are beneficial in some cases of FMS. Aerobic exercise for 20 minutes three times a week helps the body release its own painkillers (endorphins) and may be equally effective.

Rolfing
Deep massage restores the body's natural alignment, helping muscle problems.

Touch & Movement Therapies

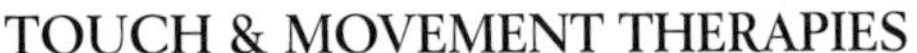

When treating muscle pain, osteopaths, chiropractors, and other practitioners use body manipulation in order to improve trigger points, stiffness in the spine, and postural problems.

Massage

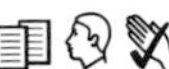

Massage stimulates the circulation and may help relax trigger points and other areas of stiffness in the muscles, easing pain. In an ongoing study at the Touch Research Institute, Miami, early evidence reports that a group receiving massage experienced greater relief than one receiving TENS therapy (see glossary). If the painful area is within reach, the affected muscle may respond to your own kneading and stroking. see pages 56–61

Aromatherapy

Aromatherapy essential oils, such as lavender and rosemary, added to a carrier oil, are thought to help relax muscles and promote a sense of well-being. see pages 62–65

Chiropractic (see Osteopathy)

Osteopathy

Evidence suggests that soft-tissue treatment focusing on muscle stretching and lengthening achieves better results than joint manipulation. see pages 70–81

Rolfing

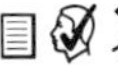

This technique, which uses vigorous manipulation to stretch muscles and to unknot deep trigger points, may help relieve pain in these areas, but the treatment itself can be uncomfortable. see pages 82–83

Acupuncture

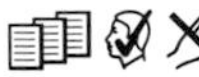

Electroacupuncture can relieve symptoms of fibromyalgia, according to a Swiss study published in 1992 in the *British Medical Journal*. see pages 90–94

Hydrotherapy

Ice packs, alternating hot and cold compresses, and warm baths with added Epsom salts may all be recommended to ease stiffness and discomfort. see pages 122–23

Caution: Avoid Epsom salts baths if elderly or frail.

Yoga

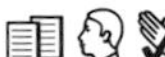

Yoga relaxes the muscles, promotes slower breathing, and calms the mind, helping to ease tension. Gentle stretching postures (known as *asanas*) are thought to be useful in alleviating FMS and correcting postural problems that may contribute to muscular pain. see pages 108–11

Medicinal Therapies

In this branch of complementary medicine, therapists work to improve circulation and induce relaxation, and to promote the body's power of self-healing.

Homeopathy

Most homeopaths prefer to diagnose and treat on the basis of a constitutional assessment. Pain that is worse on first movement and better for heat might be helped by the remedy *Rhus tox*. see pages 126–30

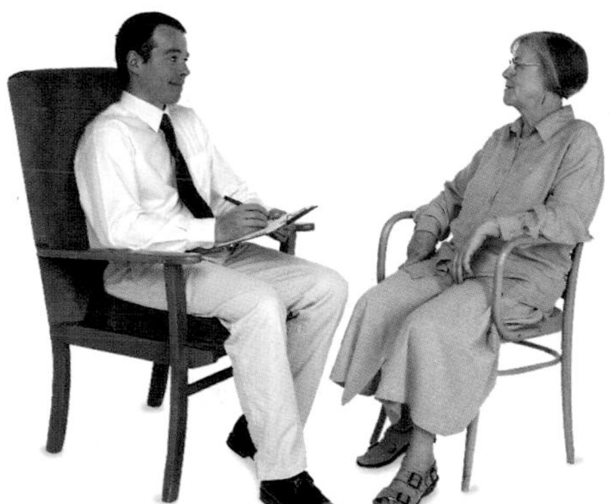

Homeopathic Assessment
Homeopathic remedies have been shown to be effective in treating fibromyalgia syndrome.

Nutritional Therapies

For long-term pain, a practitioner may recommend that you adopt a temporary raw-foods or fruit diet to help "detoxify" the system. Muscle pain has been linked to a lack of serotonin, a chemical which influences mood, helping to explain why antidepressants relieve certain instances of FMS. To help the body manufacture serotonin, your practitioner may prescribe supplements of B vitamins or magnesium. see pages 148–52

Mind & Emotion Therapies

Relaxation therapies may prove helpful in reversing muscle pain.

Psychotherapy & Counseling

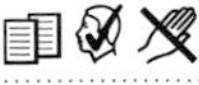

Cognitive behavioral therapy can help break cycles of depression and inactivity that can contribute to muscle pain. see pages 160–65

Hypnotherapy

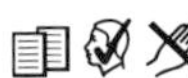

In a 1991 trial, patients with FMS who had not responded to touch therapies said that they felt less pain, fatigue, and stiffness after hypnotherapy. see pages 166–67

TENDINITIS & TENNIS ELBOW

TENDINITIS (AN INFLAMED TENDON) causes pain and tenderness, as well as limited movement in the affected area. Most susceptible is the Achilles tendon, which connects the calf muscle to the heel bone, and the tendons in the shoulder, thumb, knee, and side of the foot. Tendinitis at the attachment of the forearm muscle and the elbow is commonly known as tennis elbow. If tendinitis is long-standing, calcium deposits may form.

Causes People who exercise irregularly or without proper warm-up are prone to tendinitis. While unusual or excessive physical activity is the most common cause, tendinitis may also arise from a bacterial infection.

Conventional Treatment Rest, painkillers, and anti-inflammatory drugs are the usual first line of care. If these do not bring relief, a doctor may bandage or splint the affected area to immobilize the joint. Local steroid injections may be given to reduce inflammation. If the pain is severe, TENS therapy (see glossary) may be advised to block pain impulses. Ultrasound therapy increases circulation and can help. Calcified tendinitis or a ruptured tendon usually requires surgery.

COMPLEMENTARY TREATMENTS

Touch therapists may work on trigger points (see page 250) as well as on the tendon itself in their effort to relieve pain. Eliminating any underlying cause of inflammation is also a priority; to this end, herbal, dietary, or homeopathic remedies may be suggested.

CHIROPRACTIC (SEE OSTEOPATHY)

OSTEOPATHY

A therapist will perform soft-tissue treatment on affected tendons, muscles, and related spinal segments to ease pain and increase mobility. SEE PAGES 76–81

ACUPUNCTURE

In a study in 1990 in *The Clinical Journal of Pain* and one in 1994 in the *British Journal of Rheumatology*, acupuncture improved tennis elbow. SEE PAGES 90–94

NATUROPATHY

Many practitioners believe that local inflammation may be a physical response to internal waste products. If the reaction is exaggerated to the point at which healthy tissues are damaged, the inflammation may become self-perpetuating. Practitioners aim to reduce inflammation through a diet that is low in animal fat and high in antioxidant nutrients (see glossary). SEE PAGES 118–21

ANTIOXIDANTS
Found in vitamin C-rich foods, they help reduce swelling.

HYDROTHERAPY

A therapist's general advice might be summed up as RICE (Rest, Ice, Compression, Elevate): rest the injured limb, apply an ice pack, compress it with a bandage to reduce swelling, and elevate it. Whirlpool baths may help in relaxing affected muscles. SEE PAGES 122–23

NUTRITIONAL THERAPIES

Like naturopaths, nutritional therapists aim to boost the body's anti-inflammatory responses. Recommended supplements may include essential fatty acids (found in flaxseed, evening primrose oil, blackcurrant oil, and fish oils) to help make anti-inflammatory prostaglandins, and antioxidants such as selenium and vitamins C and E, which reduce swelling and enhance production of collagen, a major component of tendon fibers. SEE PAGES 148–52

OTHER OPTIONS

Massage	SEE PAGES 56–61
Aromatherapy	SEE PAGES 62–65
Homeopathy	SEE PAGES 126–30
Western Herbalism	SEE PAGES 134–39

REPETITIVE STRAIN INJURY (RSI)

TENDINITIS AND TRIGGER POINTS (see page 250) may both be factors in repetitive strain injury (RSI), a condition marked by pain and weakness in the forearm, wrist, and hand (see also Carpal Tunnel Syndrome, page 206). RSI stems from overuse, and is a recognized occupational hazard for musicians and people who operate computer keyboards. Stress, poor posture, and psychological factors are thought to aggravate it.

Conventional Treatment Rest, painkillers, bandaging, and anti-inflammatory drugs are the first line of treatment. To encourage healing in stubborn cases, a doctor may also suggest supporting the affected wrist with splints or plaster.

Self-Help If you use a keyboard, invest in a wrist rest. Be sure to stand and stretch every 20 minutes, and massage forearms and hands on a regular basis.

COMPLEMENTARY TREATMENTS

Movement therapies that improve posture may bring marked improvement, as may learning to cope with stress and avoiding bad working positions.

MASSAGE

Massage can stimulate the blood supply, warming and relaxing the affected area, and may help prevent RSI. SEE PAGES 56–61

THE ALEXANDER TECHNIQUE

Teachers look for clues about occupational, postural, and personal stresses and teach you to become aware of how these affect your body. SEE PAGES 86–87

BODY AWARENESS
Alexander technique teachers correct alignment.

ACUPRESSURE

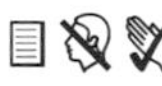

Your therapist will show you how to press on specific acupoints, for instance on the Triplewarmer meridian just above the wrist joint. SEE PAGE 95

PSYCHOTHERAPY & COUNSELING

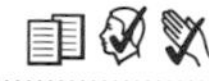

Counseling and cognitive therapy may help you improve your work habits and learn how to cope with stress, which may be causing muscle tension. SEE PAGES 160–65

RELAXATION & BREATHING

Techniques to encourage deep, even breathing and mental and physiological relaxation may reduce anxiety and ease muscle tension. SEE PAGES 170–73

OTHER OPTIONS

Acupuncture	SEE PAGES 90–94
Yoga	SEE PAGES 108–11
Naturopathy	SEE PAGES 118–21

BURSITIS

A BURSA IS A THIN, FLUID-FILLED SAC that cushions points of pressure or friction. They are found where a tendon or a muscle rubs against another muscle or bone, for example at the kneecap, elbow, or shoulder. Bursae enhance free movement, but if they are inflamed or injured, fluid may accumulate, causing pain and swelling. Housemaid's knee, in which the bursa over the kneecap becomes inflamed due to constant kneeling, is an example of bursitis. Less commonly, bursitis develops due to an injury, or as a result of bacterial infection. **Conventional Treatment** Infections generally respond to antibiotic drugs. Bursitis due to mechanical causes is usually treated with rest, painkillers, bandaging, anti-inflammatory drugs, or withdrawal of the fluid with a syringe (aspiration). If these do not help, steroid injections or surgery may be advised.

COMPLEMENTARY TREATMENTS

Therapists will seek to ease pain and reduce swelling in the affected joint. Among the many possible approaches are manipulating the soft tissues in the area, or treating them with healing medicinal substances.

AROMATHERAPY 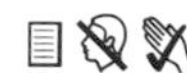

Essential oil of lavender, either added to a bath or diluted and massaged into the skin, is one of the oils that may soothe inflamed tissues. SEE PAGES 62–65

ACUPUNCTURE 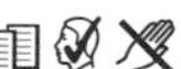

An acupuncturist will stimulate appropriate acupoints in an attempt to reduce pain, improve the healing process and increase mobility in the affected area. SEE PAGES 90–94

HYDROTHERAPY 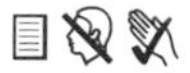

The application of alternate hot and cold compresses might be recommended to help bring down the swelling and relieve pain. SEE PAGES 122–23

HOMEOPATHY 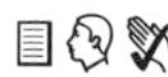

Bryonia 6c is a standard preparation that may be advised if the condition worsens with movement. *Rhus tox. 6c* is given if the first movements of the day are worse. SEE PAGES 126–30

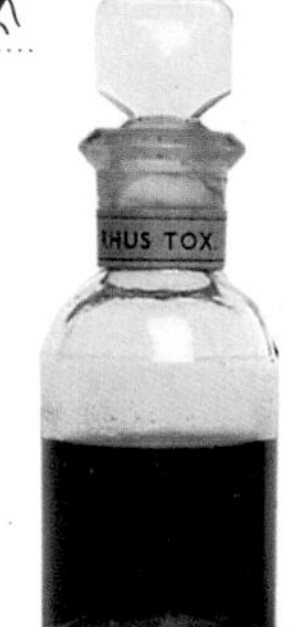

RHUS TOX.
This homeopathic remedy, made from poison ivy, is often used for musculoskeletal complaints.

WESTERN HERBALISM 

A herbalist may recommend applying compresses made with comfrey or slippery elm, which are thought to help reduce inflammation. SEE PAGES 134–39

OTHER OPTIONS

Massage SEE PAGES 56–61
Chiropractic SEE PAGES 70–75
Osteopathy SEE PAGES 76–81
Hydrotherapy SEE PAGES 122–23
Nutritional Therapies SEE PAGES 148–52

FROZEN SHOULDER

THIS IS A CONDITION in which the lining of the capsule surrounding the shoulder joint becomes inflamed, causing severe pain and stiffness. Moving the arm sideways is especially difficult, making dressing an ordeal. As pain discourages movement, stiffness increases, the muscles weaken and contract and, eventually, the fluid lubricating the capsule interior dries up. The lining sticks together in what is medically known as adhesive capsulitis. Those affected are usually between 50 and 70 years old. The condition is often triggered by a minor injury, bursitis (see above), or tendinitis (see opposite). **Conventional Treatment** A doctor will first recommend gentle exercise, painkillers, and anti-inflammatory drugs. If the condition persists, steroid injections, ultrasound therapy, or even remobilization of the joint under anesthetic may be advised. Full recovery is possible, but slow, perhaps taking 12–18 months. **Self-Help** Keep the shoulders supple with exercise, especially at the first sign of pain. Swimming at an easy pace may help to keep the joints mobile.

COMPLEMENTARY TREATMENTS

Touch therapists will try to keep the joint mobile and, at the same time, attempt to relieve pain. Medicinal remedies or therapies that stimulate circulation may also help.

MASSAGE 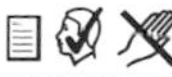

Vigorous massage of trigger points – secondary points of tension near the afflicted shoulder – may increase mobility, which in turn will help speed recovery. SEE PAGES 56–61

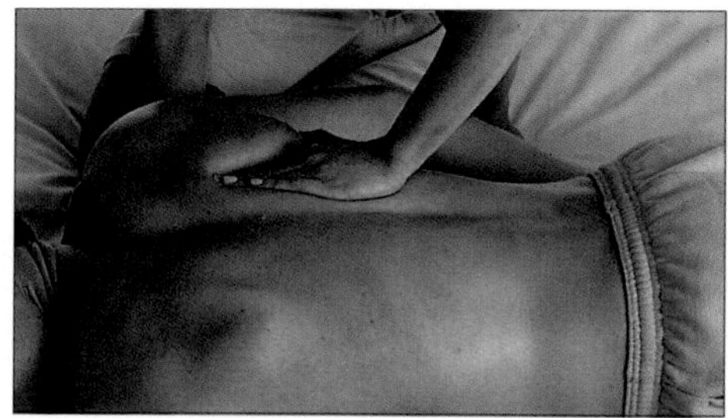

RELEASING MUSCULAR TENSION
Practitioners will seek to release trigger points or areas of muscle tension.

AROMATHERAPY

Massage with the essential oils of rosemary and sage in a carrier oil may improve circulation to the affected area. SEE PAGES 62–65

CHIROPRACTIC (SEE OSTEOPATHY) 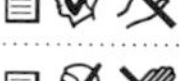

OSTEOPATHY 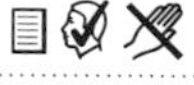

Your practitioner will focus on improving mobility in the shoulder by giving deep soft-tissue treatment, stretching the muscles and manipulating the spine. Particular attention will be paid to trigger points and to any associated contraction of muscle fibers. SEE PAGES 70–81

ACUPUNCTURE 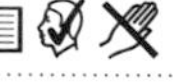

Traditional Chinese Medicine associates shoulder pain with weak *yang qi* (see glossary) and "external cold and damp." Practitioners work on stimulating appropriate acupoints located around the shoulder and on related meridians elsewhere. SEE PAGES 90–94

WESTERN HERBALISM 

Massaging the joint with a lotion of yarrow and St. John's wort – both herbs with anti-inflammatory properties – may help bring down swelling within the joint capsule. SEE PAGES 134–39

OTHER OPTIONS

Hydrotherapy SEE PAGES 122–23
Homeopathy SEE PAGES 126–30
Chinese Herbalism SEE PAGES 140–43
Magnetic Therapy SEE PAGE 156

BACKACHE

AS MANY AS 60% of adults in the West may experience acute, or sudden, back pain during their lifetime, and in 33% the condition is persistent or recurring. Back pain accounts for more lost working hours than any other ailment and is the main cause of disability for people under 45. Some people are more prone than others: manual workers and office workers are more susceptible to backache, as are sportsmen and women, tall people, the overweight, and the elderly. After a few weeks, even severe cases will usually get better with little treatment. But relapse is common and, if back pain is recurring or persistent, professional help should be sought. This complaint is the one most often seen by osteopaths and chiropractors.

CAUSES & SYMPTOMS

Surprisingly few back problems are due to a prolapsed ("slipped") disk (see page 256). Backache more commonly occurs when a facet joint, which connects two vertebrae, is strained by lifting heavy objects. Pregnancy, tense muscles, strained ligaments, and poor posture can also cause back problems, as can damaged or aging joints, infections, gallstones, kidney stones, stress, or being overweight. Occasionally, psychological factors or serious conditions, including cancer, may be responsible.

PREVENTION

Improving your posture will help prevent many kinds of recurring back problems, as will regular exercise such as swimming. Make sure your chair supports the small of your back, and buy backrests for car seats and a supportive mattress for your bed. If lifting heavy objects, bend at the hips and knees, keeping your back straight.

CONVENTIONAL TREATMENT

Traditionally, rest and painkillers are prescribed for back pain, but current expert opinion advises against more than 2–3 days in bed, preferring gentle exercise, rehabilitation, and manipulation. A physiotherapist may use mobilization techniques backed by ultrasound, laser, or heat treatment. If the problem is severe and there is no improvement after several weeks, X rays and possibly an MRI scan (see glossary) may be suggested. Treatment can include anti-inflammatory and muscle-relaxant drugs, traction, a collar or surgical corset, painkilling epidural anesthetic injections, antidepressants, TENS (see glossary) or, in the case of a prolapsed disk, surgery.

PRECAUTIONS

- **Consult a doctor if back pain is accompanied by nausea, vomiting, fever, muscle weakness, pain down an arm or leg, or bowel or bladder disturbances, or if pain is unrelieved by 2–3 days of rest.**

TOUCH & MOVEMENT THERAPIES

Most Western therapies focus on the musculoskeletal structure, aiming to relax tense muscles, correct posture, and restore mobility. Manipulative therapies such as chiropractic or osteopathy have an impressive reputation for treating short-term back pain. Long-term back pain may be helped by acupuncture, but will probably also require commitment to exercise, rehabilitation, and postural change.

MASSAGE

Massage can help relax tense muscles and relieve aches and pains. Your practitioner may use firm stroking movements up either side of the spine, fanning across the shoulders; circular thumb movements over the small muscles on either side of the spine may also ease discomfort. For the occasional, mild backache, a friend could massage you in a similar manner. However, massage should not be undertaken unless your practitioner rules out a prolapsed disk or a spinal problem, which deep massage could worsen. SEE PAGES 56–61

CHIROPRACTIC

According to practitioners, misalignment of the vertebrae in the spine can cause the joints to press on the spinal nerves, leading to direct pain in the back and possibly "referred" pain in other parts of the body. Your practitioner will carry out tests, including X rays, if necessary, to establish the cause of the pain, and will follow this with manipulation of the joints and vertebrae in the back and neck to restore their mobility. A substantial body of evidence exists in support of chiropractic. In the UK, a Medical Research Council study in 1990 suggested that improvement in back-pain patients treated with chiropractic was greater than that of patients referred for hospital physiotherapy. In 1994, the UK's Clinical Standards Advisory Group recommended that the National Health Service refer more patients to practitioners specially trained in manipulation. In several US studies, chiropractic was found to be so effective in relieving acute back pain that its use for this condition was endorsed in 1994 by the Federal Agency for Health Care Policy and Research. SEE PAGES 70–75

ALIGNING THE VERTEBRAE
Practitioners use special manipulative techniques to bring the vertebrae in the back and neck into alignment.

OSTEOPATHY

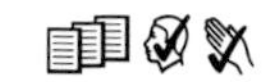

Osteopaths and chiropractors use many of the same diagnostic techniques and treatment methods: osteopaths use manipulation and specific thrusts similar to chiropractic to restore mobility to the musculoskeletal structure of the body. Diagnostic techniques are also similar to those of chiropractic. Methods for treating acute or chronic back pain depend on the cause of the problem, and range from gentle massage to ease muscle tension, to pressure and stretching techniques to restore mobility to the joints. Several studies have shown that osteopathy can aid recovery from lower back pain. SEE PAGES 76–81

THE ALEXANDER TECHNIQUE

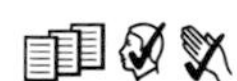

An Alexander teacher will train you to become more aware of how you move and hold yourself, and reeducate you to correct your posture. This realignment of the musculoskeletal structure eases areas of muscle tension and nerve pressure in the neck and back, and allows the body to move more effectively. SEE PAGES 86–87

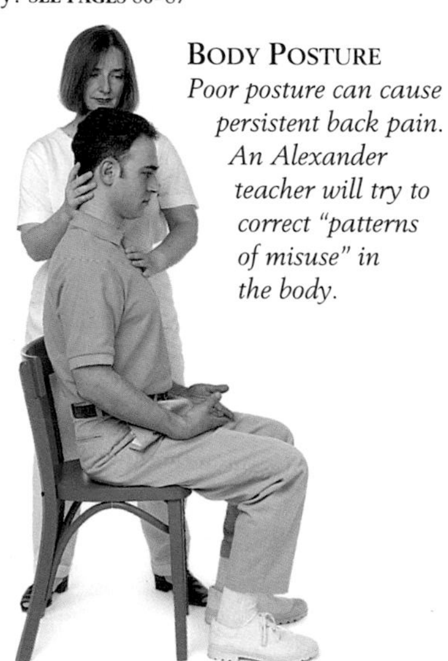

BODY POSTURE
Poor posture can cause persistent back pain. An Alexander teacher will try to correct "patterns of misuse" in the body.

ACUPUNCTURE

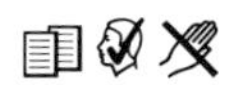

Practitioners use needles, moxibustion, or cupping to stimulate acupoints on the *yang* (see glossary) channels that flow down the back and legs, such as the Small Intestine, Kidney, and Bladder meridians, to relieve pain and restore the circulation of *qi* ("life energy"). Many British pain clinics now use acupuncture routinely, which can sometimes be helpful in dealing with persistent back pain. In the 1980s, researchers at the University of California, Los Angeles, found that acupuncture restored blood flow, relaxed muscle spasms, and strengthened weak muscles. In other US studies, published in 1980 and 1982, patients receiving acupuncture for back and neck pain improved more than control groups. SEE PAGES 90–94

ACUPRESSURE

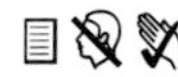

To treat persistent lower back pain, firm pressure may be applied to acupoints on the Bladder and Gallbladder meridians, relieving pain and stimulating the flow of *qi*. SEE PAGE 95

QIGONG

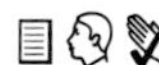

This ancient Chinese system of exercises combines movement and "mindfulness" – a form of meditation that includes focusing on breathing and body awareness – to relax the muscles and ease stresses on the body. In 1996, the Maryland School of Medicine in the US incorporated qigong into a program for managing chronic lower back pain. SEE PAGE 99

YOGA

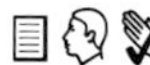

Yoga breathing exercises (*pranayama*) gently work the muscles of the upper back. A qualified teacher can tailor a specific yoga program to your needs. Lying flat on your back (the Corpse posture) is helpful for releasing tension and relieving pain, rotating the back (the Spinal Twist) eases tension in the upper back and shoulders, and back rolls (the Cat Stretch or Cobra) can increase the flexibility of the spine. In a 1985 survey published in a US magazine, 96% of respondents who practiced yoga reported relief from persistent back pain, compared to 23% who were seeing neurosurgeons. SEE PAGES 108–11

OTHER OPTIONS

Aromatherapy	SEE PAGES 62–65
Reflexology	SEE PAGES 66–69
Rolfing	SEE PAGES 82–83
Hellerwork	SEE PAGE 84
The Feldenkrais Method	SEE PAGE 85
Tragerwork	SEE PAGE 88
Shiatsu	SEE PAGES 96–97
Do-in	SEE PAGE 98
Thai Massage	SEE PAGE 98

MEDICINAL THERAPIES

Practitioners seek to reduce inflammation that may be contributing to back pain. You may be prescribed medicines to take internally or soothing creams and other preparations to apply to the area.

HYDROTHERAPY

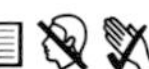

For sudden back pain, a practitioner may advocate applying alternate hot and cold compresses to the painful area – three minutes for the hot compress, one minute for the cold, repeated every 20 minutes. The hot compress will increase blood flow to the area and relax the muscles, while the cold compress helps reduce inflammation. SEE PAGES 122–23

WESTERN HERBALISM

Practitioners may recommend a massage with cramp bark essential oil to reduce muscle spasm in the back. You may be advised to take anti-inflammatory herbs, such as white willow or devil's claw, to ease painful joints, and lavender and St. John's wort to soothe nervous tension. SEE PAGES 134–39

Caution: Do not take devil's claw during pregnancy.

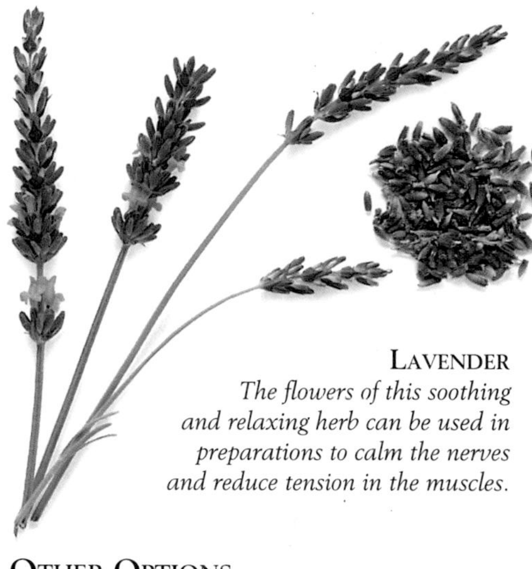

LAVENDER
The flowers of this soothing and relaxing herb can be used in preparations to calm the nerves and reduce tension in the muscles.

OTHER OPTIONS

Homeopathy	SEE PAGES 126–30
Chinese Herbalism	SEE PAGES 140–43

MIND & EMOTION THERAPIES

Persistent pain is stressful and tiring. Backache can be caused by posture problems related to emotional states, or by stress-related conditions leading to muscle tension.

PSYCHOTHERAPY & COUNSELING

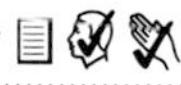

Cognitive behavioral therapy techniques may help you to understand how thoughts and emotions are linked to long-term pain. SEE PAGES 160–65

BIOFEEDBACK

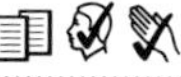

Training makes you aware of habitual muscle contraction that may be causing persistent pain, and helps you to relax the area. SEE PAGE 169

RELAXATION & BREATHING

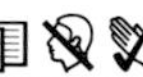

Learning to relax and breathe properly can reduce the impact of stress. A 1986 US study found relaxation techniques better at reducing pain and muscle tension than biofeedback or any placebo treatment. SEE PAGES 170–73

OTHER OPTIONS

Hypnotherapy	SEE PAGES 166–67
Visualization	SEE PAGES 178–79

PROLAPSED DISK

THE SPINAL VERTEBRAE are separated by intervertebral disks – thick pads that act as shock absorbers and help the spine flex and bend. If a disk weakens or splits, its soft center may protrude through its fibrous shell and press on a spinal nerve: a condition known medically as a prolapsed disk. The pain may be sudden and severe and is generally one-sided, radiating along the nerve. The muscles the nerve supplies may become weak (see Sciatica, below). Often the back becomes locked because the muscles contract to prevent further movement. Slipped disks usually happen to people under 50.

Causes The cause may be either a sudden strain or a fall. Pain and stiffness are often severe and persist for several weeks with little improvement, unlike simple short-term back pain, which generally settles gradually within 4–6 weeks.

Conventional Treatment This ranges from painkillers, anesthetic injections, anti-inflammatory drugs, muscle relaxants, and physiotherapy to surgery.

Cautions: Consult a doctor if you suspect you have a slipped disk. Immediately after the onset of pain, lie flat with a pillow under your knees. If pain is accompanied by weakness, tingling, or loss of bladder or bowel control, or if the pain does not ease when lying down, call emergency help, as the nerves at the end of the spinal cord may be compressed and at risk of permanent damage.

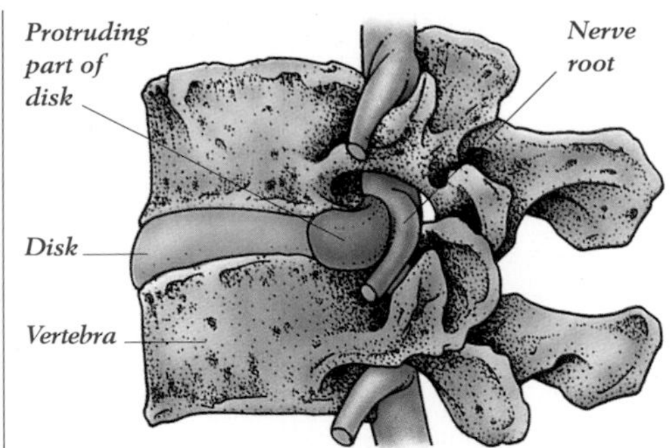

SLIPPED DISK
The disk between the vertebrae ruptures and protrudes, putting pressure on a spinal nerve.

COMPLEMENTARY TREATMENTS

Pain relief is the primary aim of treatment. Touch therapists also seek to restore mobility to the spine with manipulation. Eastern therapists try to improve the flow of qi, the "life energy" they believe circulates through and animates the body. Medicinal therapists will support the body's healing abilities with plant and other substances.

CHIROPRACTIC (SEE OSTEOPATHY) 

OSTEOPATHY

Manipulation of the spine cannot "reposition" a prolapsed disk, but it may help to restore spinal mobility while the healing process is taking place. Practitioners will examine the spine and make a series of adjustments. SEE PAGES 70–81

ACUPUNCTURE 

Practitioners aim to relieve pain and balance the flow of *qi* by stimulating local acupoints and those along the Bladder and Gallbladder meridians. SEE PAGES 90–94

HYDROTHERAPY 

A practitioner may advise applying alternate hot and cold compresses to the affected area to stimulate blood flow and relieve pain. SEE PAGES 122–23

HOMEOPATHY 

Practitioners may recommend self-treatment with *Arnica 6c* to help overcome the shock of severe pain. SEE PAGES 126–30

BACH FLOWER REMEDIES 

Rescue Remedy, comprising cherry plum, clematis, impatiens, star of Bethlehem, and rock rose, is recommended for the shock of sudden, agonizing pain caused by a slipped disk. SEE PAGES 132–33

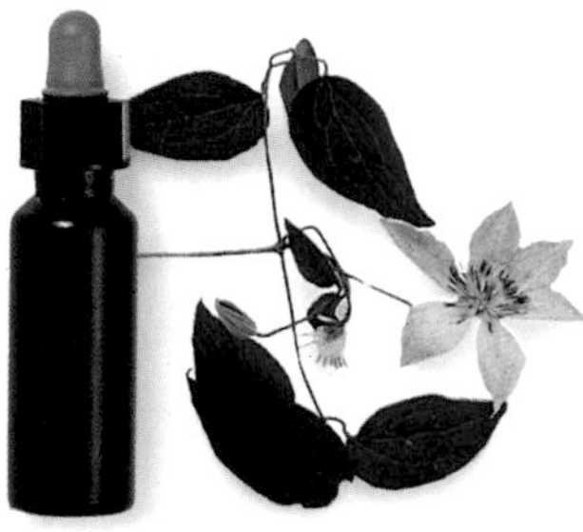

RESCUE REMEDY
This remedy is prepared by infusing flower heads in spring water for three hours.

OTHER OPTION

Acupressure SEE PAGE 95

SCIATICA

SCIATICA IS SIMPLY A LABEL for leg pain. It is thought to be caused by pressure on or irritation of the sciatic nerve (the main nerve in the leg). The pain is felt along the nerve's path, through the buttock, thigh, and sometimes down to the foot. In severe cases, the pain is accompanied by muscle weakness. The source of the pressure may be a slipped disk (see above), lower back strain, or muscle spasm. In rare cases, pressure can also arise from a blood clot, tumor or abscess. Sciatica in young adults may be the result of a sports injury or, in late pregnancy, a ligament strain.

Conventional Treatment This varies depending on the cause, but it is largely aimed at reducing pain, which generally persists from a few days to several weeks.

COMPLEMENTARY TREATMENTS

Therapists will aim to find and treat the cause of sciatica and at the same time focus on giving pain relief.

CHIROPRACTIC (SEE OSTEOPATHY)

OSTEOPATHY

Manipulation can help if there is tension in the lower back region or a strain in one of the sacroiliac ligaments linking the spine to the pelvis. Practitioners will work to release trigger points (see page 250) in the buttock muscle, which are a common cause. SEE PAGES 70–81

ACUPUNCTURE 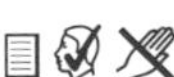

A practitioner might needle trigger points along the Bladder and Gallbladder meridians in the lower back, buttocks, and thighs. SEE PAGES 90–94

SHIATSU

This deep and penetrating soft-tissue technique may help free stiff and painful areas, especially if trigger points are involved. SEE PAGES 96–97

RELAXATION & BREATHING 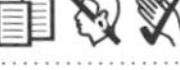

Deep breathing and relaxation techniques may help to lower anxiety and relieve muscle tension that can contribute to pain. SEE PAGES 170–73

OTHER OPTIONS

Reflexology SEE PAGES 66–69
The Alexander Technique SEE PAGES 86–87
Tragerwork SEE PAGE 88
Acupressure SEE PAGE 95
Healing SEE PAGES 104–105
Hydrotherapy SEE PAGES 122–23
Western Herbalism SEE PAGES 134–39
Visualization SEE PAGES 178–79

OSTEOPOROSIS

OSTEOPOROSIS, A CONDITION in which bones lose mass and density and become weak and brittle, is responsible for about 1.5 million fractures a year in the US and more than 200,000 in the UK. Osteoporosis is not easily detected in its early stages, and the first indication may be a fracture after a minor fall, typically in the spine, hip, or wrist. As the condition progresses, the vertebrae may compress to the point where the spine shortens and becomes humped. As many as one in four post-menopausal women have some degree of bone loss, and 89% of women past the age of 75 are osteoporotic. Men are usually not affected until their 70s.

Causes Bone loss is a natural part of aging, but in osteoporosis the process accelerates, particularly in women after menopause. This is because the ovaries stop producing estrogen, a hormone that helps the body absorb calcium from the diet and incorporate it in the bones. Other risk factors are a family history of the condition, being white or of Asian descent, experiencing menopause before the age of 45, having a low lifetime intake of calcium, smoking, excessive alcohol, and caffeine intake, lack of exercise, and prolonged treatment with steroid drugs.

Conventional Treatment After the extent of bone loss is determined, treatment focuses on preventing further breakdown. In women, hormone replacement therapy (HRT) can improve calcium absorption, restoring strength to the bones. Its benefits last only as long as the hormones are taken, however, and there can be side effects. Other drugs, such as biphosphonates, show promise.

Self-Help Osteoporosis is best prevented before menopause with a diet rich in calcium and vitamin D (necessary for calcium absorption). Afterward, women not taking HRT benefit from calcium supplements.

STRENGTHENING BONES
Weightbearing exercise – for example brisk walking, is ideal for strengthening bones.

TOUCH & MOVEMENT THERAPIES

The stiffness and pain that can accompany osteoporosis may often be helped by touch and movement therapies.

T'AI CHI CH'UAN 

This Chinese movement therapy uses breathing techniques and sequences of slow, graceful movements to improve the flow of *qi* ("life energy"). In addition to providing gentle exercise, t'ai chi benefits the posture and increases flexibility in the joints.
SEE PAGES 100–101

YOGA 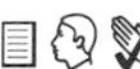

A teacher will show you particular postures (*asanas*) that will help build strength, increase flexibility, and improve your overall sense of well-being. SEE PAGES 108–11

OTHER OPTIONS

Reflexology	SEE PAGES 66–69
Chiropractic	SEE PAGES 70–75
Osteopathy	SEE PAGES 76–81
Acupuncture	SEE PAGES 90–94
Qigong	SEE PAGE 99

MEDICINAL THERAPIES

Therapists focus on preventing further loss of bone density, utilizing an array of plant and other natural remedies.

HOMEOPATHY 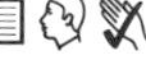

Practitioners claim that constitutional treatment, following an assessment of homeopathic type, can reduce bone loss. They may also suggest standard preparations, such as *Calc. carb.* 6c and *Calc. phos.* 6c.
SEE PAGES 126–30

WESTERN HERBALISM 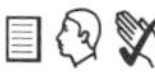

Practitioners may recommend herbs that are rich in calcium, such as parsley, horsetail, dandelion leaf, and nettle. Herbalists may also prescribe plants containing compounds similar to estrogen, such as Chinese angelica (*dang gui*), licorice, false unicorn root, black cohosh, blue cohosh, wild yam, and sage. These are said to be less powerful than synthetic hormones but have fewer side effects. You may be advised to take herbs that aid absorption of minerals, such as dandelion root.
SEE PAGES 134–39

Cautions: Do not take Chinese angelica, licorice, false unicorn root, black cohosh, blue cohosh, wild yam, and medicinal doses of sage or parsley during pregnancy. Do not take licorice if you are anemic or if you have high blood pressure.

CHINESE HERBALISM 

The health of the bones is associated with the Kidney, and treatment aims to enhance the flow of *qi* along the Kidney channels. Remedies may include Chinese angelica (*dang gui*). SEE PAGES 140–43

Caution: Do not take Chinese angelica during pregnancy.

AYURVEDA 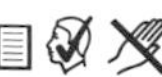

An Ayurvedic practitioner might recommend a traditional formula incorporating sesame seeds, shatavari (the main Ayurvedic rejuvenating herb for women), ginger, and sugar, all thought to stem the progress of osteoporosis.
SEE PAGES 144–47

Caution: Do not take ginger if you have a peptic ulcer.

NUTRITIONAL THERAPIES 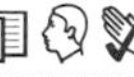

You will be advised to eat foods rich in calcium and boron (which protects against calcium loss), and to avoid foods such as sodas, spinach, and bran that inhibit calcium absorption. Calcium citrate supplements may be given. Extra vitamin C and bioflavonoids may strengthen collagen, the cell-binding protein found in bone. A practitioner may prescribe vitamins B_6 and B_{12}, folic acid, and vitamin K to help bone formation.

CALCIUM
Canned fish, cheese, and other dairy products help build up the body's stores of calcium.

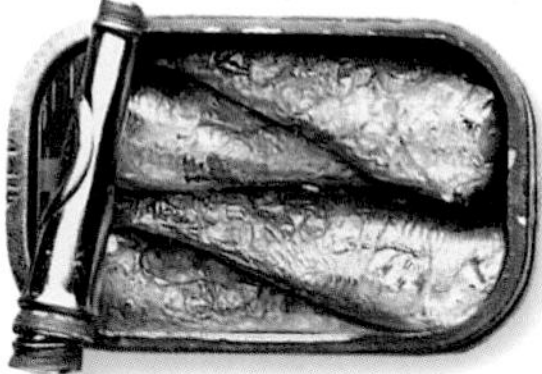

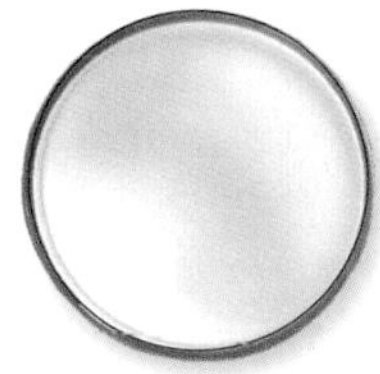

Magnesium, a mineral that plays a role in bone production, is said to be lacking in those with osteoporosis, and supplements may be prescribed. In a US study published in 1990, vegetarians showed less bone loss than those who ate meat, which may be due to their higher dietary levels of calcium.
SEE PAGES 148–52

MAGNETIC THERAPY 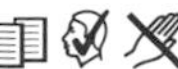

In a research study at the University of Hawaii, pulsating electromagnetic fields improved bone density in osteoporotic women. Whether this can be replicated with equipment outside a medical setting has not yet been demonstrated. SEE PAGE 156

OSTEOARTHRITIS

THIS IS THE MOST COMMON FORM of joint disease, occurring in 80% of people over 50, particularly women after menopause. In osteoarthritis, the cartilage that protects the ends of bones at their point of contact degenerates, and bony outgrowths may form. The symptoms range from mild pain, stiffness, swelling, and "creaking" to a total loss of joint function. In severe cases, the surrounding muscles may waste and the bones may distort. Osteoarthritis tends to strike the large joints that bear weight, such as the hips and knees, as well as small joints in the feet, hands, and fingers, and the vertebrae in the neck and lower back.
Causes Osteoarthritis can result from age-related degeneration, overuse of the joint, or previous injury. It may also follow inflammation caused by rheumatoid arthritis (see page 260) or gout (see opposite). Excess weight may be a factor in the onset of the condition, and so may repetitive impact on the joints caused by strenuous exercise.
Conventional Treatment While there is no cure for osteoarthritis, painkillers, anti-inflammatory drugs, heat treatment, and physiotherapy can relieve pain and maintain mobility. In advanced cases, occasional steroid injections may be advised. Joint replacement surgery is a final option if the cartilage loss is severe.
Self-Help Keep weight down to relieve pressure on the joints. Gentle exercise such as swimming will strengthen the muscles supporting them. Avoid activities that put pressure on joints, such as lifting or walking over rough terrain.

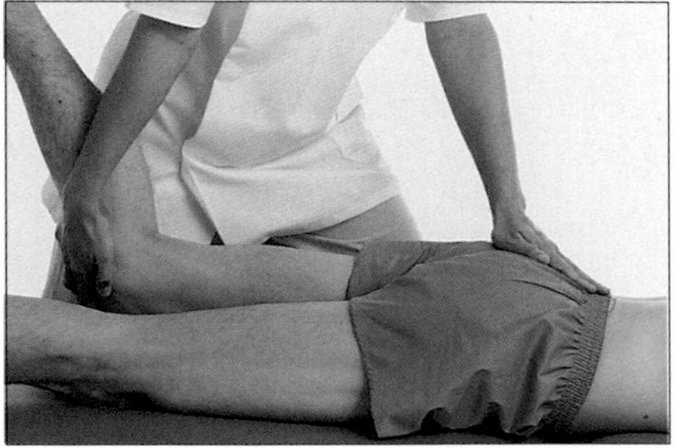

OSTEOPATHIC MANIPULATION
By stretching the soft tissues, the practitioner seeks to increase the mobility of the affected joint, to increase circulation, and to treat any related muscle tension.

TOUCH & MOVEMENT THERAPIES

Osteoarthritis may not be curable, but practitioners believe that the degeneration may be slowed and made less painful with massage, manipulation, and gentle exercise.

CHIROPRACTIC (SEE OSTEOPATHY)

OSTEOPATHY

A practitioner will encourage the relaxation of the surrounding tissues, and improve the circulation and mobility of the affected joint with manipulation. Trigger points (see page 250) may develop in related muscles, which practitioners will treat using soft-tissue techniques and stretching. **SEE PAGES 70–81**

ACUPUNCTURE

According to the World Health Organization, osteoarthritis is one of the 104 conditions that acupuncture can treat effectively. Your practitioner will stimulate appropriate acupoints with needles or moxibustion to relieve pain and inflammation. **SEE PAGES 90–94**

YOGA

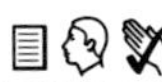

A teacher will show you gentle stretching *asanas*, or postures, to strengthen the muscles that protect joints, increase flexibility, and improve circulation. The Single-leg Raising posture, for example, is thought to be especially helpful for pains in the knee, and the Embryo posture for pains in the hip. **SEE PAGES 108–11**

OTHER OPTIONS

Massage	SEE PAGES 56–61
Aromatherapy	SEE PAGES 62–65
Hellerwork	SEE PAGE 84
Acupressure	SEE PAGE 95
Shiatsu	SEE PAGES 96–97
T'ai Chi Ch'uan	SEE PAGES 100–101

MEDICINAL THERAPIES

Some practitioners believe that diet and nutrition are significant in the onset and progress of osteoarthritis. They seek to rectify nutritional deficiencies and thereby help the body overcome obstacles to well-being.

NATUROPATHY

A practitioner will advise general dietary measures designed to improve overall nutrition, digestion, and elimination. These usually include cutting down on highly refined processed foods, saturated animal fats, sugar, and salt, and eating more whole-grain cereals, fresh fruits, and vegetables. **SEE PAGES 118–21**

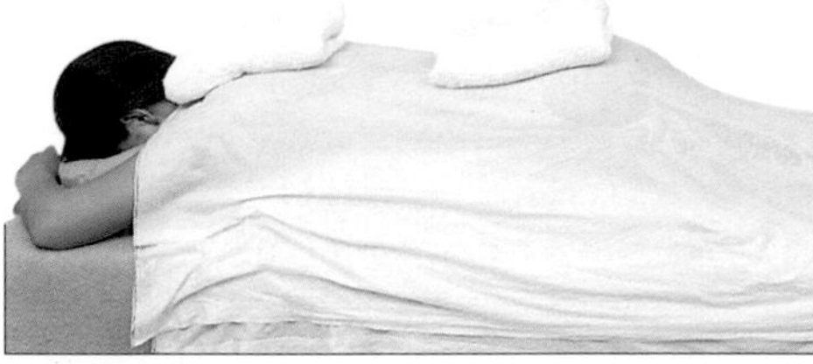

HYDROTHERAPY
Compresses or packs may be advised by therapists to reduce inflammation and dull pain.

HYDROTHERAPY

If you are generally healthy, a practitioner may advise applying cold compresses for 4–8 hours to relieve pain and swelling, or alternate hot and cold compresses to boost circulation and ease stiffness. Gentle exercise in warm water may also be recommended. **SEE PAGES 122–23**

WESTERN HERBALISM

To reduce swelling, a practitioner may suggest infusions of celery seed, lignum vitae, juniper, and devil's claw. Circulatory stimulants such as cinnamon may also be advised. **SEE PAGES 134–39**
Caution: Do not take juniper, devil's claw, or medicinal doses of celery seed or cinnamon during pregnancy.

NUTRITIONAL THERAPIES

Some researchers claim the essential amino acid methionine may reduce swelling more effectively than the drug ibuprofen. Studies indicate that glucosamine sulfate, a major component of joint fluid, may be helpful as a supplement. Chondroitin, vitamins E and C (which are often deficient in the elderly), and pantothenic acid are reported to have positive effects on cartilage. Supplements of vitamins A and B_6, zinc, and magnesium, involved in the production of the structural protein collagen, may also be recommended. **SEE PAGES 148–52**

OTHER OPTIONS

Homeopathy	SEE PAGES 126–30
Chinese Herbalism	SEE PAGES 140–43

MIND & EMOTION THERAPIES

Therapists believe that the mind can be harnessed to ease pain.

RELAXATION & BREATHING

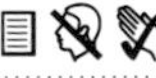

Relaxation can help counteract the muscle tension that often accompanies stiff and painful joints. **SEE PAGES 170–73**

OTHER OPTION

Visualization	SEE PAGES 178–79

CERVICAL SPONDYLOSIS

IN THIS TYPE of osteoarthritis, which mainly affects middle-aged and elderly people, joints and disks between the neck vertebrae degenerate, causing pain and stiffness. The condition is part of the aging process and affects virtually everyone to some degree, but most people show few or no symptoms. If the affected structures press on adjacent nerves, however, tingling, numbness, pins and needles, or pain in the hands and legs may result. Other symptoms, generally caused by pressure on neighboring blood vessels, include headaches, double vision, dizziness, or unsteadiness when the neck is turned.

Conventional Treatment Neck exercises, physiotherapy, painkillers, and a cervical collar may all be recommended as part of conventional treatment. Some form of physiotherapy, perhaps including ultrasound treatment and exercise, may also be proposed. In rare cases, surgery may be advised to deal with pressure on the nerve.

Caution: Consult a doctor if you have symptoms of cervical spondylosis.

COMPLEMENTARY TREATMENTS

Chiropractors and osteopaths may be able to help by easing pressure on the affected nerves and joints. The stimulation of acupoints by practitioners of Eastern therapies is another option that may be effective in relieving pain.

MASSAGE

A therapist may use firm stroking movements down the neck and back to alleviate muscle tension and enhance blood supply in the affected area. SEE PAGES 56–61

AROMATHERAPY

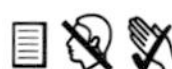

Massage with diluted lavender oil and warm baths incorporating the essential oils of rosemary, cedarwood, or the vanilla-scented benzoin may help increase flexibility.
SEE PAGES 62–65

CHIROPRACTIC (SEE OSTEOPATHY)

OSTEOPATHY

A study reported in the *British Medical Journal* in 1991 concluded that manipulative therapies produced slightly better results than physiotherapy over a period of 12 months.
SEE PAGES 70–81

ACUPUNCTURE

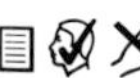

Neck and shoulder pain is attributed to an invasion of "cold and damp" or an imbalance in *qi* ("life energy"). The stimulation of appropriate acupoints, such as those along the Gallbladder meridian, will help rebalance *qi* and reduce inflammation and pain.
SEE PAGES 90–94

ACUPRESSURE

Firm stimulation of acupoints along the Gallbladder and Large Intestine meridians may help alleviate pain. SEE PAGE 95

HOMEOPATHY

To relieve symptoms, a practitioner might suggest remedies such as *Arnica 6c* if the pain is worse in heat and after prolonged movement, or *Rhus tox. 6c* for pain that is worse in cold, wet weather, after rest, and upon rising.
SEE PAGES 126–30

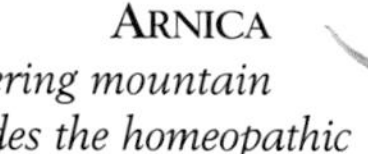

ARNICA
This flowering mountain plant provides the homeopathic remedy of the same name.

GOUT

GOUT IS A FORM of arthritis in which uric acid crystals – a waste product of protein breakdown – build up in a joint, causing it to become inflamed and very painful for a few days. These symptoms are often accompanied by fever. Attacks generally strike the big toe first and most painfully, then recur at decreasing intervals, possibly spreading to the knees, knuckles, and elbows. Most sufferers are men over 35 years of age. The precise causes are unknown, but gout often runs in families and may lead to kidney stones (see page 241). Blood disorders, obesity, and certain drugs increase its likelihood, and rich food and alcohol may be factors in the onset of an attack.

Conventional Treatment At the outset, a doctor will prescribe painkillers (except aspirin, which exacerbates gout) and anti-inflammatory drugs, followed by others that reduce uric acid levels. Drinking plenty of water may also prevent the buildup of uric acid.

COMPLEMENTARY TREATMENTS

Therapists will seek to use the body's natural eliminative processes, perhaps in conjunction with medicinal substances, homeopathic remedies, or dietary changes, to reduce uric acid levels in the body.

NATUROPATHY

As in all chronic inflammatory conditions, a naturopath will look for an underlying problem related to your digestion and elimination and treat accordingly. You will be advised not to eat foods high in purines (oily fish, shellfish, organ meats, game, poultry, legumes, caffeine, and alcohol) that increase levels of uric acid in the blood. Unsubstantiated clinical observation indicates that fresh or canned cherries, eaten regularly, may help lower blood levels of uric acid.
SEE PAGES 118–21

CHERRIES
Eating ½ lb (225 g) of cherries a day may help people with gout.

HOMEOPATHY

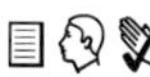

Homeopaths prefer to treat patients on the basis of their constitutional type, but the following standard remedies may be recommended: *Ledum 6c* for joint pain eased by cold, *Colchicum 6c* if joints are especially painful at night, *Arnica 6c* if joints feel bruised, *Urtica 6c* if joints burn or itch, and *Pulsatilla 6c* if the pain moves between the joints. *Urtica urens* tincture is thought to help eliminate uric acid. SEE PAGES 126–30

WESTERN HERBALISM

Celery seed is believed to increase the elimination of uric acid. The efficacy of devil's claw as an anti-inflammatory is debatable, but trials indicate that it may relieve pain and reduce blood levels of uric acid and cholesterol.
SEE PAGES 134–39

Caution: Do not take devil's claw or medicinal doses of celery seed during pregnancy.

OTHER OPTIONS

Acupuncture	SEE PAGES 90–94
Hydrotherapy	SEE PAGES 122–23
Ayurveda	SEE PAGES 144–47
Nutritional Therapies	SEE PAGES 148–52

RHEUMATOID ARTHRITIS

IN RHEUMATOID ARTHRITIS, the membrane that lines a joint capsule becomes painfully swollen and the joint becomes stiff, particularly after a night's sleep.

Symptoms The first indications may be a vague muscular ache and a general feeling of malaise, with joint pain and swelling occurring later. In other instances, the onset is sudden and severe. Small joints, such as the knuckles and toes, are most susceptible, but the wrists, ankles, knees, and neck may also be affected. Mild anemia usually accompanies the disorder. In severe cases, the inflammation spreads to the neighboring cartilage and bone, causing deformity and disability. Occasionally, the lungs, eyes, bowel, and other organs are also affected. The condition generally strikes between the ages of 40 and 50; women are at three times greater risk than men.

Causes Unlike osteoarthritis (see page 258), rheumatoid arthritis is an autoimmune disease, where the immune system attacks the body's own tissues (see Immune System, pages 308–309). The specific cause is unknown, but factors such as viral infection, stress, diet, and bacterial overgrowth in the gut have been considered as possible contributors.

Conventional Treatment Diagnosis relies upon a thorough physical examination and blood tests to establish the presence of a substance called rheumatoid factor. X rays will also be taken to determine the extent of joint damage. Treatment may include physiotherapy, heat treatment, painkillers, and anti-inflammatory drugs. In serious cases, a doctor may advise steroid or gold injections, or immunosuppressant drugs taken under close supervision. If the joint is severely damaged, joint replacement surgery may be suggested.

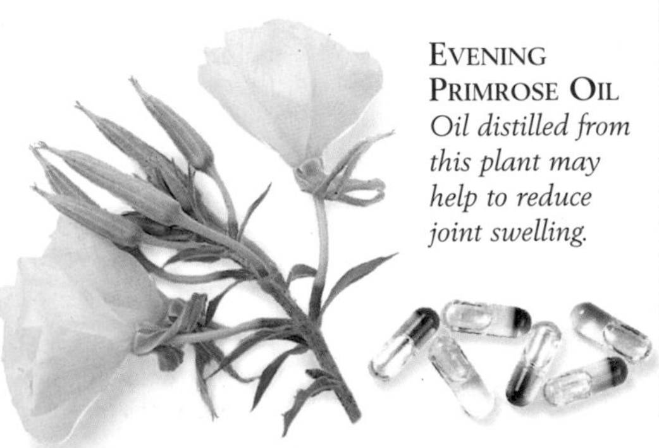

EVENING PRIMROSE OIL *Oil distilled from this plant may help to reduce joint swelling.*

TOUCH & MOVEMENT THERAPIES

Gentle movement therapies and manipulation can help to maintain mobility in the affected joints.

MASSAGE 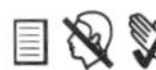

A practitioner may use a light cream or oil to massage the tissues around a joint. Employing gentle strokes toward the heart, the masseur will aim to stimulate circulation in and around the affected joint, thereby promoting the removal of waste products. SEE PAGES 56–61

AROMATHERAPY

Massage with rosemary, benzoin, German chamomile, camphor, juniper, or lavender essential oil may help relieve pain. The essential oils of cypress, fennel, lemon, and wintergreen in particular, are said to detoxify and may reduce inflammation. SEE PAGES 62–65

Caution: Do not use German chamomile, juniper, or cypress essential oils during pregnancy.

ACUPUNCTURE 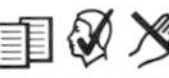

Chronic inflammatory diseases are thought of as deep-seated problems, so practitioners will consider the individual's overall pattern of disharmony prior to beginning treatment. The stimulation of appropriate acupoints may offer effective pain relief. SEE PAGES 90–94

CHIROPRACTIC (SEE OSTEOPATHY)

OSTEOPATHY 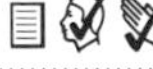

While joint manipulation is not an appropriate treatment for rheumatoid arthritis, stretching and careful trigger point therapy (see page 250) may improve overall mobility. SEE PAGES 70–81

MEDICINAL THERAPIES

Complementary therapists believe that nutrition plays a significant role in the onset and progress of rheumatoid arthritis. They may suggest changing your diet or adding food supplements as a way of boosting the immune system and counteracting symptoms.

NATUROPATHY

A naturopath will generally recommend a diet high in whole grains, vegetables, and fiber, and low in sugar, animal-derived foods, and refined carbohydrates. Evidence reported in *The Lancet* in 1991 indicates that food sensitivities and dietary fat can help to cause rheumatoid arthritis. Common suspects include eggs, dairy products, and cereal grains. To detect culprit foods, your practitioner may suggest applied kinesiology (see pages 196–97) and other diagnostic tests, or an exclusion diet, which is probably the most reliable approach. Evidence reported in the *British Journal of Rheumatology* in 1993 showed that fish oils have an anti-inflammatory effect. Other published evidence attributes this property to evening primrose oil, soybeans, and New Zealand green-lipped mussels. There is some evidence that sufferers are deficient in copper. Copper bracelets are said to transfer minute amounts of this trace element through the skin, which, at least one study suggests, helps to relieve arthritis pain and stiffness. These claims, however, are controversial. SEE PAGES 118–21

HYDROTHERAPY 

A practitioner might recommend a program that includes exercising the affected joints in warm water to increase mobility. SEE PAGES 122–23

HOMEOPATHY 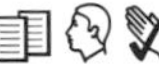

A 1980 Scottish trial found that homeopathic treatment compared favorably with aspirin or a placebo. A practitioner will give an individual assessment and prescribe suitable remedies. SEE PAGES 126–30

WESTERN HERBALISM 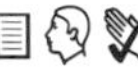

Bupleurum root, turmeric, and Chinese skullcap are well-established anti-inflammatory herbs that might be prescribed to combat swelling. SEE PAGES 134–39

CHINESE HERBALISM 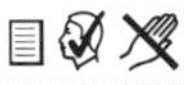

Rheumatoid arthritis is often associated both with "excess internal cold" and the "stagnation of *qi* ('life energy'), blood, and cold-damp." Among the restorative formulas that might be advised is Chinese Angelica Zi Yi Tonic, which includes Chinese angelica (*dang gui*), licorice, ginger, and cinnamon, among other ingredients. Practitioners may also attribute painful joints to "wind cold." Cinnamon may be recommended to release *qi*, along with aconite, angelica root, and ginger to relieve "cold" and "damp." SEE PAGES 140–43

Cautions: Do not take Chinese angelica, aconite, licorice, medicinal doses of cinnamon, or angelica root during pregnancy. Do not take licorice if you are anemic or if you have high blood pressure. Do not take ginger if you have a peptic ulcer.

NUTRITIONAL THERAPIES 

Flavonoids, pancreatic enzymes, and bromelain, an enzyme found in pineapple, may be recommended for their anti-inflammatory properties. In one study, reported in *The Lancet* in 1976, patients taking zinc supplements reported less swelling and discomfort. SEE PAGES 148–52

ANKYLOSING SPONDYLITIS

AN AUTOIMMUNE DISEASE (see glossary) that mostly develops in young men, ankylosing spondylitis strikes the joints of the spine and those between the spine and pelvis, causing inflammation, pain, and stiffness. Eventually, the joints may stiffen permanently and the spine may curve. The condition generally begins with a persistent lower backache and stiffness, especially after resting. Affecting more men than women, it strikes mostly between the ages of 20 and 40.

Cause The cause of the disorder is unknown, but heredity is an important factor. Research at King's College Hospital, London, also implicates an overgrowth of bacteria in the gut.

Conventional Treatment While there is no cure, early diagnosis and treatment are important to help keep the spine supple. To decrease pain and increase mobility, a doctor will prescribe painkillers, anti-inflammatory drugs, and physiotherapy. Gentle daily exercise, especially in water, will be advised.

COMPLEMENTARY TREATMENTS

Manipulation of the body to encourage mobility can help at every stage of the disease. Many practitioners will also attempt to slow down the progress of the disorder with diet, remedies, or supplements.

YOGA STRETCH
Stiffening of the spine may be offset by postures such as this, which encourage flexibility.

THE FELDENKRAIS METHOD

In this therapy, which seeks to improve health by "reprogramming" movement patterns, a practitioner will develop exercises that suit your particular needs. SEE PAGE 85

THE ALEXANDER TECHNIQUE

A practitioner will show you how to be more aware of your body, enabling you to adjust your posture to relieve pain, ease stiffness, facilitate breathing, and combat any tendency toward curvature of the spine. SEE PAGES 86–87

ACUPUNCTURE

Relief from the pain of ankylosing spondylitis may be gained through the stimulation of appropriate acupoints with needles or with moxibustion. SEE PAGES 90–94

YOGA

A qualified teacher will instruct you in gentle stretching postures (*asanas*) that will improve your flexibility and suppleness. Practiced regularly, they may counteract progressive stiffness in the spine.
SEE PAGES 108–11

RELAXATION & BREATHING

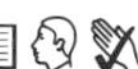

A practitioner will show you breathing and stretching exercises to release the diaphragm and open the rib cage. This helps to counteract stiffness and release tension, especially in the upper body. SEE PAGES 170–73

OTHER OPTIONS

Massage	SEE PAGES 56–61
Aromatherapy	SEE PAGES 62–65
Chiropractic	SEE PAGES 70–75
Osteopathy	SEE PAGES 76–81
Naturopathy	SEE PAGES 118–21
Western Herbalism	SEE PAGES 134–39
Nutritional Therapies	SEE PAGES 148–52

SPORTS INJURIES

SUDDEN INJURIES TO JOINTS, muscles, tendons, and ligaments are common in sporting activities (see also Muscle Pain, page 251, and Tendinitis, page 252). They may be accompanied by bleeding, bruising, swelling, and pain.

Conventional Treatment To ensure swift and complete recovery, treatment should be immediate. If there is no broken bone, a doctor will recommend that you cease activity and apply ice for ten-minute periods over the next 24 hours to help keep swelling to a minimum. The affected area should be raised and compressed with a bandage. Painkillers, anti-inflammatory drugs, and physiotherapy, especially ultrasound, may help. A doctor will also advise you to resume gentle movement as soon as it is no longer painful. Warming up the muscles before sports activities by jogging in place and then stretching, and stretching again afterward, may prevent many such injuries.

Caution: If the pain is severe, an X ray is essential.

COMPLEMENTARY TREATMENTS

When treating muscle pain caused by sudden injury, most therapists will recommend plenty of rest, foods that encourage tissue repair, and the application of appropriate medicinal substances to the affected area.

MASSAGE

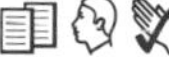

Gentle massage starting a few days after the injury will improve circulation to the damaged tissues, warming them and helping to speed healing. SEE PAGES 56–61

ACUPUNCTURE

If a sports injury has been slow to heal and is an ongoing source of pain, the stimulation of appropriate local acupoints and trigger points (see page 250) may help to ease discomfort.
SEE PAGES 90–94

HYDROTHERAPY

In addition to the application of ice packs or cold compresses, a practitioner may recommend exercise in a hydrotherapy pool to help restore strength and flexibility in the injured area. SEE PAGES 122–23

NUTRITIONAL THERAPIES

In studies performed in the 1960s, the recovery time of sports injuries was halved when patients were given supplements of citrus bioflavonoids, substances that help maintain body structures. A practitioner may also propose supplements of bromelain, an enzyme present in fresh pineapple that is thought to accelerate tissue repair and is frequently recommended for treating sports injuries. Essential fatty acids and the antioxidant vitamins C and E may also be suggested.
SEE PAGES 148–52

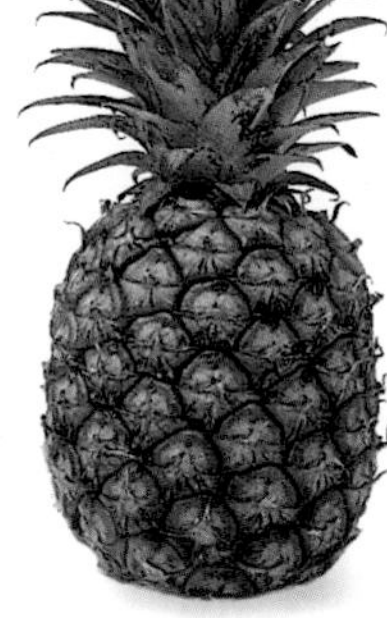

PINEAPPLE
Bromelain, an enzyme in pineapple, may prove useful in repairing soft-tissue damage.

OTHER OPTIONS

Chiropractic	SEE PAGES 70–75
Osteopathy	SEE PAGES 76–81

Hormones

The human body has an immense ability to cope successfully with environmental change, stressful demands, and fluctuating amounts of sleep and food. This is due largely to the interaction of the brain, nervous system, and the endocrine (hormonal) system. The endocrine glands secrete chemicals, known as hormones, into the bloodstream to regulate different body functions. They keep blood sugar levels constant, for example, and orchestrate the metabolism, blood clotting, response to stress, and the menstrual cycle. An imbalance of hormones is linked to a wide range of problems, including diabetes.

Key to Symbols

Evidence	Practitioner
Good scientific trials with positive results	Essential
Some research studies	Recommended
Anecdotal	Not essential
	Self-Help
	Self-help possibilities
	No self-help

Complementary Approaches

Complementary therapies take an indirect approach to the treatment of hormone disorders. Rather than directly stimulating or counteracting the output of hormones, practitioners encourage the immune system to function in a harmonious fashion. They may advocate lifestyle changes, gentle exercise, and natural remedies to promote and maintain the good health of all the internal organs.

Conventional Approaches

The development of treatments for hormone disorders is one of the great successes of conventional medicine. Effective medication is now available for diseases that previously had been uncontrollable, such as diabetes and thyroid gland disorders.

Caution: Before seeking treatment, see page 204.

How the Endocrine System Works

The hypothalamus in the brain controls the pituitary gland, which produces hormones and orchestrates all hormonal activity. The thyroid gland in the neck produces a hormone that regulates the metabolism (see glossary). The adrenal glands coordinate the body's response to stress, physical injury, and infection. The outer layer produces male sex hormones (androgens) in both men and women, as well as hormones that affect the metabolism and control blood volume and pressure. The interior produces the stress hormones epinephrine and norepinephrine. One of the functions of the pancreas, an organ in the upper abdomen, is to secrete insulin, a hormone that regulates blood sugar levels. In women, ovaries on either side of the uterus produce the female sex hormones estrogen and progesterone; in men, the testes produce the hormone testosterone. Other sources of hormones include the pineal gland in the brain, which produces melatonin, affecting body rhythms, and the thymus in the chest, part of the immune system.

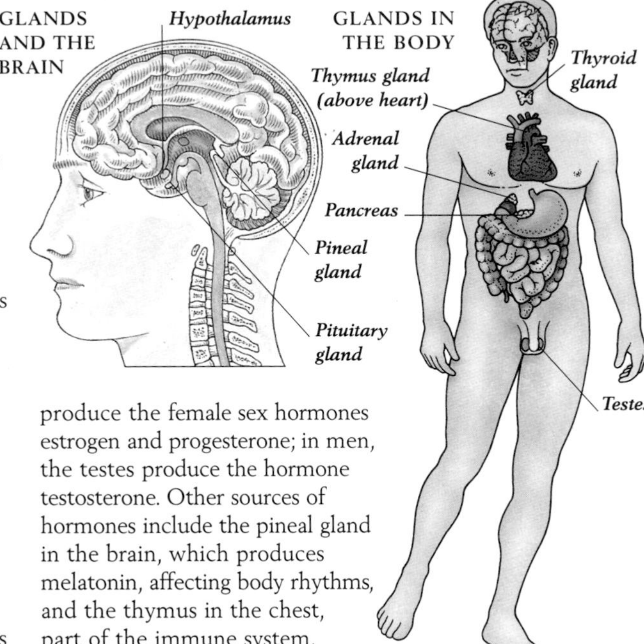

Hypothyroidism

An underactive thyroid results in inadequate production of the hormone that regulates the metabolism. Symptoms may include a goiter (enlargement of the thyroid gland at the front of the neck), lethargy, constipation, low body temperature, dry skin and hair, weight gain, depression, loss of libido, heavy menstrual periods, and arrested development in children. A doctor will prescribe supplements of the thyroid hormone thyroxin.

Caution: Consult a doctor before undertaking any complementary treatments.

Complementary Treatments

Dietary advice may complement conventional treatments to restore thyroid function.

Naturopathy

A practitioner will recommend iodine-rich foods, such as seaweed, sea fish, eggs, and milk, since iodine is needed by the thyroid for hormone production. You may be told to avoid raw cabbage, turnips, rutabagas, peanuts, and mustard, which interfere with the body's ability to absorb iodine. A practitioner will also suggest foods rich in B vitamins and selenium. SEE PAGES 118–21

Western Herbalism

Kelp and sea vegetables have a high iodine content and are regarded by practitioners as an almost universal tonic for the thyroid. SEE PAGES 134–39

Caution: Do not eat kelp during pregnancy or if breastfeeding.

Seaweed
This is one of the best sources of iodine.

DIABETES MELLITUS

INSULIN, A HORMONE produced by the pancreas, helps body cells absorb glucose (a sugar) from the blood. If insulin is deficient or absent, diabetes mellitus results, a condition in which blood glucose levels remain high and the tissues may not receive enough sugar. Symptoms include thirst and frequent urination, fatigue, weight loss, and recurrent infections. Problems with vision and circulation may develop. If untreated, very high blood sugar levels may lead to coma and death.

Conventional Treatment There is no cure, but treatment can control symptoms. Diagnosis includes a urine test for excess glucose and monitoring of blood sugar levels. There are two main forms of diabetes. Insulin-dependent diabetes mellitus (IDDM) usually begins in childhood. Noninsulin-dependent diabetes mellitus (NIDDM) develops later and may be treated with insulin and other drugs, or dietary control alone may be sufficient. All diabetics require a controlled diet to regulate blood sugar levels and annual checkups to detect damage to the eyes, nerves, and blood vessels.

Caution: If you have diabetes, consult your doctor before beginning a course of complementary therapy, and do not stop taking any prescribed medication.

COMPLEMENTARY TREATMENTS

Stress, poor diet, and lack of exercise all have a destabilizing effect on blood sugar levels. These factors may be remedied with therapies that promote a healthy lifestyle.

YOGA 

As well as being a good form of exercise, yoga may facilitate diet control, reduce stress, and enhance pancreatic function. A yoga teacher may particularly recommend postures such as the Boat, Fish, Half Wheel, and Backward and Forward Bend. SEE PAGES 108–11

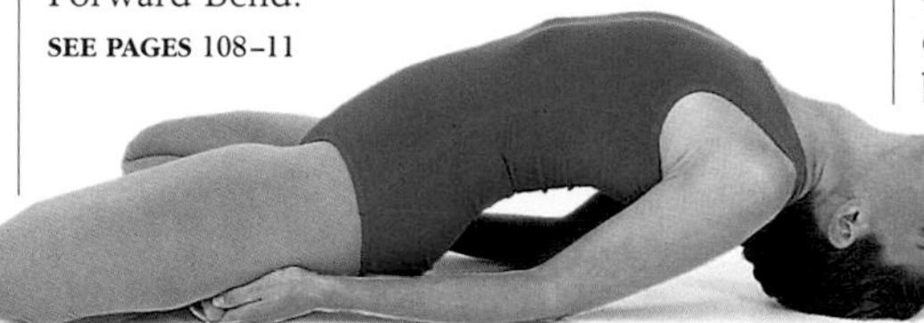

FISH POSE
This variation of the fish posture expands the lungs fully and helps to relieve stress.

NATUROPATHY 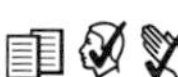

A practitioner will devise a diet that is high in complex carbohydrates (starchy foods such as bread and pasta) and fiber, and low in sugar and fat to encourage steady blood sugar levels. Diabetics are more prone to heart disease, and olive oil, garlic, and vitamin E may be advised to protect against this. Other recommended foods include oats to stabilize sugar levels, chromium to help normalize the metabolism of blood sugar, and onion and garlic, which contain a substance that helps to lower blood sugar levels. Some diabetics develop neuropathy, a nerve condition that causes numbness and tingling in the hands or feet (see page 207). It may be treated specifically with a special diet. SEE PAGES 118–21

AYURVEDA 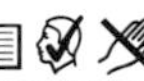

A practitioner may recommend *panchakarma,* a purification process thought to cleanse the digestive tract and increase vitality. You will also be advised to follow a diet that is high in complex carbohydrates (starchy foods such as bread and pasta) and low in fat. "Bitter" foods, such as green bananas, are considered helpful. SEE PAGES 144–47

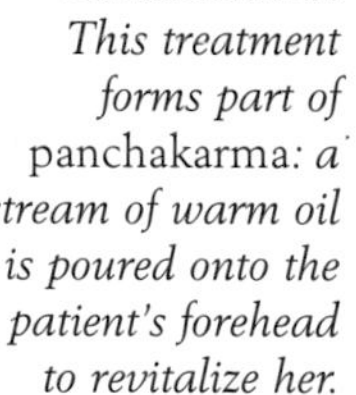

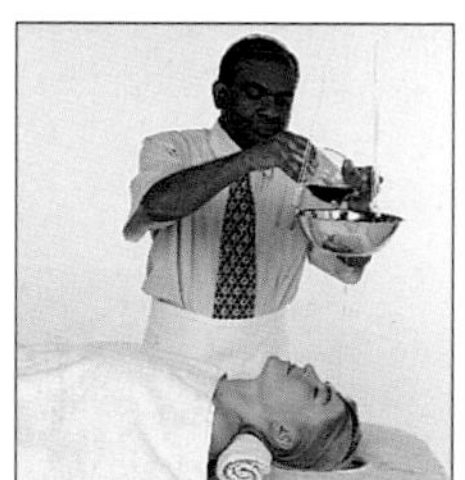

SHIRODHARA
This treatment forms part of panchakarma*: a stream of warm oil is poured onto the patient's forehead to revitalize her.*

OTHER OPTIONS

Western Herbalism SEE PAGES 134–39
Chinese Herbalism SEE PAGES 140–43
Nutritional Therapies SEE PAGES 148–52
Biofeedback SEE PAGE 169
Relaxation & Breathing SEE PAGES 170–73

OBESITY

A VERY HIGH PROPORTION of body fat (obesity) is a common problem in developed countries and is a major health risk, particularly if it is distributed mainly around the waist. If more calories are eaten than are burned off, they are stored as fat. Obesity may be caused by a number of factors besides overeating, including lack of exercise, a hormone deficiency such as hypothyroidism, psychological conditions, such as depression, that result in "comfort eating," and heredity – children of obese parents are ten times more likely than others to be overweight. A doctor will suggest a calorie-restricted, low-fat diet and regular exercise. Appetite suppressants may help; jaw-wiring is an extreme option.

Caution: Do not follow a strict diet for long periods without medical supervision.

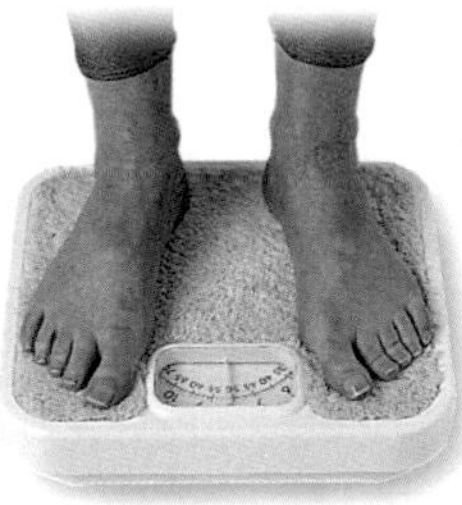

MONITORING WEIGHT LOSS
Weigh yourself once a week, at the same time of day. Slow, steady weight loss is best: aim to lose 2 lb (1 kg) a week.

COMPLEMENTARY TREATMENTS

Therapies such as counseling boost self-esteem, and acupuncture may reduce cravings.

AURICULAR ACUPUNCTURE

Practitioners tape tiny pins to acupoints on the ear to help regulate the appetite. SEE PAGE 94

NATUROPATHY 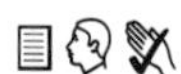

Naturopaths aim to change eating habits to encourage long-term weight loss. You will be told to eat plenty of fruits, vegetables, and complex carbohydrates (bread and pasta), and to avoid fats and sugar. Practitioners believe that unstable blood sugar levels and cravings may in some cases suggest food intolerances (see page 303), and they may advise an exclusion diet to reveal the culprit foods. SEE PAGES 118–21

PSYCHOTHERAPY & COUNSELING 

Group therapy may resolve emotional problems that are expressed through overeating. Cognitive behavioral therapy can help change attitudes toward food. SEE PAGES 160–65

HYPNOTHERAPY 

Hypnotherapy is effective in improving motivation to follow a diet. SEE PAGES 166–67

OTHER OPTIONS

Western Herbalism SEE PAGES 134–39
Nutritional Therapies SEE PAGES 148–52

WOMEN'S HEALTH

THE FEMALE REPRODUCTIVE ORGANS are the uterus (womb), ovaries, fallopian tubes, vagina, cervix, and vulva. The uterus is a pear-shaped organ in which a baby grows when the woman's egg (ovum) is fertilized by a man's sperm. The ovaries, two small glands at the ends of the fallopian tubes, store the lifetime's supply of eggs with which a woman is born, and produce the female hormones estrogen and progesterone. The hormones' healthy interaction governs the dramatic changes in a woman's body over the average lifespan, from the onset of menstruation through conception, pregnancy and labor, and finally to menopause.

KEY TO SYMBOLS

EVIDENCE	PRACTITIONER
Good scientific trials with positive results	Essential
Some research studies	Recommended
Anecdotal	Not essential
	SELF-HELP
	Self-help possibilities
	No self-help

COMPLEMENTARY APPROACHES

Practitioners aim to insure hormone balance and healthy circulation. Herbal tonics, hormone-balancing herbs, nutritional supplements, and muscle relaxants may be useful. Relaxing and calming techniques are often effective in tackling stress-related symptoms.

CONVENTIONAL APPROACHES

Powerful hormone-based treatments can control many kinds of menstrual and menopausal problems. Hysterectomy (surgical removal of the uterus) is now performed less frequently. Regular cervical smear tests can detect the early stages of cervical cancer.

Caution: Before seeking treatment, see page 204.

HOW THE FEMALE REPRODUCTIVE SYSTEM WORKS

In each menstrual cycle, the pituitary gland at the base of the skull produces follicle-stimulating hormone (FSH), which triggers an egg to develop in one of the ovaries. Estrogen levels begin to rise dramatically. After about 12 days, another hormone, luteinizing hormone (LH), triggers ovulation, when the egg leaves the ovary and travels along the fallopian tube to the uterus. After ovulation, progesterone levels rise to encourage the uterus lining to thicken. If the egg is fertilized, it will attach itself to the uterine lining and begin to develop into a baby. If unfertilized, the egg will disintegrate and progesterone levels drop. The remains of the egg and the uterine lining are flushed out during menstruation.

FEMALE REPRODUCTIVE ORGANS

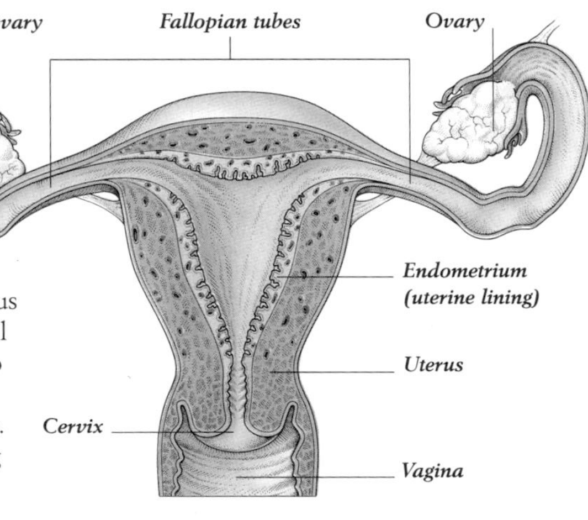

PREMENSTRUAL SYNDROME (PMS)

IN THE DAYS LEADING UP to menstruation, many women experience some form of discomfort, which may include physical problems (such as headaches, breast tenderness, and fluid retention) as well as emotional distress (anxiety, depression, and irritability). There is a variety of conventional treatments, ranging from oil of evening primrose and vitamin B_6 supplements (deficiency of B_6 can produce an imbalance between estrogen and progesterone) to progesterone treatment, estrogen implants, diuretics, painkillers, and antidepressants. Moderate exercise is recommended, particularly in the week before menstruation, since this improves the circulation, relieves fluid retention, and reduces stress levels.

COMPLEMENTARY TREATMENTS

A healthier diet and relaxation techniques can have a dramatic effect on PMS.

REFLEXOLOGY

A US study reported in the journal *Obstetrics and Gynecology* in 1993 found reflexology effective in relieving PMS symptoms.
SEE PAGES 66–67

NATUROPATHY

As women with PMS tend to eat too much sugar and refined carbohydrates, they may have a deficiency of vitamin B complex. You may be advised to reduce intake of refined carbohydrates, saturated fats, and salt, and to eat food high in protein every three hours if you suffer from cravings. Some practitioners test for food intolerances. SEE PAGES 118–21

WESTERN HERBALISM

A practitioner may prescribe agnus castus, thought to balance hormones, cramp bark, a traditional cramp remedy, dandelion, a diuretic herb, and calendula and cleavers, said to relieve breast swelling.
SEE PAGES 134–39

CHINESE HERBALISM

Symptoms may be associated with imbalances of the Spleen, Kidney, and Liver meridians. You may be advised to avoid "cold" foods (such as salads), "hot" foods (such as spicy curries), greasy foods, and red meat between ovulation and menstruation. SEE PAGES 140–43

OTHER OPTIONS

Massage SEE PAGES 56–61
Yoga SEE PAGES 108–11
Psychotherapy & Counseling SEE PAGES 160–65

MENSTRUAL PAIN

MENSTRUAL PAIN (DYSMENORRHEA) is characterized by dull aches in the lower back, often with cramps and headaches, for two or three days. Primary dysmenorrhea starts soon after puberty and ends around the age of 25. Causes include an excess of, or sensitivity to, prostaglandins (see glossary). Unprecedented painful periods are termed secondary dysmenorrhea. Causes include pelvic infection, an IUD (intrauterine contraceptive device), fibroids, endometriosis, or constipation. **Conventional Treatment** Primary dysmenorrhea can be treated with drugs to relax muscles or inhibit uterine contractions, and to inhibit secretion of hormones. Secondary dysmenorrhea is treated according to the cause.

Caution: Consult a doctor if you suspect secondary dysmenorrhea.

COMPLEMENTARY TREATMENTS

Therapies aim to normalize circulation in the uterus or to lower prostaglandin levels.

CHIROPRACTIC (SEE OSTEOPATHY)

OSTEOPATHY

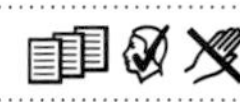

Trials have shown that these therapies can help menstrual pain. SEE PAGES 70–81

ACUPUNCTURE

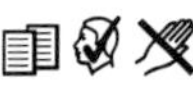

In 1987, the UK journal *Obstetrics and Gynaecology* published a trial in which 91% of subjects had less pain after acupuncture. SEE PAGES 90–94

YOGA

Yoga is said to relieve stress, normalize hormone balance, relax muscles, and tone the pelvis. Postures to release tension in the lower abdomen may be recommended. SEE PAGES 108–11

SHOULDERSTAND
This pose is believed by some to help ease menstrual pain.

NATUROPATHY

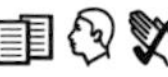

A practitioner may suggest essential fatty acids, found in oily fish and evening primrose oil, which inhibit prostaglandins. Some practitioners advise avoiding meat, dairy products, and eggs. These contain arachidonic acid, which promotes prostaglandin manufacture. SEE PAGES 118–21

HYDROTHERAPY

Alternate hot and cold sitz baths are said to improve uterine blood supply and relieve pelvic congestion. SEE PAGES 122–23

Caution: Avoid alternating hot and cold baths or showers if you have a heart condition.

OTHER OPTIONS

The Alexander Technique — SEE PAGES 86–87
Shiatsu — SEE PAGES 96–97
Western Herbalism — SEE PAGES 134–39

IRREGULAR PERIODS

PERIODS MAY BE ABSENT or irregular during pregnancy, breastfeeding, or menopause, or because of fluctuations in weight, hormonal imbalances, too much exercise, or serious illness such as a thyroid problem. If the condition is caused by a failure to ovulate, doctors may advise the hormone clomiphene.

Caution: Consult a doctor if you experience bleeding between periods or after sexual intercourse.

COMPLEMENTARY TREATMENTS

Diet and lifestyle may contribute to the problem. Therapies aim to improve both.

AROMATHERAPY

You may be massaged with essential oils believed to help induce menstruation, such as basil, clary sage, and fennel. SEE PAGES 62–65

Caution: Consult a qualified practitioner if you suspect you may be pregnant.

NATUROPATHY

See Heavy Periods, below. SEE PAGES 118–21

WESTERN HERBALISM

A practitioner may recommend the herbs shatavari, agnus castus, and sage to help regulate the menstrual cycle. SEE PAGES 134–39

Caution: Do not take sage if you may be pregnant.

OTHER OPTION

Chinese Herbalism — SEE PAGES 140–43

HEAVY PERIODS

HEAVY MENSTRUAL PERIODS may be due to an IUD (intrauterine contraceptive device) or to hormonal imbalances, fibroids, endometriosis, or pelvic infection, among other more rare conditions. Conventional treatment depends on the cause, although often no obvious reason can be identified. Hormone treatments may be prescribed to lessen bleeding, with antibiotics if the cause is an infection. You may be advised to have a D&C (dilation and curettage), an operation in which the uterine lining is scraped away. Iron supplements may be prescribed to prevent and treat anemia.

Caution: Consult a doctor if you have heavy periods.

COMPLEMENTARY TREATMENTS

Diet and herbal remedies can sometimes help to relieve heavy periods.

NATUROPATHY

Practitioners will suggest improving your diet and lifestyle. You may be advised to include iron-rich foods, such as green leafy vegetables, dried apricots, sardines, or liver, in the diet. Citrus bioflavonoids, found in the pith of citrus fruits, help iron absorption and balance hormone levels. SEE PAGES 118–21

WESTERN HERBALISM

Remedies will include herbs thought to balance hormones, such as agnus castus, and uterine tonics like false unicorn root. Goldenseal may help control the shedding of the uterine lining. Limeflower may counter anemia. SEE PAGES 134–39

Cautions: Do not take false unicorn root, goldenseal, or yarrow if you suspect you may be pregnant. Do not take goldenseal if you have high blood pressure.

LIMEFLOWER
This may help if blood loss is heavy.

OTHER OPTIONS

Acupuncture — SEE PAGES 90–94
Acupressure — SEE PAGE 95
Chinese Herbalism — SEE PAGES 140–43
Nutritional Therapies — SEE PAGES 148–52

INFERTILITY

INFERTILITY IS DEFINED as the inability to conceive after a year or more of intercourse without contraception. The problem is quite common and probably affects at least one in eight couples. Pollution of the environment may be a factor in the recent rise in infertility rates. Usually there is a specific problem in either the man (see Male Infertility, *page 277) or the woman. Sometimes both partners are infertile, and in 10% of cases no obvious reason is found. Infertility in women may be caused by factors such as ill health, a hormonal imbalance, stress, or blocked fallopian tubes. If there is no specific cause, a woman can learn to identify when she ovulates, since this is when she is most fertile, and increase frequency of intercourse at this time.*

CAUSES

In women, infertility may be caused by hormonal problems, which can lead to a failure to ovulate regularly, and to irregular or no menstrual periods (see page 265). The approach of menopause or coming off the contraceptive pill will also affect ovulation. If too little progesterone is produced, the uterine lining does not thicken sufficiently to allow implantation of a fertilized egg. The fallopian tubes or ovaries may be scarred or blocked by untreated infections arising from termination, sexually transmitted diseases, or the use of an IUD (intrauterine contraceptive device). Other causes of infertility include genetic factors, ovarian cysts, hypothyroidism, endometriosis, fibroids, poor nutrition, and environmental chemicals. Psychological factors, such as stress or subconscious feelings of fear or anger, may also play a role. Sperm may be unable to reach the uterus because mucus in the cervix is too sticky, too acidic, or because it contains spermicidal antibodies.

SELF-HELP

If your menstrual cycle is regular, have intercourse on the 13th, 14th, and 15th days before your next period. Sperm production decreases if a man has sex too often, so apart from these days, have intercourse no more than once every 30–36 hours. If your periods are irregular, take your temperature first thing every morning with a basal thermometer: a rise of 0.3–1°F (0.2–0.5°C) will indicate that you are ovulating. You can also detect ovulation with special urine-testing kits.

When making love, avoid using artificial lubricants, which can inhibit sperm movement. Use butter if lubrication is necessary, and do not douche afterward. The best position for conception is the "missionary position," with your partner on top and facing you, and with a pillow under your hips. His penis should remain inside your vagina until it has gone limp. It takes about 20–30 minutes for the sperm to reach the uterus, so lie on your back with your knees raised for the next half hour.

CONVENTIONAL TREATMENT

Investigations to diagnose the cause of infertility include blood tests to check hormone levels, an ultrasound scan of the ovaries, an X ray of the uterus, a sperm count, and sperm assessment. The uterus, ovaries, and fallopian tubes may be examined with a laparoscope, an illuminated viewing tube, and drugs may be given to stimulate ovulation. Surgery to clear blocked fallopian tubes and various kinds of "test-tube," or *in vitro*, fertilization techniques are a last resort. The drug clomiphene may be prescribed: it stimulates the ovaries to produce more eggs. Multiple births may occur as a result of taking the drug.

TOUCH & MOVEMENT THERAPIES

Worrying about failure to conceive creates tension, which can have an adverse effect on fertility. Massage-based techniques and movement therapies help to break the vicious circle by encouraging relaxation.

AROMATHERAPY

A practitioner may recommend relaxing essential oils of lavender, geranium, or rosemary to relieve stress and tension. Rose and lemon balm are believed to have a particular affinity with female sex organs and are especially useful for stress-related conditions. Cinnamon, peppermint, and ginger oils act as tonics, warming the body and increasing circulation to all organs. They may be massaged in a carrier oil, added to the bath or inhaled.

SEE PAGES 62–65

ACUPUNCTURE

A practitioner will give you an individual assessment and stimulate certain acupoints believed to improve hormonal balance and increase energy flow.

SEE PAGES 90–94

T'AI CHI CH'UAN

A teacher will show you a series of movements that may be useful in lowering stress levels. The gentle exercises are thought to encourage the flow of *qi* ("life energy") and to restore natural harmony.

SEE PAGES 100–101

T'AI CHI MOVEMENT
Practitioners teach a sequence of t'ai chi movements to perform daily, which may ease anxiety about conceiving.

OTHER OPTIONS

Massage SEE PAGES 56–61
Qigong SEE PAGE 99
Yoga SEE PAGES 108–11

MEDICINAL THERAPIES

Fertility levels may be low due to a wide range of factors other than physical causes, including stress, environmental pollution, and lack of particular nutrients. Medicinal therapies aim to boost general health and support the body's healing processes with dietary supplements and herbal remedies.

AGNUS CASTUS
One of many herbs used to boost fertility, agnus castus is said to stimulate ovulation.

NATUROPATHY

A healthy, balanced diet; regular, moderate exercise; and a positive attitude are essential for general health and fertility. A practitioner may advise you to avoid caffeine, which is suspected of interfering with ovulation, to maintain a normal weight, and to eat only organic fruits and vegetables, grown without the use of potentially toxic chemical pesticides.

You will also be told to restrict alcohol, since excessive amounts increase the hormone prolactin, which may disturb the menstrual cycle. Smoking is also seen as harmful, reducing blood flow to the cervix and inhibiting the action of cilia, the tiny hairs in the fallopian tubes that guide the egg toward the uterus. Splashing hot and cold water alternately on the genital area helps to stimulate local circulation. Your practitioner will advise you not to take a hot bath before sexual intercourse, as sperm need cool temperatures in order to survive. SEE PAGES 118–21

HOMEOPATHY

Practitioners prefer to treat you according to your constitutional type but may recommend *Sabina 6c* if you have miscarriages before 12 weeks, or *Sepia 6c* for irregular periods, or if you feel chilly, weepy, irritable, and averse to sex. SEE PAGES 126–30

WESTERN HERBALISM

Herbs often recommended for infertility are agnus castus, said to act on the pituitary gland to stimulate hormones involved in ovulation, and false unicorn root, which stimulates the ovaries themselves. Wild yam is traditionally linked with the regulation of female hormones and the health of the reproductive organs. A liver remedy, such as rosemary, may also help maintain hormone balance. Herbs such as German chamomile may be suggested to ease stress and promote relaxation. SEE PAGES 134–39
Caution: Do not take wild yam or false unicorn root if you suspect you may be pregnant.

CHINESE HERBALISM

In Traditional Chinese Medicine, infertility is often seen as an expression of "disharmony," associated with "damp heat" and an imbalance of *yin* and *yang* (see glossary). Blood and hormonal tonics may be given, as may remedies containing Chinese angelica (*dang gui*) or ginseng. SEE PAGES 140–43
Caution: Do not take Chinese angelica or ginseng if you suspect you may be pregnant, or ginseng if you have high blood pressure.

AYURVEDA

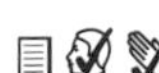

In Ayurveda, shatavari root is considered the most important rejuvenative tonic for women, and is used for infertility. Asparagus, fenugreek, garlic, onion, and licorice are said to invigorate the reproductive organs. SEE PAGES 144–47
Caution: Do not take licorice or fenugreek if you suspect you may be pregnant.

NUTRITIONAL THERAPIES

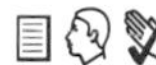

Although there is little scientific evidence supporting nutritional therapy's effect on infertility, nutritionists say that slight vitamin and mineral deficiencies, and exposure to chemical toxins, interfere with sperm and egg production and can encourage miscarriage.

A practitioner may recommend alkaline foods, such as bean sprouts, peas, and milk, to offset acidity in the cervical mucus, which can inhibit sperm. You will be told to avoid acidic foods, such as red meat and tea. Foods rich in vitamin E, like vegetable oils, nuts, and eggs, may be advised to protect fatty tissues (thought to be important for fertility). Foods containing essential fatty acids, such as seeds, legumes, and oily fish, are also recommended, as well as supplements such as evening primrose oil, starflower oil, linseed oil, borage seed oil, and blackcurrant oil. Folic acid and vitamin B_{12} supplements may be suggested, since deficiencies can lead to anemia, associated with infertility. Some practitioners also claim that supplements of vitamin B_6 may raise levels of progesterone in women with irregular or absent periods. SEE PAGES 148–52

VITAMIN E DIET
Foods rich in vitamin E, including liver, sunflower oil, and pumpkin seeds, may counter infertility.

MIND & EMOTION THERAPIES

These therapies can help you cope with stress, which may be affecting your ability to conceive. Mind therapies may also reveal unconscious fears, and help those unable to conceive to come to terms with this.

PSYCHOTHERAPY & COUNSELING

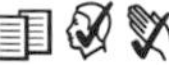

It is possible that unconscious feelings about starting a family, such as fear of childbirth or unresolved anger toward your partner, may contribute to infertility. Therapy and counseling can help you explore and deal with these issues. SEE PAGES 160–65

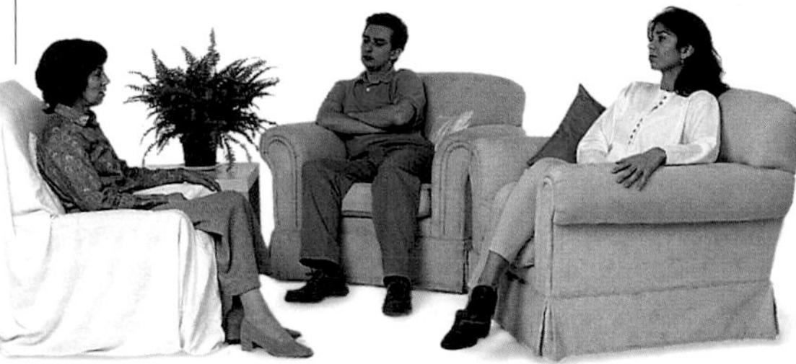

FERTILITY ISSUES
Talking to a counselor, either on your own or with your partner, may resolve underlying fears.

HYPNOTHERAPY

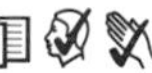

Research at the Chelsea and Westminster Hospital in London, UK, in 1994 showed that hypnotherapy can reduce stress levels and help some women to conceive. Hypnotherapy may also help to uncover fears about labor, motherhood, hospitals, or the child as a threat to your relationship. SEE PAGES 166–67

AUTOGENIC TRAINING

This method of deep relaxation is believed to allow the body and mind to rest and restore themselves to health. "Emotional discharges" sometimes happen, during which you briefly reexperience repressed memories or emotions. They are considered part of the healing process. SEE PAGE 168

RELAXATION & BREATHING

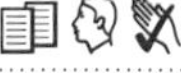

Not being able to conceive is stressful, especially where there is no detectable reason. In animals, adverse conditions can halt reproductive activity, and stress may have the same effect in humans. Although little research has been done, there is some evidence that reducing stress may lower levels of prolactin (a hormone that, in excessive amounts, can inhibit fertility), and help some women to become pregnant. Relaxation and breathing techniques to reduce anxiety and ease muscle tension may be useful. SEE PAGES 170–73

OTHER OPTIONS

Meditation SEE PAGES 174–77
Visualization SEE PAGES 178–79

PREGNANCY

PREGNANCY IS A TIME when it is essential to be as healthy and relaxed as possible. Women planning to conceive should take the opportunity to optimize good health, attempt to remedy any dietary or lifestyle imbalances and medical disorders, and avoid unnecessary medication. While pregnancy and childbirth are completely natural processes, modern medicine has tended,

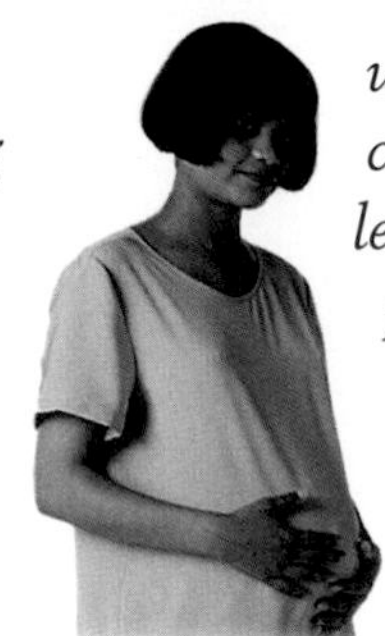

until quite recently, to treat them as medical conditions. Today there is a movement toward a less clinical approach – a trend that complementary practitioners applaud. As well as relieving specific ailments, many complementary therapies, such as yoga, visualization, and massage, are useful for all pregnant women, because they calm the mind and encourage a sense of being in control.

COMPLEMENTARY APPROACHES

Since the 1960s, there has been a landslide of opinion in the West in favor of the "low-tech, natural" approach to pregnancy and labor. To ensure a peaceful birth and successful breastfeeding, complementary practitioners focus on prenatal nutrition, well-being, and fitness in pregnancy, and natural methods to help the mother cope with the physical and emotional aspects of labor.

CONVENTIONAL APPROACHES

Doctors examine both mother and baby throughout pregnancy to monitor their well-being. Regular checks ensure that the baby is developing normally, and highlight any problems that the mother may be experiencing, such as fluid retention, high blood pressure, or poor placental growth. The trend toward less intervention during pregnancy and childbirth, with minimal monitoring and drugs, is growing worldwide. However, "high-tech" obstetrics will always have an important place in childbirth, saving the lives of mothers and their babies.

SELF-HELP

Once you know you are pregnant, pay attention to your diet, and get regular exercise and plenty of rest. Use techniques such as visualization to concentrate on positive feelings about your baby, and try to enjoy art, music, and the beauty of nature. It helps to share practical advice and experiences with other parents, and to prepare for the birth and parenthood by talking it through with your partner, your family, and your doctor.

PRECAUTIONS

- **Avoid anyone with German measles, or get vaccinated at least three months before trying to conceive.**
- **Do not take herbs in medicinal doses in the first three months of pregnancy, and consult a trained medical herbalist thereafter.**
- **Do not take essential oils internally, and do not use thyme or German chamomile essential oils externally during pregnancy.**
- **Seek immediate medical advice for the following: prolonged nausea and inability to eat properly, frequent urination for more than two days, especially if accompanied by pain, prolonged flulike illness, fluid retention that has not decreased after three days.**

MORNING SICKNESS

HALF OF ALL PREGNANT WOMEN experience nausea and vomiting in the first three or four months of pregnancy, and not just in the mornings. Although the cause has not been firmly established, low blood sugar, food sensitivities, poor diet, and emotional factors are thought to contribute. Small, regular meals are advised. In severe cases intravenous fluids may be given to prevent dehydration.

SELF-HELP
A dry biscuit eaten first thing in the morning can help reduce nausea.

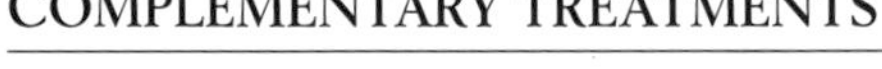

COMPLEMENTARY TREATMENTS

Morning sickness may be allayed with dietary adjustments, gentle herbal remedies, or stimulation of appropriate acupoints.

ACUPRESSURE

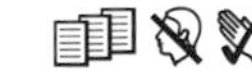

A practitioner will show you how to stimulate an acupoint located just below the wrist on the Pericardium meridian. Clinical trials have shown that this can relieve nausea in early pregnancy. A wristband with a stud over the acupoint has also proved effective for some women. SEE PAGE 95

WESTERN HERBALISM

In a clinical trial, ginger was found to reduce nausea and vomiting attacks. Practitioners may also advise sipping small quantities of an herbal tea, such as German chamomile or lemon balm, throughout the day to settle the stomach. SEE PAGES 134–39

Caution: Do not take ginger if you have a peptic ulcer.

CHINESE HERBALISM

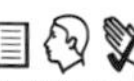

Nausea in early pregnancy is linked to "excess cold" and weakness of the Stomach. "Hot" foods, such as chili peppers, may be recommended, and "cold" foods, such as bananas, discouraged. SEE PAGES 140–43

OTHER OPTIONS

Acupuncture	SEE PAGES 90–94
Naturopathy	SEE PAGES 118–21
Homeopathy	SEE PAGES 126–30
Nutritional Therapies	SEE PAGES 148–52
Psychotherapy & Counseling	SEE PAGES 160–65
Hypnotherapy	SEE PAGES 166–67

LABOR

SMALL CONTRACTIONS of the uterus may occur days before labor begins in earnest. At this point, the mucous plug blocking the cervix may be expelled, and the amniotic sac surrounding the baby may rupture, commonly known as the "breaking of the waters." As contractions get stronger and more regular, the cervix widens and the baby descends into the vagina. The process can be very painful. **Conventional Treatment** Hospital labor wards offer pain relief through nitrous oxide gas, narcotic injections, and epidural (spinal) anesthesia. TENS (see glossary) may be used by some practitioners to block pain transmission. If labor is prolonged, or if there are complications, the baby may be delivered surgically by cesarean section.

COMPLEMENTARY TREATMENTS

Massage, breathing techniques, and acupuncture all help to ease tension and relieve pain, possibly reducing the need for conventional drugs.

MASSAGE

A practitioner will demonstrate pressure techniques to use on the back and buttocks that will help alleviate the pain of contractions. Directed by the mother herself, this can be very effective. SEE PAGES 56–61

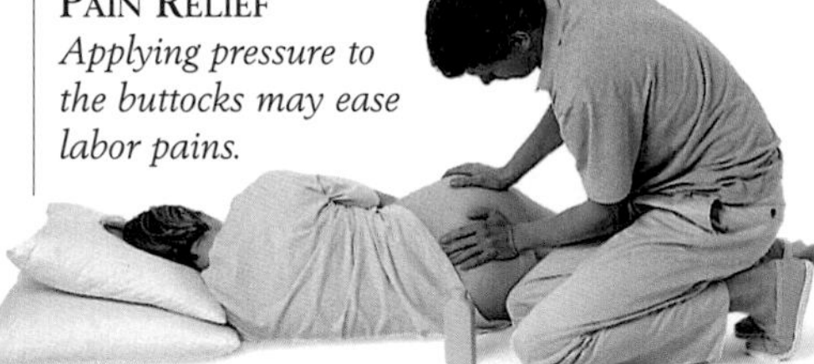

PAIN RELIEF
Applying pressure to the buttocks may ease labor pains.

OSTEOPATHY

Reports indicate that women treated with osteopathy during pregnancy may experience less pain during labor. SEE PAGES 76–81

ACUPUNCTURE

Acupuncture relieves pain in some women. In one study, it was found to increase contractions in women past their due dates. SEE PAGES 90–94

WESTERN HERBALISM

In the last weeks of pregnancy, a practitioner may suggest raspberry leaf tea, which is thought to tone the uterine muscles. SEE PAGES 134–39

Caution: Do not take raspberry leaf during the first three months of pregnancy.

RELAXATION & BREATHING

There are several techniques based around relaxation and breathing that overcome the tension that is a natural, but unhelpful, reaction to pain during labor. SEE PAGES 170–73

BREASTFEEDING PROBLEMS

PROBLEMS WITH BREASTFEEDING include insufficient milk production, breast engorgement, sore or cracked nipples, and mastitis (blocked milk ducts leading to infection). Exhaustion, anxiety, tension, and an inadequate fluid intake can all play a role. Conventionally, mastitis is treated with painkillers and antibiotics. A doctor will check that the baby is feeding in the correct position and provide reassurance and practical help.

COMPLEMENTARY TREATMENTS

Herbal remedies address the specific problem, and mind therapies improve your confidence to help overcome breastfeeding difficulties.

WESTERN HERBALISM

A practitioner may suggest goat's rue to improve breast milk production and advise you to apply calendula cream or wheat germ oil to prevent and treat sore nipples.
SEE PAGES 134–39

VISUALIZATION

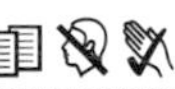

A practitioner will guide you to imagine a positive outcome (for example, your baby feeding contentedly). One study of new mothers reported that the majority produced 63% more breast milk after listening to a 20-minute guided imagery tape.
SEE PAGES 178–79

OTHER OPTIONS

Naturopathy SEE PAGES 118–21
Homeopathy SEE PAGES 126–30

POSTNATAL DEPRESSION

GIVING BIRTH is a dramatic, powerful moment in a woman's life, but it is also exhausting. Mood swings (the "baby blues"), involving weepiness, feelings of inadequacy, anxiety, resentment, guilt, and anger, are common after delivery but generally settle down within a few weeks. Postnatal depression is triggered by hormonal changes and fatigue. Emotional or financial strains are contributing factors. If prolonged, doctors may prescribe antidepressants and hormonal drugs, and suggest counseling. Severe cases may require hospitalization.

Caution: Consult a doctor if negative feelings about your baby persist.

COMPLEMENTARY TREATMENTS

Depression and exhaustion may respond to uplifting oils and nutritional supplements.

AROMATHERAPY

A practitioner may massage you with essential oils of clary sage and jasmine, said to have antidepressant properties. SEE PAGES 62–65

JASMINE
Aromatherapists use jasmine essential oil to aid relaxation and help lift postnatal depression.

CRANIAL OSTEOPATHY

Cranial osteopathy is said to release strain patterns caused by childbirth that affect the body and mood. SEE PAGE 81

NATUROPATHY

Foods rich in magnesium, zinc, vitamins B_2, and B_6 may help normalize hormone levels, and unrefined carbohydrates, such as whole-grain bread, may be advised to maintain blood sugar levels. SEE PAGES 118–21

WESTERN HERBALISM

St. John's wort, proven to have antidepressant properties, may be suggested. SEE PAGES 134–39

OTHER OPTION

Psychotherapy & Counseling SEE PAGES 160–65

MENOPAUSE

MENOPAUSE IS THE CESSATION of menstruation and the term is also used to describe the "change of life" experienced as a woman's childbearing years end. Menopause usually takes place between 45 and 55, but it may happen as early as 35. Hormonal changes leading up to and beyond this event occur over several years and may bring on a number of symptoms, although many women experience none at all. Problems can include circulatory disturbances, mental and emotional difficulties, skin changes, and aches and pains. Psychological symptoms, such as depression, may have more to do with a woman's sense of changing identity as her family grows up than with physical processes, and those with a positive attitude to aging seem to suffer fewer symptoms.

CAUSES & SYMPTOMS

Decreasing levels of estrogen during a woman's forties mean that eggs mature less regularly, and so less progesterone is produced. In response, the lining of the uterus thickens less and periods become increasingly erratic and eventually stop. A hysterectomy accompanied by removal of the ovaries will result in menstrual periods stopping at once. Fluctuating blood levels of estrogen disturb the circulation and can lead to breast lumpiness (see Fibrocystic Breast Disease, page 272). The lower estrogen levels also cause reduced bone calcification, which can result in osteoporosis (see page 257) and an increased risk of bone fractures. Menopausal symptoms are wide-ranging. Common mental and emotional difficulties include poor concentration and memory, depression, and loss of self-esteem and libido. The hormonal changes can result in vaginal dryness, skin problems, hot flashes, sweating, and itching.

SELF-HELP

A diet rich in calcium and vitamin D (for calcium absorption) helps ward off osteoporosis. Regular exercise aids relaxation and relieves stress; weightbearing activities, such as walking, dancing, or tennis, are particularly helpful because they strengthen the bones. Eating a healthy low-fat, high-fiber, whole-foods diet with plenty of vegetables and fruits improves general health, and foods rich in natural estrogens (phytoestrogens) may help protect against osteoporosis, heart disease, and breast cancer. Soy is a particularly rich source of phytoestrogens. Artificial lubricants, such as KY Jelly or cocoa butter, may counteract vaginal dryness during intercourse.

CONVENTIONAL TREATMENT

Specific problems, such as depression, insomnia, and bladder infections, can be treated and, with the exception of osteoporosis, most disappear once menopause is over. Some symptoms may be alleviated with hormone replacement therapy (HRT), in the form of pills, skin implants, slow-release skin patches, and vaginal creams. HRT replaces estrogen and progesterone, the hormones lost during the menopause, so that hot flashes and vaginal dryness are relieved and brittle bones can be prevented. There is increasing evidence that HRT may reduce the risk of heart disease and stroke and protect against Alzheimer's disease. The risk factors associated with long-term use of HRT, such as breast cancer, are still unclear.

PRECAUTIONS

• Consult a doctor if you begin to bleed again after your periods have ceased, if periods are very prolonged or heavy, or if you have abdominal pain or distension, or a persistent change in bowel habits.

TOUCH & MOVEMENT THERAPIES

Massage-based therapies aid relaxation and acupuncture helps to lessen symptoms by rebalancing the hormonal system.

MASSAGE

A regular massage using gentle stroking techniques may ease symptoms, relieve tension, and restore self-esteem. SEE PAGES 56–61

AROMATHERAPY

Many women find essential oils effective in relieving the symptoms associated with menopause. A practitioner may suggest a massage with German chamomile, sandalwood, or rose essential oil, diluted in a carrier oil. They are believed to help even out mood swings and ease hot flashes. SEE PAGES 62–65

Caution: Do not use German chamomile oil if you may be pregnant.

ROSE

Rose oil, also known as attar of roses, is commonly used as a massage oil for its antidepressant effect.

REFLEXOLOGY

Stimulation of points on the feet associated with the pelvic organs may ease symptoms and relieve tension. SEE PAGES 66–69

ACUPUNCTURE

Practitioners believe that acupuncture balances the hormonal system and alleviates pain. Moxibustion may also be advised. SEE PAGES 90–94

YOGA

The harmony of mind and body required for yoga *asanas* (postures) relieves anxiety and restores emotional stability. Gentle stretching encourages flexibility, which is especially important as women age. SEE PAGES 108–11

MEDICINAL THERAPIES

Menopause, many practitioners believe, is a process that should be gradual and trouble-free. Problems are a sign of an underlying condition, such as poor diet or stress. Naturopaths and nutritionists focus on diet and lifestyle, and herbal practitioners provide remedies to encourage the body to adapt smoothly to the hormonal change.

NATUROPATHY 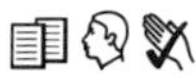

Many naturopaths attribute menopausal symptoms to the poor elimination of waste products, lack of exercise and essential nutrients, and an inability to manage stress. They believe that menopause should be a slow, gentle process, during which the adrenal glands and fatty tissues increase their output of estrogen to offset the ovaries' decline in production. Severe menopausal symptoms are seen as a sign that the adrenal glands are not functioning properly, which may be due to poor diet, low blood sugar levels, and stress. You are likely to be encouraged to avoid refined carbohydrates, salt, sugar, caffeine, alcohol, and stress, and so avoid "adrenal overstimulation." Eating a number of small meals a day, instead of two or three large ones, can help prevent low blood sugar.

A practitioner may specifically recommend foods rich in calcium, vitamin D, magnesium, and phosphorus, such as dairy products, green leafy vegetables, and oily fish, to slow down loss of bone mass. You may also be advised to avoid tea, coffee, and salt, all of which promote calcium excretion. Boron, a mineral found in beans, vegetables, and fruit (such as prunes, strawberries, and cabbage), appears to increase estrogen retention. Other dietary recommendations include plants containing natural estrogens, called phytoestrogens, which may help ward off osteoporosis, heart disease, and breast cancer. These include carrots, corn, apples, and oats, and especially soy and soy-based products.

Linseed, sunflower seeds and oil, pumpkin seeds, and evening primrose oil supplements may also be advised. They contain essential fatty acids needed to help maintain hormone balance, lower blood pressure, and reduce sodium and water retention. SEE PAGES 118–21

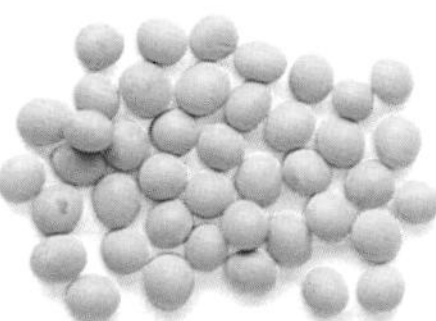

SOYBEANS & TOFU
Foods derived from the soy plant, such as soybeans and tofu (bean curd), are especially rich in natural estrogens.

HOMEOPATHY 

Menopausal problems are thought to represent long-standing imbalances within the body. A practitioner will assess you in order to diagnose your "constitutional type" correctly, but the following standard remedies may be useful: *Sepia 6c* for poor memory, mood changes, anxiety, irritability, vaginal dryness, and night sweats; *Sulfur 6c* for hot flashes that become worse in a warm room, poor memory, and depression; *Natrum mur. 6c* for depression, weepiness, vaginal dryness, weariness, and faintness; *Calcarea 6c* for irritability, panic attacks, mood changes, anxiety, hot flashes, and a tendency to put on weight; *Graphites 6c* for overexcitability and for difficulty in concentrating, irritability, weepiness, fearfulness, and feeling faint in a warm room.
SEE PAGES 126–30

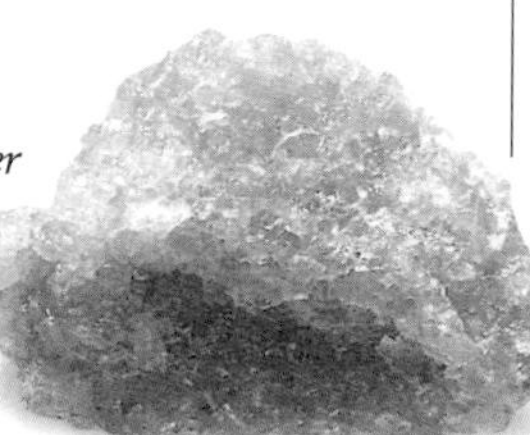

ROCK SALT
The remedy Natrum mur.*, which may counter despondency during menopause, is derived from rock salt.*

WESTERN HERBALISM 

Practitioners try to encourage the hormonal changes to proceed as smoothly as possible. False unicorn root is a well-known ovarian tonic. Black cohosh, blue cohosh, agnus castus, hops, and wild yam have an action similar to that of estrogen and may be given for hot flashes, night sweats, and flooding. Sage and motherwort also have an estrogenlike action and may be prescribed as a tea for vaginal dryness, perhaps with calendula cream to be applied directly to the vagina.

If the practitioner thinks that your symptoms may be due to stress inhibiting the adrenal glands' production of estrogen, calming herbs such as skullcap and vervain may be prescribed. If depression is a problem, St. John's wort (one of the best proven herbal remedies for depression) may be suggested, and adding a few drops of lavender, rose, or ylang ylang essential oils to a bath may be recommended to encourage relaxation. Lemon balm and wild oats may restore the nervous system and ease anxiety and mood changes.
SEE PAGES 134–39

Caution: If you may be pregnant, do not take false unicorn root, wild yam, black cohosh, blue cohosh, motherwort, or vervain, or medicinal doses of sage.

CHINESE HERBALISM 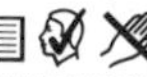

Menopausal symptoms are associated with "weakness of the Kidney," "deficient Blood," and "imbalance between the Kidney and Liver." A practitioner may prescribe remedies containing Chinese angelica (*dang gui*), ginseng, rehmannia, peony, and thorowax root.
SEE PAGES 140–43

Cautions: Do not take any of the above if you may be pregnant. Do not take ginseng if you have high blood pressure.

NUTRITIONAL THERAPIES 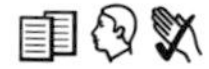

Nutritionists consider that higher levels of certain vitamins and minerals are necessary for well-being and energy as women age, particularly vitamins B_6, B_{12}, D, and E, and folic acid, magnesium, chromium, and zinc. Vitamin B_6 is thought particularly important because it is diuretic, helping to rid the body of toxins, and also supports the manufacture of prostaglandins, the chemicals that help maintain hormone balance. Studies show that menopausal symptoms, such as vaginal dryness, hot flashes, sweats, dizziness, and fatigue, improve with supplements of vitamin E.

Hydrochloric acid in the stomach assists the digestion and absorption of minerals such as calcium, but tends to decline with age and appears to be absent in some postmenopausal women. A practitioner may recommend papaya, which is rich in hydrochloric acid, or supplements. Evening primrose oil, rich in essential fatty acids, is often prescribed to relieve menopausal symptoms, although the results of research into its effectiveness are inconclusive. SEE PAGES 148–53

MIND & EMOTION THERAPIES

Mind and emotion therapies can help to reduce stress, which exacerbates menopausal symptoms, and help women adjust psychologically to a new stage in life.

PSYCHOTHERAPY & COUNSELING 

Some women see the menopause in a negative way: it can be a reminder of increasing age, loss of fertility, and a sense of transition from "mother" to "elder." Hormonal changes often coincide with the "empty nest" syndrome, a mother's perceived loss of identity as children grow up and leave home. Counseling may help resolve these issues and promote a more positive self-image. SEE PAGES 160–65

RELAXATION & BREATHING

Stress, whether from overwork or emotional problems, can make menopausal symptoms worse. Stress management techniques that relieve tension and promote relaxation may help. SEE PAGES 170–73

OTHER OPTIONS

Meditation SEE PAGES 174–77
Visualization SEE PAGES 178–79

BREAST PAIN

SWOLLEN, TENDER BREASTS (mastalgia) can occur just before a menstrual period or in pregnancy, or in women starting oral contraceptives or hormone replacement therapy. Women in their forties, particularly if they have "lumpy" breasts (see below), may feel short, stabbing pains, unrelated to their cycle, in one breast.

Cause The pain is caused by fluid trapped in the fatty parts of the breasts, causing them to swell. This is triggered by raised levels of the female hormone estrogen and of the hormone aldosterone, responsible for sodium and water retention. Mastitis, a bacterial infection, can also result in painful breasts.

Conventional Treatment Doctors often prescribe diuretics if breast pain is caused by fluid retention before menstruation. Hormone antagonists, such as danazol and bromocriptine, may be suggested to balance the level of estrogen. Antibiotics will usually be given to fight an infection.

Caution: Consult a doctor if you find a breast lump.

COMPLEMENTARY TREATMENTS

Therapies aim to stimulate the lymphatic system and correct hormone imbalances in order to relieve the fluid retention that is causing discomfort.

AROMATHERAPY

A full body massage with geranium essential oil a few days before menstruation may relieve pain by increasing blood and lymph circulation and easing fluid retention. SEE PAGES 62–65

NATUROPATHY

A practitioner will aim to reduce excess levels of estrogen and aldosterone by improving the diet. A healthy low-fat diet, with lots of fresh fruit and vegetables, is recommended. You will be asked to reduce your caffeine, salt, and alcohol intake, as these encourage fluid retention. Fatty foods may increase estrogen levels and should be avoided. You may be advised to bathe your breasts with cold water once a day. SEE PAGES 118–21

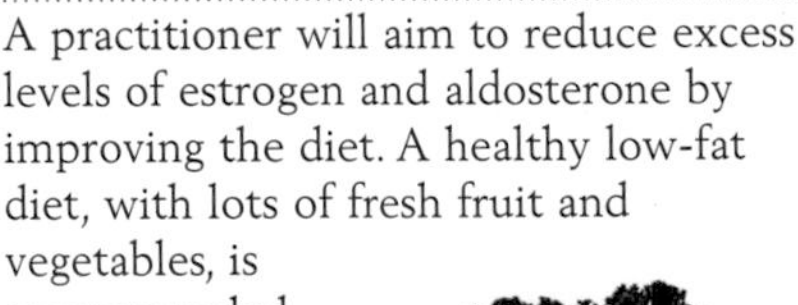

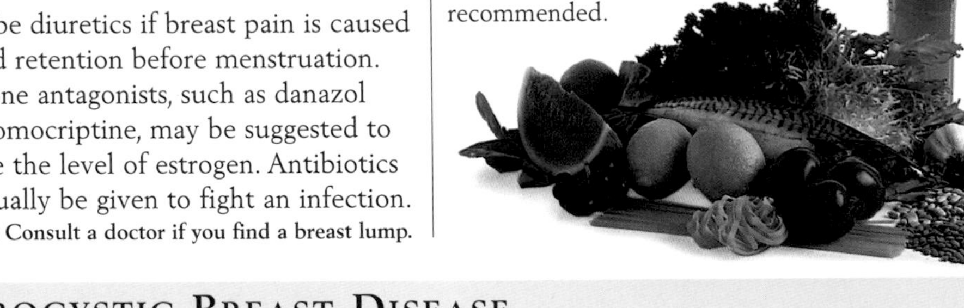

HEALTHY DIET
A low-fat, low-salt diet, including plenty of fresh fruit and vegetables, may help balance hormone levels.

WESTERN HERBALISM

Your practitioner may recommend that you eat cabbage to relieve fluid retention. You may also be told to ease breast pain by placing a clean, fresh and softened cabbage leaf in a bra against your breasts. SEE PAGES 134–39

NUTRITIONAL THERAPIES

Supplements of vitamin E are often advised, although there is no scientific evidence to support its use. In one study, women with breast pain found that evening primrose oil was as useful in relieving pain as the drug bromocriptine, and reported fewer side effects. SEE PAGES 148–52

FIBROCYSTIC BREAST DISEASE

BREAST LUMPINESS, known as fibrocystic breast disease, begins as part of premenstrual syndrome (see page 264), but can become a persistent condition. Cysts and strands of fibrous tissue form in one or both breasts, accompanied by anything from mild discomfort to severe pain. The condition is very common, affecting as many as 40% of pre-menopausal women.

Cause Fibrocystic breast disease is due to overstimulation of breast tissue by the hormones estrogen and prolactin. It has been associated with stress, which destabilizes the hormone balance.

Conventional Treatment Breast lumps are always investigated to rule out cancer. There is no specific treatment for fibrocystic breast disease, but cysts may be drained of liquid, and diuretics may be prescribed to reduce symptoms.

Self-Help Self-examination of breasts every month after a menstrual period can help you detect changes that require investigation.

Caution: Consult a doctor if you find a breast lump.

COMPLEMENTARY TREATMENTS

As well as treating hormonal imbalances, practitioners may use nutrient supplements for suspected deficiencies, or devise an exclusion diet to deal with food intolerances.

NATUROPATHY

Treatment aims to reduce excess estrogen and other hormones and restore a natural balance. A low-fat, high-fiber diet is usually suggested to encourage excretion of estrogen. You may be advised to avoid coffee, tea, cola and chocolate, since these contain methylxanthines, which are said to stimulate production of cyst fluid. A practitioner may suggest that you eat organic meat to avoid hormone residues (non-organically reared animals are given hormones to increase growth). You may also be recommended evening primrose oil and fish oils, because they contain essential fatty acids that are considered vital for hormonal balance. Some practitioners believe that women with fibrocystic breast disease, especially if they also have constipation, may be suffering from a food intolerance, which they will treat with an exclusion diet. SEE PAGES 118–21

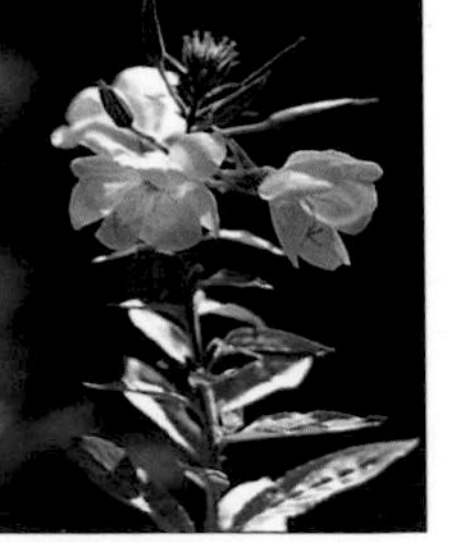

EVENING PRIMROSE
The seed oil of evening primrose contains essential fatty acids said to help maintain hormonal balance.

WESTERN HERBALISM

A practitioner will aim to restore hormonal balance with herbs such as agnus castus and false unicorn root, and to support the liver and help elimination of excess estrogen and toxins with herbs such as burdock, dandelion and yellow dock. Calendula may encourage lymphatic drainage. SEE PAGES 134–39

Caution: do not take yellow dock or false unicorn root during pregnancy.

NUTRITIONAL THERAPIES

Recommended supplements include vitamin E, which may reduce breast pain, evening primrose oil, vitamin B^6 to help metabolism of essential fatty acids and reduce premenstrual symptoms, vitamin A (as beta-carotene), and magnesium. Zinc is also advised, particularly for women with PMS or with high prolactin levels that may inhibit zinc uptake by the body. SEE PAGES 148–52

YEAST INFECTIONS

VAGINAL YEAST INFECTIONS produce a curdlike, white discharge with a strong vinegary or yeastlike odor. They are usually accompanied by soreness and itching of the vulva, the skin around the opening of the vagina.

Cause Yeast infections are caused by *Candida albicans*, a common yeastlike microorganism that lives in the vagina, mouth, and gut (see also Candidiasis, page 235). It is normally held in check by "friendly" bacteria in the vagina but lowered immunity, nutritional deficiencies, oral contraceptives, and drugs such as antibiotics may allow it to multiply. Factors such as allergies and overuse of douches, spermicides, and bath products can also encourage overgrowth. Yeast infections are a common problem during pregnancy, sometimes indicating the presence of sugar in the urine.

Conventional Treatment Antifungal tablets, vaginal suppositories, or creams are available. Women with recurrent yeast infections may be referred to a specialist. A partner may also be infected and so will need to be treated at the same time.

COMPLEMENTARY TREATMENTS

Practitioners see persistent bouts of yeast infection as evidence of poor immunity. Dietary improvements and the application of healing remedies may be recommended.

AROMATHERAPY

A practitioner may advise massaging your lower back and abdomen with antiseptic and antifungal oils, such as lavender, sandalwood, or tea tree, or suggest adding a few drops to a bath. SEE PAGES 62–65

TEA TREE OIL
The antiseptic and antifungal properties of tea tree oil are well established.

NATUROPATHY

Practitioners believe that *Candida albicans* overgrowth in the vagina indicates that the condition is also present in the intestines. Nutritional advice will follow that for candidiasis (see page 235). Apple cider vinegar douches and *Lactobacillus* yogurt suppositories or tampons may encourage "friendly" bacteria in the vagina. SEE PAGES 118–21

WESTERN HERBALISM

Herbs with an antifungal action, such as calendula or thyme, may be suggested for use as douches, in the form of infusions or decoctions. If a hormonal imbalance is suspected, herbs such as false unicorn root may be prescribed. SEE PAGES 134–39

Caution: Do not take false unicorn root during pregnancy.

CHINESE HERBALISM

Practitioners of Traditional Chinese Medicine associate yeast infections with "excess damp" and "damp heat." Chinese wormwood and gentian may be recommended. SEE PAGES 140–43

Caution: Do not take Chinese wormwood during pregnancy.

RELAXATION & BREATHING

If you suffer repeated yeast infections, a practitioner may suggest a series of breathing exercises to induce relaxation. Reducing stress enhances the immune system's ability to fight harmful microorganisms. SEE PAGES 170–73

OTHER OPTIONS

Yoga SEE PAGES 108–11
Nutritional Therapies SEE PAGES 148–52

VAGINITIS & VULVITIS

VAGINITIS IS INFLAMMATION of the vagina. It can cause irritation, redness, odor, abnormal discharge, and pain during intercourse or urination. Inflammation of the vulva is known as vulvitis and causes itchiness and discomfort.

Causes Injury, a forgotten tampon, and chemicals found in medication and hygiene products can all inflame the vaginal area. Vaginitis and vulvitis may also be symptoms of infections such as *Trichomonas vaginalis*, *Candida albicans*, *Gardnerella vaginalis*, *Herpes simplex*, or gonorrhea. In menopausal and postmenopausal women, lack of estrogen can thin the walls of the vagina, leaving them more susceptible to soreness.

Conventional Treatment A doctor will take swabs for examination. Depending on the cause, vaginitis and vulvitis are treated with soothing creams, antibiotics, and antiviral and antifungal drugs.

COMPLEMENTARY TREATMENTS

The vagina is normally protected from infection by "friendly" bacteria and its own slight acidity. Therapies aim to restore these to natural levels, boost the immune system, and destroy any bacteria causing infection.

AROMATHERAPY

A few drops of tea tree essential oil, which has antibacterial and antifungal properties, may be helpful added to a bath. SEE PAGES 62–65

NATUROPATHY

A practitioner will aim to restore the normal ecology of the vagina, enhance the immune response, and cleanse and detoxify the digestive tract. Recommendations may include a raw-foods diet, eating garlic and onion, which have antibacterial, antiviral, and antifungal properties, and drinking cranberry juice to help resist infection. You will be advised to reduce your intake of coffee and sugar, which may upset the normal acidity of the vagina and encourage infection, and to avoid alcohol and tobacco, which may suppress the immune system. A practitioner may advocate "live" yogurt douches or *Lactobacillus* suppositories to help restore friendly bacteria. Apple cider vinegar, added to a bath, may help reacidify the vagina. SEE PAGES 118–21

WESTERN HERBALISM

A practitioner may recommend goldenseal, echinacea, myrrh, or calendula to fight infection, thyme or cleavers to cleanse and detoxify the reproductive organs, and burdock to cleanse the digestive tract. For a heavy discharge, astringent herbs like lady's mantle or beth root are often given. Goldenseal, calendula, rosemary, myrrh, or thyme, as creams or douches, may be suggested. Goldenseal is particularly helpful: it soothes inflammation and contains berberine, an important antibacterial agent. SEE PAGES 134–39

Cautions: Do not take myrrh, goldenseal, lady's mantle, or beth root during pregnancy. Do not take goldenseal if you have high blood pressure.

OTHER OPTION

Nutritional Therapies SEE PAGES 148–52

FIBROIDS

FIBROIDS ARE NONMALIGNANT growths in or on the muscular wall of the uterus. They can be symptomless but, if large, they may cause extended and heavy menstrual bleeding, cramps, back pain, painful intercourse, and pressure on the bladder or bowel. Fibroids seem to be linked to higher estrogen levels and may be encouraged by oral contraceptives. If symptoms are a problem or are preventing conception, or if bleeding is so severe that anemia results, fibroids can be removed surgically. If fibroids are very large or numerous, a hysterectomy may be advised.

Caution: Consult a doctor if menstrual bleeding becomes heavier than usual.

COMPLEMENTARY TREATMENTS

Herbal and other treatments may reduce heavy bleeding and improve circulation.

YOGA

Postures that encourage circulation in the pelvic region, such as the Pelvic Lift, Triangle, or Moon, may ease symptoms. SEE PAGES 108–11

NATUROPATHY

Obesity and a diet high in fat are linked to excess estrogen production, which seems to be a factor in fibroid growth. A naturopath may suggest a diet that is low in fat and high in fiber to encourage elimination of excess estrogen. You will also be advised to eat iron-rich foods to prevent and treat anemia. SEE PAGES 118–21

WESTERN HERBALISM

A practitioner may recommend false unicorn root, thought to balance hormones, uterine tonics, like blue cohosh, relaxants for pain, such as cramp bark, and detoxifying herbs – for example, dandelion. SEE PAGES 134–39

Caution: Do not take false unicorn root or blue cohosh during pregnancy.

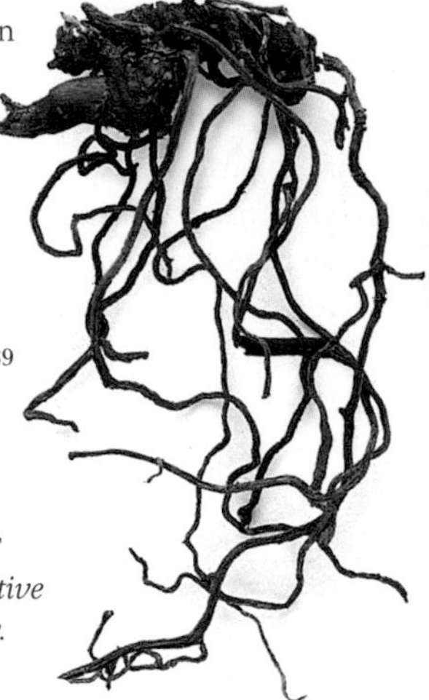

BLUE COHOSH ROOT
This is a traditional Native North American remedy.

PELVIC INFLAMMATORY DISEASE

IN PELVIC INFLAMMATORY DISEASE (PID), the uterus, fallopian tubes, and ovaries become infected, usually by sexually transmitted microorganisms, such as chlamydia, or by bacteria introduced during surgery or via an intrauterine contraceptive device (IUD). Symptoms include lower abdominal, back, and leg pain, irregular and heavy bleeding, vaginal discharge, painful sex, fever, nausea, and diarrhea. If untreated, PID can lead to scarring and infertility. A doctor will prescribe painkillers, anti-inflammatory drugs, and antibiotics.

Caution: Consult a doctor if you suspect PID.

COMPLEMENTARY TREATMENTS

Alongside the necessary conventional treatment, complementary therapies may help boost recovery from infection.

AROMATHERAPY

You may be given a lower abdominal massage with essential oils of lavender, rosewood, rosemary, and geranium. SEE PAGES 62–65

NATUROPATHY

Treatment seeks to detoxify the system and strengthen immune function. A cleansing fast may be followed by a healthy, whole-foods diet. SEE PAGES 118–21

HYDROTHERAPY

Alternate hot and cold sitz baths are thought to help reduce pelvic "congestion." SEE PAGES 122–23

Caution: Avoid alternate hot and cold baths or showers if you have a heart condition.

NUTRITIONAL THERAPIES

Practitioners recommend vitamins and minerals to strengthen immune function and heal tissues. Some studies have shown that vitamin E supplements may increase resistance to chlamydial infection. SEE PAGES 148–53

OTHER OPTIONS

Western Herbalism SEE PAGES 134–39
Chinese Herbalism SEE PAGES 140–43

ENDOMETRIOSIS

SOMETIMES TISSUE from the endometrium (uterine lining) grows in or on other organs in the pelvic cavity. The tissue responds to the woman's hormonal cycle, bleeding each month, and the discharge collects because it has no escape route. The woman may experience heavy, painful menstruation and back pain. The cause is unclear, but it has been linked to selenium deficiency, the use of tampons, excess estrogen production, delayed first pregnancy, early puberty, and stress. Doctors may give drugs to suppress the hormonal cycle and surgery may be necessary.

Caution: Consult a doctor if you have unusual pain with your periods.

COMPLEMENTARY TREATMENTS

Therapies that can relieve pain and reduce stress would be appropriate.

NATUROPATHY

Normal hormone balance is encouraged with a healthy high-fiber whole-foods diet, including essential fatty acids, found in evening primrose oil, linseed, and oily fish. SEE PAGES 118–21

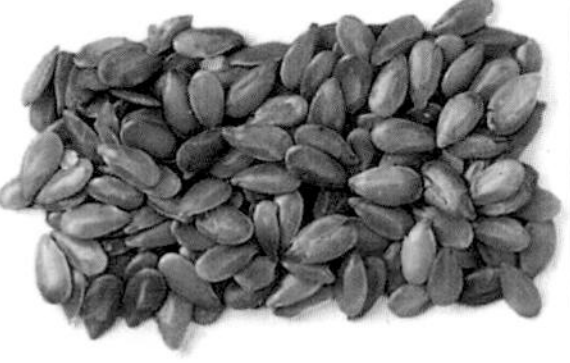

GOLDEN LINSEED
Taken internally, linseed provides essential fatty acids that help balance hormone levels.

WESTERN HERBALISM

A practitioner will prescribe herbs to regulate the hormone balance and promote liver function. Some practitioners believe that saw palmetto can block the action of the hormone that triggers the thickening of the uterine lining. SEE PAGES 134–37

RELAXATION & BREATHING

Stress appears to contribute to the hormonal imbalances that may lie behind endometriosis. Techniques to induce relaxation can help you to cope with pain. SEE PAGES 170–73

OTHER OPTIONS

Acupuncture SEE PAGES 90–94
Chinese Herbalism SEE PAGES 140–43
Nutritional Therapies SEE PAGES 148–52

Cystitis

Cystitis is usually caused by a bacterial infection inflaming the lining of the bladder and urethra. Symptoms include a burning or stinging sensation (dysuria) when passing urine, wanting to pass urine more frequently, lower abdominal pain, and unpleasant-smelling urine. There may also be blood in the urine, and a chill or fever. More than 20% of women have an attack once a year, and many cases go on to cause a kidney infection.

Cause Bacteria from the anus and vagina infect the bladder and urethra. Women are more susceptible than men because the urethra, which carries urine from the bladder, is shorter and its opening is closer to the anus. Various factors increase the likelihood of infection, including incomplete bladder emptying in pregnancy, spermicidal gels, contraceptives that irritate or put pressure on the bladder, and hormone deficiency during and after menopause. Stress, oral contraceptives, and poor diet lower resistance to infection.

Conventional Treatment Highly effective antibiotics are usually given, but can lead to yeast infections. If attacks are frequent, a gynecological examination, kidney X ray, and bladder examination through a viewing tube may be carried out.

Self-Help Avoid foam baths, scented soap products, and vaginal deodorants. Use lubrication during sex to avoid bruising and pass urine afterward. Drink lots of water and urinate regularly. Avoid tight-fitting or synthetic-fiber clothing.

Complementary Treatments

Recurrent attacks of cystitis indicate reduced resistance to infection. Therapies seek to boost the body's natural healing powers with changes in diet, nutritional supplements, and soothing herbs.

Acupressure 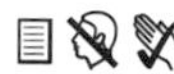

A practitioner will show you how to gently stimulate acupoints along the Stomach meridian, which may bring relief. SEE PAGE 95

Naturopathy 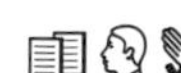

A practitioner will aim to reduce susceptibility to infection by improving digestion and elimination. Tests for food intolerances or candidiasis may be given if attacks are recurrent. You will be told to eat a healthy, whole-foods diet, with onion and garlic to fight infection. Tea, coffee, alcohol, sugar, and other refined carbohydrates, as well as spicy and acidic foods, such as tomatoes, strawberries, and spinach, should be avoided. In an attack, to reduce the urine's acidity so that it does not sting, drink ½ pt (250 ml) of water containing a tablespoon of bicarbonate of soda every 20–30 minutes. Studies carried out in the US in 1991 and 1994 show that drinking unsweetened cranberry juice can help prevent bacteria from adhering to the urinary tract. SEE PAGES 118–21

Cranberries *Research shows that regular intake of cranberry juice helps reduce the likelihood of bacterial infection in the urinary tract.*

Homeopathy 

A remedy suited to your constitutional type is recommended, but the following standard remedies may also bring relief: *Cantharis 6c* for excruciating pain before, during, and after frequent urination, *Sarsaparilla 6c* for burning pain after urination, and *Merc. cor. 6c* for painful passing of urine that contains blood. SEE PAGES 126–30

Western Herbalism 

Herbalists aim to cleanse and soothe the urinary tract and relieve pain. Along with large quantities of water and fruit juice, you will be advised to take herbs that have soothing and urinary disinfectant properties, such as buchu and cornsilk. They may be combined with dandelion leaves, which have a diuretic effect, echinacea to boost the immune system, and skullcap or lavender to help relieve pain. SEE PAGES 134–39

Caution: Do not take buchu during pregnancy.

Skullcap *This herb may offer relief during attacks of cystitis.*

Chinese Herbalism 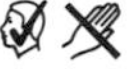

Cystitis is associated with "damp heat"; restorative herbal remedies may include plantain seeds. SEE PAGES 140–43

Nutritional Therapies

Nutritional therapists believe that poor nutrition is at the heart of many diseases. A practitioner will recommend high doses of vitamin C, as well as other supplements, to treat and prevent infection. SEE PAGES 148–53

Prolapse

The ligaments that support the uterus can stretch in old age or during childbirth, allowing it to drop from its usual position and put pressure on the bladder and rectum. Symptoms include a dragging sensation in the pelvis, backache, and incontinence. The uterus may protrude through the vaginal opening, causing soreness and encouraging infection. Prolapse is exacerbated by a persistent cough, straining with persistent constipation, or obesity. Physiotherapy can help strengthen the pelvic floor, and surgery can repair the supporting tissues.

Complementary Treatments

Stimulating treatments and herbal remedies can help to strengthen the uterine muscles.

Acupuncture 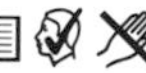

Prolapse is attributed to deficiency of *qi* ("life energy"). Stimulating points on the Conception Vessel meridian may help tone the supporting soft tissues. SEE PAGES 90–94

Naturopathy 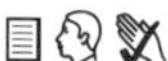

Sitting in cold water for 30 seconds daily is advised to tone muscles. Practitioners will also try to treat constipation if it is present. SEE PAGES 118–21

Western Herbalism 

Traditional uterine tonics like lady's mantle or raspberry leaf may be advised. Pelvic ligaments can atrophy after menopause because of lack of estrogen, so herbs with an estrogen-like action, such as sage or wild yam, may be prescribed. Astringents such as bayberry may help prevent inflammation. SEE PAGES 134–39

Caution: Do not take lady's mantle, wild yam, bayberry, or medicinal doses of sage during pregnancy, or raspberry leaf in the first three months of pregnancy.

Other Options

Aromatherapy SEE PAGES 62–65

Acupressure SEE PAGE 95

Chinese Herbalism SEE PAGES 140–43

MEN'S HEALTH

AT THE ONSET OF PUBERTY, increased secretion of the male sex hormone testosterone stimulates the maturation of the reproductive organs. A complex assembly of erectile tissue, glands, and tubules, the system is located both inside and outside the pelvic area. The male genitals are subject to ailments ranging from infection and impaired sperm production to testicular cancer. Even when they do have symptoms, many men do not seek medical advice. Most conditions are readily treated, and some can threaten fertility and sexual function, so it is important to consult a doctor.

KEY TO SYMBOLS

EVIDENCE	PRACTITIONER
Good scientific trials with positive results	Essential
Some research studies	Recommended
Anecdotal	Not essential
	SELF-HELP
	Self-help possibilities
	No self-help

COMPLEMENTARY APPROACHES

Men's sexual activity and interest can be life-long. Good general health makes this potential more likely and complementary therapies emphasize a balanced diet and stress management techniques as the foundation for sexual health.

CONVENTIONAL APPROACHES

The process of erection and ejaculation depends on the health of nerve and circulatory tissue. Many sexual and erectile problems have a treatable physical cause and should not be dismissed as due to the aging process alone, or regarded as purely psychological. This is especially true for men with diabetes or related circulatory disorders or those on regular medication, which can interfere with sexual arousal or ejaculation.

Caution: Before seeking treatment, see page 204.

HOW THE MALE REPRODUCTIVE SYSTEM WORKS

The testes, two rounded glands tucked within the scrotum, produce sperm cells and the sex hormone testosterone. The testes are located outside the body cavity because sperm production is optimal slightly below body temperature. After about three months' development, the sperm travel to the epididymes, sacs on the back of each testis, for an additional 1–3 weeks' maturation. With sexual excitement, blood rushes to spongy reservoirs within the penis, causing it to stiffen, ready for sexual intercourse. Muscles at the base of the penis swell to prevent blood leaving so that the erection is maintained. If the loose foreskin over the glans or head of the penis has not been removed (circumcision), it retracts as the penis swells.

Shortly before climax, the sperm are shunted through the vas deferens to the seminal vesicles, which bathe the cells in a nutrient-rich seminal fluid. The prostate gland, situated just below the bladder, contributes additional fluid before a powerful surge causes ejaculation, when rhythmic contractions send an average of 250 million sperm out through the urethra.

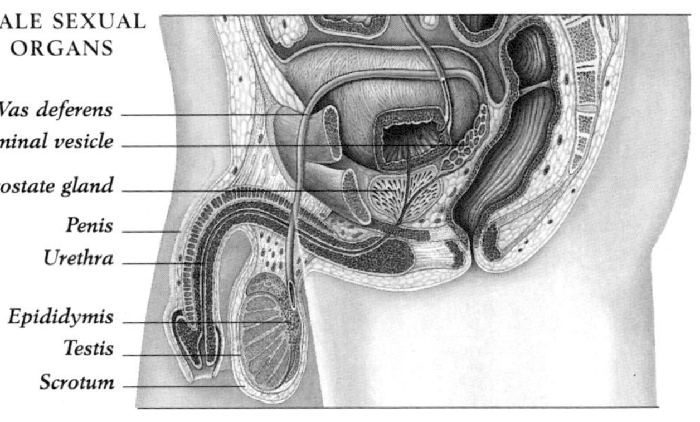

MALE SEXUAL ORGANS

BALANITIS

THIS ITCHY INFLAMMATION of the head of the penis and foreskin in uncircumcised men may be caused by a bacterial or fungal infection, or by chemical irritants. It is often associated with an abnormally tight foreskin. Diabetic men are prone to balanitis, as sugar in the urine encourages the growth of micro-organisms under the skin. Doctors advise keeping the penis clean and dry. If a bacterial infection is the cause, antibiotics will be prescribed. Circumcision may also be advocated.

Caution: Check symptoms with your doctor. Inflammation may indicate a more serious condition.

COMPLEMENTARY TREATMENTS

Therapists focus on reducing the source of irritation and stimulating the body's own responses in order to speed healing.

NATUROPATHY

If candidiasis infection (see Yeast Infections, page 273) is the cause, eating or applying "live" yogurt to the area may be advised to help keep the microorganism in check. Practitioners may suggest a fast followed by a whole-foods diet to improve the function of the immune system. Reducing sugar and "yeasty" foods (mushrooms, blue cheese, wine) may also be advised. SEE PAGES 118–21

WESTERN HERBALISM

To encourage tissue repair, a practitioner may suggest washing the area with an extract of calendula flowers. Aloe-vera gel applied afterward may also help to soothe and heal. A few drops of antiseptic and antifungal tea tree essential oil added to the bath may be suggested. SEE PAGES 134–39

NUTRITIONAL THERAPIES

If balanitis is caused by a candidiasis infection, your practitioner may prescribe supplements of the yeast-countering *lactobacillus* bacteria. Antioxidant (see glossary) vitamin and mineral supplements may also be recommended to boost immunity. SEE PAGES 148–52

PROSTATITIS

AN INFLAMMATION or infection of the prostate is marked by aches, fever, pain upon urination, and blood in the urine. Usually traceable to an infection (see Nonspecific Urethritis, page 240), prostatitis may also be caused by sexually transmitted diseases or blood-borne infections. A doctor will advise antibiotics. In severe cases, the pus may be drained surgically.

COMPLEMENTARY TREATMENTS

Plant remedies and nutritional supplements may help combat infection and stimulate the body's self-healing abilities.

WESTERN HERBALISM

A practitioner may prescribe urinary antiseptics, such as uva-ursi, or urine-increasing herbs, such as pipsissewa. SEE PAGES 134–39

UVA-URSI
This evergreen shrub is a natural urinary antiseptic.

CHINESE HERBALISM

Prostatitis is associated with an excess of "damp heat." Your practitioner may recommend Dianthus Formula, a patent remedy for this condition. SEE PAGES 140–43

NUTRITIONAL THERAPIES

Zinc, said to be important for prostate function, may be prescribed as a food supplement, as may garlic, and vitamins C and E, and essential fatty acids. SEE PAGES 148–52

OTHER OPTION

Naturopathy SEE PAGES 118–21

PROSTATE ENLARGEMENT

USUALLY OCCURRING in men over 50, this condition is gradual and symptomless until the prostate gland presses on the urethra, leading to difficulty in urinating, frequent urination, and possible abdominal pain. The cause is unknown, but testosterone may play a role. If symptoms are mild, conventional treatment may be delayed. Otherwise, options include diathermy (see glossary), laser techniques, drugs to shrink the gland, or surgical removal.

Caution: Check symptoms with your doctor to rule out a more serious condition.

COMPLEMENTARY TREATMENTS

To discourage enlargement, practitioners will focus on improving your general health.

YOGA

Your teacher may suggest the Triangle posture to help open up the urethra. SEE PAGES 108–11

NATUROPATHY

Increased dietary zinc (found in lean meat, grains, legumes, and seafood) may reduce an enlarged prostate. Alternate hot and cold compresses applied behind the scrotum may help boost blood flow. SEE PAGES 118–21

WESTERN HERBALISM

A study in the *British Journal of Clinical Pharmacology* confirmed saw palmetto berries' reputation to improve urinary flow impaired by prostate enlargement. Rye-grass pollen extract is less well researched, but in German trials described in *Complementary Therapies in Medicine* in 1996, two-thirds of patients showed improvement. In France, the foremost conventional treatment is an extract of the bark of pygeum, an African tree. SEE PAGES 134–39

OTHER OPTIONS

Chinese Herbalism SEE PAGES 140–43
Nutritional Therapies SEE PAGES 148–52

MALE INFERTILITY

A MAN'S FERTILITY is said to be impaired when the number of sperm present in a milliliter of ejaculate is less than 20 million, or if the sperm are slow moving or misshapen. Overheated or undescended testes, tube blockage, infection, and weight problems are among the causes of a low sperm count. Poor sperm quality may result from a hormonal imbalance, smoking, and various drugs. An inability to achieve erection or ejaculation is another cause (see Erectile Dysfunction, page 295). **Conventional Treatment** If a couple has not conceived after a year of trying, a doctor will examine a semen sample. Some cases may respond to lifestyle changes or to hormone injections. Others may require surgery. Artificial insemination is a last-resort solution. (See also Female Infertility, pages 266–67.)

COMPLEMENTARY TREATMENTS

Remedies help combat infection and other factors that may impair sperm production.

WESTERN HERBALISM

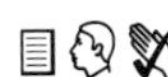

Herbs traditionally considered beneficial for men, such as ginseng and saw palmetto, may be prescribed. A practitioner may suggest a cleansing remedy, such as red clover, to improve general health. SEE PAGES 134–39

Caution: Do not take ginseng if you have high blood pressure.

WATERCRESS
This plant is a rich source of vitamin C and other nutrients.

NUTRITIONAL THERAPIES

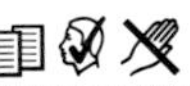

According to practitioners, vitamin C decreases sperm abnormalities and increases sperm number and quality. In an Italian study reported in *Fertility and Sterility* in 1993, folinic acid was successfully used in certain cases of male infertility. Zinc, found in the seminal fluid, increases sperm count and mobility, and blood testosterone levels. For mild cases, practitioners may recommend supplements of argenine, a nutrient found in the heads of sperm. SEE PAGES 148–52

AUTOGENIC TRAINING

Learning to relax by this method has been shown to improve the sperm count. SEE PAGE 168

OTHER OPTIONS

Naturopathy SEE PAGES 118–21
Chinese Herbalism SEE PAGES 140–43
Psychotherapy & Counseling SEE PAGES 160–65

CHILDREN'S HEALTH

CHILDREN HAVE A NATURAL VITALITY AND RESILIENCE, provided they enjoy a healthy diet, plenty of exercise, and a caring environment. Most childhood ailments get better of their own accord, but the symptoms may fluctuate dramatically, alarming both child and parent. A child can be playing at noon, become listless and feverish in the evening, and be back to normal by the next morning. Yet symptoms should not be ignored, since serious illness can develop rapidly. Infants and young children need an especially watchful eye. Diarrhea, for example, particularly in hot weather, can quickly dehydrate babies and the very young.

KEY TO SYMBOLS

EVIDENCE	PRACTITIONER
Good scientific trials with positive results	Essential
Some research studies	Recommended
Anecdotal	Not essential
	SELF-HELP
	Self-help possibilities
	No self-help

COMPLEMENTARY APPROACHES

Complementary practitioners believe that common childhood illnesses help to strengthen the immune system. Treatment is largely a matter of rest and care to encourage the healing process. Gentle remedies are considered best for children, and homeopaths claim that their remedies are particularly effective.

CONVENTIONAL APPROACHES

Modern pediatrics increasingly accepts practices such as low-intervention childbirth, breastfeeding, and less use of antibiotics. Many parents are concerned about the safety of immunization, although doctors strongly advise vaccinating children against such diseases as measles.

Caution: Before seeking treatment for a child, see page 204.

HOW A CHILD GROWS

A newborn baby's head does not increase much in size, but his body changes proportion dramatically over the next 12 years. By the age of two, the baby has become a child and is able to stand upright and walk. The child continues to slim down and his body elongates gradually, until the prepubescent years, at around nine years old, when hormones begin to trigger body changes and the child begins to develop into an adult.

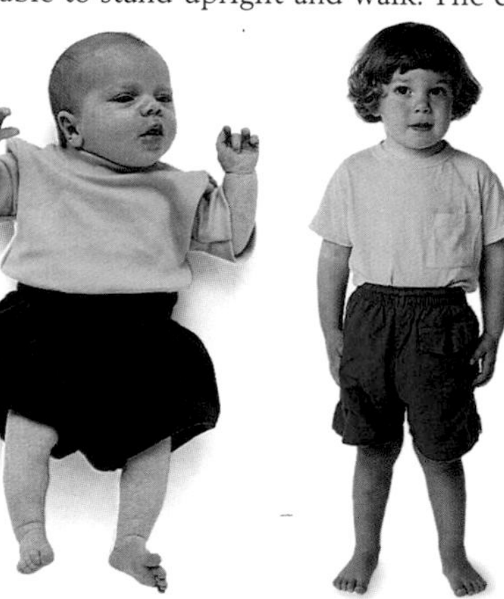

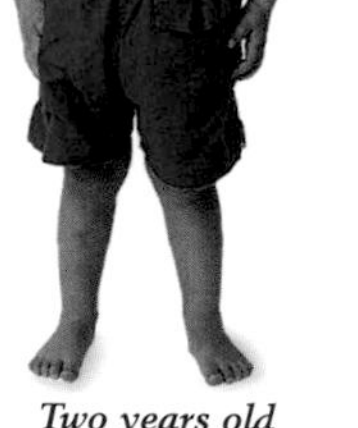

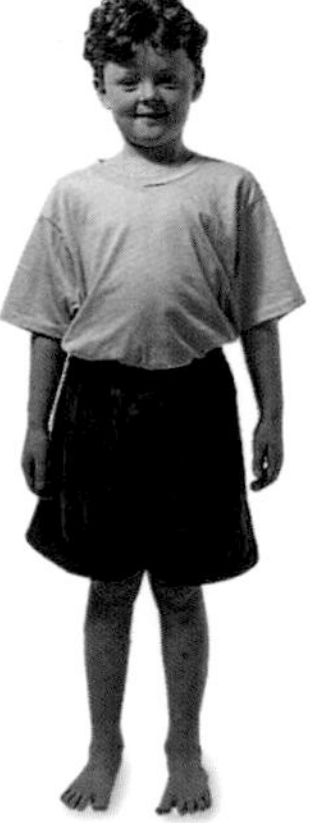

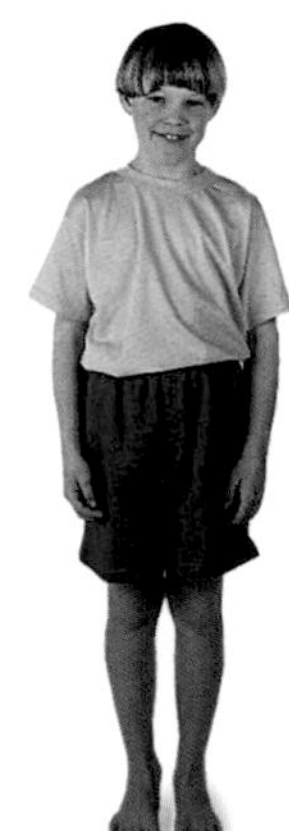

Two months old *Two years old* *Four years old* *Seven years old* *12 years old*

DIAPER RASH

REDDENED, SORE SKIN under the diaper affects most babies to some degree. The rash may involve a few raised spots, or an extensive and intense irritation of the whole diaper area. Bottlefed babies may be more susceptible, babies wearing disposable diapers slightly less so. Causes include the ammonia in stale urine, fecal toxins, detergent, or prolonged wetness.

Conventional Treatment Keeping the skin as clean and dry as possible, perhaps with waterproof barrier creams, will help. In severe cases, corticosteroid or antifungal creams may be prescribed if eczema or candidiasis is suspected.

COMPLEMENTARY TREATMENTS

Plant-derived remedies are a gentle means of soothing the irritation of diaper rash.

AROMATHERAPY

A practitioner may suggest adding 6–8 drops of antiseptic tea tree essential oil to the final rinse to help medicate cloth diapers.
SEE PAGES 62–65

NATUROPATHY

Goat's milk may be advised if the baby is allergic to cow's milk. If you are breastfeeding, a practitioner will advise that you eat plenty of vegetables, and avoid potentially "toxic" substances, such as those in citrus and fruit juices, tomatoes, spices, alcohol, coffee, and junk food, which can pass to the baby and may irritate the skin after elimination. Traditional remedies include washing the affected area with well-diluted vinegar, and applying protective layers of egg white.
SEE PAGES 118–21

WESTERN HERBALISM

To prevent and treat diaper rash, practitioners may recommend washing the baby's bottom regularly with a soothing, healing, and cleansing infusion of lavender, thyme, German chamomile, calendula, or rose water. Afterward, a cream of German chamomile, calendula, or chickweed may be applied for further protection. SEE PAGES 134–39

COLIC

THE INTERMITTENT PAINS of colic cause a baby to cry or scream, draw up its legs, and possibly refuse comfort. Colic usually strikes babies at 1–3 months.

Causes The precise cause is unknown, but intestinal spasms seem to be a major factor. These may be due to the baby swallowing air while feeding, overfeeding, tension on the part of the caregiver, or an allergy to milk or other foods.

Conventional Treatment Doctors advise soothing physical stimuli, such as a warm, wrapped water bottle on the stomach, continuous vibratory noises, such as a vacuum cleaner, or rocking. It helps if the parent is relaxed when feeding, especially breastfeeding.

COMPLEMENTARY TREATMENTS

Therapies that help the baby and the parents relax will prove the most helpful.

CRANIAL OSTEOPATHY

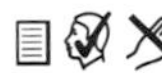

Cranial osteopaths suspect that a "colicky" tendency results from the baby's position in the uterus and from the stress of birth. Gentle manipulation of the baby's skull by a trained practitioner is thought to ease the resulting irritability. SEE PAGE 81

NATUROPATHY

Because diet affects your breast milk, a practitioner will suggest that you exclude dairy products, wheat, eggs, and citrus fruits.

CABBAGE
This vegetable is a useful source of calcium in lieu of dairy products.

You may also be advised to drink goat's milk and eat other calcium-rich foods, such as leafy vegetables. If your baby is weaned, you will be told not to give legumes, cow's milk, wheat, or other foods that might be difficult to digest until the child is at least one year old. Non-cow's milk products (goat's milk, soy milk or synthetic breast milk formulas) may be less irritating for babies who have an intolerance to cow's milk. SEE PAGES 118–21

WESTERN HERBALISM

Giving the baby drops of a weak infusion of dill or fennel, both of which help relieve gas, is a traditional herbal remedy.
SEE PAGES 134–39

OTHER OPTIONS

Aromatherapy SEE PAGES 62–65
Acupressure SEE PAGE 95
Homeopathy SEE PAGES 126–30
Nutritional Therapies SEE PAGES 148–52

CROUP

IN CROUP, WHICH OCCURS mainly in children under five, an inflamed trachea becomes narrowed by mucus, causing a barking cough, hoarseness, and a grunting noise when the child inhales. Croup usually arises from a viral or bacterial infection. Attacks generally begin at night and are usually mild, but they can become serious if fear provokes coughing spasms. Staying calm and taking the child into a steamy bathroom (turn on the hot water) should help ease breathing.

Caution: Consult a doctor urgently if croup is distressing or persists for more than 60 minutes.

COMPLEMENTARY TREATMENTS

Simple home remedies such as aromatic inhalations and herbal infusions may help relieve the symptoms and allay fear.

AROMATHERAPY

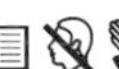
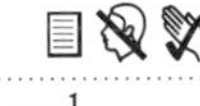

Essential oils diluted in a carrier oil and rubbed on to the child's chest, or diffused in a vaporizer, may help soothe coughing and distress. Commonly suggested oils include eucalyptus and thyme, which are antiseptic; German chamomile, an anti-inflammatory; or lavender, which has soothing properties.
SEE PAGES 62–65

HOMEOPATHY

These typical croup remedies can be tried in succession every 20 minutes: *Aconite 6c* in the early stages to allay fear, *Hepar sulf. 6c* for coughing spells that are worse in a cold atmosphere, and *Spongia 6c* if the child wakes up after midnight with a loud, rough cough.
SEE PAGES 126–30

WESTERN HERBALISM

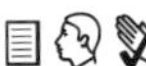

Herbal practitioners make syrups and infusions from plants such as mullein, licorice, wild cherry, or white horehound to ease coughing. Others made with German chamomile or catnip help sedate the child.
SEE PAGES 130–39

TEETHING

MILK TEETH ERUPT in children from the age of six months to three years, often leading to fretfulness, crying, drooling, poor appetite, sleep difficulties, and clinginess. A doctor may advise teething gels containing antiseptics and painkillers. In severe cases, infant acetaminophen may be recommended.

Self-Help Chewing a chilled teething ring may bring relief. Rubbing the gums gently with a finger may also help.

Cautions: Consult a doctor if teething is accompanied by diarrhea, fever, or a rash.

COMPLEMENTARY TREATMENTS

Practitioners tend to focus on calming and painkilling remedies.

NATUROPATHY

Practitioners believe digestive problems can exacerbate symptoms and may advise you to wean the baby onto easily digestible foods, such as baby rice, and to avoid added sugar.
SEE PAGES 118–21

HOMEOPATHY

Homeopaths advise *Chamomilla 6c* if the baby is frantic, *Aconite 6c* for acute discomfort and fever, and *Pulsatilla 6c* if the baby is weepy and wants constant cuddling. SEE PAGES 126–30

WESTERN HERBALISM

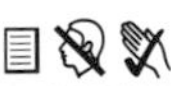

Marshmallow syrup may be advised to reduce swelling. A drop of clove oil in pasteurized honey rubbed on the gums may also help.
SEE PAGES 134–39

HONEY
This has antiseptic properties and makes pain-numbing clove oil palatable.

HEAD LICE

HEAD LICE ARE PINHEAD-SIZED, blood-sucking parasites that live in the hair, causing reddening of the scalp and persistent itching. Lice spread by crawling from one head to another, or are picked up from infested bedding, mattresses, and towels. Infestation is common among schoolchildren. Doctors advise washing the whole family's hair with an antilouse preparation, allowing it to dry, and then using a fine-toothed metal comb to remove the dead nits (eggs). Clothes and other items that may be sheltering lice should be washed in hot water, or put aside for a week until the creatures die off.

COMPLEMENTARY TREATMENTS

Plant-based remedies offer a useful alternative to chemical treatments for lice. Reinfestation is common and many parents are unhappy about repeatedly applying strong insecticides to children's heads. Furthermore, lice are becoming increasingly resistant to chemical treatments.

AROMATHERAPY

A blend of the essential oils of tea tree, geranium, rose, eucalyptus, lemon, and lavender may be suggested as a remedy, to be rubbed into the scalp and left overnight before washing out and carefully combing the hair. SEE PAGES 62–65

WESTERN HERBALISM

A practitioner may recommend lavender and olive oil rubbed into the scalp then rinsed with vinegar to help remove the nits, but re-infestation may occur if the lice are not killed as well. Common wormwood scattered among clothes and bed linen is said to kill lice and fleas, but it is toxic if eaten and should be used with great care near small children. SEE PAGES 134–39

COMBING
After an herbal shampoo, combing helps remove nits.

ADENOIDS

THE ADENOIDS ARE TWO GLANDS found at the back of the nasal cavity that produce infection-fighting white blood cells. The hard-working adenoids of children often become enlarged, blocking the nasal passage or the eustachian tubes, which run from the ears to the throat. As a result, breathing, speech, or hearing may be impaired. Trapped secretions may also lead to conditions such as glue ear (see below). If enlargement persists after antibiotic drug treatment, doctors may recommend that the glands be removed.

COMPLEMENTARY TREATMENTS

Enlargement of the adenoids most usually affects children aged between five and seven. Several therapies aim to protect the glands by preventing infection and allergies.

NATUROPATHY

A naturopath may concentrate on strengthening the child's digestive and immune systems. Exercise and a whole-foods diet high in vitamin C may be recommended, possibly with vitamin and mineral supplements. Cutting out dairy products and sugar or an elimination diet may also be advised. SEE PAGES 118–21

HOMEOPATHY

Treatment is based on constitutional type. Practitioners may suggest *Pulsatilla 6c* if the child is tearful and has a yellow nasal discharge, or *Calc. phos. 6c* for inflamed adenoids in a slender child. SEE PAGES 126–30

WESTERN HERBALISM

Red-sage gargle is believed to treat infection and soothe the throat. A steam inhalation containing Friar's balsam may clear congestion. An infusion of cleavers is said to reduce inflammation and "tone" the lymphatic system. SEE PAGES 134–39
Cautions: Friar's balsam inhalations are not advised for asthmatics. Do not give sage to epileptic children.

GLUE EAR (MIDDLE EAR EFFUSION)

"GLUE," OR MUCUS in the middle ear, is caused by a blockage in the eustachian tube, which links the middle ear to the throat. It may be the result of persistent ear infections. Research also implicates bottlefeeding, finding that the shorter nipples on bottles do not exercise a muscle that opens the ear tubes, allowing mucus to drain. This may be why breast-feeding appears to protect against glue ear. **Conventional Treatment** If decongestant medication does not help, doctors may surgically insert a drainage tube called a grommet. Some specialists now believe the ear should clear of its own accord. Antibiotics seem not to be effective.

COMPLEMENTARY TREATMENTS

Manipulation of the skull, plant medicines, and dietary adjustment are among the possible approaches to treatment.

CRANIAL OSTEOPATHY

By gently manipulating the skull, the practitioner seeks to improve drainage of mucus through the middle ear. SEE PAGE 81

MANIPULATION
Cranial osteopaths aim to treat glue ear by gently pressing the skull.

NATUROPATHY

A food intolerance (see page 303) may be thought responsible for producing excess mucus. A practitioner will suggest that nursing mothers and weaned children avoid dairy products and sugar in order to reduce mucus production. Cod liver oil and vitamin C supplements may be advised to help the immune system. SEE PAGES 118–21

WESTERN HERBALISM

Goldenseal tincture is believed to reduce mucus, and an herbalist may recommend that you give this to your child for several months. It may be added to a mixture of echinacea, licorice, elderflower, and cleavers, herbs that are thought to boost immunity.
SEE PAGES 134–39

CHILDREN'S FEVERS

FEVER MEANS THAT the body temperature is over 98.6°F (37°C). Fever may be accompanied by shivering, thirst, aches and pains, and hot skin. Depending on the child's age and the severity and rapidity of onset of the fever, delusions, convulsions, or coma may occur.

Causes Fever is a symptom of many diseases and conditions. It is most often a sign that the body is fighting a bacterial or viral infection, but environmental conditions, emotional disturbances, or shock can all raise body temperature, especially in babies.

Conventional Treatment General advice is to keep garments light, monitor the temperature regularly, and give plenty of fluids. Tepid sponge baths and children's acetaminophen are generally advised if the fever reaches 102.2°F (39°C), especially if the child has previously had fever-related convulsions.

CONSULT A DOCTOR IF:

- The temperature of a baby under six months old is over 102.2°F (39°C)
- The temperature of an older infant or child is 104°F (40°C) or more
- The fever lasts more than three days
- The fever is accompanied by drowsiness, confusion, a stiff neck, persistent vomiting, a rash, severe headaches, back and joint pain, discomfort from bright lights, or convulsions
- Do not give aspirin to children under the age of 12

COMPLEMENTARY TREATMENTS

Complementary practitioners see fever as a sign of healing as the body temperature rises to destroy microorganisms and eliminate waste products. If the child is over six months old and the temperature is under 102.2°F (39°C), practitioners generally advise against fever-suppressing drugs. Many therapists, especially herbalists and naturopaths, say that fever is an opportunity to "flex" and strengthen the child's defenses. Treatment concentrates on helping the body cope effectively over the course of the illness.

NATUROPATHY 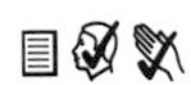

If a child's temperature rises above 102°F (38.8°C) taken orally or in the armpit, practitioners advise sponging with tepid water or applying cool compresses. Rest is important and a 24-hour water-only fast may be advised. Pasteurized honey and orange or lemon drinks are beneficial if no other nourishment can be kept down. When the fever has fallen, a healthy diet including lots of fruits and vegetables, especially vegetable juices such as carrot and beet juice, will be advised to build up strength. SEE PAGES 118–21

TAKING THE TEMPERATURE
Since a young child may bite a thermometer that is put into her mouth, it is safer to insert it under her armpit.

HOMEOPATHY 

The following are standard remedies for fever in children: *Aconite 6c* at the onset of a fever accompanied by thirst, chills, dry burning skin, and restlessness, *Belladonna 6c* for high fever, with dry burning skin, red face, dilated pupils, and swollen tender glands, *Arsen. alb. 6c* if the child is restless and agitated, anxious, hot and cold alternately, thirsty for small amounts of fluid, and worse after midnight, *Bryonia 6c* if the child is shivery and sweating, very thirsty at long intervals and experiencing headaches and pain, and *Ferrum phos. 6c* for a mild fever of slow onset, frequent bouts of sweating, shivering, and headaches.
SEE PAGES 126–30

WESTERN HERBALISM 

Fever management is an expert skill and requires a qualified medical herbalist. If the temperature rises above 102°F (38.8°C), a practitioner may advise bathing the child in tepid infusions of herbs such as limeflower, elderflower, yarrow, or German chamomile, all thought to help "normalize" body systems. Infusions or tinctures of catnip, hyssop, lemon balm, and vervain may be given. These herbs help to lower the temperature, increase perspiration, and calm the system. Infusions of German chamomile, lavender, and limeflower are considered relaxing and will encourage rest. Echinacea and garlic may be suggested to fight infection. SEE PAGES 134–39

OTHER OPTIONS

Aromatherapy	SEE PAGES 62–65
Acupressure	SEE PAGE 95
Biochemic Tissue Salts	SEE PAGE 131
Bach Flower Remedies	SEE PAGES 132–33
Nutritional Therapies	SEE PAGES 148–52

GERMAN MEASLES

ALSO KNOWN AS RUBELLA, German measles is an infectious, mild viral illness. Symptoms include fever, and possibly swollen glands and a pink rash. It has serious implications for unborn babies under 16 weeks, whose eyes and ears may be damaged. The illness usually lasts 4–5 days and the patient is infectious from five days before the fever until five days after it is gone. Doctors generally advise bed rest, fluids, and possibly children's acetaminophen.

Caution: Women in the first 16 weeks of pregnancy should consult a doctor immediately if exposed to German measles.

COMPLEMENTARY TREATMENTS

Since German measles is usually a mild illness in children, the worst symptom is likely to be a fever. Practitioners will advise fever management (see above).

AROMATHERAPY 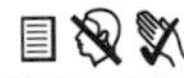

To soothe a fever, practitioners recommend cool compresses to which a couple of drops of peppermint oil have been added. SEE PAGES 62–65

NATUROPATHY 

Practitioners will suggest that you make sure the child has plenty of rest. You will be recommended to apply cool compresses or to sponge the child's skin with tepid water to bring relief from fever. Vegetable juices and a healthy diet will help reinforce the body's natural defenses. SEE PAGES 118–21

HOMEOPATHY 

See Children's Fevers, above. SEE PAGES 126–30

WESTERN HERBALISM 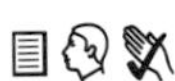

To treat a mild fever, an herbalist may recommend infusions made with yarrow or elderflower, which stimulate sweating. Catnip has a gentle action and is particularly suitable for treating childhood fevers.
SEE PAGES 134–39

MEASLES

ONCE A COMMON childhood infection, measles has become quite rare since immunization was introduced. The illness begins with flulike symptoms, followed by white spots in the mouth and a rash of raised reddish-purple spots covering the body. High fever, a swollen face, sensitivity to light, coughing, stomach pains, vomiting, and diarrhea may also occur, as may chest and ear infections, a temporary loss of hearing and, in about 1 in 1,000 cases, brain inflammation (encephalitis), a complication that can lead to seizures, coma, and even to death.

Cause The measles virus causes the illness, spread via direct contact or airborne droplets. The incubation period is 8–14 days, and the child is infectious for up to 7 days after symptoms appear.

Conventional Treatment Doctors advise acetaminophen and plenty of fluids, and, for chest or ear infections, antibiotics.

Prevention Measles can be dangerous. A vaccination is routine for children aged 12–18 months. It offers up to 95% protection, but the need for a booster at 4–5 years old has recently been suggested.

Caution: Call a doctor if your child has a high fever.

COMPLEMENTARY TREATMENTS

Many complementary practitioners believe that childhood illnesses serve a purpose by strengthening the immune system. Treatment aims to control fever (see also page 281), support the body's self-healing ability, and soothe discomfort.

NATUROPATHY

Practitioners will advise managing the fever with a light diet consisting mainly of fluids, followed by vegetables when the temperature falls. Tepid baths with baking soda may help soothe the rash. SEE PAGES 118–21

HOMEOPATHY

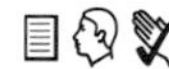

Homeopathy is based on the principle that "like cures like." A minute amount of a substance that causes illness in larger doses is thought to "immunize" against the disease. There is no evidence that homeopathic "immunization" is effective, although the following remedies may be helpful for the coldlike symptoms and fever that accompany measles: *Aconite 6c, Belladonna 6c,* and *Euphrasia 6c.* SEE PAGES 126–30

WESTERN HERBALISM

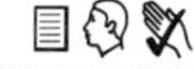

A practitioner may advise you to bathe your child with a tepid, weak infusion of German chamomile to reduce the fever. Infusions of lavender and witch hazel, applied as a wash, help to ease itching. Reddened eyes may be bathed with an infusion of eyebright. Expectorant herbs, such as hyssop, loosen phlegm, and echinacea may be suggested to help the immune system fight infection.
SEE PAGES 134–39

CHINESE HERBALISM

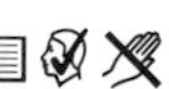

In Traditional Chinese Medicine, measles is associated with "excess heat in the Blood and Stomach." Cooling herbal remedies might include safflower, peppermint, and honeysuckle. SEE PAGES 140–43

Caution: Do not give peppermint to children under five.

NUTRITIONAL THERAPIES

A practitioner may recommend vitamin A because measles is reported to respond to large doses of this vitamin. In a study published in 1993 in the *Journal of the American Medical Association,* in trials undertaken in developing countries involving children hospitalized with measles, death rates declined when they were treated with vitamin A.
SEE PAGES 148–52

OTHER OPTIONS

Aromatherapy SEE PAGES 62–65
Bach Flower Remedies SEE PAGES 132–33

MUMPS

MUMPS IS AN INFECTION of the main salivary glands (parotids), located at the sides of the face. Symptoms include uncomfortable swelling, fever, headaches, and difficulty in swallowing. While complications are unusual, inflammation of the pancreas or the brain membranes (meningitis) can occur. After adolescence, the testes may be affected, occasionally leading to infertility.

Cause The mumps virus spreads in airborne droplets. The child should be isolated until the seventh day after the swelling has subsided.

Conventional Treatment Doctors advise bed rest, cool compresses, fluids, and children's acetaminophen for discomfort. Corticosteroid drugs may be prescribed for male teenagers. A vaccination is available for children over 12 months old.

Caution: Call a doctor if your child has a severe headache, or is sensitive to light, drowsy, or confused.

COMPLEMENTARY TREATMENTS

Treatment will focus on fever management (see page 281), relieving discomfort and boosting immunity.

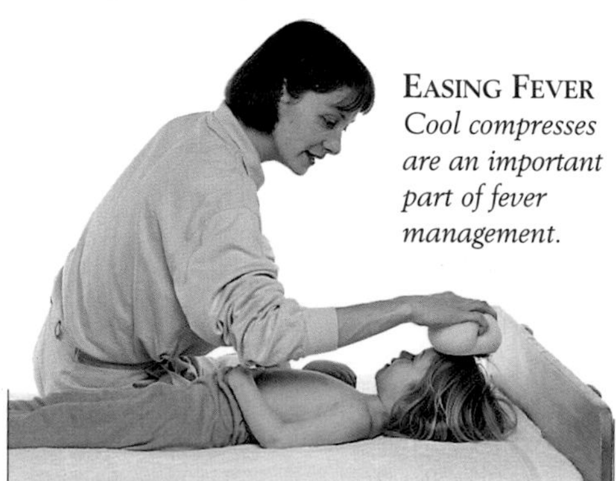

EASING FEVER *Cool compresses are an important part of fever management.*

HOMEOPATHY

The following remedies may be helpful: *Rhus tox. 6c* and the nosode (see glossary) *Parotidinum* if the disease is recognized very early on, *Aconite 6c* for pain and the onset of fever, *Belladonna 6c* for fever and throbbing glands, *Lachesis 6c* if there is difficulty in swallowing liquids, and *Merc. sol. 6c* for a stiff neck, swollen glands, and profuse saliva.
SEE PAGES 126–30

WESTERN HERBALISM

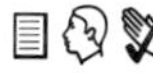

Practitioners seek to promote lymphatic drainage and to enhance immunity. Herbs that may be recommended include cleavers and calendula. An antiseptic gargle with tincture of thyme may also be recommended, with the addition of echinacea to help fight infection. SEE PAGES 134–39

CHINESE HERBALISM

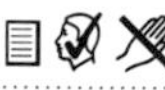

Mumps is associated with "wind and damp heat." Practitioners may prescribe cooling herbal remedies that include dandelion, honeysuckle, skullcap, and Chinese rhubarb.
SEE PAGES 140–43

OTHER OPTIONS

Aromatherapy SEE PAGES 62–65
Biochemic Tissue Salts SEE PAGE 131

CHICKEN POX

THIS VERY INFECTIOUS ILLNESS begins with a mild fever followed by a rash of spots on the head and body that turn into itchy blisters, which then burst and form scabs. If scratched, they may become infected and leave scars. The first attack gives immunity, but the virus lies dormant in nerve tissue and may reappear later in life as shingles (see page 217). While an infected child can activate shingles, shingles does not cause chicken pox.

Cause The varicella-zoster virus spreads in airborne droplets. After a 14–21 day incubation period, the child is infectious from about two days before the rash until seven days after the last spot appears.

Conventional Treatment Doctors advise children's acetaminophen to lower fever, and calamine lotion dabbed on the rash to ease discomfort.

Caution: Call a doctor if fever is high, the child is distressed, or has a headache with drowsiness.

COMPLEMENTARY TREATMENTS

Practitioners will focus on fever management (see page 281) and relieving the discomfort of itchy spots.

AROMATHERAPY

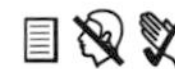

You may be advised to use essential oils of lavender, tea tree, or bergamot very well diluted in chamomile tea, dabbed onto the skin. This has a soothing and possibly antiviral effect. Lavender, bergamot, or chamomile oil may be added to the bath. **SEE PAGES 62–65**

USING ESSENTIAL OIL
Diluted essential oils may allay the discomfort of chicken pox.

NATUROPATHY

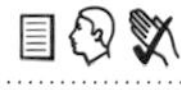

To soothe itching, practitioners advocate giving the child tepid baths with added starch, baking soda, cider vinegar, or oatmeal. If chicken pox is only suspected, a hot bath may be advised to bring out a latent rash. The traditional thought is that this hastens the progress of the illness.
SEE PAGES 118–21

HOMEOPATHY

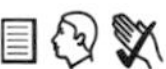

If exposure to chicken pox is likely, a practitioner will suggest "preventive" remedies such as *Rhus tox.* 6c and *Varicella 30c.* During the illness, the following may help: *Antim. tart.* 6c if the child is peevish, *Pulsatilla 6c* if the child is whiny and clinging, *Aconite 30c* for the initial fever, *Sulfur 6c* if the child is thirsty and hungry but won't eat, and *Mercurius iodatus* 6c during recovery. **SEE PAGES 126–30**

WESTERN HERBALISM

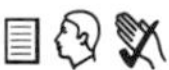

Chickweed is traditionally recommended, applied as a lotion or a wash to irritated skin. Soothing infusions of elderflower, witch hazel, rosemary, or calendula may also be suggested.
SEE PAGES 134–39

OTHER OPTIONS

Bach Flower Remedies **SEE PAGES 132–33**
Chinese Herbalism **SEE PAGES 140–43**

WHOOPING COUGH

FITS OF VIOLENT COUGHING, punctuated with a characteristic "whoop" as the child inhales, can distress both parent and child. Whooping cough begins with fatigue, phlegm, sneezing, sore eyes, mild fever, and coughing. The coughing may become severe enough to cause nosebleeds, burst blood vessels in the eyes, vomiting, and blue lips, fingers, and toes. Possible complications may include pneumonia, convulsions, and brain damage.

Causes Whooping cough is caused by the *Bordetella pertussis* bacterium, which inflames the respiratory tract and is spread via airborne droplets. Symptoms manifest after a period of 1–3 weeks. The cough can last for up to 14 weeks (in China, it is known as "hundred-day cough").

Conventional Treatment A doctor will advise you to stay calm and give the child small frequent meals and plenty to drink. Antibiotics may be prescribed if the illness is diagnosed before severe coughing starts. In the US, immunization has virtually wiped out this disease.

Caution: Call an ambulance if the child cannot breathe, has a high fever, or vomits continually.

COMPLEMENTARY TREATMENTS

In general, the approach is to try to enhance the child's defenses while limiting the most distressing aspects of the illness.

AROMATHERAPY

A practitioner may advocate essential oil of lavender, which can have a soothing effect, and the essential oils of rosemary and eucalyptus, which are thought to fight off infection. A few drops may be diffused in a vaporizer.
SEE PAGES 62–65

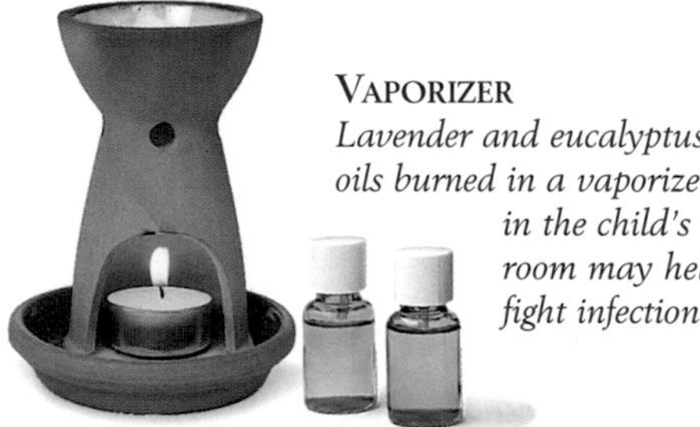

VAPORIZER
Lavender and eucalyptus oils burned in a vaporizer in the child's room may help fight infection.

NATUROPATHY

Practitioners may advise feeding the child a light diet of fruit juice, vegetable juice, and broth when the illness is at its peak. Garlic and foods rich in zinc and vitamins C and A may be suggested to fight infection.
SEE PAGES 118–21

HOMEOPATHY

It is important to consult a qualified, experienced homeopath for whooping cough. He or she may prescribe the nosode (see glossary) *Pertussin.* Although many claim that it is effective as an "immunization" against whooping cough, this has not been proven. Standard remedies include *Aconite 6c* in the early stages for a dry, hard cough, fever, thirst, hot skin, rapid pulse, and anxiety, *Belladonna 6c* for a barking repetitive cough that is worse at night, with hot red dry skin, crying, and restlessness, *Drosera 6c* for violent and spasmodic coughs, and *Ipecac. 6c* if the cough causes vomiting. **SEE PAGES 126–30**

WESTERN HERBALISM

Your practitioner may prescribe expectorant herbs, such as elecampane, wild cherry, mullein flowers, and hyssop, to loosen the cough, and antiseptic and antispasmodic herbs, such as thyme, flavored with honey and licorice, to relax the bronchial tubes. Some practitioners recommend wild lettuce as a calming sedative if anxiety aggravates coughing spasms. **SEE PAGES 134–39**

Caution: Do not give unpasteurized honey to children under one year old.

OTHER OPTION

Bach Flower Remedies **SEE PAGES 132–33**

HYPERACTIVITY

THE SYMPTOMS of hyperactive behavior include overactivity, restlessness, inattention, impulsiveness, disruptiveness, and lack of control. Hyperactivity is now widely accepted as part of a syndrome called Attention Deficit Disorder (ADD). About 3% of school-aged children are said to be affected.

Causes There is no single cause. Hyperactivity seems to result from a combination of biological, neurological, psychological, and environmental factors. Nutritional deficiencies, food intolerances, food additives, caffeine, excessive sugar, learning difficulties, environmental pollution, and an unstable home life have all been blamed, but research studies have found no universal links with any of them.

Conventional Treatment Some children seem to improve when processed foods and caffeine are removed from their diet. Doctors may also prescribe an amphetamine-type drug, but many feel this is inappropriate, in part due to potential adverse side effects. Researchers now advise psychological and educational approaches, possibly in combination with medication.

COMPLEMENTARY TREATMENTS

Some practitioners seek to identify nutritional or environmental factors that may lead to hyperactivity. Others try to pinpoint psychological triggers.

NATUROPATHY

A practitioner will advise a whole-foods diet with mineral water, and suggest avoiding processed foods and additives such as tartrazine (E101) and benzoic acid (E210–219). Possible food sensitivities will be investigated, especially to salicylates (chemicals found in aspirin and many foods, including apples, almonds, apricots, peaches, tomatoes, berries, and raisins), which may trigger hyperactivity. Dr. Benjamin Feingold in the US claimed in the early 1980s that 70% of hyperactive children improved when food coloring, preservatives, sugar, additives, and salicylates were removed from their diet. Subsequent studies have not always supported this, but additives may be relevant in combination with social and psychological factors. SEE PAGES 118–21

WESTERN HERBALISM 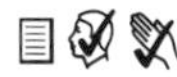

Practitioners will suggest relaxing herbal infusions made with vervain or German chamomile. If necessary, they may also use "detoxifying" herbs such as red clover, kelp, nettle, or self-heal. SEE PAGES 134–39

NUTRITIONAL THERAPIES 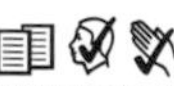

Some hyperactive children have been found to be deficient in essential fatty acids, zinc, vitamin C, vitamin B_6, and niacin. Practitioners may recommend supplements if necessary. If environmental pollution is thought to be a factor, kelp supplements may be advised to "detoxify" the system. SEE PAGES 148–52

PSYCHOTHERAPY & COUNSELING 

A number of therapies, including cognitive and behavioral therapy, child therapy, and family counseling, may help to resolve any psychological factors, social factors, or educational difficulties that may play a role in hyperactivity. SEE PAGES 160–65

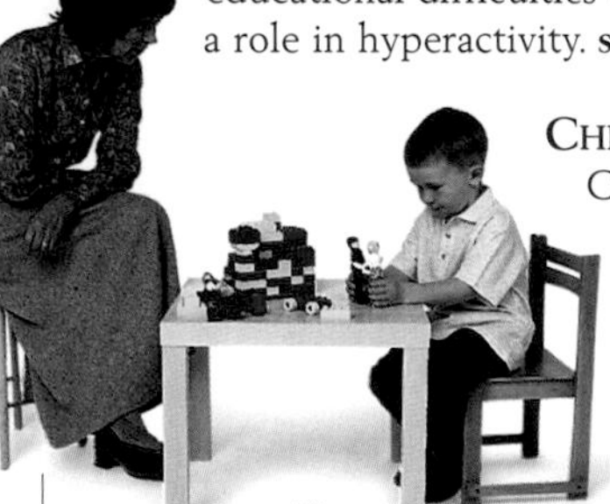

CHILD THERAPY *Constructive play may help to improve a hyperactive child's attention span.*

OTHER OPTIONS

Cranial Osteopathy SEE PAGE 81

Homeopathy SEE PAGES 126–30

Relaxation & Breathing SEE PAGES 170–73

SLEEP PROBLEMS

IN A BABY under six months old, sleeplessness may be due to hunger, gas, a dirty diaper, diaper rash, colic, a raised temperature, or feeling cold after kicking off bedclothes. Older children can be kept awake by overexcitement and restlessness, an irregular bedtime, caffeine, fear of the dark, lack of exercise and fresh air, an overheated or cold bedroom, or illness. A doctor will ask about underlying causes.

Self-Help Check that the child is comfortable and does not require a clean diaper, for example. Keep to a regular bedtime and avoid stimulating activities beforehand. Give a warm drink (not cocoa, which contains caffeine) and follow a settling-down ritual such as story-telling. Allay any fears with cuddles, and go back once or twice if the child calls, but set limits on how often you return.

COMPLEMENTARY TREATMENTS

Having a child who refuses to go to sleep can be distressing. Among the approaches practitioners may advise are calming foods and herbal remedies given before bedtime, or aromatic essential oils to relax and calm the child.

AROMATHERAPY 

Practitioners recommend a few drops of essential oil of German chamomile, lavender, rose, neroli, or geranium added to a bath to induce calm. Lavender essential oil diffused in a vaporizer may be soothing. SEE PAGES 62–65

NATUROPATHY

To avoid overstimulating the child, a practitioner will advise against foods that contain sugar or additives. Instead, a bedtime snack of a banana, lettuce sandwich, or a milk drink may be suggested. These foods contain tryptophan, vitamin B, and calcium, substances used by the body to make serotonin, a brain chemical that induces sleep. SEE PAGES 118–21

WESTERN HERBALISM

Infusions of calming herbs, such as catnip, lemon balm, lavender, or hops, help promote restful sleep when given as teas before bedtime. German chamomile, limeflower, or skullcap infusions are said to relieve nervous tension, and rosemary to allay bad dreams. Herbal "sleep" pillows, filled with hops and lavender, are available. SEE PAGES 134–39

OTHER OPTIONS

Homeopathy SEE PAGES 126–30

Bach Flower Remedies SEE PAGES 132–33

BED-WETTING

CHILDREN ARE LIKELY to wet the bed until they are about three or four; one in ten do so until they are five, and some continue into their teens. In time, almost all outgrow it. Bed-wetting is largely due to a child's nervous system being too immature for total bladder control, but it can also be triggered by anxiety.

Conventional Treatment Some doctors prescribe antidepressant drugs, but they do not always work, and if they do they are effective only for as long as they are taken. Automatic buzzers, activated when the bed starts to become wet so that the child wakes and can go to the toilet, may also help.

Self-Help It is important not to be angry with the child. Discouraging large drinks before bedtime may help. Star charts or other reward systems that highlight dry nights can help the child feel a sense of achievement.

COMPLEMENTARY TREATMENTS

Complementary therapists seek to support and strengthen the urinary tract with medicinal remedies and dietary aids.

CHIROPRACTIC (SEE OSTEOPATHY)

OSTEOPATHY

Some practitioners claim that "spinal dysfunction" can disrupt nerve impulses between the brain and bladder, and will treat the child accordingly. SEE PAGES 70–81

ACUPUNCTURE

Two Italian studies undertaken in 1981 and 1991 show that acupuncture can help children with bed-wetting problems. SEE PAGES 90–94

HOMEOPATHY

The following standard remedies may help: *Plantago 6c* if the bed is wet early in sleep, *Lycopodium 6c* if later in sleep, *Pulsatilla 6c* if the child is clingy, and *Causticum 6c* if bedwetting is worse with a cough. SEE PAGES 126–30

WESTERN HERBALISM

Practitioners may prescribe a relaxant such as St. John's wort if bed-wetting appears to be caused by anxiety. Gentle diuretics, such as couch grass, cornsilk, and marshmallow, may help to encourage a more regular bladder rhythm. SEE PAGES 134–39

CORNSILK
Drinking cornsilk tea in the day stimulates urination before bedtime.

PSYCHOTHERAPY & COUNSELING

Practitioners will focus on any underlying causes of stress, and work to defuse anxiety about bed-wetting itself. They will also encourage the child to establish realistic goals. SEE PAGES 160–65

OTHER OPTION

Cranial Osteopathy SEE PAGE 81

STAMMERING

ABOUT 1 IN 10 YOUNG CHILDREN stammer. It is three times more likely to affect boys than girls, and all but 20% outgrow it. Recent research indicates that the brain's speech coordination processes may be involved, and that genetic, emotional, and psychological factors also contribute. As stammering is difficult to treat, early referral to a speech therapist is advised. Many techniques are used, sometimes in combination with family counseling.

COMPLEMENTARY TREATMENTS

Therapies that improve relaxation, breathing, and confidence may prove to be most helpful.

PSYCHOTHERAPY & COUNSELING

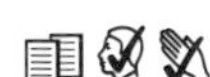

One-to-one counseling may enhance social skills and confidence. Counseling can also take place in a group with other young stammerers, or with the family, to explore sources of stress and try to address possible tension in the child's surroundings. SEE PAGES 160–65

HYPNOTHERAPY

Suggestions made to the child when he or she is in a relaxed state have been successful in certain cases. SEE PAGES 166–67

RELAXATION & BREATHING

Techniques to reduce anxiety and muscle tension may help stammering. SEE PAGES 170–73

MUSIC THERAPY

Exploring a range of expression may help. Stammerers rarely hesitate when singing or reciting in chorus. SEE PAGE 181

TEMPER TANTRUMS

FURIOUS OUTBURSTS are relatively common in children aged one to five, but most eventually outgrow them. Family tension, the birth of a sibling, and inconsistent discipline can all contribute to the behavior. Doctors advise trying to ignore outbursts, unless the situation is dangerous. Diverting a child's attention is preferable to punishment, but avoid using "bribes." If temper tantrums continue past the age of five, or if the child is particularly manipulative, family therapy or child psychology may be suggested.

COMPLEMENTARY TREATMENTS

Naturopaths determine whether food allergies make the problem worse, while mind therapies try to help parents cope.

NATUROPATHY

Practitioners believe that food sensitivities can affect mood and will suggest an elimination diet. SEE PAGES 118–21

HOMEOPATHY

An assessment of your child is advisable, followed by appropriate treatment. *Nux vomica 6c* may be suggested for irritability, especially after overeating. SEE PAGES 126–30

NUX VOMICA
These seeds are the source of a homeopathic remedy for irritability.

PSYCHOTHERAPY & COUNSELING

As well as helping the child, family therapy may improve parents' ability to cope with temper tantrums. SEE PAGES 160–65

MIND & EMOTIONS

SINCE THE 1980S, PET SCANS (see glossary) and other advances in brain imaging have revealed that certain areas of the brain are associated with specific emotions and mental functions. This technology is helping neuroscientists understand more about brain activity and psychiatric illness. The body and the mind and emotions appear to be closely interrelated, particularly through the part of the brain known as the limbic system, which influences emotions and controls the hormones. Thoughts and emotions have a direct impact on this area, thereby affecting circulation, digestion, and musculoskeletal bearing.

KEY TO SYMBOLS	
EVIDENCE	**PRACTITIONER**
Good scientific trials with positive results	Essential
Some research studies	Recommended
Anecdotal	Not essential
	SELF-HELP
	Self-help possibilities
	No self-help

COMPLEMENTARY APPROACHES

Touch therapies concentrate on relieving muscle tension. Medicinal therapies may improve the function of brain and nerve chemicals. Relaxation and psychological therapies calm the mind, reduce internal conflict, and ease physical tension.

CONVENTIONAL APPROACHES

Developments in behavioral therapies (see page 164) have helped doctors treat psychological conditions such as phobias and anxiety. The use of brain surgery and electroconvulsive therapy has declined.

Caution: Before seeking treatment, see page 204.

THE ROLE OF THE LIMBIC SYSTEM

The key connection between the mind and the body is the limbic system. Structures such as the cingulate gyrus, fornix, and hippocampus moderate instincts and emotions and control the nervous and hormonal systems. The limbic system also orchestrates neurotransmitters, which act as chemical "messengers" throughout the body. One neurotransmitter, serotonin, appears to enhance mood, while a deficiency may lead to depression. Some mental illness may be due to disturbed brain chemistry. Studies also indicate that changing someone's outlook with psychological therapies can change their brain chemistry.

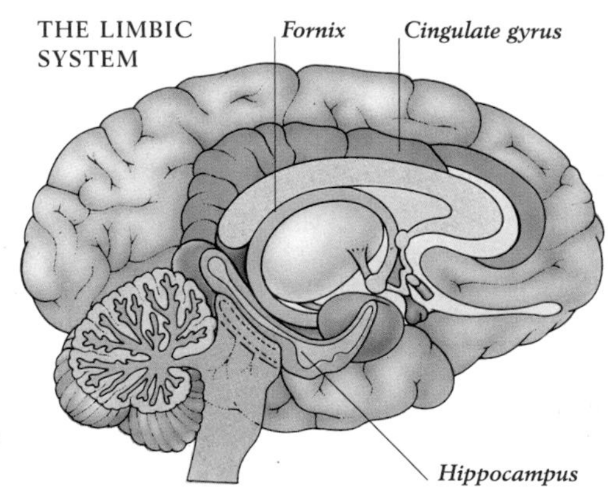

PHOBIAS

A PHOBIA IS AN IRRATIONAL FEAR of an object or a situation, causing anxiety, panic attacks, and possibly depression. Some phobias, such as fear of open spaces (agoraphobia), can severely restrict everyday life. Other common phobias are fear of enclosed spaces (claustrophobia), and of specific animals, such as spiders. A phobia may follow a bad experience in the past or the behavior of a parent or sibling who has a similar fear. Subsequent anxiety and hyperventilation (rapid breathing) can make it worse.

Conventional Treatment A doctor will usually suggest cognitive behavioral therapy. Antidepressants can be helpful but may take 4–6 weeks to work.

Self-Help Learn to control your reactions by using stress management techniques such as relaxation and breathing.

COMPLEMENTARY TREATMENTS

Mind therapies aim to help people gain control over their fears. Homeopathy is also a popular therapy for emotional problems.

HOMEOPATHY

Standard remedies that may be suggested include *Aconite 6c* for agoraphobia, *Argent. nit. 6c* for claustrophobia and fear of heights, and *Phos. 6c* for fear of the dark. SEE PAGES 126–30

NUTRITIONAL THERAPIES

Some practitioners claim agoraphobia can be triggered by a deficiency of omega-3 fatty acids, although this is unproved. Fish-oil supplements may be prescribed. SEE PAGES 148–52

PSYCHOTHERAPY & COUNSELING

Exposure therapy, which is a form of behavioral therapy, is particularly useful. You will be helped to face the object of your phobia, gradually increasing your exposure until anxiety diminishes, while using stress management techniques to control your reactions. Cognitive behavioral therapy can help you to adopt more positive ways of thinking and behaving. Practitioners of Neurolinguistic Programming claim theirs is a fast, effective method of curing phobias. SEE PAGES 160–65

RELAXATION & BREATHING

A practitioner will teach progressive muscle relaxation and diaphragmatic breathing, which may help you control anxiety and prevent hyperventilation when faced with the object or situation that you fear. SEE PAGES 170–73

ART THERAPY

Expressing irrational fears through drawing or painting may reduce their hold over the imagination. SEE PAGES 182–83

OTHER OPTIONS

Hypnotherapy SEE PAGES 166–67
Biofeedback SEE PAGE 169

ANXIETY

ANXIETY IS PART of the "fight-or-flight" response to stress (see pages 290–91) and is a normal reaction to certain situations, for example if a child is late coming home from school. However, sometimes anxiety becomes so intense that it can interfere with ordinary life. Overanxious people are irritable, cannot concentrate, sleep badly, tire easily, and often become depressed. Muscle tension leads to headaches, pain in the neck and back, and an inability to relax. Anxiety can manifest in other physical ways, for example as palpitations, chest pains, and digestive disturbances. Physically and emotionally draining in the long term, anxiety may compromise the immune system and also lead to disorders such as high blood pressure and irritable bowel syndrome.

Causes It is often difficult to pinpoint the exact cause. Some people tend to become anxious more easily than others. This may be partly genetic. Those with a tendency toward pessimism or neuroticism are particularly likely to suffer from anxiety when under stress. Bad experiences in the past and family behavior patterns are also important factors.

Conventional Treatment A doctor may prescribe a short course of beta-blockers (see glossary) or antidepressants, sometimes alone but more often in combination with psychotherapy and counseling.

Self-Help Talking about your concerns may help you achieve a more balanced perspective. Try to think positively and view the source of anxiety as a challenge, rather than a problem. Get plenty of exercise: a number of studies since the 1970s have shown that exercise has a "tranquilizing" effect on anxiety, reducing muscle tension, and releasing mood-enhancing endorphins.

ROMAN CHAMOMILE
Massage with the essential oil of this plant is soothing.

TOUCH & MOVEMENT THERAPIES

The therapeutic benefit of touch is well documented. Many people find that therapies of this type help them cope with stress that contributes to anxiety.

MASSAGE 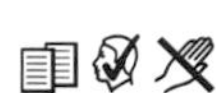

Regular massage can relieve muscle tension and reduce stress and anxiety. In a 1992 study by the Touch Research Institute in Miami, 30 minutes of daily massage was found to be more effective than a relaxation video. SEE PAGES 56–61

AROMATHERAPY 

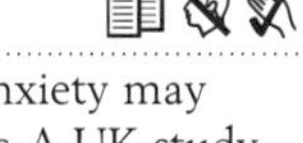

Aromatherapists believe that anxiety may be relieved with calming aromas. A UK study in 1995 found that a massage with Roman chamomile essential oil was more effective in reducing anxiety in cancer patients than a massage with a carrier oil. SEE PAGES 62–65

Caution: The use of Roman chamomile essential oil is subject to restriction in some countries.

ROLFING 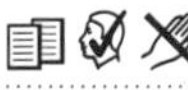

In one US study reported in 1979, people undergoing the firm pressure and manipulation used in Rolfing were shown to be less anxious than another group following a program of exercises. SEE PAGES 82–83

THERAPEUTIC TOUCH 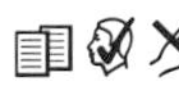

In this therapy, a practitioner places her hands close to the patient to "rebalance" the flow of energy. Several studies have shown that Therapeutic Touch reduced anxiety in hospital patients more effectively than either ordinary touching or conversation. SEE PAGE 106

OTHER OPTIONS

Bioenergetics	SEE PAGE 89
Acupressure	SEE PAGE 95
Qigong	SEE PAGE 99
Healing	SEE PAGES 104–105
Yoga	SEE PAGES 108–11

MEDICINAL THERAPIES

An improved diet and homeopathic remedies may help to relieve anxiety.

NATUROPATHY 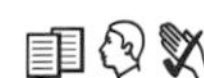

A practitioner will ensure that your diet contains adequate nutrients and complex carbohydrates (such as bread and pasta), which help stabilize blood sugar levels. Some cases of anxiety are attributed to hypoglycemia (low blood sugar). This is associated with depression, panic attacks, and mood swings. Stimulants such as caffeine and alcohol should be avoided. An exclusion diet may be advised to identify any food intolerances that could affect mood. SEE PAGES 118–21

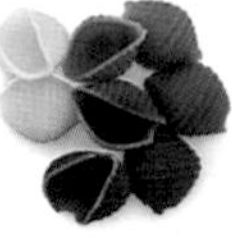
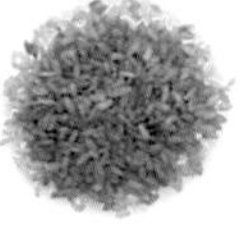
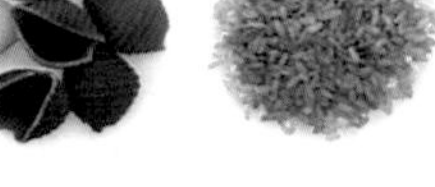
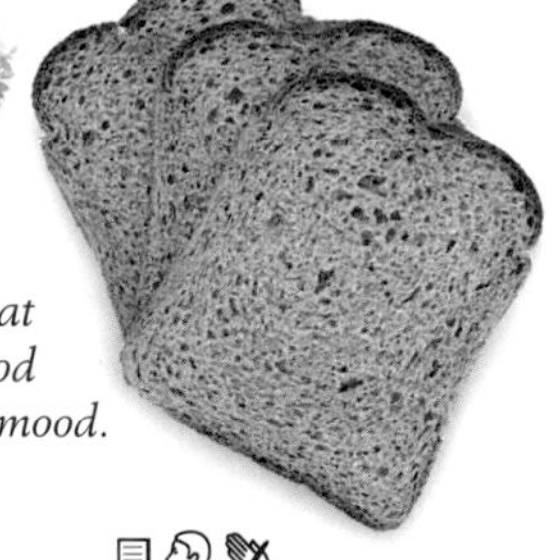

STARCHY FOODS
Pasta, rice, and whole-wheat bread help to stabilize blood sugar levels and enhance mood.

HOMEOPATHY 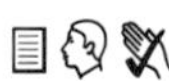

A practitioner will recommend remedies tailored to your constitution. Standard remedies include: *Gelsemium 6c* if you are fearful of future events, *Arsen. alb. 6c* for persistent anxiety with restlessness, *Phos. 6c* if you are oversensitive and needing reassurance, and *Argent. nit. 6c* if anticipation upsets the digestion. SEE PAGES 126–30

MIND & EMOTION THERAPIES

Overanxious people often have a "victim" mentality. Mind and emotion therapies aim to boost self-esteem and teach how to control reactions that may be unhelpful.

PSYCHOTHERAPY & COUNSELING 

Psychotherapy may help you to recognize, understand, and come to terms with the reasons for your anxiety. Cognitive behavioral therapy has been found especially successful in helping people change patterns of thinking and behavior that reinforce anxiety. SEE PAGES 160–65

HYPNOTHERAPY 

Hypnotherapy can be particularly helpful in undoing conditioned physiological responses, such as nausea or hyperventilation (rapid breathing). It may also help to allay fear to do with exams or public speaking. SEE PAGES 166–67

RELAXATION & BREATHING 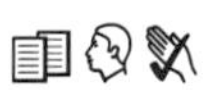

Learning to release muscle tension and breathe with the diaphragm can help bring anxiety under control. SEE PAGES 170–73

MEDITATION 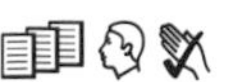

In 1992, US researchers found that patients using a *Vipassana*, or "mindfulness meditation" program, were less anxious and depressed than before. Three years later, those who were still meditating showed continued improvement. SEE PAGES 174–77

PANIC ATTACKS & HYPERVENTILATION

SUDDEN SURGES of intense anxiety (panic attacks) can occur seemingly at random, or be prompted by a certain situation, such as traveling on a crowded train, in which case it is diagnosed as a "phobia" (see page 286). Symptoms of panic attacks include chest pains, breathing problems, palpitations, and dizziness. Hyperventilation is rapid, shallow breathing. It causes the level of carbon dioxide in the blood to drop, leading to faintness, numbness, and muscle tension. **Conventional Treatment** A doctor will treat panic attacks with cognitive behavioral therapy, possibly together with beta-blocker drugs (see glossary) to help control physical symptoms. **Self-Help** Don't fight the attack; try to remind yourself that it will soon pass. If you are hyperventilating, breathing into a paper bag can help because it raises the levels of carbon dioxide in the body.

COMPLEMENTARY TREATMENTS

Practitioners may be able to suggest physical and psychological self-help methods to bring quick relief during an attack.

AROMATHERAPY

A practitioner may suggest putting a few drops of clary sage, lavender, sandalwood, or rose essential oil on a handkerchief to inhale during an attack. SEE PAGES 62–65

HOMEOPATHY

The following remedies may be suggested for an acute panic attack: *Arnica 6c* as a first resort; *Aconite 6c* after sudden shock, with chest pains and fear of dying; *Gelsemium 6c* if weak and shaky afterward. SEE PAGES 126–30

PSYCHOTHERAPY & COUNSELING

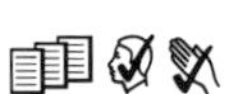

Cognitive behavioral therapy can be highly effective in helping dispel the fear associated with panic attacks and hyperventilation.
SEE PAGES 160–65

RELAXATION & BREATHING

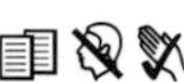

Muscle relaxation techniques practiced daily and before a stressful event may help reduce tension. SEE PAGES 170–73

MEDITATION

By helping you to concentrate on your breathing and to think positively early in an attack, *Vipassana* ("mindfulness meditation") may prevent further panic.
SEE PAGES 174–77

INNER CALM
Focusing on breathing or on an object of meditation is calming.

OTHER OPTIONS

Yoga SEE PAGES 108–11
Naturopathy SEE PAGES 118–21
Bach Flower Remedies SEE PAGES 132–33
Hypnotherapy SEE PAGES 166–67
Autogenic Training SEE PAGE 168

OBSESSIVE-COMPULSIVE DISORDER

PHOBIAS MAY MANIFEST as obsessive thoughts, or compulsive rituals that must be performed again and again as a way of fending off anxiety and panic attacks. The most common obsessions are about dirt, disorder, or violence. Some people, for example, have an abnormal fear of germs and have to wash their hands repeatedly. Doctors usually recommend a form of behavioral therapy and sometimes antidepressants. Conventional treatment can be highly effective.

COMPLEMENTARY TREATMENTS

Practitioners will suggest techniques to help you understand and change your patterns of behavior. These can help when faced with a problematical situation.

PSYCHOTHERAPY & COUNSELING

Exposure therapy, which is a form of behavioral therapy, may be successful. You will be taken into the situation that triggers your compulsive rituals and helped to resist the urge to carry them out.
SEE PAGES 160–65

HYPNOTHERAPY

When you are in a deeply relaxed state, the hypnotherapist will suggest ways of dealing with situations you find difficult. SEE PAGES 166–67

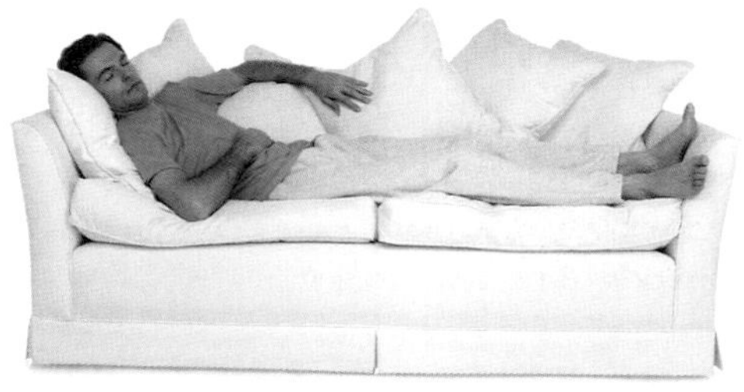

SELF-HYPNOSIS
Learning to relax deeply at will can allay fears.

POST-TRAUMATIC STRESS DISORDER

THOSE WHO HAVE ENDURED extreme experiences, such as war or rape, may continue to feel anxious long after the event. This can manifest as disturbed sleep, flashbacks, hallucinations, and a variety of physical disorders. Panic attacks and hyperventilation (see above) are also common. A doctor will usually advise counseling.

COMPLEMENTARY TREATMENTS

Psychological approaches and therapies that use touch may help people cope with the aftermath of a traumatic experience.

CRANIOSACRAL THERAPY

Practitioners apply corrective pressure to the cranium and spine. They claim that this approach helps to "unwind body memories" of the event that may otherwise keep the patient in a persistent state of shock. SEE PAGE 81

PSYCHOTHERAPY & COUNSELING

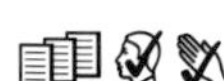

Cognitive behavioral therapy is widely used in the treatment of this condition. Some psychologists report interesting results with a controversial treatment called "eye movement desensitization and reprocessing," in which eye movements replicate the information-processing function of REM sleep (see page 39), a process that may help the patient move on psychologically.
SEE PAGES 160–65

INSOMNIA

INSOMNIA, THE PERSISTENT INABILITY to sleep, is a common problem, particularly as people grow older: around half of those aged between 40 and 55 suffer at least occasionally from insomnia. Sleeplessness falls into three categories: not being able to go to sleep; waking frequently; and waking too early in the morning. A minimum amount of sleep is essential for many body functions; too little can lead to fatigue and irritability.

Causes Psychological factors are the most common causes. Trouble in falling asleep is associated with anxiety, while difficulty in remaining asleep is linked to illness, depression, persistent pain, or changes in circadian (daily body-clock) rhythms due to jet lag or shift work. Lack of exercise, substances such as caffeine, alcohol, and nicotine, or a change in surroundings can also affect sleep rhythms.

Conventional Treatment Doctors will try to address the cause of the insomnia with counseling or relaxation techniques and may prescribe antidepressants if you are depressed. As a last resort, sleeping pills may be suggested as a very short-term solution. Sleep restriction, which limits patients to six hours in bed a night until exhaustion forces new sleep patterns, has been successful for some people.

Self-Help A number of simple, practical measures may help ensure a good night's sleep. These include sensible eating and drinking habits, regular exercise, and periods of relaxation (see also page 39).

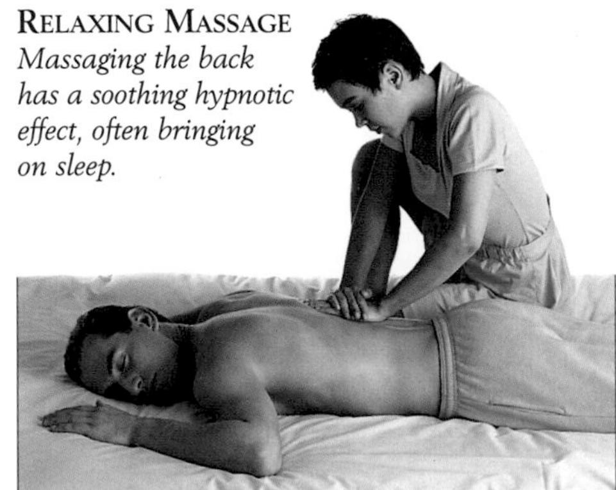

RELAXING MASSAGE
Massaging the back has a soothing hypnotic effect, often bringing on sleep.

COMPLEMENTARY TREATMENTS

Touch therapies that induce relaxation help insomnia by encouraging the brain to produce sleep-promoting chemicals. Other therapies, such as naturopathy, can help relieve sleeplessness if an underlying cause, for example a digestive problem, is disrupting sleep.

MASSAGE 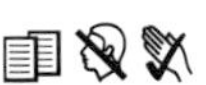

A massage as close as possible to bedtime can relieve muscle tension, reduce anxiety, and boost sleep-enhancing brain chemicals. SEE PAGES 56–61

AROMATHERAPY 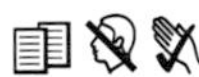

Hospital nurses in the UK have reported that lavender essential oil used before bedtime, whether inhaled, added to a hot bath, or massaged in a carrier oil, helped to induce and enhance sleep. SEE PAGES 62–65

ACUPUNCTURE 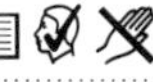

Stimulation of appropriate meridians with acupuncture may help insomnia by encouraging the release of endorphins, the body's natural mood-enhancing chemicals. SEE PAGES 90–94

NATUROPATHY 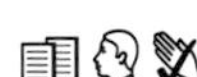

A healthy diet, fresh air, and exercise are basic naturopathic recommendations for a good night's sleep. A practitioner will check for any food intolerances or digestive problems that can interfere with sleep patterns. He or she may also recommend a warm bath shortly before bedtime. This improves the circulation, relaxes muscles, and is almost as effective in encouraging deep sleep as exercise, according to research carried out in the UK in 1987 and the US in 1995. SEE PAGES 118–21

HOMEOPATHY 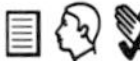

A practitioner will prescribe a remedy suited to your constitution. The following may also help: *Coffea 6c* if your mind is overactive at night; *Arnica 6c* if you are wakeful due to exhaustion; and *Arsen. alb. 6c* if you are restless and waking in the early hours. SEE PAGES 126–30

WESTERN HERBALISM 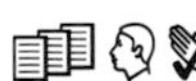

A practitioner will suggest gentle herbs to restore the nervous system and aid relaxation, and will resort to more strongly sedative herbs if necessary. European studies reported in 1982, 1989, and 1994 showed that valerian can induce sleep more quickly and enhance its quality better than placebos, and that it works as well as small doses of barbiturates and benzodiazepines. SEE PAGES 134–39

Caution: Do not take valerian if you are taking other sleep-inducing drugs.

CHINESE HERBALISM 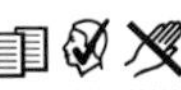

Practitioners associate insomnia with deficiency of *qi* ("life energy") in the Kidney and "heat" in the Heart, which drive out *shen*, the power that stabilizes the mind and emotions. Herbal remedies may include poria, fleeceflower, and wild jujube. SEE PAGES 140–43

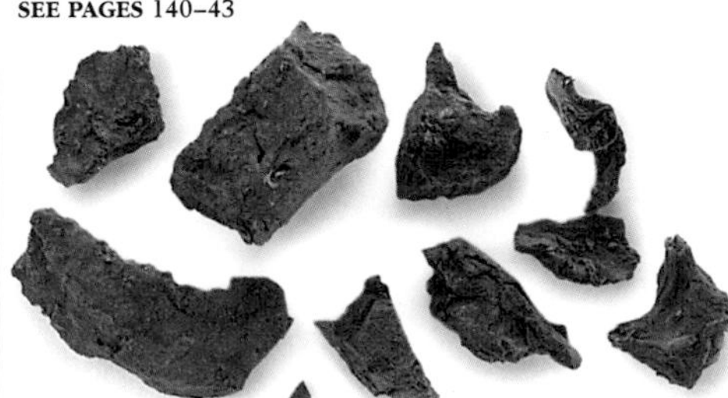

FLEECEFLOWER
In Traditional Chinese Medicine, the root is considered "cooling" and is given to clear toxins.

NUTRITIONAL THERAPIES 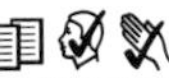

A practitioner may suggest supplements of magnesium, calcium, and vitamins B_6 and B_{12}, which are thought to calm the nerves. Supplements of melatonin, the hormone produced during darkness to promote sleep, may be suggested, but studies in the UK in 1993 and 1995 showed that it did not increase the amount of sleep. SEE PAGES 148–52

CLINICAL ECOLOGY 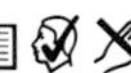

Practitioners will check for evidence of heavy-metal toxicity or allergies, which may be disrupting sleep. SEE PAGES 154–55

PSYCHOTHERAPY & COUNSELING 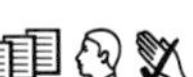

A practitioner may suggest setting aside a particular time of day in which to worry, so that the mind can be cleared at night. SEE PAGES 160–65

RELAXATION & BREATHING 

Progressive muscle relaxation and diaphragmatic breathing before going to bed help release muscle tension, relieve anxiety, and calm the mind. SEE PAGES 170–73

OTHER OPTIONS

Acupressure SEE PAGE 95
Shiatsu SEE PAGES 96–97
Qigong SEE PAGE 99
Yoga SEE PAGES 108–11
Bach Flower Remedies SEE PAGES 132–33
Hypnotherapy SEE PAGES 166–67
Autogenic Training SEE PAGE 168
Biofeedback SEE PAGE 169
Meditation SEE PAGES 174–77
Visualization SEE PAGES 178–79
Light Therapy SEE PAGE 188

STRESS

STRESS HAS BEEN DESCRIBED as the pressure we experience in situations that threaten well-being or tax our resources. Much of the time it is a positive force: it prompts us to get out of the way of a runaway car, for example, or to study hard for exams. However, stress can be a problem for those who feel overwhelmed and unable to cope with the challenges faced.

An individual's perception of a situation and the amount of stress already being handled is important: two people faced with a stressful event, such as being late for an important appointment, may react completely differently. Complementary therapies can be particularly good at relieving stress-related symptoms and helping people cope with pressure in a more relaxed way.

CAUSES & SYMPTOMS

The body's reaction to an emergency (a "stressor") is known as the "fight-or-flight response." Stress hormones flood the system, the heart pumps faster, muscles tense, and the breathing rate increases. This reaction anticipates physical activity, which dispels the stress hormones. In modern life, stress is often mental or emotional. The strain of being in a constant state of alert, without the release that physical action brings, leads to problems such as back pain, headaches, raised blood pressure, indigestion, sweating, palpitations, irritability, and anxiety. In addition, stress contributes to, or directly causes, a variety of complaints, from cold sores to heart disease. Stressors can be "external" – events over which we have little control, for example traffic jams, financial hardship, or bereavement; or "internal" – our personality traits and emotions. Our reaction to these external and internal pressures is governed by the amount of control we *feel* we have. Chemical substances such as alcohol, caffeine, nicotine, sugar, additives, drugs, and environmental toxins, are further sources of stress. These all put a strain on body systems and deplete energy levels.

CONVENTIONAL TREATMENT

As many as 80% of visits to the doctor are for stress-related complaints. Attempts are made to identify the cause of the stress and to find ways of dealing with it.

PREVENTION & SELF-HELP

The self-assessment questionnaire on page 28 may give you an idea of the amount of stress in your life and how it is affecting you. Explore various stress management options (such as meditation, relaxation, or breathing techniques) to find one that appeals to you and follow it. Try to avoid resorting to alcohol, drugs, or nicotine. There are a number of steps you can take, such as organizing your time differently, talking through problems, and getting regular exercise, that may help you cope with stress and stop it from getting out of control (see page 38). Above all, it is important to recognize and deal with the source of the stress. If you are exhausted, time off, such as a complete break from work and home, may be essential. "Toughing it out" will not help, and you are unlikely to change for the better unless you have a chance to recuperate.

TOUCH & MOVEMENT THERAPIES

Therapies such as aromatherapy and massage can help break the stress spiral by aiding relaxation. Eastern therapies aim to improve the flow of qi ("life energy") around the body.

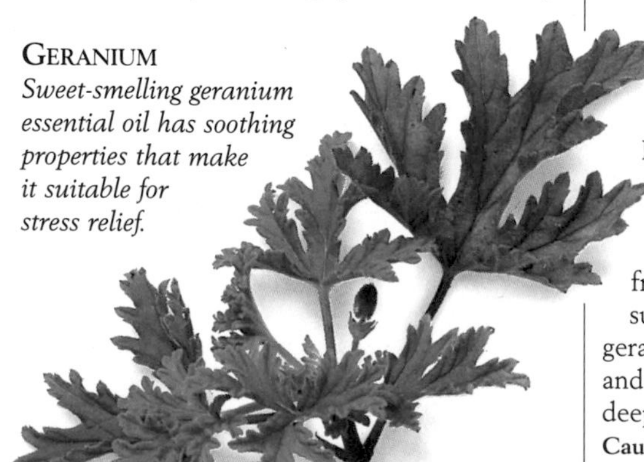

GERANIUM
Sweet-smelling geranium essential oil has soothing properties that make it suitable for stress relief.

MASSAGE

A regular massage is most beneficial for stress. A practitioner will use techniques such as rubbing, kneading, and pummeling. These increase blood circulation, reduce pain, and relieve muscle tension. They also help to release endorphins, substances that have a mood-enhancing effect. SEE PAGES 56–61

AROMATHERAPY

Lavender essential oil may reduce anxiety and tension when diluted in a carrier oil and used in massage, added to the bath, or inhaled from a vaporizer or from a tissue. A practitioner may also suggest using rose, German chamomile, and geranium essential oils to induce relaxation, and frankincense essential oil to calm and deepen breathing. SEE PAGES 62–65

Caution: Do not use German chamomile essential oil during pregnancy.

ACUPUNCTURE

Practitioners consider stress to be a factor in the development of many diseases, causing tensions that disrupt the flow of *qi*. Acupuncture may restore harmony and can induce a state of deep relaxation. SEE PAGES 90–94

QIGONG

Part of Traditional Chinese Medicine, qigong is a combination of gentle movement, controlled breathing, and meditation. Practiced regularly, it is said to enhance the flow of *qi* in the body, improving the circulation and reducing stress. SEE PAGE 99

T'AI CHI CH'UAN

This popular Chinese movement therapy has been described as "meditation in motion." A teacher will show you sequences of exercises that coordinate the body and mind, relax the muscles, and "switch off" stressful thoughts.

T'AI CHI CH'UAN *continued*

In a US study reported in the *Journal of Psychosomatic Research* in 1992, regular practitioners of t'ai chi subjected to mental and emotional stress showed lower levels of stress hormones and of mood disturbance than nonpractitioners. SEE PAGES 100–101

YOGA

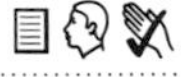

A practitioner trained in therapeutic yoga will guide you through a series of postures (*asanas*) to flex the body, and will teach you relaxation and breathing techniques. The exercises aim to integrate mind and body, relieve muscle tension, and improve physical function. The Corpse posture is particularly effective. Alternate nostril breathing, practiced regularly, is said to cleanse and strengthen the body, and calm and steady the mind. SEE PAGES 108–11

OTHER OPTIONS

Reflexology SEE PAGES 66–69
Rolfing SEE PAGES 82–83
Hellerwork SEE PAGE 84
The Feldenkrais Method SEE PAGE 85
Acupressure SEE PAGE 95
Shiatsu SEE PAGES 96–97
Reiki SEE PAGE 107

MEDICINAL THERAPIES

Continual stress undermines a healthy constitution, which in turn creates more stress. Medicinal therapies aim to break the vicious circle.

NATUROPATHY

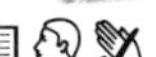

Practitioners believe that one of the most harmful effects of stress is that it interferes with digestion, leading to nutrient deficiencies, fluctuating blood sugar levels, candidiasis, and food intolerances – ailments that create more stress. A practitioner will emphasize the importance of fresh air, plenty of exercise, and regular meals, eaten slowly. He or she will suggest a healthy diet based on whole foods and will ask you to limit your intake of chemical "stressors," such as caffeine, alcohol, saturated fats, food additives, and sugar. He or she will also devise a treatment regime to boost immunity, improve digestion and elimination, correct nutritional deficiencies, and promote restful sleep. SEE PAGES 118–21

HOMEOPATHY

A practitioner will prescribe a remedy that is best suited to your constitution to boost your "vital force." The following standard remedies may also help: *Ignatia 6c* for emotional stress, grief, and disappointment; *Nux vomica 6c* for high expectations, overwork, and irritability; and *Sepia 6c* if you are unable to cope, weepy, and irritable. SEE PAGES 126–30

WESTERN HERBALISM

A practitioner may suggest ginseng, since various studies have shown it can help the body withstand stress. He or she will also suggest a combination of other herbs according to your individual pattern of symptoms. A prescription may include herbs to support and restore the nervous system, such as vervain, skullcap, damiana, and oats; antispasmodics to soothe nerves and muscles, for example German chamomile, limeflower, and passionflower; remedies to aid the digestion, like cinnamon, goldenseal, parsley, and thyme; and echinacea to improve the function of the immune system. SEE PAGES 134–39
Cautions: Do not take ginseng, vervain, goldenseal, or medicinal doses of cinnamon during pregnancy. Do not take ginseng or goldenseal if you have high blood pressure. Do not take valerian if you are already taking sleep-inducing drugs.

OATS
Oat grains and straw are traditional remedies for many kinds of nervous disorders.

NUTRITIONAL THERAPIES

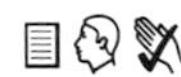

Practitioners take the view that certain nutrients are used up more rapidly when the body is under stress. You may be asked to take supplements of B vitamins to support the nervous system, and of vitamin C and zinc to increase resistance to infection. Magnesium and pantothenic acid may also be suggested to support the adrenal glands, which play a crucial part in the stress response. You may be advised to increase your uptake of complex carbohydrates, such as bread and pasta, to boost energy levels. SEE PAGES 148–52

OTHER OPTION

Chinese Herbalism SEE PAGES 140–43

MIND & EMOTION THERAPIES

Mind therapies combine mental techniques with breathing and relaxation to reverse the "fight-or-flight" response.

PSYCHOTHERAPY & COUNSELING

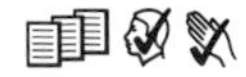

A cognitive behavioral therapist can help you change the way you perceive pressure by working out what events, thoughts, and feelings trigger the stress response in you and by helping you to identify warning signs. He or she may also help you modify personality traits that make you prone to stress. The people most vulnerable are those who are impatient and hostile, or who are obsessive, silent worriers. A practitioner can teach you to intervene in a negative stress cycle by stopping your thoughts, breathing to release tension, reflecting on why you are stressed, and choosing a more appropriate response. Keeping a diary in which you describe stressful situations and how you felt, thought, and behaved can help you change your attitudes and behavior. SEE PAGES 160–65

KEEPING A DIARY
Recording daily thoughts and feelings helps identify stress patterns.

HYPNOTHERAPY

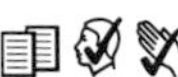

A hypnotherapist can take you into a state of deep relaxation, which you may be able to recreate when faced with stressful situations. SEE PAGES 166–67

AUTOGENIC TRAINING

Autogenic training can help switch off the stress response with a program that includes elements of relaxation, self-hypnosis, yoga, and meditation. SEE PAGE 168

BIOFEEDBACK

Biofeedback enables you to monitor your reactions to stress and, used in conjunction with techniques such as relaxation and meditation, can help you learn to control them. SEE PAGE 169

RELAXATION & BREATHING

A practitioner will show you techniques of slow diaphragmatic breathing and muscle relaxation. These are the keys to managing stress, calming the body so that the mind has a chance to deal with the situation. SEE PAGES 170–73

MEDITATION

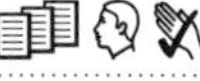

Clinical trials show that regular meditation induces a state of deep physical relaxation and mental awareness. It also reduces stress, as measured by a slower pulse rate, lower blood pressure, lower levels of stress hormones in the blood, and an increase in alpha brain waves, associated with relaxation. SEE PAGES 174–77

MUSIC THERAPY

Music can be soothing. In one study, reported in the *Journal of the American Medical Association* in 1994, surgeons performed stressful tasks better when listening to a favorite piece of music. SEE PAGE 181

DEPRESSION

MOST PEOPLE EXPERIENCE some degree of depression. The term is used to describe a spectrum of negative feelings that ranges from mild, temporary "blues" to "clinical" or "major" depression, which is thought to affect as many as 30% of the population at some stage in their lives.

Symptoms Depression often has physical symptoms, including disturbed sleep and appetite, mood swings, restlessness, unexplained aches and pains, fatigue, and loss of interest in sex. It may manifest as drug dependency or behavioral problems, or simply as a constant feeling of dejection. Thoughts of suicide are common in clinical depression.

Causes Both everyday and clinical depression can strike for no apparent reason. Triggers, however, can include worries related to finances, work, and health, relationship problems, or bereavement. Physical illness can affect the mental state, as can hormonal changes, such as those of menstruation and childbirth. One in ten women who have recently given birth experience postnatal depression (see page 269). In addition, some personalities, especially pessimists, seem more vulnerable.

Conventional Treatment In mild and moderate cases, exercise and psychotherapy or counseling may help. If you are severely depressed, a doctor will suggest antidepressants, but it may take several weeks before improvements are felt.

Self-Help For those experiencing mild to moderate depression or recovering from clinical depression, the following suggestions may help. Do not bottle up your feelings or brood on problems – talk them through with someone close to you. Keep active mentally and physically: studies show a link between moderate exercise and feeling less anxious and depressed. Try to eat sensibly, and resist the temptation to resort to alcohol or drugs.

Caution: Consult a doctor if you feel suicidal or if symptoms last for longer than two weeks.

COMPLEMENTARY TREATMENTS

Many complementary treatments can help people with depression. Benefits include an increased sense of well-being and control.

MASSAGE 

Massage can help to relieve the symptoms of depression and boost self-esteem.
SEE PAGES 56–61

AROMATHERAPY 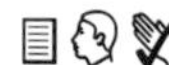

A practitioner may massage you with one of the following essential oils that aid relaxation and lift mood: bergamot, lavender, rose, clary sage, neroli, and ylang ylang. SEE PAGES 62–65

Caution: Do not use clary sage oil during pregnancy.

CRANIAL OSTEOPATHY 

A practitioner will gently handle your head. This procedure is said to relieve depression caused by post-traumatic stress disorder, shock, childbirth, or chronic pain. SEE PAGE 81

TA'I CHI CH'UAN 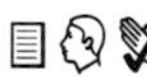

The flowing exercises of this Chinese therapy are believed to increase vitality and improve the function of both mind and body.
SEE PAGES 100–101

NATUROPATHY 

Practitioners advocate stress management techniques, exercise, and a healthy diet, with plenty of whole grains, lean meat, oily fish, shellfish, eggs, fresh fruits, and vegetables. These foods are rich in nutrients that seem to be involved in brain chemistry. A number of other foods, including turkey, bananas, nuts, and milk, may also be suggested because they contain tryptophan. This amino acid stimulates the production of serotonin, a chemical that has a positive effect on mood. Small amounts of chocolate may also enhance mood. You will be advised to avoid caffeine, which exacerbates depression, and alcohol, which suppresses the appetite. SEE PAGES 118–21

HOMEOPATHY

Constitutional assessment is best, but standard remedies include: *Ignatia 6c* for grief, *Aurum met. 6c* if feeling suicidal and worthless, *Pulsatilla 6c* if tearful and in need of reassurance, *Natrum mur. 6c* if weepy and bottling up emotions, and *Sulfur 6c* if depressed or despairing. SEE PAGES 126–30

PASQUE FLOWER
Homeopaths extract the juice of this delicate European plant to make the remedy Pulsatilla.

WESTERN HERBALISM 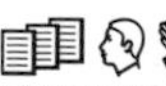

A practitioner may recommend St. John's wort. Recent scientific research, including a study reported in *The Lancet* in 1996, confirms the efficacy of this herb as an antidepressant.
SEE PAGES 134–39

CHINESE HERBALISM 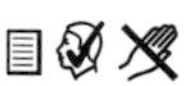

Depression is associated with "stagnation" of Liver *qi* ("life energy"). Practitioners will attempt to counter the condition with herbal remedies, perhaps including Chinese angelica (*dang gui*), peony, licorice, and thorowax.
SEE PAGES 140–43

Cautions: Do not take Chinese angelica or licorice during pregnancy. Do not take licorice if you have high blood pressure.

NUTRITIONAL THERAPIES 

Practitioners may recommend supplements of vitamins and minerals that are considered important for brain chemistry. Vitamin B_6 and magnesium may help premenstrual depression. Supplements of the amino acid phenylalanine may also be suggested, although the scientific evidence for its efficacy is inconclusive. SEE PAGES 148–52

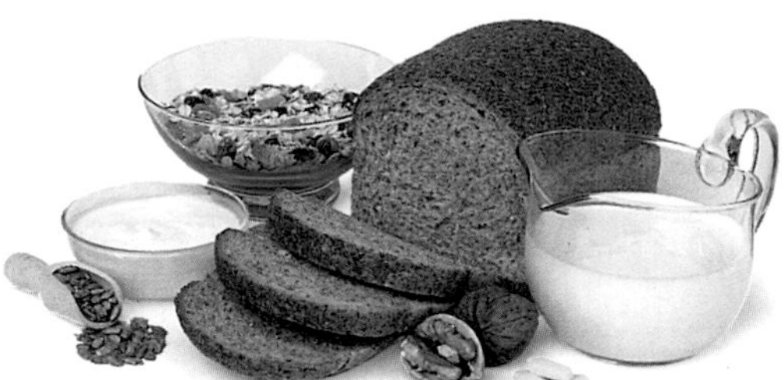

FOODS TO FIGHT DEPRESSION
Magnesium-rich foods, such as dairy products, nuts, and whole-grain cereals, may improve mood.

PSYCHOTHERAPY & COUNSELING 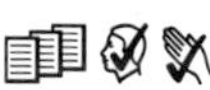

Cognitive behavioral therapy can be as effective as antidepressant drugs in relieving mild to moderate depression. Your practitioner will teach you to identify pessimistic and self-deprecating thoughts and show you how to change them to more positive ways of thinking. SEE PAGES 160–65

RELAXATION & BREATHING

Diaphragmatic breathing and progressive muscle relaxation can help relieve tension and anxiety, which may be contributing to depression.
SEE PAGES 170–73

OTHER OPTIONS

Yoga	SEE PAGES 108–11
Hypnotherapy	SEE PAGES 166–67
Meditation	SEE PAGES 174–77
Art Therapy	SEE PAGES 182–83

GRIEF

GRIEVING IS THE NATURAL RESPONSE to the loss of someone or something we love. First reactions are usually numbness and a sense of unreality, followed by yearning and often anger or guilt. Such feelings are increasingly interspersed with periods of sadness and depression. Psychologists believe that unless grief is expressed in a way that enables people to come to terms with their loss, long-term depression and illness may follow.

Conventional Treatment Doctors may prescribe antidepressants, but these should be used only for a short time. It is better to be in touch with your emotions, however difficult this may be.

Self-Help Do not be afraid to express emotions that seem overwhelming. Talk to friends and family about the person you have lost and about how you feel, and seek help from the clergy, doctors, or organizations that offer support to the bereaved.

COMPLEMENTARY TREATMENTS

Therapies that treat depression and stress, support body systems, and strengthen coping mechanisms are all appropriate for helping those who are bereaved.

HOMEOPATHY

An individual assessment to ascertain the best treatment is advised, but there are standard remedies for various stages of grief: *Arnica 6c* for the initial shock, *Aconite 6c* if fearful and about to collapse, *Nux vomica 6c* if angry and critical, *Pulsatilla 6c* for helpless weeping and insomnia, *Natrum mur. 6c* if grief is suppressed, and *Ignatia 6c* for uncontrollable grief.
SEE PAGES 126–30

BACH FLOWER REMEDIES

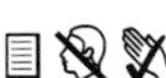

Practitioners believe that flowers have healing properties that can help emotional problems. A recommended mixture for grief includes star of Bethlehem for shock, gentian to give optimism and perseverance, honeysuckle for nostalgic loss, and sweet chestnut for anguish and bereavement. Pine for guilt, holly for anger, and willow for resentment and bitterness may also be recommended.
SEE PAGES 132–33

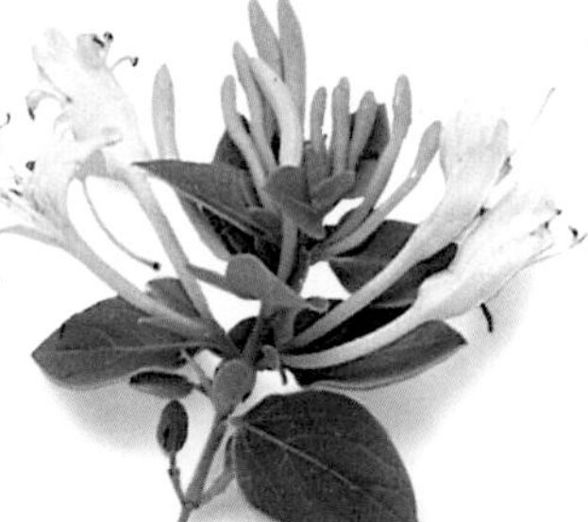

HONEYSUCKLE
Flowers are infused in pure springwater to make the honeysuckle remedy, used to treat grief.

PSYCHOTHERAPY & COUNSELING

Psychotherapists, bereavement counselors, and support groups can help people acknowledge and talk about difficult feelings and find ways to express their grief. SEE PAGES 160–65

ART THERAPY

Painting, sculpting, and drawing can all help the bereaved to express their emotions.
SEE PAGES 182–83

OTHER OPTION

Relaxation & Breathing SEE PAGES 170–73

SEASONAL AFFECTIVE DISORDER (SAD)

SEASONAL AFFECTIVE DISORDER (SAD) is a type of depression brought on by the decrease in daylight in winter. It is thought to affect about 2% of the population, and another 20% experience a milder form known as "winter blues." The symptoms of SAD include sleep problems, lethargy, loss of libido, depression, irritability, anxiety, mood changes, and a craving for carbohydrates. People with SAD may be more vulnerable to infections, gastrointestinal problems, and other illnesses in winter.

Causes Lack of light causes the condition, but exactly how is unknown. It may be linked to faulty production of serotonin (a substance that helps control mood). SAD may also be caused by increased levels of melatonin, a hormone released by the pineal gland during darkness that makes us sleep. Levels of melatonin are higher in winter in people with SAD.

Conventional Treatment Light therapy, antidepressants (particularly SSRIs – selective serotonin reuptake inhibitors, such as Prozac), psychotherapy, and counseling have all been found helpful.

COMPLEMENTARY TREATMENTS

Both conventional and complementary practitioners agree that light therapy benefits people with SAD. In addition, therapies that aid relaxation and improve overall well-being will help.

AROMATHERAPY

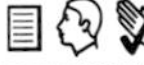

A practitioner will massage you with uplifting and relaxing essential oils, such as ylang ylang, rose, neroli, and lavender. SEE PAGES 62–65

PSYCHOTHERAPY & COUNSELING

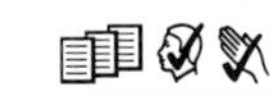

Talking over problems can help you to relax and cope. Cognitive therapy in particular helps to restore self-esteem and lift the sense of failure that accompanies depression.
SEE PAGES 160–65

LIGHT THERAPY

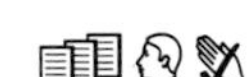

Daily exposure to strong light appears to relieve symptoms in 85% of those with SAD. The length of exposure varies from 20 minutes to two hours a day. Beneficial effects are usually felt within three or four days, but wear off if treatment is not continued. Specially designed light boxes and visors are also available for home use, providing either full-spectrum light (the equivalent of natural daylight) or bright white light, which does not include ultraviolet (UV) rays.
SEE PAGE 188

Cautions: Do not take vitamin D supplements when undergoing light therapy. Overexposure to UV radiation can be harmful.

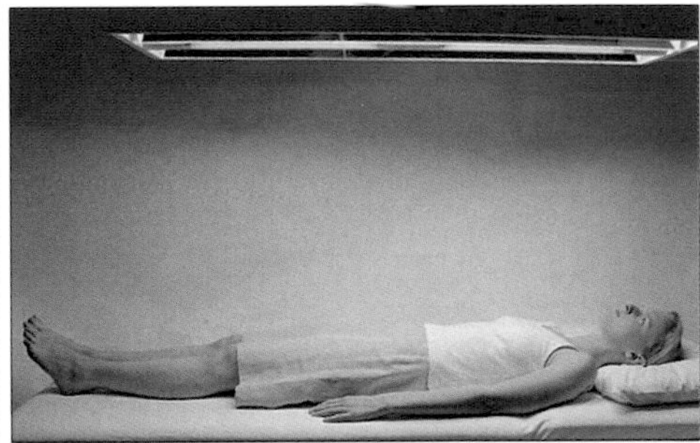

LIGHT TREATMENT
Lying under a therapeutic light source is a fast and effective treatment for SAD.

OTHER OPTIONS

Reflexology SEE PAGES 66–69
Acupuncture SEE PAGES 90–94
Yoga SEE PAGES 108–11
Homeopathy SEE PAGES 126–30
Hypnotherapy SEE PAGES 166–67
Relaxation & Breathing SEE PAGES 170–73

LACK OF SEX DRIVE & INABILITY TO ACHIEVE ORGASM

A LOSS OF LIBIDO (interest in sex) or an inability to achieve orgasm may have physical or psychological causes. Lack of sex drive may be due to a depletion in testosterone (the male sex hormone, also produced by women in small amounts), which plays an important part in sexual arousal in both sexes. Testosterone levels fall naturally with age, but also may be lowered by a physical disorder. In women, hormonal disturbances can send libido plummeting before menstruation, after childbirth or gynecological surgery, and if using oral contraceptives or hormone replacement therapy. Stress, depression, alcohol, and drugs, including medication such as antidepressants, are passion-killers for both sexes. Emotional factors that can cause lack of desire and an inability to climax include bad sexual experiences in the past, painful intercourse, and lack of communication.

Conventional Treatment Testosterone implants to increase libido are given to menopausal women in a growing number of countries, but some degree of masculinization can result. Testosterone injections for men are also available. Psychosexual therapy or marriage counseling is often recommended.

Self-Help Try to vary the time and place of lovemaking. Exercise regularly to encourage the production of endorphins, hormones that can enhance sensuality and raise testosterone levels. Try arousing yourself with masturbation. Talk to your partner: communication is the key to healthy and happy sex.

COMPLEMENTARY TREATMENTS

Therapies that promote relaxation, correct hormonal imbalance, and encourage the enjoyment of sensual stimuli may all help to restore libido.

MASSAGE 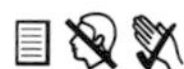

Massage by your partner can relieve stress and arouse desire by stimulating the erogenous zones (lips, nipples, genitalia), where sensory nerve endings are concentrated. SEE PAGES 56–61

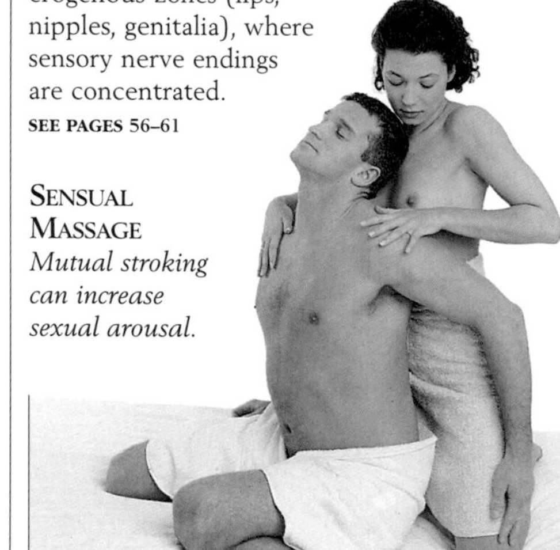

SENSUAL MASSAGE *Mutual stroking can increase sexual arousal.*

ACUPUNCTURE 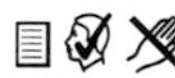

Practitioners associate loss of sex drive with "deficiency of Kidney *qi* ('life energy')" or "stagnation of Liver *qi*," and will stimulate appropriate acupoints. SEE PAGES 90–94

NATUROPATHY 

Practitioners believe that eating meat from cattle that were fed estrogen (a hormone that helps fatten them) can dampen sexual desire. Organic meat or a vegetarian diet would be advised. Cold showers and baths are said to increase the metabolic rate and therefore increase production of testosterone. SEE PAGES 118–21

Caution: Avoid cold showers and baths if you have a heart condition.

WESTERN HERBALISM 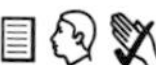

Ginseng and the Ayurvedic herb ashwagandha are widely regarded as aphrodisiacs. Raspberry leaf, agnus castus, and false unicorn root may be prescribed to relax female reproductive organs and restore hormonal imbalances. There has been interest in yohimbe, a West African herb traditionally used as a male aphrodisiac, but it must be taken under professional supervision. SEE PAGES 134–39

Cautions: Do not take ginseng or false unicorn root during pregnancy. Do not take ginseng if you have high blood pressure. Do not take raspberry leaf in the first three months of pregnancy.

NUTRITIONAL THERAPIES 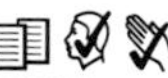

Lack of zinc, important for the metabolism of sex hormones, may affect libido and erectile function. Zinc-rich foods include seafood, red meat, peanuts, and sunflower seeds. Vitamin E supplements are widely reputed to enhance sex drive, but there is no scientific evidence for this. SEE PAGES 148–52

PSYCHOTHERAPY & COUNSELING 

A practitioner specializing in sex therapy may recommend the "sensate focusing" technique, in which you concentrate on communication and the enjoyment of sensual touch, rather than on penetration. You may also be encouraged to identify and resolve emotional problems and past experiences that may be a factor in your current sex life. SEE PAGES 160–65

OTHER OPTION

Aromatherapy SEE PAGES 62–65

PAINFUL SEXUAL INTERCOURSE

PAIN DURING SEXUAL INTERCOURSE may be due to lack of lubrication in the vagina. Stimulation of the clitoris or vulva induces the vaginal glands to secrete mucus, which eases penetration. Insufficient mucus may mean that a woman is not sexually aroused. After the menopause, vaginal dryness may be caused by a depletion of female hormones. Pain may be be an aftereffect of childbirth, or caused by an infection or cysts, which are conventionally treated with antibiotics.

COMPLEMENTARY TREATMENTS

Touch therapies and psychological approaches may help ease physical tension.

AROMATHERAPY 

Essential oils are a means of alleviating the tension that may contribute to painful intercourse. Jasmine essential oil may be used to arouse sensuality, rose to overcome anxiety, and ylang ylang to increase libido. They may be diluted and used for massage, added to a bath, or diffused in a vaporizer. SEE PAGES 62–65

CHIROPRACTIC (SEE OSTEOPATHY) 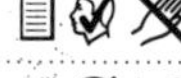

OSTEOPATHY 

Practitioners will determine whether back problems or tension in the pelvic muscles is contributing to painful sexual intercourse, and treat accordingly. SEE PAGES 70–81

PSYCHOTHERAPY & COUNSELING 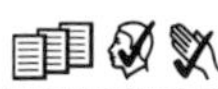

The "sensate focusing" technique increases attentiveness to mutual arousal, which may help if lack of lubrication is causing pain. SEE PAGES 160–65

VAGINISMUS

DURING SEX, muscles around the vagina can go into spasm, making any kind of penetration difficult or impossible. A woman's legs may straighten and come together to prevent entry. Fear of intercourse, due to an earlier traumatic sexual experience, guilt, or painful childbirth, may be the source of the problem. Professional help should be sought and some form of counseling will usually be recommended.

COMPLEMENTARY TREATMENTS

Therapies that help you to relax physically and emotionally may be most useful.

AROMATHERAPY 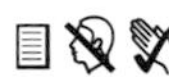

Regular sensual massage (but avoiding the genital area) by a partner using essential oils of ylang ylang, rose, jasmine, sandalwood, or rosemary blended in a carrier oil may help relaxation and build trust. SEE PAGES 62–65

ROSEMARY
Believed to improve zest for life, rosemary has uplifting properties that may help counter the tension underlying vaginismus.

PSYCHOTHERAPY & COUNSELING 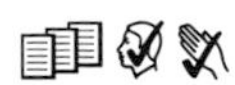

If a woman is in a relationship, sexual counseling usually involves both partners. It may include education about sexual responses, examination of the vagina, and vaginal exercises. Techniques used may include "sensate focusing," which emphasizes sensual touch and pleasure rather than penetration, or relaxation exercises, visualization, and perhaps hypnotherapy. Psychotherapy may help identify and resolve emotional problems that result from past experiences. SEE PAGES 160–65

ERECTILE DYSFUNCTION

THE INABILITY to achieve or maintain an erection can be caused by a physical disorder (see page 276), but is often a psychological problem, caused by factors such as stress, depression, or lack of confidence. If it persists, it can lead to long-term anxiety. Any underlying physical problem should be investigated. If the cause is psychological, a doctor may advise sex counseling or psychosexual therapy, along with stress management techniques.

COMPLEMENTARY TREATMENTS

Therapies that encourage relaxation and sexual confidence help erectile dysfunction.

MASSAGE 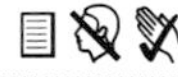

Your partner may help to arouse you by massaging your erogenous zones. SEE PAGES 56–61

ACUPRESSURE

A practitioner may show you how to stimulate an acupoint on top of the head, on the Governing Vessel meridian, which is said to help erectile problems. SEE PAGE 95

PSYCHOTHERAPY & COUNSELING 

A psychosexual therapist will teach you "sensate focusing," which aims to take the pressure off performance. You will be asked to concentrate on showing affection in words, touch, and massage (avoiding the genitals). You will be told to avoid having intercourse for an agreed period of time. SEE PAGES 160–65

PREMATURE EJACULATION

EJACULATION before or very soon after penetration is common among overeager and inexperienced young men, but may occur at any age. It may be due to stress or anxiety over sexual performance, and if it recurs can lead to problems. The woman is left dissatisfied and the man's sense of inadequacy may result in erectile dysfunction or loss of libido.

Conventional Treatment A doctor will check to see if there is a physical cause, such as the side effect of prescribed medication, or urethritis, prostatitis, or a nervous disorder. He or she will suggest counseling or psychosexual therapy to alleviate the problem if it has a psychological cause.

COMPLEMENTARY TREATMENTS

Practitioners will recommend techniques that give you more control over your body to aid sexual performance.

YOGA 

Practitioners of Tantric yoga use breathing techniques to prolong sexual arousal without ejaculation. Qualified teachers are essential but not easy to find. SEE PAGES 108–11

PSYCHOTHERAPY & COUNSELING 

A therapist will probably recommend the "squeeze" technique to help gain control. The man's partner stimulates him manually until he is about to ejaculate, then squeezes the end of the penis for several seconds to stop the climax. Other suggestions may include concentrating on sensual touch and massage without attempting penetration. SEE PAGES 160–65

RELAXATION & BREATHING 

Practicing relaxation techniques before and during intercourse can help reduce the stress and anxiety that may lead to loss of control. Slow diaphragmatic breathing during intercourse may help delay orgasm.
SEE PAGES 170–73

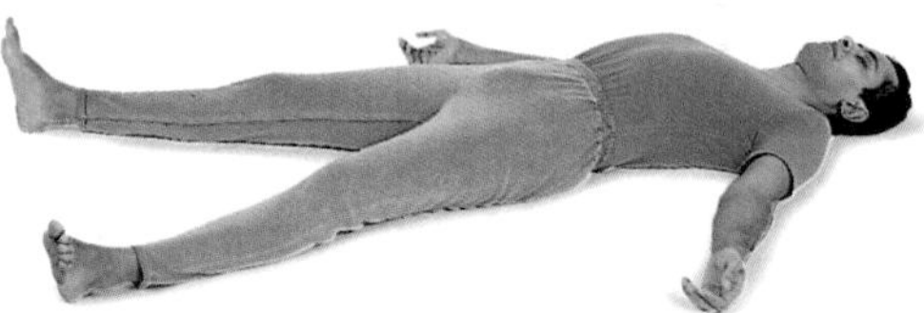

PROGRESSIVE RELAXATION
Systematically relaxing the body before sex releases tension and may help performance.

OTHER OPTIONS

Acupressure — SEE PAGE 95
Hypnotherapy — SEE PAGES 166–67
Autogenic Training — SEE PAGE 168
Visualization — SEE PAGES 178–79

ADDICTIONS

ADDICTION IS A PHYSICAL and psychological dependence on a substance or activity that takes over a person's life, affecting personality, work, and relationships. Dependency is particularly associated with alcohol, drugs such as tranquilizers and heroin, nicotine, and gambling. All addicts suffer unpleasant withdrawal symptoms if they try to give up. These may be physical, as in the sweating and nausea of the drug addict's "cold turkey" and coffee drinker's headaches, or psychological, such as cravings.

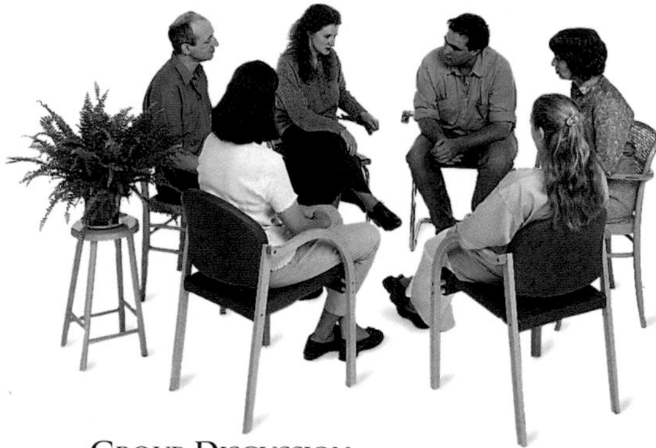

GROUP DISCUSSION
Listening and talking to others with the same addiction can be an immense source of strength.

Causes Addictions were once blamed on lack of willpower, but evidence now indicates that neurological, social, dietary, and environmental factors are involved, as well as genetic predisposition. Scientists are investigating the theory that someone becomes addicted because the part of the brain that controls habitual behavior has been "reprogrammed."

Conventional Treatment In heroin addiction, the brain chemistry becomes dependent on the substance, so oral methadone, a substitute drug, may be given. A doctor will advise counseling; there are a number of organizations that run programs to help people overcome dependency. As depression is often a symptom of addiction, antidepressants may be prescribed. In severe cases, drug addicts may need hospital care.

Self-Help The first step in overcoming an addiction is to recognize that you have a problem and be prepared to seek help. It is important to take one day at a time and not to set overly ambitious goals that you are unlikely to reach.

COMPLEMENTARY TREATMENTS

Touch and movement and medicinal therapies have a key role in the initial phase of treatment for addiction, when withdrawal symptoms are severe. Mind therapies provide support that is necessary for a long-lasting recovery.

MASSAGE

Touch is a gesture of support, and massage may boost self-esteem, helping addicts face up to problems, and feel more at peace with themselves. Massage is one of the therapies offered to addicts in "harm-reduction centers" in the US. In unpublished studies at the Touch Research Institute in Miami in 1996, smokers taught to massage their ears and hands when they craved a cigarette smoked 40% fewer cigarettes after one month. SEE PAGES 56–61

ACUPUNCTURE

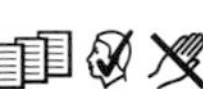

Acupuncture is probably the most widely accepted complementary treatment for addiction to alcohol, heroin, cocaine, and nicotine. It is available in conventional addiction clinics and is the subject of a study by the US National Institute of Drug Abuse. US studies reported in the *International Journal of the Addictions*, 1980, and the *Journal of Psychoactive Drugs*, 1984, showed it to be equal to, or better than, methadone in helping to ease withdrawal symptoms from heroin, such as insomnia, aching muscles, sweating, and nausea. In 1994, the *Journal of Substance Abuse Treatment* reported that acupuncture could relieve depression, cravings, and fatigue during withdrawal from cocaine, and diarrhea, seizures, and high blood pressure during withdrawal from alcohol.

A practitioner will work with acupoints on the ear, which is thought to stimulate the production of natural pain-relieving substances. So far, there is less evidence of acupuncture's success in preventing relapses, although practitioners say that the reduction in stress, depression, and cravings can help people deal with issues underlying their addiction. SEE PAGES 90–94

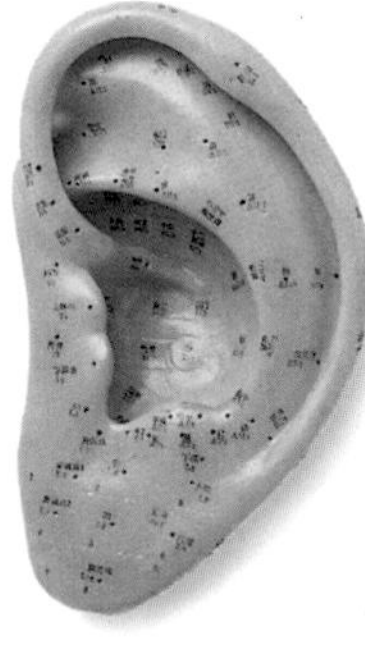

ACUPUNCTURE ON THE EAR
The meridians channeling "life energy" converge on the ears. Acupuncture here is especially helpful for painful withdrawal symptoms.

YOGA

The psychological and physical discipline of yoga helps to foster feelings of control and self-esteem, possibly making withdrawal easier. A trial at the Harvard Medical School (reported in *Psychology Today* in 1996) found that hatha yoga was as effective as group therapy in treating heroin addicts receiving methadone. Some practitioners claim that certain yoga postures may help disperse toxins that build up in the liver and kidneys as a result of substance abuse. SEE PAGES 108–11

NUTRITIONAL THERAPIES

A practitioner will seek to correct any vitamin and mineral deficiencies, which are common among addicts. A balanced diet is important to insure adequate production of the brain chemicals involved in regulating mood and behavior: endorphins (natural painkillers) and the neurotransmitters norepinephrine and serotonin. Some practitioners prescribe intravenous vitamin C to aid detoxification, and amino acid supplements and a high-carbohydrate diet to boost tryptophan, which the body needs to make serotonin. Chromium, niacin, and magnesium may be given to help stabilize erratic blood sugar levels, frequently found in alcoholics and users of hard drugs. The amino acid glutamine is said to reduce cravings for alcohol. SEE PAGES 148–53

PSYCHOTHERAPY & COUNSELING

Doctors will often advise psychotherapy and counseling alongside other treatment programs. Cognitive behavioral therapy, group therapy, and methods such as 12-Step Programs are widely used in dependency clinics. SEE PAGES 160–65

HYPNOTHERAPY

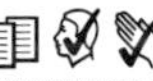

Hypnotherapy is said to help alleviate anxiety and depression associated with addiction, and to help addicts cope with temptation. The treatment is most widely accepted for nicotine addiction, but its efficacy is still in question. SEE PAGES 166–67

BIOFEEDBACK

In one study, alcoholics who learned by way of computer monitors to increase alpha brain waves, associated with a state of relaxation, and theta waves, associated with deep meditation, were shown to become less depressed during the withdrawal period. SEE PAGE 169

OTHER OPTIONS

Western Herbalism SEE PAGES 134–39
Chinese Herbalism SEE PAGES 140–43
Meditation SEE PAGES 174–77

EATING DISORDERS

Anorexia Terrified of becoming fat and obsessed with losing weight, anorexics can starve themselves to the point of emaciation and even death. Anorexia usually starts in the mid-teens and affects about one in every 150 teenage girls. Like bulimia, it is less common among men. Symptoms of starvation include weight loss, lack of menstrual periods, severe constipation, insomnia, abdominal pain, increased body hair, dizziness, extreme sensitivity to cold, and depression.

Bulimia This condition is characterized by binging on exceptionally large amounts of food, followed by self-induced vomiting and large doses of laxatives. It affects three out of every 100 women, usually between the ages of 15 and 30. Sufferers have often had eating or weight problems as children or adolescents. Anorexics may develop bulimic symptoms during or after their anorexia.

Causes Anorexia and bulimia share a number of causes. Some experts believe they may be triggered by biochemical imbalances; for example, in bulimics, binging on carbohydrates may be an attempt to increase levels of serotonin, a mood-enhancing substance. Other experts believe binging is an attempt to ease emotional tension; thinking obsessively about food, particularly for bulimics, may be a reaction to a traumatic event, such as the end of a relationship. Anorexia can also provide a refuge from emotions, in the sense that dieting may produce a feeling of control. Fear of sexuality plays a part for some anorexia sufferers, and weight loss at puberty can delay breast development and the onset of menstruation. Personality is also a factor. Perfectionism and obsessiveness are common among anorexics and bulimics. Adolescence is a time of intense physical and emotional changes, and the desire to conform to an ideal shape is very strong.

Conventional Treatment Treatment is usually provided by a psychiatrist or psychologist specializing in eating disorders, and includes dietary control, antidepressants, and behavioral psychotherapy. Hospital care may be necessary as a last resort.

COMPLEMENTARY TREATMENTS

Complementary therapies can help those struggling to overcome eating disorders by improving self-esteem and releasing hidden emotions.

MASSAGE

Massage encourages relaxation and may help people with eating disorders to accept and "get in touch" with their bodies. In an unpublished US study at the Touch Research Institute in Miami, teenagers having hospital treatment for anorexia and bulimia were less depressed and had a better body image after a course of massage. SEE PAGES 56–61

UPLIFTING MASSAGE
Massage may counter the poor self-esteem that many people with eating disorders experience.

AROMATHERAPY

A growing body of research has shown that odors can strongly influence mood. Depression and anxiety are often symptoms of eating disorders, and a practitioner may try to improve your mood by massaging you with uplifting and relaxing essential oils, such as bergamot, clary sage, lavender, neroli, and ylang ylang. You may be advised to use the same oils in a vaporizer or add a few drops to bathwater. SEE PAGES 62–65

Cautions: Do not use clary sage oil during pregnancy.

ACUPUNCTURE

Eating disorders may be associated with a deficiency of *qi* ("life energy") in the Stomach and Spleen, and a deficiency of Blood. Practitioners stimulate appropriate acupoints. SEE PAGES 90–94

DANCE THERAPY

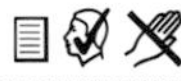

Practitioners believe that dance is a way of bypassing the conscious mind and making contact with inner emotions. You will be encouraged to feel aware of your body and to move freely to express your feelings. SEE PAGES 112–13

NUTRITIONAL THERAPIES

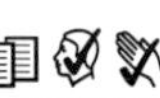

Vitamin and mineral deficiencies are said to be a factor in anorexia and bulimia, and practitioners will prescribe supplements. Anorexia is thought to be a symptom of pellagra (niacin deficiency), and lack of zinc is thought to erode the appetite. Some bulimics have responded favorably to a nutrient-dense, sugar-free diet with tryptophan and vitamin B_6 supplements. SEE PAGES 148–52

PSYCHOTHERAPY & COUNSELING

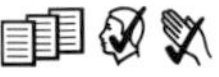

Behavioral therapy is the mainstay of residential programs for eating disorders, with rewards for eating normally and disincentives for starving or binging, reinforced by group therapy sessions. The aim is to help those with eating disorders come to terms with the problems and pressures driving their behavior. Cognitive behavioral therapy can help change sufferers' attitudes toward food and other factors contributing to their condition. Support groups can provide a forum for sharing feelings and experiences. Neurolinguistic Programming (NLP) may help people with eating disorders to recognize and adapt distorted perceptions of themselves and their world. Some therapists use a form of 12-Step Program to help those with eating disorders overcome detrimental behavior. SEE PAGES 160–65

HYPNOTHERAPY

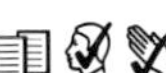

Practitioners say that hypnotherapy can encourage positive responses to other forms of psychotherapy. SEE PAGES 166–67

OTHER OPTIONS

T'ai Chi Ch'uan SEE PAGES 100–101
Meditation SEE PAGES 174–77
Art Therapy SEE PAGES 182–83

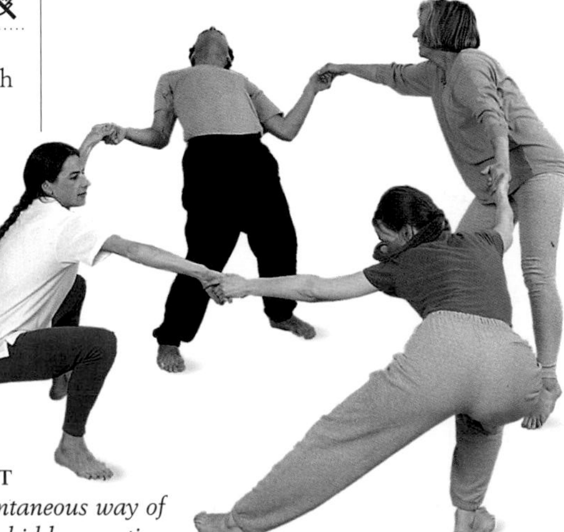

THERAPEUTIC MOVEMENT
Dancing in a group is a spontaneous way of communicating and releases hidden emotions.

ALLERGIES

AN ALLERGY DEVELOPS when the immune system reacts to a harmless substance as if it were harmful. The substance may be in food, in the air we breathe, in contact with the skin, injected as an insect sting, or ingested as a drug. Reactions are quick and take the form of various named disorders, including allergic rhinitis, hay fever, asthma, hives (urticaria), atopic eczema, and food allergies. One person in five in developed countries has some kind of allergy, and numbers are increasing, especially among children. No one knows exactly why this is so, but pollutants, food additives, and stress have all been blamed.

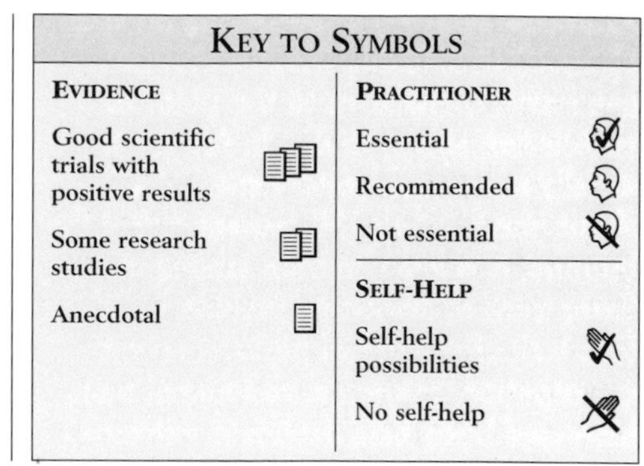

COMPLEMENTARY APPROACHES

Practitioners see allergies as a sign that the processes of digestion and elimination are overburdened, possibly as a result of poor diet, pollution, and stress. Practitioners first try to reduce the patient's exposure to environmental and dietary irritants, and to stimulate the body's innate healing processes. They also attempt to identify allergens and encourage the patient to avoid them. Medicinal therapies seek to strengthen the digestion and overall metabolic function, to eliminate waste products, and to repair any damage they may have caused.

CONVENTIONAL APPROACHES

Practitioners seek to identify the allergen (see Diagnosis, below). They may also prescribe medicines that reduce the effects of an allergic reaction. These include antihistamines, steroid ointments, oral steroids, and for severe reactions, steroid injections. Desensitization therapy, in which the patient is exposed to gradually increasing doses of a given allergen, may prove helpful, but the treatment carries a risk, as it may set off a dangerous anaphylactic reaction (see page 302).

Caution: Before seeking treatment, see page 204.

DIAGNOSIS

In conventional medicine, two principal methods are used to identify an allergen: skin tests, in which substances are injected under or applied onto the skin, and the RAST (Radio Allergosorbent Test), which analyzes antibody formation in the blood. Complementary diagnostic methods are found on pages 191–201.

HOW THE BODY RESPONDS TO ALLERGENS

To protect the body from viruses, bacteria, and other harmful microorganisms, the immune system produces proteins in the blood known as antibodies. In people with allergies, an antibody known as IgE (immunoglobulin E) is triggered in response to substances that are harmless for most people. These substances are known as allergens.

After formation, IgE antibodies attach to specialized immune cells called mast cells. If the allergen is reencountered, antibodies bind to it and cause the mast cells to release chemicals that trigger the allergic response. Histamine is one of the main chemicals. It causes smooth muscles to contract, blood vessels to enlarge, and capillaries to become more "leaky," causing local swelling. Antihistamine drugs are mainstays in allergy treatment. In asthma, the lung airways become inflamed and contract in response to histamine release. Steroids and antispasmodic drugs are prescribed to ease breathing.

Why people are susceptible to allergies is unclear. A predisposition to produce IgE, known as "atopy," tends to run in families, so a mother may suffer from hay fever, her son from eczema, and her daughter from asthma.

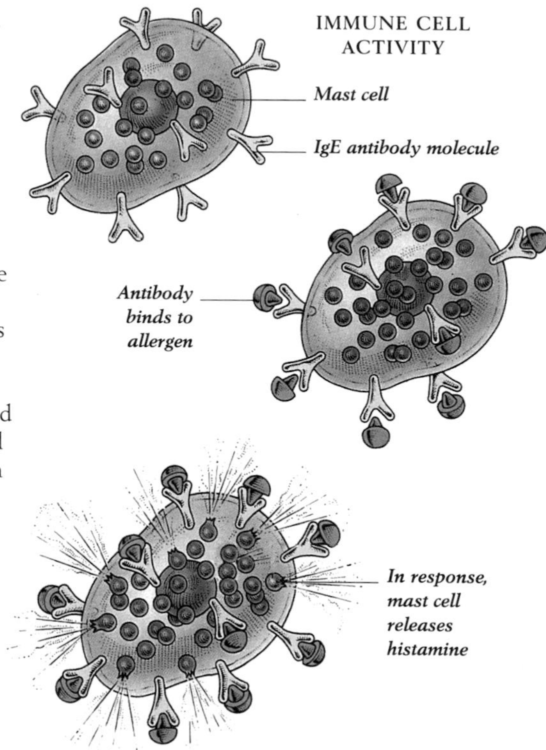

Skin Tests The *skin-prick test* is most reliable for detecting allergies to inhaled substances, such as pollen. Practitioners inject an extract of the suspect substance under the skin. If there is an allergy, weals will form. The *patch test* is used to detect allergies that develop upon contact with a particular substance, for example a rash caused by contact with a chemical. In this test, a number of suspected allergens are taped to the skin with adhesive patches. After the patches are removed, any reddening, blistering, or rash is noted.

RAST (Radio Allergosorbent Test) This is the most reliable test for detecting allergies to food substances. A sample of the patient's blood is drawn and the clear fluid serum, which contains antibodies (see above and page 308), is separated out. It is then added to an extract of the suspected allergen. If the serum is prearmed with antibodies against the allergen, they will bind to it. This activity is revealed by radioactive or colored markers, indicating the presence of an allergy-causing substance.

ALLERGIC RHINITIS & HAY FEVER

THE BODY REACTS to airborne allergens by releasing histamine, a substance that causes inflammation of the mucous membranes lining the nose, throat, and sinuses. This increases the production of mucus and causes sinus congestion. Depending on the allergen, symptoms may be year-round or seasonal (when the disorder is commonly known as "hay fever"). Symptoms may include a blocked or runny nose, itchy, red, and watering eyes, sneezing, a heavy head, inability to concentrate, drowsiness, and a sore throat. Often associated with asthma and eczema, allergic rhinitis may be made worse by psychological factors such as stress and tension.

Causes Dust mites, mold, animal dander (scales from skin, hair, or feathers), and inhaled particles of dust can all cause allergic reactions at any time of year. Pollen shed by grasses, trees, and other plants during spring and summer causes hay fever.

Conventional Treatment Allergic rhinitis and hay fever can usually be treated with antihistamine preparations. Doctors may also prescribe anti-inflammatory nasal sprays and eyedrops, with or without steroids. Nasal decongestant sprays may bring relief, but prolonged use should be avoided as they can damage the delicate mucous membranes.

Self-Help Try to stay indoors when the pollen count is high, and keep doors and windows closed, particularly in the mid-morning and afternoon. Regularly dust and vacuum household surfaces, and keep pets out of bedrooms. Special bed linen and sprays are available to reduce exposure to dust mites.

Caution: Always consult a pharmacist when buying hay fever treatment. The prescription medication terfenadine can cause serious and even fatal reactions if taken with grapefruit juice, or with certain other medications.

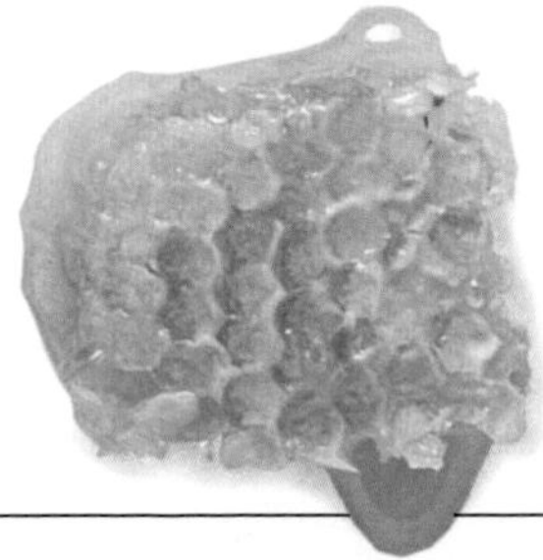

HONEYCOMB
Naturopaths believe that eating honeycomb in winter will help ward off hay fever in spring.

COMPLEMENTARY TREATMENTS

Some practitioners aim to soothe the symptoms of allergic rhinitis and hay fever. Others, especially herbalists and naturopaths, may try to build up the body's natural defenses. Psychological techniques to lessen the effects of stress may help to reduce the number or severity of attacks.

AROMATHERAPY 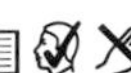

Practitioners advise massaging the under-eye sinus area with diluted lavender oil, or inhaling a few drops of lemon balm, German chamomile, lavender, or eucalyptus essential oil from a tissue. SEE PAGES 62–65

Caution: Do not use German chamomile essential oil during pregnancy.

CHIROPRACTIC (SEE OSTEOPATHY) 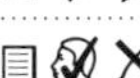

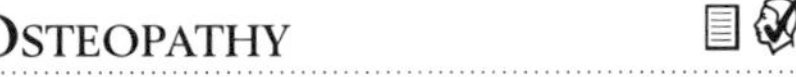

OSTEOPATHY

Soft-tissue manipulation or cranial osteopathy may help ease chronic congestion.
SEE PAGES 70–81

ACUPUNCTURE 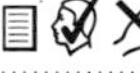

In Traditional Chinese Medicine, hay fever is regarded as an invasion of "heat" and "wind." Practitioners will work with acupoints on the appropriate meridians to restore "harmony."
SEE PAGES 90–94

ACUPRESSURE 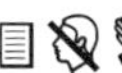

A practitioner will show you how to apply pressure to an acupoint known as Yintang, found between the eyebrows, and on points on the Large Intestine meridian, to restore the flow of *qi* ("life energy") and so boost the immune system. SEE PAGE 95

NATUROPATHY 

Eating garlic, or honeycomb in winter, may be suggested to enhance immunity. Raw onion may ease breathing, and a drink of warm lemon juice and honey can soothe a sore throat. Practitioners may advise a 48-hour fast with water and fruit juice to eliminate waste products, followed by a raw-foods diet.
SEE PAGES 118–21

HYDROTHERAPY 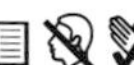

Bathing the eyes and face in cold water can ease symptoms; a sitz bath may relieve inflammation.
SEE PAGES 122–23

HOMEOPATHY 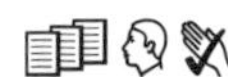

The most common standard remedy for hay fever symptoms is *Allium 6c*. Others that might be recommended include: *Euphrasia 6c*, *Arsen. alb. 6c*, *Natrum mur. 6c*, *Nux vomica 6c*, and *Kali iod. 6c* for runny eyes and nose; and *Calc. sulf. 6c* and *Hepar sulf. 6c* for thick catarrh. In a Scottish study reported in *The Lancet* in 1986, a homeopathic mixture of grass pollens reduced symptoms.
SEE PAGES 126–30

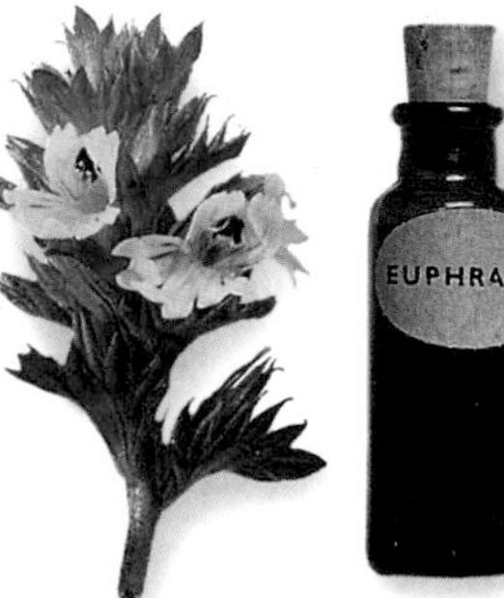

EUPHRASIA
This wildflower, named after the Greek word for "gladness," has had long use as a homeopathic and herbal remedy for eye complaints.

WESTERN HERBALISM 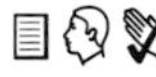

Taking echinacea before the pollen season may boost the immune system. An herbalist may advise tincture of nettle to clear phlegm, inhalation of diluted peppermint essential oil to clear congestion, and plantain-leaf syrup to suppress mucus production. SEE PAGES 134–39

Caution: do not use peppermint as an inhalant over a long period.

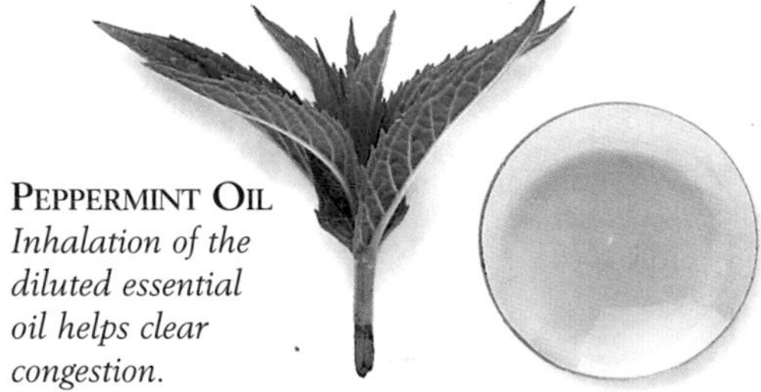

PEPPERMINT OIL
Inhalation of the diluted essential oil helps clear congestion.

NUTRITIONAL THERAPIES

Supplements of vitamin C and bioflavonoids (see glossary) may be advised to stop a runny nose or unblock a congested nose. Pantothenic acid, one of the B vitamins, may ease stress reactions. Research suggests that vitamin E may reduce histamine reactions. SEE PAGES 148–52

CLINICAL ECOLOGY 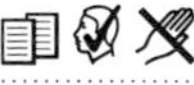

Practitioners believe that changing the diet reduces demands on the body's self-regulating mechanisms, thereby lessening the severity of symptoms. Diets that are free from additives, wheat, or dairy products are among those that may be suggested. SEE PAGES 154–55

Caution: Restricted diets may lead to malnutrition.

HYPNOTHERAPY 

Hypnosis has been successful in averting allergy attacks. A practitioner may also demonstrate breathing techniques that can help to ease symptoms. SEE PAGES 166–67

Asthma

More than 200 million people around the world suffer from asthma, an intermittent narrowing of the airways in the lungs that leads to shortness of breath, coughing, and wheezing. The condition is becoming common, and is diagnosed five times more frequently in industrialized countries than in developing ones. The same inhaled allergens responsible for allergic rhinitis (see page 299) are largely to blame, but other triggers include diet, drugs, stress, and pollution. Asthma can start at any age, and the severity of attacks varies, but about a quarter of sufferers feel that it has a major impact on their lives. Severe attacks, characterized by a racing pulse, sweating, and breathlessness, are very frightening and can be dangerous if untreated.

Causes & Symptoms

When asthmatics inhale allergens or irritants, the muscles in the bronchial tubes (airways) contract and the membranes lining the tubes become inflamed, restricting airflow and making it a struggle to breathe out. Common allergens include dander (particles of animal hair, skin, and feathers), dust mites, pollen, mold, tobacco smoke, and exhaust fumes. Viral infections may also trigger asthma. The food additive monosodium glutamate may trigger an attack, and so may physical and emotional stress. Electromagnetic radiation from cellular telephones, televisions, and computers is now also a suspected factor. Research suggests that a diet high in polyunsaturated oils may predispose some people to asthma.

Conventional Treatment

Sodium cromoglycate or corticosteroid drugs, which suppress the release of histamine (a chemical that contracts the lung airways), may be given. Nebulizers or inhalers containing drugs that dilate the airways (bronchodilators) may be used during an attack. RAST or skin-prick tests (see page 298) may help to identify an allergen.

Prevention & Self-Help

You can protect against the most common allergen, the dust mite, by using synthetic bedding with special covers, choosing short-pile synthetic carpets or none at all, and using an anti-allergy vacuum cleaner. Don't keep pets, and avoid tobacco smoke. Stay away from areas of long grass in spring, and keep windows closed, particularly between mid-morning and late afternoon or early evening, when the pollen count is highest. Regular exercise, especially aerobic exercise such as swimming, helps to increase lung capacity and strengthen the heart. Use humidifiers indoors, and avoid very cold or polluted air. If you are exposed to allergens at work (in a paint shop, garage, or hairdressing salon, for example) you may need to consider changing your job. The airways can become increasingly sensitive if constantly exposed to irritants.

Precautions

- **Always keep emergency medicines to hand. If an attack does not respond quickly to self-administered bronchodilator drugs, call a doctor or go to a hospital immediately.**
- **Use steam inhalations with care if you have asthma.**

Touch & Movement Therapies

Practitioners aim to improve lung function with exercises, by correcting poor posture, stimulating "energy flow," and manipulating joints and muscles.

Aromatherapy

To ease breathing, practitioners recommend eucalyptus essential oil, either inhaled from a tissue (not in steam inhalations) or massaged onto the chest in a carrier oil. **See pages 62–65**

Chiropractic (see Osteopathy)

Osteopathy

A practitioner will use manipulation techniques and soft-tissue massage to try to relax and stretch the chest muscles, to promote mobility and easier breathing. Treatment of the thoracic vertebrae, at the back of the chest and the rib cage, may be particularly beneficial. Some practitioners claim these manipulations also calm oversensitivity of the airways. **See pages 70–81**

The Alexander Technique

Some asthmatics make the problem worse by hunching the shoulders and sinking the neck into the chest. Teachers of the Alexander technique can help by showing how to stand and move with minimum strain. Correcting the posture allows the chest to expand fully, relieves strain, and improves breathing. **See pages 86–87**

Improving Lung Function
An Alexander teacher will give individual instruction on how to improve posture in order to clear the airways of the lungs and increase lung capacity.

ACUPUNCTURE

According to various reports, described in the UK journals *The Lancet* (1986) and *Thorax* (1991) among others, there is some evidence that needling appropriate acupoints to treat the Lung, Kidney, and Spleen meridians may relieve asthma symptoms (if only temporarily). SEE PAGES 90–94

ACUPRESSURE

A practitioner will demonstrate a range of acupressure techniques to improve the flow of *qi* ("life energy") around the body, helping to relieve symptoms. SEE PAGE 95

YOGA

Yoga breathing and stretching postures are used to increase respiratory stamina, relax the chest muscles, expand the lungs, raise energy levels, and calm the body. During an attack, controlled breathing (*pranayama*) may help reduce panic. Several studies show that yoga may be helpful for asthma. For example, at City Hospital, Nottingham, UK, asthmatics practiced yoga exercises that focused on better breathing twice a day for two weeks. They subsequently found themselves to be less dependent on inhalers and to have a reduced reaction to histamine. SEE PAGES 108–11

OTHER OPTIONS

Massage	SEE PAGES 56–61
Reflexology	SEE PAGES 66–69
Rolfing	SEE PAGES 82–83
Shiatsu	SEE PAGES 96–97

MEDICINAL THERAPIES

The causes of asthma vary from one sufferer to another. Practitioners will attempt to identify underlying factors, and will also prescribe remedies to control the symptoms.

NATUROPATHY

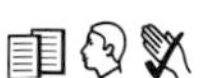

Practitioners often recommend occasional fasting and a "low-allergy diet," avoiding cow's milk, and eating foods such as garlic, onion, and citrus fruits, to reduce mucus formation. Practitioners will test for food allergies, and may advise you to avoid processed foods and artificial preservatives, additives, and coloring. Sulfites, salts once used for preserving raw fruits and vegetables but blamed for a number of fatal asthma attacks, may still be present in low levels in meat products, jams, processed vegetables, cider, and wine. It is wise to avoid these foods when it is not possible to check the labeling, for example when eating out. Oily fish and fish-oil supplements may be recommended, since they are a rich source of omega-3 fatty acids, thought to have an anti-inflammatory effect. Some asthmatics may be deficient in vitamin B, particularly vitamin B_6 (which helps the body counter stress) and B_3 (niacin, used by the cells to produce energy). Eating foods rich in these nutrients, such as fish and poultry, may help asthmatics who experience stress-provoked attacks. Foods containing antioxidants (see glossary), especially vitamins E and C, found in wheat germ and citrus fruits, may also be advised. They are believed to help strengthen the lungs against damage by free radicals (see glossary), generated as part of the asthmatic response to allergens.

A study undertaken in 1994 at Nottingham University, UK, linked low levels of magnesium with asthma, which suggests that foods rich in this trace element may help relax the airways. Caffeine expands the air passages. In an emergency, drinking two cups of strong coffee may bring relief. Some practitioners apply hot compresses to the chest and back to ease lung congestion and to help restore free breathing during attacks. Daily breathing exercises will also be advised. SEE PAGES 118–21

Caution: Avoid caffeine if you take medication that contains theophyline or chemically similar substances.

MACKEREL
Oily fish such as this provide vitamins that may offset asthma attacks triggered by stress.

HOMEOPATHY

Practitioners will seek to identify the specific allergen in order to prescribe it as a remedy at a homeopathic potency. In a study described in *The Lancet* in 1994, asthmatics who were given homeopathic remedies to regulate their immune responses showed greater improvement after 3–4 weeks than those who were given a placebo. SEE PAGES 126–30

WESTERN HERBALISM

Practitioners will try to reduce sensitivity of the bronchial tubes to allergens. Herbs that have an antispasmodic effect, such as coltsfoot, and sedative properties, such as hyssop and pill-bearing spurge (euphorbia), may be given to help ease symptoms. Some studies indicate that mullein leaf, ginkgo, aloe vera, and khella may also help ease constriction. In German clinical studies published in 1986 and 1993, the Ayurvedic herb *Coleus forskholii* was shown to dilate the bronchial tubes almost as powerfully as conventional medication. SEE PAGES 134–39

HYSSOP
This herb's mildly sedative effect may help relieve attacks.

NUTRITIONAL THERAPIES

Taking nutritional supplements while avoiding potentially allergenic foods may bring good results. Practitioners may advise supplements of vitamin A (beta-carotene), C, E, B-complex (especially B_6 and B_{12}), niacin, calcium, selenium, magnesium, manganese, and zinc to support the immune system and maintain mucous membranes. Some asthmatics are said to have low levels of gastric hydrochloric acid (see page 232), and a course of hydrochloric acid capsules with pepsin may be suggested to counter the deficiency. According to one study, intramuscular injections of vitamin B_{12} prevented attacks in four out of five sulfite-sensitive asthmatic children. In a trial reported in the *Journal of the American Medical Association* in 1989, magnesium supplements appeared to improve breathing in people with asthma. SEE PAGES 148–52

MIND & EMOTION THERAPIES

Cognitive behavioral therapy and relaxation techniques such as autogenic training and biofeedback can help asthmatics feel in control and prevent the panic that can exacerbate an attack.

PSYCHOTHERAPY & COUNSELING

Cognitive behavioral therapy has been found helpful in reducing the frequency of attacks in children. Patients are encouraged to develop ways of dealing with attacks. SEE PAGES 160–65

HYPNOTHERAPY

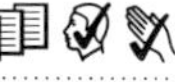

Several research studies published in the *British Medical Journal* have found that by helping the patient to relax and cope with the unpleasant sensations of an attack, hypnosis can both relieve symptoms and significantly reduce the need for asthma medication. SEE PAGES 166–67

RELAXATION & BREATHING

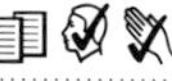

Relaxing muscle tension, especially in the shoulders and abdominal region, while simultaneously breathing calmly from the diaphragm, can help improve lung function. These skills can be particularly effective during an asthma attack. To help reduce the rate of respiration, some practitioners advise drawing air slowly into the nose, holding the breath for about half the length of time it took to inhale, then just as slowly exhaling. In the Buteyko breathing method, asthma is attributed to hyperventilation (rapid breathing). Patients are taught to alternate shallow breathing with holding the breath. SEE PAGES 170–73

FOOD ALLERGIES

CERTAIN FOODS PROVOKE a reaction in some people, which may be defined as an allergy or as an intolerance (see opposite). The symptoms of a food allergy are more sudden and severe than those of an intolerance. Allergies also differ from intolerances in that they are triggered by the immune system, which reacts to the food as though it were a harmful substance invading the body.

Symptoms Food allergies can trigger allergic disorders – allergic rhinitis, eczema, asthma, and hives – as well as stomach cramps, diarrhea, and headaches. Symptoms may be mild, but for some people, an extreme reaction, known as anaphylaxis, can be caused by eating even a morsel of the allergen (the food that provokes the attack). Within minutes, a rash, wheezing, vomiting, and swelling of the lips, mouth, and tongue may develop. In severe cases, collapse (anaphylactic shock) can result, and even death. Not all anaphylactic reactions occur immediately: some may take several hours, but can be equally as violent as reactions of swifter onset.

Causes Nuts – especially peanuts – cause some of the most extreme food allergies. One in 20 people with peanut allergy will also react to soy, peas, and beans. Other common culprits include dairy products; gluten (see Celiac disease, page 235); eggs; fish, especially cod, sole, and smoked fish; shellfish; preservatives, especially benzoic acid; colorings, particularly tartrazine; and other additives.

Conventional Treatment A skin-prick test or RAST (see page 298) will usually identify the allergen. Anaphylaxis is treated with injections of cortisone and epinephrine.

Self-Help A food allergy generally lasts for life, so it is important to avoid the foods that are responsible. Those at risk of anaphylaxis should take meticulous care with their diet, particularly when eating out, and should wear a medical alert tag.

Cautions: Call an ambulance immediately if you suspect an anaphylactic reaction. Consult a doctor if any of the following symptoms develop an hour or two after a meal: itching or swelling in the mouth or over the whole body, nausea, stomach pains, sneezing, a runny nose, diarrhea, or weakness of the muscles.

COMPLEMENTARY TREATMENTS

A food allergy may be a contributing factor in conditions such as eczema (see page 218), which are often broadly termed "allergic," but the specific cause may be more difficult to pin down. In these situations, complementary methods focus on "detoxifying" and strengthening the digestive system, improving the elimination processes, and increasing overall well-being.

YOGA

Mild or undiagnosed food allergies can disturb digestive processes and cause a general feeling of malaise. To help support the digestion, yoga teachers may emphasize postures (*asanas*) such as the Half Shoulderstand or the Relaxation pose, and breathing exercises (*pranayama*). SEE PAGES 108–11

NATUROPATHY

To pinpoint the cause of a mild food allergy, a practitioner may advocate the skin-prick test or RAST, but is more likely to suggest an elimination diet. You will be advised to cut out all suspect foods from the diet for at least two weeks, or until there are signs of improvement. Once symptoms are no longer present, you reintroduce foods one by one, stopping if any of them causes a reaction. Practitioners may also recommend undertaking occasional juice-and-water fasts and raw-foods diets to help eliminate waste products from the body. SEE PAGES 118–21

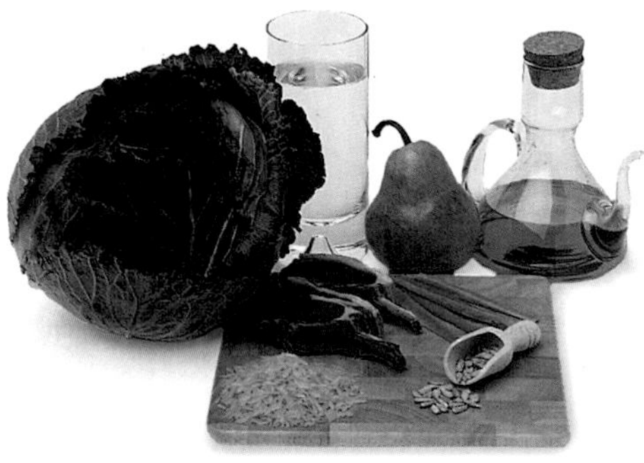

ELIMINATION DIET
By systematically eliminating food groups from the diet and observing how this affects symptoms, naturopaths are often able to detect culprit foods.

HOMEOPATHY

The homeopathic practitioner's approach will be guided by your particular constitutional type and the symptoms of your allergy. "Homeopathic immunotherapy" may be recommended. This is a form of treatment in which you take extremely diluted preparations that have been made from the relevant allergen. SEE PAGES 126–30

WESTERN HERBALISM

To complement an elimination diet, herbalists may recommend slippery elm and marshmallow to soothe the digestive tract, dandelion root to support the liver, hops, buckbean, and white horehound to stimulate digestion, and echinacea and red clover to strengthen the immune system. Astringent herbs such as calendula and goldenseal may be prescribed if damage to the gut wall is suspected. Nettle soup may be suggested to calm an allergic response.
SEE PAGES 134–39

Cautions: Do not take goldenseal during pregnancy or if you have high blood pressure. Do not take hops if you have clinical depression.

RED CLOVER
This common herb is given to boost immunity.

NUTRITIONAL THERAPIES

Nutritional supplements to boost the body's regenerative powers will be advised. These may include selenium and zinc to support the immune system, pantothenic acid, thought to have an antihistamine effect (see page 300), vitamin C, which is antioxidant (see glossary), and magnesium and manganese, said to be deficient in some people with food allergies.
SEE PAGES 148–52

CLINICAL ECOLOGY

Practitioners use controversial diagnostic methods, including cytotoxic tests, pulse testing, hair analysis, Vega testing, and applied kinesiology (see pages 191–201). Many researchers and doctors doubt their accuracy. Treatment may take the form of Enzyme Potentiated Desensitization (EPD), in which an enzyme and a dilute mixture of common allergens are injected into the patient. This is said to work by "reprogramming" white blood cells that have been reacting unnecessarily to food substances. SEE PAGES 154–55

RELAXATION & BREATHING

Hyperventilation (rapid breathing) stimulates the release of the chemical histamine. Learning to regulate breathing can help reduce the severity of the allergic response. SEE PAGES 170–73

FOOD INTOLERANCES

STRESS & FOOD INTOLERANCES

Inability to cope with stress is thought to contribute to poor digestion. The undigested food irritates the gut wall, causing it to become "leaky." Food molecules and toxic substances are believed to pass through to the bloodstream, affecting the liver, kidneys, and ultimately the immune system, leaving the body vulnerable to illness.

Toxin-induced ailments lead to more stress

STRESS

Effect on gut:
- fewer digestive enzymes
- poor circulation
- irregular peristalsis (see glossary)

Food is not properly broken down or absorbed

May lead to:
Leaky gut: Toxins from poorly digested food "leak" from the gut into the bloodstream.
Dysbiosis: Poorly digested food in the gut encourages overgrowth of unfriendly gut bacteria (for example, candidiasis).

Toxins cause problems in other parts of the body (for example, joints, skin)

Toxins overload the liver and kidneys

UNLIKE FOOD ALLERGIES, food intolerances do not appear to produce IgE antibodies (see page 298) in the body. Some intolerances seem to disappear if the food is avoided for a few months, and people often report cravings for the very foods to which they are sensitive. While there is much debate over the symptoms, those most often linked with intolerances include headaches, migraines, fatigue, depression, anxiety, hyperactivity, canker sores, muscle soreness, water retention, and skin, digestive, and joint disorders.

Causes Apart from conditions related to deficiencies in enzymes (such as lactase, needed to digest milk), many doctors find the idea of food intolerance unconvincing. But according to practitioners of nutritional medicine, factors such as stress, "dysbiosis" – the overgrowth of unfriendly gut bacteria (see also Candidiasis, page 235, and the diagram above) – and "liver congestion" may result in poor digestion, causing toxins to "leak" into the blood. This in turn is said to cause ill-effects elsewhere in the body.

Conventional Treatment Those doctors who do accept that food intolerances play a part in at least some cases of long-term illness usually suggest an elimination diet to identify the culprit food.

COMPLEMENTARY TREATMENTS

With such a wide range of symptoms, food intolerance is notoriously difficult to diagnose. A battery of tests (see pages 191–201) helps practitioners pinpoint the culprit food. Stress appears to make food intolerance worse, and counseling and mind/body techniques may improve the ability to cope.

NATUROPATHY

According to naturopaths, inadequate digestion causes irritation of the gut lining. Incompletely digested food molecules (see above) eventually permeate the mucous membrane. The naturopath will almost certainly advocate an elimination diet, in which suspect food groups are cut out for two weeks or until there is some sign of improvement. Initially, symptoms may sometimes get worse, but if they subsequently improve, foods are reintroduced one by one and stopped if there is a reaction. Research published in *The Lancet* in 1985 suggested that elimination diets relieved symptoms in people with inflammatory bowel disease by successfully identifying food intolerances. SEE PAGES 118–21

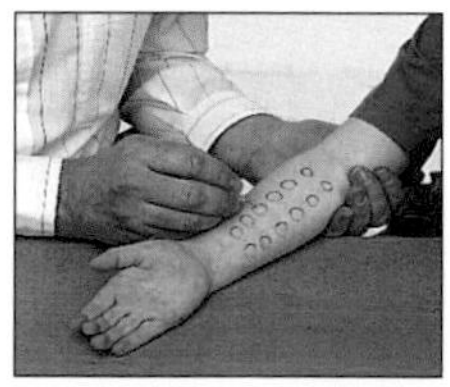

SKIN-PRICK TEST
Some practitioners use a modified skin-prick test to identify the intolerance.

NUTRITIONAL THERAPIES

According to practitioners, the "leaky" gut that results from irritation caused by poorly digested food leads in turn to loss of essential nutrients, especially magnesium and zinc. Treatment is tailored to the individual, but recommended nutritional supplements may include: vitamin A (as beta-carotene) to mend the intestinal wall; vitamin B-complex to support the function of the adrenal glands, which affect the body's metabolic rate and response to stress; vitamin C, which supports the adrenal glands and is an antioxidant (see glossary); vitamin E and calcium to reduce the allergic response; selenium, magnesium, and zinc to support the immune system; essential fatty acids to counteract inflammation; and digestive enzyme supplements. If dysbiosis is a problem, kelp, bifidobacteria, *lactobacillus* supplements, and live yogurt, all of which contain beneficial bacteria to normalize gut flora, may be suggested. SEE PAGES 148–52

CLINICAL ECOLOGY

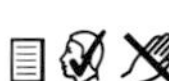

Practitioners say that anyone eating an average Western-style diet is likely to ingest over 100 synthetic chemicals a day in food and water, and that these can encourage food intolerances. A number of controversial diagnostic tests may help identify the culprit; in addition, a practitioner will devise an elimination diet. You may also be advised to filter tap water and take antioxidant (see glossary) supplements. The practitioner may suggest an EPD injection (see Clinical Ecology, opposite) or a treatment called provocation neutralization, in which a tiny amount of the irritant food is injected as a vaccine.
SEE PAGES 154–55

PSYCHOTHERAPY & COUNSELING

Stress and emotional problems seem to play a role in triggering food intolerances. People may also become obsessed by their ailment, conditioning themselves to expect symptoms. Psychotherapy and counseling may help them to "unlearn" these responses. SEE PAGES 160–65

RELAXATION & BREATHING

Symptoms attributed to food intolerances appear to be made worse by stress, and many people who have intolerances also have difficulty in coping with stress. Some also tend to hyperventilate (breathe too rapidly). Stress management techniques may be used to promote deep, slow breathing, reduce muscle tension, and relieve anxiety. SEE PAGES 170–73

CANCER

CANCER OCCURS WHEN CELLS in certain tissues multiply uncontrollably. The second biggest killer after heart disease in developed countries, it is often the diagnosis that people dread most – even though some forms are relatively mild and have a 100% survival rate. It most commonly affects the breasts, lungs, bowel, skin, stomach, ovaries, pancreas, prostate, bladder, and lymph glands. About a third of people in the developed world will develop cancer in their lifetime, but it is estimated that as many as 70% of cases could be prevented by avoiding trigger factors, such as tobacco, ultraviolet light, and certain foods.

KEY TO SYMBOLS

EVIDENCE

Good scientific trials with positive results

Some research studies

Anecdotal

PRACTITIONER

Essential

Recommended

Not essential

SELF-HELP

Self-help possibilities

No self-help

COMPLEMENTARY APPROACHES

In the past, complementary medicine has claimed various "miracle" cures for cancer, which have since proved ineffective or even fraudulent. However, a promising way forward lies in integrating conventional and complementary therapies; this approach has been adopted at leading cancer treatment centers and hospices and by self-help groups. Gentle therapies such as massage, relaxation, and healing play a major role in palliative care (symptom relief). Rather than trying to effect cures, complementary practitioners aim to ease pain and alleviate the side effects of conventional treatment, helping patients to come to terms with their situation and enjoy whatever time is left. Enhancing emotional and spiritual well-being in this way may itself prolong life.

CONVENTIONAL APPROACHES

There are three approaches to treating cancer, which are sometimes used individually, but more often in combination. Surgery removes the tumor, radiotherapy (treatment with X rays or other forms of radiation) kills any remaining cancer cells, and chemotherapy (treatment with drugs) destroys cancer cells that have traveled to other parts of the body (metastasized). These methods have varying degrees of success, depending on the type of cancer. Conventional approaches are invasive, do not always work, and have unpleasant side effects. Nevertheless, the stakes are so high that treatment using these methods is an essential part of the fight against cancer.

HOW CANCERS GROW

There are more than 200 forms of cancer, but they all have one thing in common: abnormal cells whose growth is out of control. All cells multiply by splitting in two, a process controlled by genes called oncogenes. Normally these genes allow just the right amount of cell division to maintain and repair tissue. But changes within a cell can plunge everything out of control, and abnormal cells divide at a very fast rate, doubling over and over. Unlike a benign tumor, as a cancerous tumor grows, its cells gradually invade and destroy neighboring tissues. Cancerous cells may also travel through the bloodstream and lymphatic system to distant parts of the body, where they form secondary tumors.

SKIN CANCER

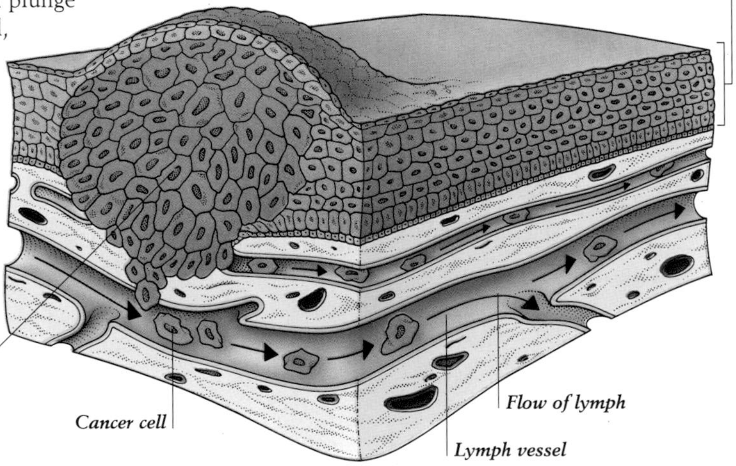

Epidermis of skin

Cluster of cancer cells

Cancer cell

Flow of lymph

Lymph vessel

PRECAUTIONS

Consult a doctor before undertaking any complementary therapy and do not stop taking conventional medication.

Cancer can cause a variety of symptoms. Consult a doctor as soon as possible if you have any of the following:

- unexplained, persistent weight loss
- a mole that changes shape, gets bigger, itches, or bleeds
- sores, scabs, or ulcers on the skin that do not heal
- a lump in the breast, discharge or bleeding from the nipple or flattening of the nipple, change in the shape or size of the breast, dimpling or puckering of the skin
- change in the shape or size of the testicles
- unexplained, severe headaches
- constant hoarseness, persistent sore throat, nagging cough, difficulty in swallowing, repeatedly coughing up blood
- persistent abdominal pain or indigestion
- blood – either red or black – in the stool or urine
- change in bowel habits, for example persistent constipation
- vaginal bleeding between menstrual periods, after sex, or after menopause.

See also page 204.

CANCER PREVENTION & TREATMENT

A TENDENCY FOR CELLS to mutate can be inherited or triggered by factors such as diet, tobacco-smoking, alcohol, pollution, radiation, industrial chemicals, or unidentified viral infections. The incidence of the various forms of cancer varies from one country and culture to another. Stomach cancer, for example, is highest in Japan, possibly due to a high salt intake and greater rates of infection with the stomach bacterium *Helicobacter pylori*.

Self-Help There are numerous steps you can take to improve your chances of avoiding many of the common cancers.

- Be familiar with your body: examine skin and breasts or testicles regularly.
- Don't smoke: smoking is a factor in cancers of the lung, mouth, throat, esophagus, pancreas, bladder, and cervix.
- Avoid becoming sunburned: ultraviolet light can trigger skin cancers.
- Practice safer sex: cervical and some anal cancers are linked to a sexually transmitted virus.
- Get daily physical exercise. Research shows that inactive people are almost twice as likely to develop cancer as those who exercise regularly.
- Learn to manage stress (see page 38): high stress levels may be linked to cancer.
- Watch your weight: cancers of the breast, uterus, and gallbladder are more common in overweight people.
- Keep alcohol intake low: in excess it may increase the risk of cancer of the mouth, esophagus, larynx, and liver.
- Eat a balanced whole-foods diet high in fresh fruits and vegetables and whole-grain cereals, but low in fat, especially saturated fat, red meat, processed meat, and smoked or salted foods. A dietary factor is suspected in a third of all cancers. A high-fat diet, for example, is linked to breast cancer.
- Eat more foods that protect against cancer (see Naturopathy, right).
- Choose organic food where possible: pesticides, additives, and other chemicals may increase susceptibility to cancer.
- Avoid charring food when grilling or barbecuing: this produces potential carcinogens (cancer-inducing agents).
- Throw moldy food away: some molds are carcinogenic.

TOUCH & MOVEMENT THERAPIES

Various forms of touch therapy can help to improve physical and emotional well-being in cancer patients. Acupuncture helps to relieve pain and counter the unpleasant side effects of conventional treatment.

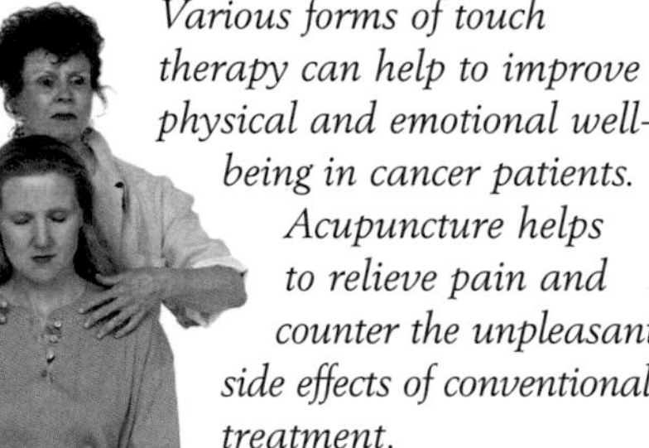

HELPING HANDS
Therapeutic Touch may help patients cope with pain and anxiety.

MASSAGE

Therapeutic massage, available in many cancer wards and hospices, can help relieve muscle pain and tension, reduce anxiety, and encourage relaxation. In a US study described in *Cancer Nursing* in 1993, therapeutic massage of cancer patients was shown to reduce the perception of pain and anxiety. Family members and friends taught to massage the patient can bring comfort and reassurance through physical touch.
SEE PAGES 56–61

AROMATHERAPY

In a 1995 study, UK cancer patients massaged with Roman chamomile essential oil reported less anxiety, fewer physical symptoms, and a better quality of life than patients massaged with an unscented oil. SEE PAGES 62–65

Caution: The use of Roman chamomile essential oil is subject to legal restrictions in some countries.

REFLEXOLOGY

According to practitioners, the feet are a mirror of the body, and applying pressure to areas on the foot that correspond to the affected organs may help to relieve symptoms such as pain, constipation, and nausea. Reflexology is increasingly available in many hospices, and is often given by nurses.
SEE PAGES 66–69

ACUPUNCTURE

Stimulation of acupoints can relieve nausea and other symptoms associated with chemotherapy, and help to alleviate pain (see also acupuncture entry in Pain, page 315). Acupuncture is believed to encourage the release of endorphins, natural painkillers that can also increase feelings of well-being. Acupressure, in which the same acupoints are stimulated by hand, may be effective in the same way, but to a lesser degree. SEE PAGES 90–94

HEALING

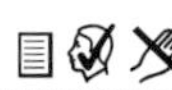

There are various forms of healing, including the laying on of hands and absent healing, in which practitioners pray for the recipient or visualize a transfer of healing energy. Doctors are skeptical about practitioners' claims for cures and spontaneous remission, but many patients and their families report that healing has given them support, strength, relief from symptoms, and spiritual solace. SEE PAGES 104–105

THERAPEUTIC TOUCH

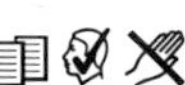

A growing number of nurses, particularly in the US, use Therapeutic Touch, which is a form of healing believed to stimulate the body's natural healing powers. Studies report that it can improve pain management.
SEE PAGE 106

MEDICINAL THERAPIES

The influence of diet and food supplements on cancer is unclear, but it does seem that some foods and dietary aids have certain protective qualities. Homeopathic and herbal practitioners use medicinal remedies to boost the body's natural regenerative powers.

NATUROPATHY

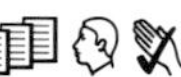

To prevent cancer, a practitioner will recommend foods rich in various substances:

Fiber Found in the bran of cereal grains, fiber aids digestion and elimination, helping to move undigested food through the bowel, so that toxins and potential carcinogens are not absorbed into the bloodstream.

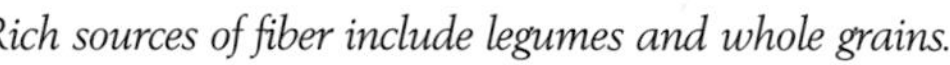

HIGH-FIBER DIET
Rich sources of fiber include legumes and whole grains.

Antioxidants Vitamins A (as beta-carotene), C, and E, the mineral selenium, and bioflavonoids (see following, page 306) are known as antioxidants. As food is turned into energy (oxidized), chemicals known as "free radicals" are produced. In excess, free radicals damage cell membranes, deplete the immune system, disrupt the hormonal and other systems, and stimulate the growth of cancer cells. Antioxidants help to check the number of free radicals produced.

NATUROPATHY *continued*

◆ *Beta-carotene* is found in red, orange, and yellow fruits and vegetables. A high intake of this nutrient reduces the risk of cancers of the bladder, breast, large bowel, larynx, stomach, cervix, and uterine lining. Beta-carotene may also protect against sunburn.

◆ *Vitamin C* helps prevent carcinogenic nitrosamines (derived from nitrates and nitrites, found in smoked and salty foods) from forming in the stomach, and enhances immune function. Citrus fruits, black currants, tomatoes, broccoli, cabbage, and potatoes are all good sources of vitamin C. Diets low in vitamin C have been linked to cancer of the stomach, esophagus, breast, and liver, and to leukemia (in which white blood cells multiply abnormally).

◆ *Vitamin E* protects the cells and boosts immunity. Good sources include wheat germ, nuts, vegetable oils, seeds, and whole-grain bread. Vitamin E may reduce the risk of oral and stomach cancers.

◆ *Selenium* is a mineral found in seafood, cereal grains, brazil nuts, and meat. It protects the cells and may inhibit cancers of the colon, cervix, breast, skin, and liver. The diet of many people is dangerously deficient in selenium, and the results of a 1996 trial in the US reported that supplements reduced death rates in a group of those who had skin cancer by 52%.

◆ *Bioflavonoids* are chemicals found in many types of fruits, including lemons, grapefruit, and cherries. As well as having antioxidant properties, they strengthen the capillaries.

Zinc Found in fish, lean meat, and peanuts, zinc is necessary for a healthy immune system.

B vitamins Vitamin B_2 (riboflavin) is found in yeast extract, dairy products, and eggs. It helps prevent cancer of the esophagus and works with vitamin B_6 (pyridoxine), found in yeast extract, whole-wheat bread, wheat germ, and bananas, to destroy possible carcinogens. A deficiency of folic acid, another B vitamin, found in wheat germ, broccoli, nuts, and yeast extract, is linked with cervical cancer, as is a lack of vitamin B_6.

Other recommended foods include garlic and onions, which contain allicin, a substance that may help prevent gastrointestinal and bladder cancer. Foods containing lycopene, such as red peppers, may lower the risk of cervical and prostate cancer. Crucifers (members of the cabbage family) contain indoles, chemicals thought to protect against breast cancer. Soy products, such as tofu, contain phytoestrogens, substances that may also help protect against breast cancer. SEE PAGES 118–21

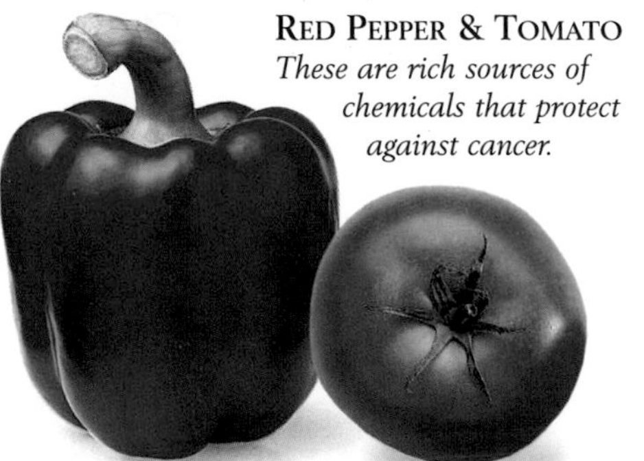
RED PEPPER & TOMATO
These are rich sources of chemicals that protect against cancer.

ANTHROPOSOPHICAL MEDICINE 

Practitioners take a holistic approach to cancer, incorporating dietary advice, counseling, and a form of dance therapy called eurythmy. Studies of Iscador, an anthroposophical medicine extracted from mistletoe, have shown that it can increase white blood cells (which fight infection) and affect the growth of cancer cells in the laboratory. However, there is as yet little conclusive evidence that it inhibits the progress of cancer in patients. SEE PAGES 124–25

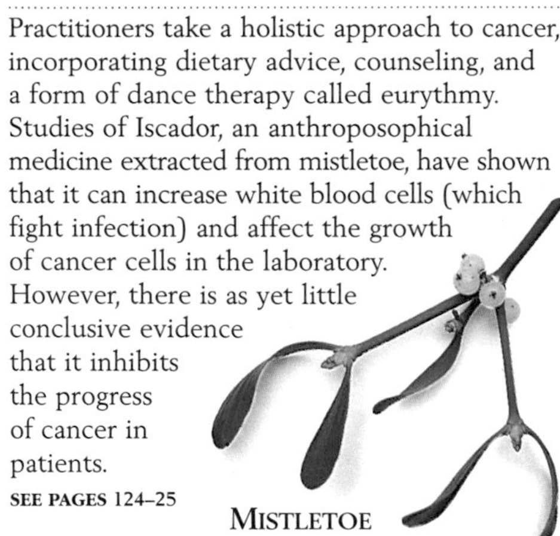
MISTLETOE
An extract is used to treat cancer.

WESTERN HERBALISM 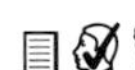

Treatment may be given alongside conventional chemotherapy and radiotherapy, and aims to boost the body's defenses. It might begin with a cleansing program, with herbs such as burdock given to help elimination. Restorative remedies usually follow, including "bitter" herbs for the liver and digestion, circulatory stimulants, and herbs for the nervous system. Canadian medical herbalists claim some success with the remedy known as Essiac, based on a Native American formula containing burdock root, sheep's sorrel, Chinese rhubarb, and slippery elm. Although Essiac is unlicensed, it is taken by a growing number of patients.

The Hoxsey therapy is based on a formula of nine herbs that includes licorice, red clover, cascara, burdock root, and queen's delight (stillingia root). Harry Hoxsey developed the formula in the US in the 1840s after watching a horse cure itself of cancer by eating medicinal herbs. Banned in the US, the therapy is still practiced in Mexico, along with many other treatments outlawed elsewhere. SEE PAGES 134–39

Caution: Take herbal remedies only under professional supervision and with the consent of your doctor.

CHINESE HERBALISM 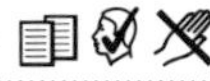

In Traditional Chinese Medicine, cancer is associated with "deficiency of *qi* ('life energy') or Blood," or an imbalance in *yin* and *yang* (see glossary). Interesting, if mixed, results are reported for Chinese herbal remedies taken to treat cancer or alleviate the side effects of chemotherapy and radiotherapy. *Fu zheng* therapy, which relies on an herbal formula that includes ginseng and astragalus, is claimed to double the life expectancy of patients with advancing cancer. In a 1988 study, astragalus was shown to boost immunity in patients receiving chemotherapy. In Korea in 1995, people taking ginseng as a powdered extract exhibited lower incidences of lung, liver, mouth, and throat cancer. In 1995, clinical studies of a Japanese formula, *Syo-saiko-to*, based on a Chinese medicine *Xiao Chai Hu Tang* (TJ-9), which contains seven herbs, showed that it could prevent or delay liver cancer in people with cirrhosis. SEE PAGES 140–43

Caution: Take herbal remedies only under professional supervision and with the consent of your doctor.

AYURVEDA 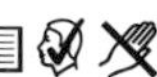

Practitioners will give an individual assessment and treat accordingly. A US study reported in *Pharmacology, Biochemistry, and Behavior* in 1990 found that an herbal formula known as Maharishi 4 could reduce the incidence of mammary-gland cancer in rats, but it has not yet been shown to treat breast cancer in humans effectively. SEE PAGES 144–47

NUTRITIONAL THERAPIES 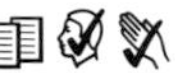

A number of different dietary therapies aim to treat cancer. Although diet is important in preventing the disease, and may offset nutritional deficiencies caused by chemotherapy and radiotherapy, there is, as yet, very little scientific evidence showing that diet can affect the course of cancer.

To rid the body of toxins, practitioners may advise fasting, eating large quantites of fruits or raw vegetables, or taking large doses of vitamins and minerals. Conventional doctors are concerned that extreme regimes – high in bulk and low in calories – may be the opposite of what many patients need, causing weight loss in people who are already underweight. The diets may lead to depression, as eating is no longer enjoyable, and failure to follow them can induce guilt. Some practitioners advise less rigid diets, emphasizing nutritious, natural, unprocessed foods to restore energy. They advise eating slowly and deliberately to aid digestion, and scheduling the main meal at midday so the body can rest at night.

The Bristol Diet Devised in the 1980s at the Bristol Cancer Help Centre in the UK, the original organic vegan diet has now been superseded by a less rigorous regime. The Centre's advice for managing cancer is tailored to meet the needs of individual patients, following guidelines issued by the Committee of Diet, Nutrition, and Cancer in the US in 1982. The emphasis is on natural, unprocessed foods: whole grains, fruits rich in vitamin C, vegetables, legumes, nuts, sesame and sunflower seeds, and filtered water. Eggs, dairy products, fish, and white meat can be eaten in moderation, but the Centre recommends that caffeine, red meat, salt, sugar, hydrogenated margarine, saturated fats, processed polyunsaturated fats, and deep-fried foods all be avoided.

Gerson Therapy Dr. Max Gerson believed that an excess of sodium in the body disrupts the function of the liver, pancreas, thyroid gland, and immune system. He devised a low-salt, organic diet, focusing on raw vegetable and fruit juices, with nutritional supplements and frequent coffee enemas to "detoxify" the liver and relieve pain. The regime demands enormous commitment from patients, and has potentially harmful side effects, including weight loss and poor resistance to disease. Improvement is not guaranteed. However, a 1995 study of cancer patients in Mexico following the Gerson therapy found that their survival rate was higher than average.

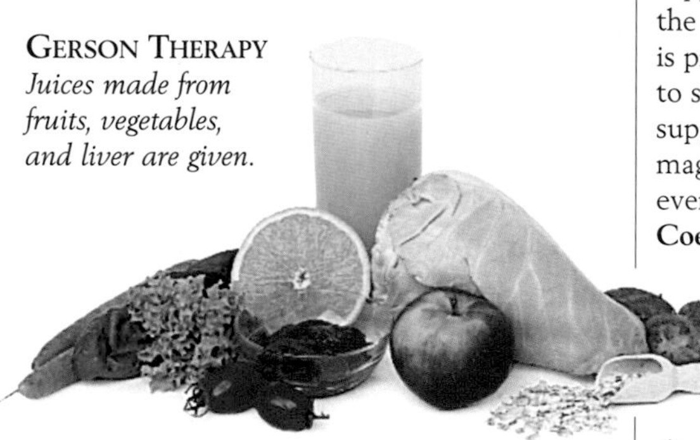

GERSON THERAPY
Juices made from fruits, vegetables, and liver are given.

Antineoplaston Therapy Adherents of this therapy believe that naturally occurring proteins, called antineoplastons, are deficient in cancer patients. Treatment consists of reintroducing them into the bloodstream, either by intravenous injection or as tablets, to normalize cell growth and shrink tumors. The treatment remains on the American Cancer Society's list of unproved methods.
Laetrile Therapy Also known as amygdalin or vitamin B_{17}, laetrile is a preparation extracted from apricot kernels. It contains cyanide, which, practitioners claim, is highly effective in destroying cancer cells. A scientific study failed to show any benefits from the use of laetrile and reported that blood levels of cyanide in patients were dangerously high.
Other Treatments Some practitioners believe various substances may help to cure cancer, but their claims have not always been proved. A 1986 Scandinavian study claimed that shark-liver oil enhanced the success of radiation therapy for uterine cancer, while Japanese studies have found that shiitake mushrooms helped prolong the life of some patients with cancers of the stomach, breast, colon, and rectum. High doses of the hormone melatonin are under investigation as a cancer treatment. According to a report in the US journal *Cancer* in 1994, in one study of patients with brain tumors, a combination of melatonin and supportive care increased survival time and slowed or stopped the growth of cancer. SEE PAGES 148–52
Caution: Follow a specialized diet only with professional supervision and with the consent of your doctor.

ORTHOMOLECULAR THERAPY

Practitioners believe that large doses of vitamins, minerals, and other substances can treat diseases. Whether such supplements can treat cancer is the subject of enormous controversy and a growing body of research. The vitamins most often given, sometimes by intravenous injection, are beta-carotene (vitamin A) and vitamins C and E. Vitamins C and E are thought to defend against carcinogens, but there is so far no conclusive evidence to support these claims. In theory, beta-carotene can destroy cancer cells, but a recent US study showed that supplements of this vitamin actually increased the risk of lung cancer. Beta-carotene in food is probably safer and more effective. Evidence to support the use of megadoses of other supplements, including vitamin B-complex, magnesium, calcium, chromium, zinc, and evening primrose oil, is sketchy.
Coenzyme Q10 Also known as ubiquinone, this organic compound is an antioxidant (see glossary) and works with enzymes to help cells produce energy. Its possible role in treating cancer has received much attention since the publication of a Danish study in 1994, in which women with breast cancer who took up to 300 mg a day showed an improvement. SEE PAGE 153
Caution: Take very large doses of supplements only with professional supervision and the consent of your doctor.

MIND & EMOTION THERAPIES

A diagnosis of cancer can stir up painful and bewildering emotions. Practitioners help patients to express their feelings and encourage a support network.

PSYCHOTHERAPY & COUNSELING

Psychotherapy and counseling are now widely used for cancer patients and their families. The role played by psychological factors in the development of cancer is highly controversial. There is no firm evidence that personality, emotions, or stress can cause the disease, nor that feelings of depression or helplessness will make tumors grow faster. There is growing evidence, however, that supportive social environments and psychological factors may improve chances of recovery or increase the survival time of cancer patients. A US study, reported in *The Lancet* in 1989, found that attending weekly support groups, coupled with relaxation techniques and self-hypnosis, doubled the length of survival of women with advanced breast cancer. In another US study in 1990, skin-cancer patients who received counseling, education about the disease, and training in relaxation and coping skills experienced less distress and were found to have more natural killer cells (see page 308) and other immune cells. SEE PAGES 160–65

HYPNOTHERAPY

Hypnotherapy may help people cope with pain and other symptoms of cancer, and with side effects of chemotherapy and radiotherapy, such as nausea and vomiting. SEE PAGES 166–67

RELAXATION & BREATHING

Patients are taught techniques to help to release muscle tension, relieve breathlessness, lessen anxiety, and encourage a greater sense of control, particularly when receiving unpleasant or stressful treatments. SEE PAGES 170–73

MEDITATION

Many people find that meditation brings physical and mental relaxation, and helps spiritual development. Australian psychiatrist Ainslie Meares developed a program for people with cancer that involved three hours of daily meditation. Deep relaxation and a spiritual state of mind likened to prayer were the aims. A few cases of apparent tumor regression were reported, but there has been no continuing research. SEE PAGES 174–77

VISUALIZATION

Patients are asked to focus on feeling stronger or better, or to picture the destruction of tumor cells while in a state of relaxation. In one technique, patients visualize various aspects of treatment, from the least frightening to the most painful, remaining calm and relaxed at each step. This method has helped patients to control nausea before chemotherapy. SEE PAGES 178–79

ART THERAPY

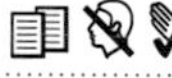

Drawing, painting, and sculpture, especially when carried out in a group environment, encourage pleasure in creativity and enable people to find a nonverbal way of expressing their feelings. SEE PAGES 182–83

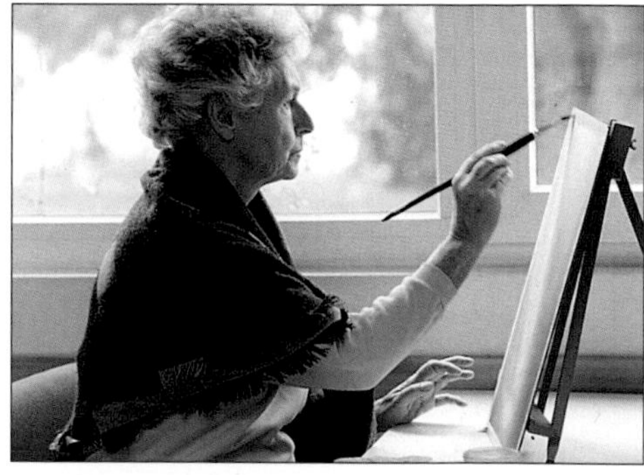

THERAPEUTIC PAINTING
Art therapy helps people express emotions that cannot easily be put into words.

THE IMMUNE SYSTEM

THE BODY'S FRONTLINE DEFENSES, the skin and mucous membranes, are sometimes breached by viruses. When this occurs, specialized cells of the immune system engulf the invaders or neutralize them with "antibody" chemicals. The immune system retains a profile of the invaders for future rapid response, enabling the body to develop immunity to certain diseases. If the system is underactive, it fails to deal with infections. If the immune response is overactive, it may be triggered by harmless substances, resulting in allergies. Autoimmune diseases occur when the immune system turns against the normal tissues of the body.

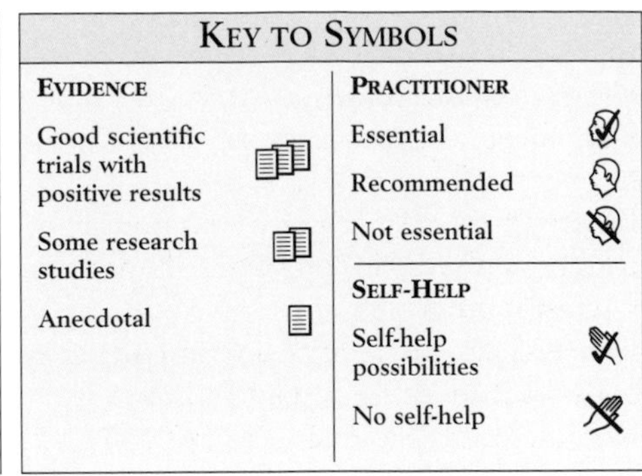

COMPLEMENTARY APPROACHES

The harmonious interaction of the brain, nervous system, and endocrine glands is important if the immune system is to function correctly. Practitioners believe that a healthy lifestyle, with a well-balanced diet, adequate sleep, and exercise, and a positive outlook on life is the best way to support the immune system. Touch and movement therapies improve the flow of lymph, vital to healthy immune function. Herbal remedies and nutritional supplements may enhance immune activity, but there are no "complementary" vaccines. Thoughts and feelings influence immune processes, so mind therapies may help long-standing conditions.

CONVENTIONAL APPROACHES

Conventional medicine can prevent certain diseases by immunization. This process, which involves putting dead or inactivated forms of a virus or bacterium into the body, causes the immune system to produce antibodies. These deal with any threatened infection by attracting killer cells (see above right) to destroy the intruder or by doing so themselves. Healthy cells are also armed against viruses with proteins called interferons, which can now be synthesized and used in the fight against leukemia, AIDS, and other disorders.

It is sometimes necessary to inhibit the immune system. Doctors prescribe corticosteroid and immunosuppressant drugs when the system overreacts (causing allergies, see pages 298–303) or starts destroying its own tissues (autoimmune diseases).

Caution: Before seeking treatment, see page 204.

HOW THE IMMUNE SYSTEM FUNCTIONS

The bone marrow, thymus gland, spleen, and lymph nodes (also called lymph glands) are the major elements of the immune system. They produce several types of white blood cells, including lymphocytes. B-lymphocytes produce antibodies to neutralize dangerous organisms at the prompting of other cells, called "helper T-cells," and stop producing antibodies when "suppressor T-cells" signal them to do so. Other lymphocytes, called "killer T-cells" or "natural killer cells," attack tumors and viruses. Lymphocytes recognize organisms that have invaded in the past, which helps them mobilize very quickly, but if an unfamiliar bacterium or virus appears, it may take a few days to produce antibodies. Swollen glands, a symptom of various illnesses, are caused by white blood cells incubating a supply of antibodies in the lymph nodes. Phagocytes, another type of white blood cell, are activated by injury or infection. Drawn into the injured area by histamine (see page 298), the cells devour microbes and debris.

ELEMENTS OF THE IMMUNE SYSTEM

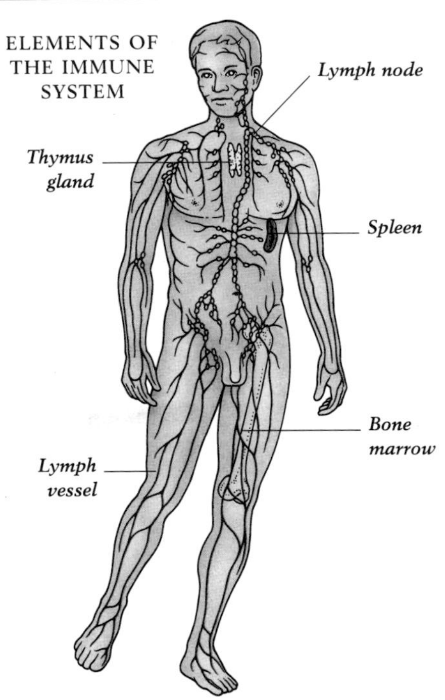

WHAT CAN GO WRONG?

Several factors can interfere with the orchestration of the immune system:

◆ In good health, the helper and suppressor T-cells are in balance, so that antibodies are produced only when needed. If suppressor cells dominate, however, the system may become "immunodeficient," or weakened. This may be due to an inherited condition or viral infection such as HIV (see pages 310–11).

◆ If helper T-cells dominate, the immune system becomes overactive, and its ability to differentiate between "self" and "invader" is lost. The immune system starts attacking body tissues, in what are generally known as autoimmune diseases. These include multiple sclerosis (see page 212) and rheumatoid arthritis (see page 260).

◆ The immune system may become hypersensitive and react against normally harmless substances, such as dust, pollen, and certain foodstuffs, causing allergic disorders, such as asthma (see pages 300–301), hay fever (see page 299), eczema (see page 218), and food allergies (see page 302).

◆ After an organ transplant, doctors deliberately suppress the immune system to keep the body from rejecting foreign tissue, but great care must be taken to avoid infection.

DEPLETED IMMUNE SYSTEM

COMPLEMENTARY PRACTITIONERS believe that people who regularly suffer from coughs, colds, and general ill-health, but who have no serious underlying condition, have a "depleted immune system." Environmental, hereditary, emotional, dietary, and lifestyle factors are all thought to contribute to the problem.

Causes Inadequate nutrition impairs the body's ability to keep its defenses in top working order. Smoking, environmental toxins, and industrial pollution may tax the system to the point where it cannot respond adequately. Excessive exercise has been shown to leave the body more vulnerable to infection. Certain hormones released in response to stress, such as epinephrine, appear to interfere with the ability of T-cells and B-lymphocytes (see opposite) to divide and multiply (while laughter seems to support their production). Lack of sleep may be another factor that impairs immune function. Singly or in combination, these influences may result in a system whose ability to cope has been overloaded. Infections and other disorders then follow.

Conventional Treatment A doctor will advocate dietary improvements, adequate sleep and exercise, giving up smoking, and reducing stress. Depending on the symptoms and cause, painkillers, antibiotics, or other drugs may be prescribed.

COMPLEMENTARY TREATMENTS

Practitioners believe that we can improve our defenses by maintaining overall health and well-being through regular exercise, a healthy diet, and relaxation.

MASSAGE 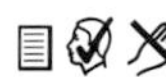

Given its ability to lower stress and induce relaxation, massage may play an important role in supporting the immune system. Practitioners also believe that certain techniques help to stimulate lymph flow and eliminate wastes from the body. SEE PAGES 56–61

WESTERN HERBALISM 

A practitioner may suggest taking echinacea, which research studies suggest may enhance immunity. Garlic, ginger, thyme, sage, and rosemary are also said to help neutralize invading organisms. SEE PAGES 134–39

Cautions: Do not take medicinal doses of thyme or sage during pregnancy. Do not take ginger if you have a peptic ulcer.

NUTRITIONAL THERAPIES 

Studies of elderly people have shown that vitamin and mineral supplements improved their immune responses. Helpful substances include vitamins A (as beta-carotene), C, E, and zinc, selenium, and bioflavonoids (see glossary). These all have an antioxidant effect, neutralizing superfluous free radicals (chemicals that can damage cell membranes). Beta-carotene also strengthens the skin and mucous membranes and increases antibody response, vitamin C helps increase antibody levels, and vitamin E protects body cells and tissues. Other advised nutrients may include vitamin D, B-complex vitamins, iron, calcium, magnesium, and manganese. SEE PAGES 148–52

CLINICAL ECOLOGY 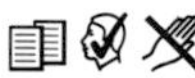

Practitioners claim that people who repeatedly suffer minor illnesses without apparent cause may be sensitive to certain foods or to environmental factors. A series of analytical tests will be carried out to determine whether this is the case. SEE PAGES 154–55

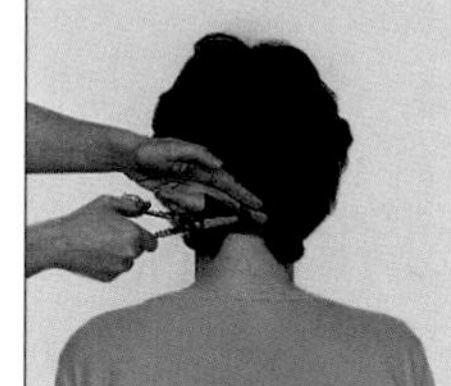

HAIR ANALYSIS
A hair sample is taken for analysis, to identify toxins in the body.

PSYCHOTHERAPY & COUNSELING 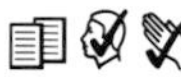

Counseling offers a supportive setting in which to uncover and explore hidden causes of stress, anxiety, or depression. Addressing these problems and developing ways of coping may improve immune-system response as well as state of mind. SEE PAGES 160–65

MEDITATION 

Practitioners believe that the calming, restorative act of meditation not only lowers heart rate and blood pressure, but also improves the ability to cope with stress, a factor that may impair immune-system function.
SEE PAGES 174–77

OTHER OPTION

Naturopathy SEE PAGES 118–21

INFECTIOUS MONONUCLEOSIS

ALSO KNOWN AS glandular fever, infectious mononucleosis usually affects young adults. Symptoms include fever, headaches, swollen lymph glands, and a severe sore throat. Caused by either the Epstein-Barr virus or the cytomegalovirus, it spreads via saliva, hence its nickname, the "kissing disease." The recovery period is usually 4–6 weeks. Doctors generally advise bed rest, fluids, and painkillers such as aspirin. Aftereffects, such as lethargy, may persist for many months.

COMPLEMENTARY TREATMENTS

Practitioners will advocate healing plant remedies to support the body through the recuperative period.

NATUROPATHY 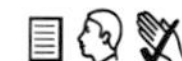

A practitioner will recommend supporting the system with easily digestible foods, such as soup, and fruit or vegetable juices. Garlic may be suggested for its antiseptic properties.
SEE PAGES 118–21

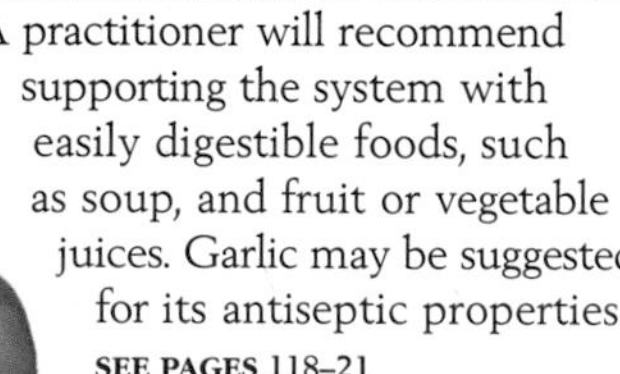

CHECKING THE GLANDS
Swollen lymph glands in the neck are a symptom of infectious mononucleosis.

HOMEOPATHY 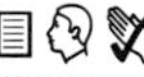

Belladonna 6c may be recommended for fever, sweating, and swollen glands. Some practitioners may suggest the mononucleosis nosode (see glossary), but there is no evidence that this will actually "immunize" against the disease. SEE PAGES 126–30

WESTERN HERBALISM 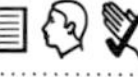

Goldenseal may increase white cell activity. A gargle made with sage, rosemary, and echinacea may help relieve sore throats. SEE PAGES 134–39

Caution: Do not take goldenseal during pregnancy or if you have high blood pressure.

NUTRITIONAL THERAPIES 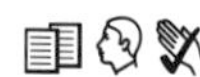

You may be advised to take vitamin B and antioxidant (see glossary) supplements, thought to increase antibody production. SEE PAGES 148–52

AIDS

ACQUIRED IMMUNODEFICIENCY SYNDROME (AIDS) is a condition in which the human immunodeficiency virus (HIV) invades and destroys infection-fighting cells called T-lymphocytes, leaving the body open to a range of fatal diseases. Usually symptomless at first, an HIV infection can take ten years or more to develop into AIDS. Despite global research, much remains unknown about the illness. Some with long-standing HIV show no signs of AIDS, and a few people who once tested positive for HIV appear to do so no longer. Some people with AIDS have tested negative for HIV. Given these anomalies and, more importantly, the lack of a cure, many people turn to complementary therapies, hoping that they will, at the very least, improve the quality of life.

CAUSES & SYMPTOMS

HIV spreads mainly through semen and blood. The vast majority of transmissions occur during sexual intercourse and blood transfusions, and when drug users share needles. As HIV weakens the immune system, viral, bacterial, protozoal, and fungal infections become more frequent. With full-blown AIDS, flulike symptoms and weight loss are followed by a range of disorders, which may include persistent herpes simplex (see page 217). Cancers, pneumonia, and wasting diarrhea are characteristic as the condition progresses. Finally, the brain may be affected by a form of encephalitis. However, there is no consistent pattern. About 28 diseases are associated with AIDS, and these differ between countries and even between those groups most typically at risk of contracting the virus.

PREVENTION

Practice safer anal, vaginal, and oral sex by using a condom. Do not share needles. Make sure that dentists, acupuncturists, tattooists, and body-piercers have adequate sterilization procedures and use disposable needles. In developing countries, carry a sterile hypodermic needle and syringe in case an injection is necessary, and avoid blood transfusions if possible.

CONVENTIONAL TREATMENT

From the time of infection, HIV takes between three weeks to three months or more to reveal itself in blood tests. The stress of testing positive means that counseling is required. As yet, there is no cure for AIDS. Antiviral, antibacterial, and antifungal drugs are used to preempt or combat infection. AZT, a drug that interferes with the reproduction of HIV cells, is the best-known approach to HIV. While this drug may prolong life, it can have unpleasant side effects: critics argue that it may be toxic and that any increase in T-lymphocytes (see page 308) is temporary. Interleukin 2, a natural protein which so far is too rare and too expensive to be widely available, can boost the production of T-cells, which are destroyed by AIDS and possibly by AZT as well. Promising new avenues of research include the recently developed protease inhibitor drugs.

A combination of three powerful antiviral drugs, including a protease inhibitor and an AZT drug, which attack HIV in different ways, was shown in 1997 to halve cancers, infections, and deaths in AIDS patients. Such drug combinations are very expensive, must be taken at the same time daily, and cause side effects. But they are capable of eliminating 99.9% of detectable HIV in body tissues, making AIDS a treatable disease.

TOUCH & MOVEMENT THERAPIES

Most therapies focus on encouraging relaxation and improving the circulation of blood and lymph. This may have a beneficial effect on the immune system.

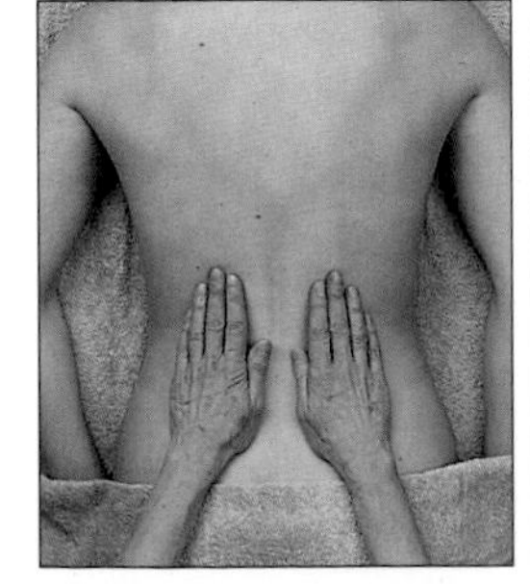

BENEFICIAL TOUCH
Regular massage comforts AIDS patients and may help body defenses by improving the circulation.

MASSAGE

An empathetic practitioner can provide the kind of caring and pleasurable touch that AIDS denies many patients, particularly those who are bedridden. Massage may bolster self-esteem and relieve distress, as well as improve circulation, lymph drainage, muscle relaxation, and joint flexibility. SEE PAGES 56–61

ACUPUNCTURE

Acupuncture is popular among people with AIDS. By encouraging the body's healing processes, it may help alleviate symptoms and increase immune function. A practitioner will stimulate appropriate acupoints to improve the flow of *qi* ("life energy"). Because of the use of needles, a highly trained practitioner must be consulted. SEE PAGES 90–94

QIGONG

This therapy combines movement, meditation, and breath control to enhance the flow of *qi*. Qigong may improve circulation and enhance immune function. SEE PAGE 99

HYDROTHERAPY

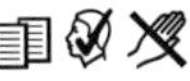

A practitioner may advise taking hot baths. Research indicates that HIV is less active when the body temperature climbs above its normal 98.6°F (37°C). SEE PAGES 122–23

Caution: Only undertake this treatment with professional supervision.

OTHER OPTIONS

Aromatherapy SEE PAGES 62–65
Reflexology SEE PAGES 66–69
Shiatsu SEE PAGES 96–97

MEDICINAL THERAPIES

Practitioners attempt to enhance the body's self-healing abilities by eliminating potentially undermining factors such as poor nutrition or environmental toxins. Many HIV-positive people and people with AIDS use homeopathy as part of a package of complementary therapies.

NATUROPATHY

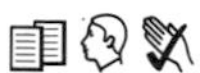

To support the immune system, the US-based Healing AIDS Research Project (HARP) advocates consuming a ratio of 65% unrefined carbohydrates, 15% protein, and 20% fat from as wide a range of foods as possible to avoid intolerances. Fruits and vegetables should be thoroughly washed to remove bacteria and chemicals, and vegetables lightly steamed to make them easier to digest. A practitioner will also advise you to avoid caffeine and reduce alcohol intake, as well as suggest that you get regular exercise and adequate sleep.
SEE PAGES 118–21

HOMEOPATHY

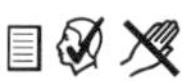

A practitioner will assess your personality, features, and many other factors to determine your constitutional type as a basis for treatment. Complex homeopathy aims to stimulate organs and tissues directly.
SEE PAGES 126–30

WESTERN HERBALISM

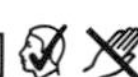

Herbal practitioners use powerful combinations of herbs to treat AIDS, and self-help is not advised. Garlic, ginger, cinnamon, cloves, and aloe-vera gel are commonly recommended for their antimicrobial properties. Extract of aloe vera, also an immune stimulant, has been used in conjunction with AZT in the hope of lowering the necessary dose of the drug, but the results of clinical trials are so far inconsistent.

Other herbs that may be prescribed to boost immunity include: goldenseal and astragalus to enhance the production of interferon, a substance that regulates immune-cell activity; licorice to normalize white-cell function and promote production of antibodies; and garlic to increase T-lymphocyte production.

Detoxifying herbs, such as red clover, cleavers, dandelion root, and milk thistle, may be suggested to strengthen the liver, which is at risk of being damaged by conventional medication. Nerve tonics such as St. John's wort may be advised, along with nutritional herbs such as nettle, which is rich in iron and other minerals. Herbs that are beneficial for the digestive system, such as celery and thyme, may also be recommended.
SEE PAGES 134–39

Caution: Take herbal remedies for AIDS and HIV only under professional supervision.

CHINESE HERBALISM

Many AIDS patients claim that Chinese herbal remedies improve their overall well-being and lessen the side effects of conventional drugs. Tonic herbs such as ginseng, and herbs that improve the circulation, such as red sage and white peony, are often used, while Chinese bitter melon and lentinan (shiitake mushrooms) are alleged to have anti-HIV effects.
SEE PAGES 140–43

Cautions: Do not take ginseng, red sage, or white peony in pregnancy. Do not take ginseng if you have high blood pressure.

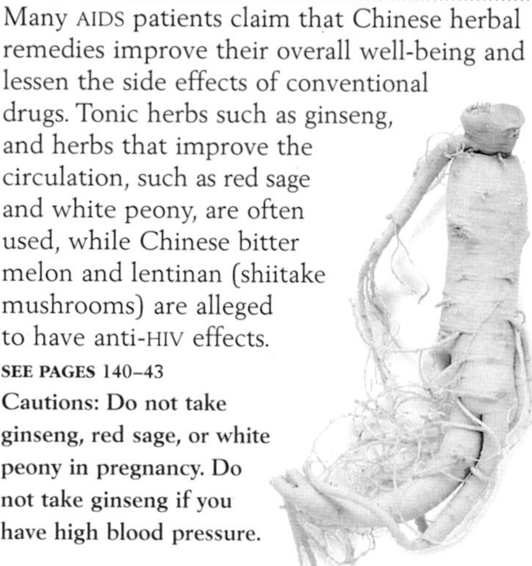

GINSENG
This tonic and restorative herb has been taken in China for around 7,000 years.

NUTRITIONAL THERAPIES

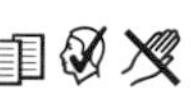

Practitioners may recommend supplements of vitamins A, B_6, and B_{12}, C, and E, as well as folic acid, selenium, zinc, and bioflavonoids (see glossary), to strengthen the immune system. According to a 1993 US study, the steroid hormone DHEA (dehydroepiandrosterone), which is found naturally in the body but decreases with age, may be deficient in people with advanced HIV. Supplements may therefore be advised. Propolis, an antiviral and antibacterial compound made by bees, may also be given to improve immunity. SEE PAGES 148–52

OZONE THERAPY

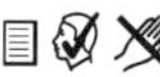

Laboratory tests have demonstrated that ozone can deactivate HIV in test tubes; critics point out that this does not mean it will have the same effect in the body or that it is safe to use. SEE PAGE 157

MIND & EMOTION THERAPIES

Coming to terms with being HIV-positive can be very difficult. Psychological therapies provide a safe and supportive setting in which to cope with strong emotions, and to develop strategies to deal with the progress of the disease.

PSYCHOTHERAPY & COUNSELING

Counseling is essential both before and after diagnosis of HIV to help prepare you for the ramifications of a positive result. Apart from providing basic information and advice on healthy living, the sessions will help you deal with difficult feelings, such as anger, fear, denial, and depression. AIDS support groups can be helpful as a forum in which to share experiences, methods of coping, and information on research and treatment. Research into mind/body medicine shows that having a good attitude about the disease and one's power to influence survival may help raise T-lymphocyte cell counts, reduce symptoms, and possibly extend lifespan. In 1996, the UK journal *Complementary Therapies in Medicine* claimed that a program that focused on the visualization of positive feelings helped to alleviate symptoms, reportedly by reducing stress and anxiety, improving physical vitality, and enhancing psychological well-being.
SEE PAGES 160–65

RELAXATION & BREATHING

By relieving stress and reducing muscle tension, relaxation may help boost the immune system. Diaphragmatic breathing improves circulation and the function of all body systems. The sense of calm that results may encourage a more positive attitude. SEE PAGES 170–73

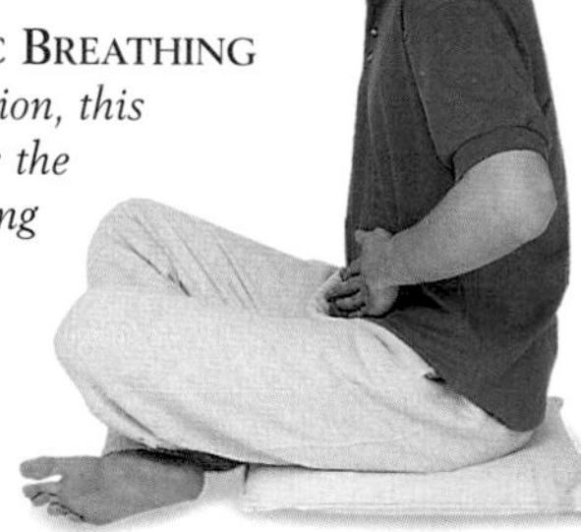

DIAPHRAGMATIC BREATHING
The key to relaxation, this technique expands the chest fully, providing the optimum amount of oxygen.

MEDITATION

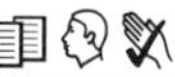

Learning to relax and simultaneously concentrate the mind through the regular practice of meditation can help lower stress levels, replenish the body's resources, and refresh the spirit, offsetting the strain of illness. SEE PAGES 174–77

VISUALIZATION

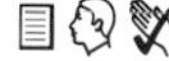

In this therapy, a practitioner will teach you how to transport yourself to an inner landscape of tranquility and beauty, or to imagine your pain or illness as an object that can be melted down or otherwise carried away or diminished. Exercises may also incorporate breathing and relaxation techniques. Preliminary research suggests that some people with AIDS may be able to use these techniques to increase immune-cell activity. The immediate and basic benefit of visualization, however, is in lessening the impact of day-to-day stress.
SEE PAGES 178–79

OTHER OPTIONS

Hypnotherapy SEE PAGES 166–67
Autogenic Training SEE PAGE 168

CHRONIC FATIGUE SYNDROME (CFS)

PROLONGED FATIGUE can be a symptom of a number of conditions, including anemia, depression, chronic infection, autoimmune disorders, and cancer. For some kinds of extreme and disabling exhaustion, however, no apparent cause can be found, even though the problem may last for years. This increasingly common condition has acquired various names, the most generally accepted being Chronic Fatigue Syndrome (CFS). CFS is gaining official recognition by the conventional medical establishments in many countries, but some doctors still dismiss it as "all in the mind." Complementary practitioners are more ready to look beyond the symptoms for possible physical and psychological contributing factors.

CAUSES & SYMPTOMS

The symptoms of CFS may appear suddenly, sometimes after a viral infection. They commonly include incapacitating and persistent fatigue, muscle and joint pain, headaches, repeated infections or mild fever, depression, inability to concentrate, memory loss, sleep disturbance, food intolerances, and heightened sensitivity to the environment. Many people with CFS insist that the cause is a physical disorder, but it seems increasingly likely that both mind and body are involved. Psychologists talk in terms of a "CFS personality profile" – a hardworking perfectionist who finds it hard to relax and is inclined to become depressed and introverted. A disproportionate number of people with CFS are young professional women.

CONVENTIONAL TREATMENT

There is no conventional treatment as such, although many medical centers in the US offer CFS clinics. Doctors recommend rest, a balanced diet, vitamin supplements, counseling, and perhaps antidepressants, since depression is often a component of the disorder. Because prolonged disuse of the muscles leads to aches and pains and stiffness, doctors may recommend some form of gentle exercise, which should be gradually increased.

PREVENTION & SELF-HELP

Medical experts now believe CFS may be the result of a complex interaction between trigger factors such as stress, viral infection, psychological problems, brain chemistry, and social attitudes. If you are under pressure at work, learn to pace yourself, allowing time to relax during the day. Look at your lifestyle for ways to ease stress and delegate commitments. If you catch a viral infection such as a bad cold or flu, get plenty of rest and do not try to "tough it out." It is normal to have minor ailments from time to time – illnesses such as coughs and colds may be nature's way of telling you to slow down for a few days. After resting, gentle exercise, such as walking or swimming, prevents muscles from wasting and stimulates the release of endorphins, the body's natural painkillers. It also improves circulation and increases the number of killer T-cells produced by the immune system to deal with infections (see page 308). Most countries have national CFS associations or societies, which can supply literature and information about clinics and support groups.

PRECAUTION

- **Tell your complementary therapist if you are taking antidepressants or other conventional medication.**

TOUCH & MOVEMENT THERAPIES

CFS is a difficult condition to treat, so it is important to be open-minded and ready to try a number of therapies until you find one that suits you, bearing in mind that any improvement could take several months. Gentle touch and movement therapies may prove useful in stimulating systems stalled by illness or exhaustion.

MASSAGE

A valuable technique for stimulating the healing processes, massage encourages relaxation by giving you time to unwind and by relieving anxiety and muscle tension. SEE PAGES 56–61

ACUPUNCTURE

Practitioners often diagnose "damp heat" as the problem at the heart of CFS, but complex patterns of disharmony are also said to be involved. A combination of acupuncture, Chinese herbalism, and tuina, the most popular form of acupressure practiced in China, may offer the best results. SEE PAGES 90–94

YOGA

Unlike some forms of exercise, which seem to make CFS worse, yoga increases energy levels through breathing exercises and by gently working the muscles. It is therefore said to counter lethargy and fatigue. SEE PAGES 108–11

YOGA POSE
The Triangle posture stretches the entire body and improves breathing.

OTHER OPTIONS

Aromatherapy	SEE PAGES 62–65
The Feldenkrais Method	SEE PAGE 85
The Alexander Technique	SEE PAGES 86–87
Tragerwork	SEE PAGE 88
Qigong	SEE PAGE 99
T'ai Chi Ch'uan	SEE PAGES 100–101

MEDICINAL THERAPIES

Complementary practitioners treating cases of CFS may look for evidence of candidiasis, nutritional deficiencies, food allergies and intolerances, and hypoglycemia (low blood sugar levels). Many complementary treatment techniques aim to "detoxify" the body by eliminating suspect substances in the diet and the environment, and by helping the elimination of waste products through the bowel. Practitioners will also attempt to enhance immunity as well as your ability to cope with stress.

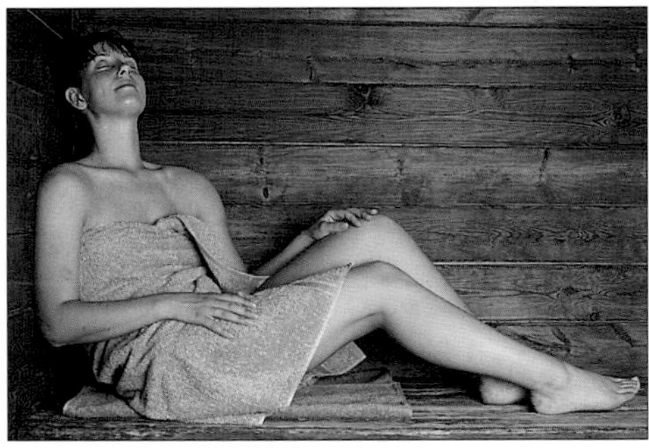

SAUNA TREATMENT
The heat of a sauna relaxes tight muscles, easing pain and increasing lung capacity.

NATUROPATHY 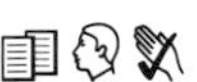

Practitioners aim to ease the strain on body systems by reducing stress and by responding to possible food allergies and intolerances. You may be advised to undertake an exclusion diet. Substances that are routinely discouraged include processed food, alcohol, caffeine, additives, and any potential food allergens. You will be told to eat fruits, vegetables, whole grains, legumes, nuts, seeds, and fish. A calcium and magnesium drink or melatonin supplement before bedtime may be suggested to help regulate sleep patterns and allow release of the growth hormone that is essential for tissue repair. Some practitioners may suggest cold baths and showers to boost the immune system, and hot baths and saunas to ease muscle pain. Mercury poisoning caused by dental fillings is sometimes said to cause CFS, but this has not been clinically proved. **SEE PAGES 118–21**

Caution: Avoid cold baths and showers if you have a heart condition.

HYDROTHERAPY 

Lowering the body temperature with cold baths seems to boost energy. Gradual acclimatization over several weeks, starting with a footbath and working up to whole-body immersions, each for a few minutes, is said to reduce fatigue.
SEE PAGES 122–23

Caution: Avoid cold baths and showers if you have a heart condition.

HOMEOPATHY 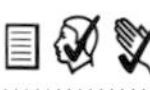

Your practitioner will give you an individual assessment that takes your symptom pattern into account and will treat you accordingly. Complex homeopathy aims to target any viral infection and to boost liver and kidney function. **SEE PAGES 126–30**

WESTERN HERBALISM 

Practitioners may recommend echinacea, yellow dock root, cleavers, wild indigo, astragalus, and goldenseal to improve immunity and help the body rid itself of waste products. Licorice, Siberian ginseng, and ginseng may be prescribed, as they are thought to support the adrenal glands. Milk thistle, barberry, and dandelion are considered beneficial for the healthy function of the liver; oats, vervain, and skullcap are said to support the nervous system. St. John's wort is not only antibacterial but an effective mood-enhancer and antidepressant. Ginkgo can benefit impaired circulation in the brain, which seems to be implicated in some people with CFS.
SEE PAGES 134–39

Cautions: Do not take yellow dock root, goldenseal, licorice, ginseng, barberry, and vervain during pregnancy. Do not take goldenseal, licorice, or ginseng if you have high blood pressure. Do not take licorice if you have anemia.

CHINESE HERBALISM 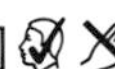

Remedies may be particularly helpful in conjunction with acupuncture. While most practitioners prefer to prescribe on the basis of an individual assessment, several standard herbal remedies may be advised, including Isatis Formula for viral infections, Astragalus, and Ganoderma Formula for deficiency of *qi* ("life energy") and *yin* (see glossary), and Anemphello and Rehmannia Formula for deficiency of *yin* with "heat."
SEE PAGES 140–43

AYURVEDA

Those with a *vata* constitution are said to be more susceptible to CFS than others. Practitioners suggest changes in diet and a cleansing or purification program to improve digestion, help eliminate waste products, and promote normal sleep patterns.
SEE PAGES 144–47

NUTRITIONAL THERAPIES 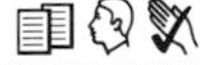

The following supplements are among those most commonly advised for CFS sufferers: beta-carotene, B vitamins (especially pantothenic acid, B_6, B_{12}, and folic acid), vitamin C, vitamin E, magnesium, zinc, selenium, molybdenum, copper, essential fatty acids, amino acids, and coenzyme Q10. Clinical studies in the early 1990s found high doses of essential fatty acid supplements (such as evening primrose oil and fish oils), or injections of magnesium, to be effective in treating CFS. Injections of vitamin B_{12}, while less well substantiated, have also produced good results. "Friendly" gut bacteria, such as *Lactobacillus acidophilus*, which help control candidiasis, may be advised if an overgrowth of this organism is suspected. **SEE PAGES 148–52**

OTHER OPTION

Bach Flower Remedies **SEE PAGES 132–33**

MIND & EMOTION THERAPIES

Depression and anxiety are associated with CFS, but it is hard to tell whether they are a cause or a result. Relaxation and coping techniques may be beneficial.

PSYCHOTHERAPY & COUNSELING 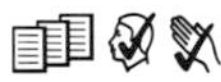

Several studies have found that CFS patients receiving cognitive behavioral therapy, which helps people change the way they think and behave, improved more quickly than those who did not. A gradual return to activity was an important part of the recommended regime. Counseling may help you reevaluate lifestyle and career goals, and manage stress. Support groups can also help, but beware of those that turn inward and focus on symptoms to the exclusion of issues that may be contributing to the condition. **SEE PAGES 160–65**

RELAXATION & BREATHING 

Hyperventilation (rapid breathing) may be part of the condition. Diaphragmatic breathing improves circulation and works to counter the tight-chestedness of many people with CFS. Relaxation reduces muscle tension and helps promote healing. **SEE PAGES 170–73**

RELAXATION EXERCISES
Simple exercises can help, particularly when practiced on a daily basis.

MEDITATION 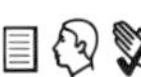

The combination of relaxing the body and focusing the mind is said to support the body's self-healing ability and to restore energy levels, self-confidence, creativity, and a sense of control over one's life. Ideally, you should meditate for twenty minutes twice a day. The discipline and rhythm of daily practice can also help restore a feeling of control. **SEE PAGES 174–77**

OTHER OPTIONS

Autogenic Training **SEE PAGE 168**
Biofeedback **SEE PAGE 169**

PAIN

SHORT-TERM, OR "ACUTE," PAIN ranges in intensity from nagging discomfort to excruciating agony. It is the body's signal that something specific is wrong. Pain may also last for months or even years. As many as 10% of the population experience this persistent, or "chronic," pain, which lasts for six months or longer. It may have a clear source – perhaps a nerve injury, shingles, or a bone tumor affecting the spine – or no apparent physical explanation. Such persistent pain may be influenced by a number of mental and physical factors, so holistic approaches are more likely to succeed than treatments directed at single causes.

KEY TO SYMBOLS

EVIDENCE		PRACTITIONER	
Good scientific trials with positive results		Essential	
Some research studies		Recommended	
Anecdotal		Not essential	
		SELF-HELP	
		Self-help possibilities	
		No self-help	

COMPLEMENTARY APPROACHES

About 75% of those who visit complementary practitioners do so because of painful conditions. Exercise, biofeedback, meditation, hypnotherapy, special diets, acupuncture, and relaxation are among the methods used to stimulate endorphin production (see right), raise pain tolerance, and help people manage their perception of pain.

CONVENTIONAL APPROACHES

For short-term pain, doctors may prescribe painkilling drugs ranging from aspirin to narcotics. Persistent joint pain may be treated with massage, vibration, physiotherapy, or heat and cold. Transcutaneous electrical nerve stimulation (TENS), in which minute impulses are applied to nerve endings, seems to block pain signals. Local anesthetics relieve pain for short periods. Nerves may be surgically severed, but this is irreversible and can mean a total loss of sensation.

Caution: Before seeking treatment, see page 204.

HOW PAIN IS TRANSMITTED

Sensory nerve endings, or receptors, are found throughout the body but are most highly concentrated in the skin. When stimulated by heavy pressure, extreme temperature, or prostaglandins – chemicals released by injured cells – they relay messages to the spinal cord and on to the brain, where they are interpreted as pain.

According to the "gate control" theory, the information carried on the limited number of pain pathways to the brain is regulated as it passes through "gates." Various factors close these gates or hold them open. Once established, a pain pathway can become facilitated, or more easily set off, long after the original problem is resolved. Endorphins, the body's natural painkillers, slot into receptors located in the brain, spinal cord, and nerve endings, blocking pain impulses. How wide the pain gates are open and how much information reaches pain receptors, depends on the level of endorphins in circulation. This level is affected by our psychological state: emotions can affect the perception of pain. This is why a soldier can keep going in the heat of battle, unaware of devastating injury. Likewise, pain may be perceived as being worse if the person experiencing it is depressed.

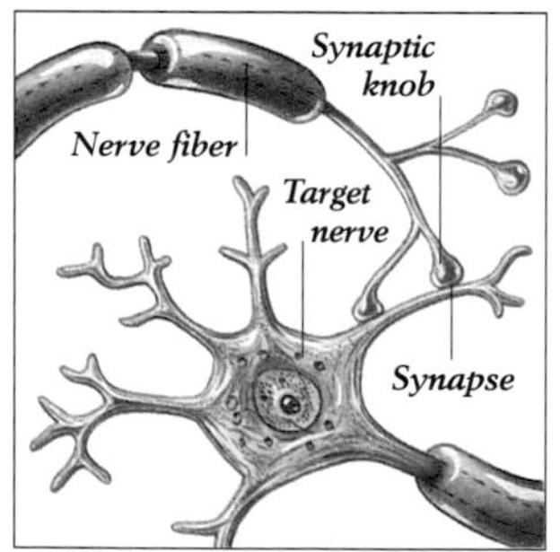

NERVE CELLS

Impulses run down the nerve fiber to the synaptic knob. At the synapse – the juncture between nerves – high endorphin levels may block transmission of a pain impulse.

Psychological states can also directly affect areas of the body that have become accustomed to sensing pain. In one experiment, just thinking about painful experiences caused the back muscles of people who complained of chronic back pain to become tense.

Simple painkillers, like aspirin, work by preventing the production of prostaglandins. Acetaminophen blocks pain impulses in the brain itself. Narcotics mimic endorphins, blocking pain impulses at specific sites.

PERSISTENT (CHRONIC) PAIN

ABOUT FIVE OUT OF SIX PEOPLE with persistent pain take painkillers, but an estimated 70% say they continue to feel severe pain. Whatever the cause, persistent pain is real and incapacitating and has enormous social and economic implications. It affects the ability to work or lead a normal life, and leaves millions permanently disabled. Increasingly, such pain is viewed not so much as a symptom but as a disorder in its own right.

Causes Cancer, neuralgia, arthritis, shingles, and muscle disorders, including myofascial pain and fibromyalgia, can all cause long-term pain. Some diseases and injuries set up a pattern of pain that lingers long after the original cause has gone. The stress and anxiety that result can cause the muscles to become tense. This may accentuate the perception of pain, creating a self-perpetuating downward spiral.

Conventional Treatment The causes of chronic pain may not be revealed by medical diagnostic tests, such as X rays, blood tests, and MRI scans (see glossary). Painkillers may be of little use in chronic pain. In addition to the techniques described in Conventional Approaches (above), many mainstream specialized pain clinics now offer a range of psychological and complementary treatments, including acupuncture and massage.

TOUCH & MOVEMENT THERAPIES

Practitioners believe that touch therapies and gentle exercise may reduce the perception of pain, stimulate the release of endorphins, and help people actively to manage their perception of pain.

MASSAGE 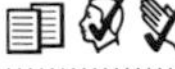

Studies have shown that massage can alleviate muscle pain, inflammatory bowel disease pain, and tissue-injury pain. The considerable psychological effects of massage may also be useful for persistent pain. SEE PAGES 56–61

AROMATHERAPY 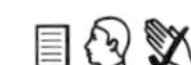

Essential oils are said to stimulate endorphin production and, when used with massage, to encourage relaxation. Eucalyptus essential oil is often suggested for muscular pain and headaches, juniper oil for arthritis, and marjoram and lavender oils for migraines and muscle cramps. According to a UK study reported in the *Journal of Advanced Nursing*, massage with lavender essential oil in a carrier oil helped relieve discomfort after childbirth, but synthetic lavender oil and an aromatic placebo were found to be equally effective. SEE PAGES 62–65

EUCALYPTUS OIL
This essential oil, diluted and rubbed onto the skin, has a warming and mildly pain-relieving effect.

CHIROPRACTIC 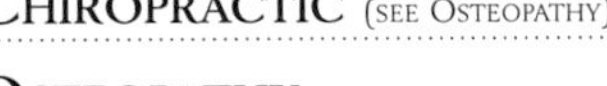 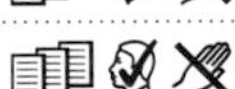

OSTEOPATHY

Manipulation of spinal joints and muscle tissues can ease neck and shoulder pain, backache, and sciatica. Numerous studies show that chiropractic and osteopathy are beneficial for short-term back pain (see pages 254–55) but are less demonstrably helpful for persistent back pain. SEE PAGES 70–81

ACUPUNCTURE 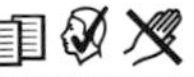

Acupuncture is said to work partly by stimulating the release of endorphins and prostaglandin-suppressing corticosteriod hormones (see glossary). The insertion of needles in appropriate acupoints may also help relieve anxiety and depression associated with persistent pain. The World Health Organization recommends acupuncture for pain caused by osteoarthritis (see page 258) and 103 other conditions. Several studies have shown acupuncture to be effective in relieving lower back and neck pain. Reports in the Journals of the Canadian Dental and Medical Associations have claimed that massage of acupoints on the hand and arm with ice reduced dental pain by half. Other studies of different kinds of pain show conflicting results, but on balance acupuncture seems to be very helpful. Practitioners note that the more persistent the pain, the more treatments may be required before the patient experiences relief. SEE PAGES 90–94

HEALING 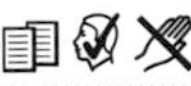

There is some clinical evidence that healing can reduce the severity of headaches. In one trial of healing for persistent pain, feelings of hopelessness decreased and patients gained a greater sense of control, although pain as such was not markedly relieved. SEE PAGES 104–105

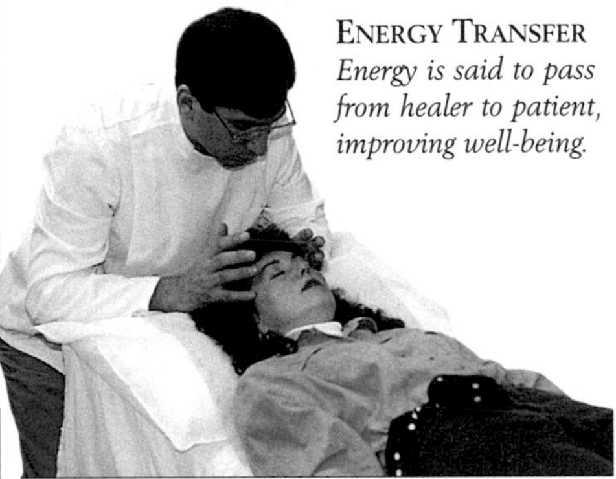

ENERGY TRANSFER
Energy is said to pass from healer to patient, improving well-being.

OTHER OPTIONS

Reflexology SEE PAGES 66–69
Rolfing SEE PAGES 82–83
The Feldenkrais Method SEE PAGE 85
The Alexander Technique SEE PAGES 86–87
Tragerwork SEE PAGE 88
Qigong SEE PAGE 99
Therapeutic Touch SEE PAGE 106

MEDICINAL THERAPIES

Practitioners believe that natural approaches – using diet and medicinal herbs, for instance – can increase vitality, helping to raise tolerance to pain.

HYDROTHERAPY 

Exercise in heated swimming pools is a powerful way to relieve joint and muscle pain. Ice packs can reduce the pain caused by inflammation, and cold compresses may dull the sensitivity of pain-sensing nerves. A study reported in the Dutch journal *Pain* in 1980 showed that massage with ice was as effective as TENS therapy in relieving lower back pain. SEE PAGES 122–23

WESTERN HERBALISM 

Qualified practitioners may use herbs such as yellow jasmine, Jamaica dogwood, and aconite to relieve pain, but they can be fatal in large doses as they depress essential body functions. California poppy and wild lettuce are safer alternatives. Applied to the skin in a cream, capsaicin, the active ingredient in chili peppers, has proved useful in clinical studies in alleviating some kinds of pain. SEE PAGES 134–39

Cautions: Take yellow jasmine or aconite only under professional supervision. Do not take Jamaica dogwood during pregnancy or if you have heart problems.

OTHER OPTIONS

Naturopathy SEE PAGES 118–21
Homeopathy SEE PAGES 126–30
Bach Flower Remedies SEE PAGES 132–33
Chinese Herbalism SEE PAGES 140–43

MIND & EMOTION THERAPIES

Psychological techniques that increase feelings of control and self-esteem may be valuable weapons in the fight against pain.

PSYCHOTHERAPY & COUNSELING 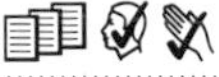

Our thoughts, beliefs, moods, and emotions have been described as a kind of "volume control," capable of turning pain up or down, and largely determining our pain tolerance. Cognitive behavioral therapy helps develop a positive attitude that encourages mastery and control. Also, because chronic pain can become so central to a person's life, counseling or psychotherapy may be advisable to identify and resolve this and other significant issues. SEE PAGES 160–65

BIOFEEDBACK 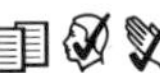

Research shows that biofeedback may help 40–60% of people with headaches or pain in the jaw from temperomandibular joint disorder (TMJ). In other studies, biofeedback has proved beneficial for persistent backache and muscle pain. SEE PAGE 169

RELAXATION & BREATHING 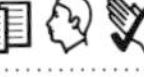

Pain feels worse when you are tense, and muscle relaxation is probably the most effective way to control it. Researchers have found this therapy to be effective in relieving tension headaches, migraines, and back pain. SEE PAGES 170–73

VISUALIZATION 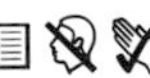

Imagery helps distract from pain, and seems to work best when used with other relaxation techniques. Approaches may include imagining yourself in peaceful, pain-free environments, or imagining that your pain has a color or shape and then visualizing another color or shape that will control it. SEE PAGES 178–79

OTHER OPTION

Hypnotherapy SEE PAGES 166–67

FIRST AID

COMPLEMENTARY REMEDIES PLAY an important role in relieving pain, calming the mind, and helping the body heal itself, and can often be used in the home to treat everyday ailments and minor accidents. It is important to remain calm so that you can assess the patient's condition and deal with it appropriately, calling expert help if necessary. A well-stocked first-aid kit is essential. The kit should be equipped with a good first-aid reference book, basic necessities such as bandages and a thermometer, conventional medication such as aspirin, emergency telephone numbers, and the complementary remedies described below.

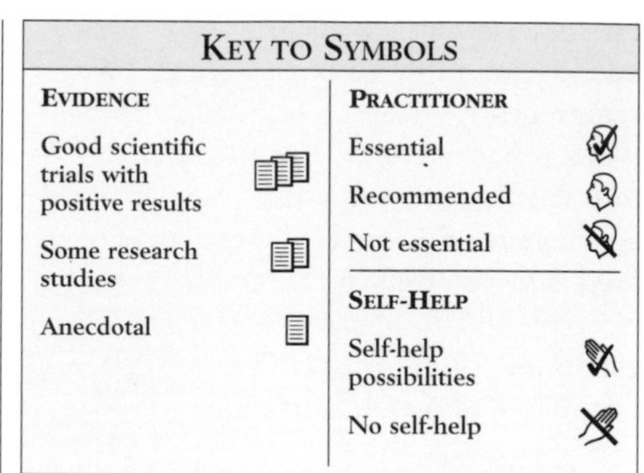

KEY TO SYMBOLS

EVIDENCE	PRACTITIONER
Good scientific trials with positive results	Essential
Some research studies	Recommended
Anecdotal	Not essential
	SELF-HELP
	Self-help possibilities
	No self-help

COMPLEMENTARY FIRST-AID KIT

Herbs: Aloe-vera gel, arnica cream, echinacea tincture or capsules, elderflower tea, garlic capsules, German chamomile tea, calendula cream, St. John's wort tincture, slippery elm powder, valerian tablets, witch hazel (see also page 139). **Essential oils**: Camphor, eucalyptus, geranium, lavender, peppermint, rosemary, tea tree (see also page 63). **Homeopathic**: (Store away from essential oils) *Arnica, Aconite, Apis, Arsen. alb., Belladonna, Bryonia, Chamomilla, Hypericum, Pulsatilla, Rhus tox., Silica, Urtica urens* cream (see also page 130). **Nutritional**: Vitamin C, vitamin E oil. **Bach Flower Remedy**: Rescue Remedy.

CONVENTIONAL FIRST-AID KIT

Antihistamine preparations, antiseptic cream, aspirin, bandages, calamine lotion, insect-sting reliever, bandages, surgical tape, thermometer, tweezers.

FIRST-AID KIT

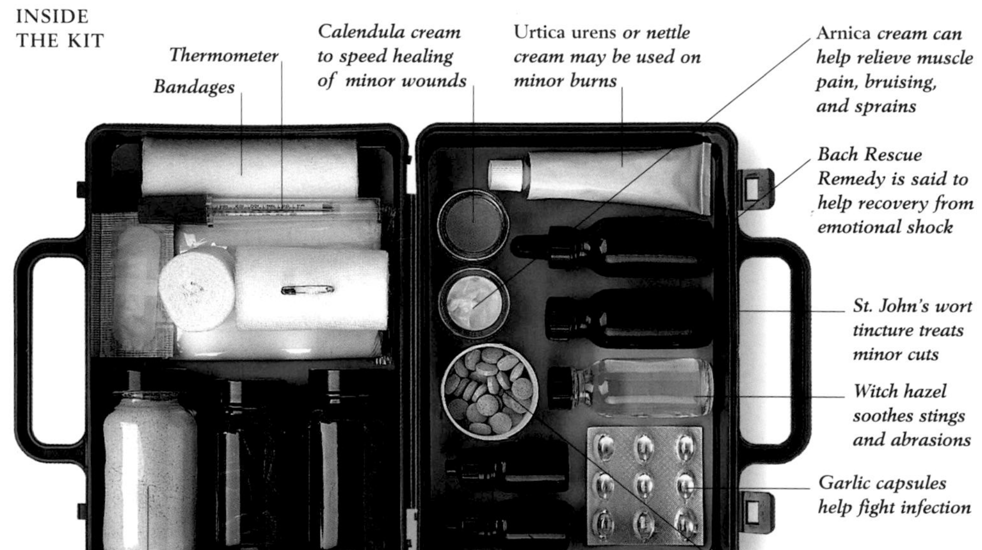

MINOR CUTS & BRUISES

First Aid Elevate the injured area (if possible) and apply firm pressure for up to ten minutes to stop any bleeding. Gently clean wounds with soap and water, wiping away from the cut. Apply an antiseptic cream and cover with a dry dressing or bandage. Apply ice packs to bruises for 15–20 minutes at a time.

Cautions: See a doctor if bleeding cannot be controlled, if the wound is deep or becomes infected, if debris cannot be removed, or if bruising persists. Check your tetanus immunization status: a booster injection is recommended every 5–10 years.

COMPLEMENTARY TREATMENTS

After general first aid has been given, complementary remedies can be used to calm the patient and help speed healing.

AROMATHERAPY

Essential oil of tea tree is a powerful antiseptic, antibacterial, antiviral, and antifungal agent that also relieves pain and aids healing. Add a few drops to water when cleaning the cut. Lavender and well-diluted geranium essential oils also have antiseptic and healing properties. SEE PAGES 62–65

HOMEOPATHY

Hypericum 6c may help if a scratch is sensitive. *Arnica 6c* (granules and cream) is used for bruises, and *Aconite 6c* for anxiety.
SEE PAGES 126–30

WESTERN HERBALISM

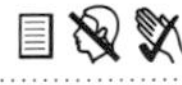

Antiseptic and astringent calendula tincture, diluted in warm water, promotes blood clotting when used as a wash. The herb may also be applied as a cream. St. John's wort, an astringent, sedative, and antimicrobial herb, may be used as a diluted tincture or ointment to help heal wounds. SEE PAGES 134–39

Bites & Stings

First Aid Consult a doctor about animal and human bites. To remove a bee sting, scrape it out with a thumbnail or blunt blade (tweezers may squeeze more poison into the flesh). Wash with soap and water, apply an ice pack, and try to keep the area raised to reduce swelling. Aspirin or acetaminophen will relieve pain. Calamine lotion or antihistamine cream can ease itching and irritation.

Caution: Allergic reactions may lead to collapse and even death. Seek medical help immediately if the lips, tongue, or throat swell, or if breathing is difficult.

COMPLEMENTARY TREATMENTS

Natural remedies of all kinds can be helpful in treating bites and stings.

Naturopathy

Bee stings and ant bites are acidic. Applying an alkali such as bicarbonate of soda helps neutralize them. Wasp and hornet stings are alkaline, and can be neutralized with an acid such as lemon juice. Applying vitamin E oil may help ease pain. For a jellyfish sting, rinse with seawater, alcohol, vinegar, or ammonia. Eating garlic and dabbing cider vinegar on the skin are said to repel insects. SEE PAGES 118–21

Western Herbalism

Practitioners recommend placing half a raw onion on a sting for about ten minutes to deactivate insect poison. Distilled witch hazel (especially for mosquito bites), crushed basil leaves, and fresh aloe-vera gel are also suggested. SEE PAGES 134–39

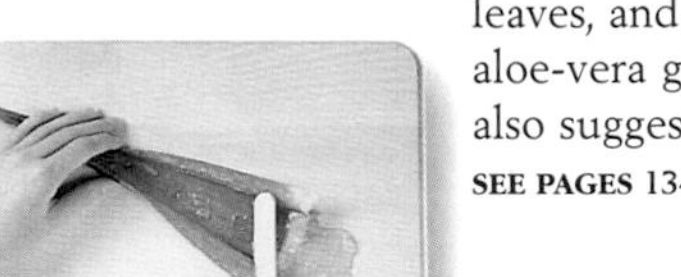

Aloe Vera
The gel may be collected by scraping a split fresh leaf.

Fainting

First Aid If you feel faint, sit with your head between your legs. Lay a person who has fainted on his back, loosen his collar and elevate his legs 1 ft (30 cm). Be sure the airways are clear: pull the jaw forward and up. (See also Dizziness, page 208.)

Caution: Call emergency help if the patient does not regain consciousness within two minutes.

COMPLEMENTARY TREATMENTS

Natural remedies can support first-aid care.

Aromatherapy

Recommended essential oils include rosemary, camphor, and peppermint. Put a few drops of an oil on a handkerchief and hold it under the nose for inhalation. SEE PAGES 62–65

Western Herbalism

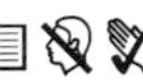

Practitioners recommend that the patient take sips of a tea made with ginger once he has regained consciousness. Teas of elderflower and rosemary made with honey and ginger are also traditional remedies. SEE PAGES 134–39

Caution: Do not give ginger if the patient has a peptic ulcer.

Shock

Physiological shock may follow an injury. Blood supply to the brain and gut is depleted, causing nausea, rapid pulse, pale clammy skin, and in some cases, loss of consciousness and even death. Emotional shock may follow bad news.

First Aid For physiological shock, call emergency help. If the patient is mobile, lay him down with legs raised 1 ft (30 cm), clear the mouth, and turn the head to one side. Keep him covered and warm.

Caution: Do not give food or drink to those in shock.

COMPLEMENTARY TREATMENTS

Complementary remedies may help after recovery but must not interfere with conventional treatment.

Rescue Remedy
One of the Bach Flower Remedies, this is said to calm and soothe after emotional shock.

Acupressure

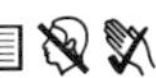

Constant pressure applied to the acupoint two-thirds of the way from the top lip to the nose on the Conception Vessel meridian is said to help revival. SEE PAGE 95

Bach Flower Remedies

For emotional shock only, four drops of Rescue Remedy should be placed on the tongue as often as required. SEE PAGES 132–33

Other Option

Homeopathy SEE PAGES 126–30

Burns

First-degree burns, such as sunburn, damage the surface of the skin, causing pain, redness, and swelling. Second-degree burns raise blisters. Third-degree burns destroy all the layers of the skin and expose the underlying tissues.

First Aid *Immediately* immerse first- and second-degree burns in cold water for at least ten minutes. Do not apply fats. Keep the area clean and cover with a sterile, nonfluffy dressing. Give plenty of fluids.

Cautions: For third-degree burns, call emergency help immediately. Do not put water on the burn or try to remove burned clothing adhering to the skin. Cover the burned area with a clean dry cloth. Call a doctor if a second-degree burn is larger than the patient's hand, if a burn is still painful after 24 hours, or if the patient is in shock or collapses.

COMPLEMENTARY TREATMENT

Natural remedies may speed healing after initial treatment and relieve pain.

Naturopathy

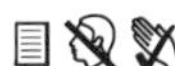

Practitioners recommend 1 g of vitamin C taken internally every hour for 2–3 hours after a bad burn. Vitamin E cream or aloe-vera gel may help speed healing. SEE PAGES 118–21

FINDING A PRACTITIONER

Establishing a sense of rapport and trust with your practitioner is an important element of therapy if any benefits are to be derived from nonconventional treatment. Another key factor is, of course, the competence of the practitioner.

Finding a good practitioner may be simply a matter of trial and error, and there are many people who prefer to rely on word-of-mouth recommendations. This approach is not necessarily infallible, however.

Training for complementary practitioners can range from as little as a correspondence course lasting only one weekend to three or four years of full- or part-time degree study. The issue of how to establish adequate standards of training, ethical practice, and disciplinary procedures has been a problem for complementary medicine for years, and is an issue that has still not been resolved for many forms of therapy. This means that you may have little means of redress if anything goes wrong during your treatment or if you are dissatisfied with the treatment you receive. At the very least, you must be able to feel confident that, should you have any serious condition that has so far remained undiagnosed, it would be recognized and you would be advised to seek professional medical help if the complementary practitioner suspected the problem lay beyond his or her expertise.

If you are planning to self-refer to any form of complementary medicine, you should first consider the following important issues.

TRAINING & CREDENTIALS

Make sure that the complementary practitioner you are considering is adequately trained and reputable, especially if the therapy is one of those that the British Medical Association calls a "discrete, clinical discipline," such as chiropractic, osteopathy, homeopathy, acupuncture, naturopathy, or any type of herbal medicine. Since therapies such as these involve the use of either physical manipulation or invasive techniques (i.e., you swallow medication or have needles inserted into you), they can be potentially harmful.

Before embarking on any course of complementary treatment you should ask your practitioner the questions outlined below:

- What are the practitioner's qualifications? What sort of training was undertaken, and for how long?
- For how many years has the practitioner been in practice?
- Does the practitioner advise your doctor of any treatment given?

PROFESSIONAL ORGANIZATIONS

Some disciplines have professional associations to regulate training, provide a code of conduct and keep a register of members. For others, particularly noninvasive therapies, standards vary greatly.

It may be helpful to ask the following questions:

- Is the practitioner registered with a recognized professional organization, and does this organization have a public directory?
- Does the organization have a code of practice, specifying the professional conduct required?
- Does the organization have a complaints system, and an effective disciplinary procedure and sanctions?
- Can the practitioner give you the address of the organization?

FINANCIAL CONSIDERATIONS

- Is treatment available on referral by your doctor? Some therapies, such as chiropractic, osteopathy, and acupuncture, are becoming accepted into mainstream medicine.
- Can you claim for the treatment through your health insurance, if you have it?
- What is the cost – both short- and long-term – of treatment?
- How many treatments might you expect to require?
- Is the practitioner covered by professional insurance so that you receive compensation if the practitioner is negligent?

RELATIONSHIP WITH THE PRACTITIONER

Avoid any practitioner who makes you feel uncomfortable. Trust and empathy are important, and treatment is unlikely to succeed without it. Treatment is often conducted on a one-to-one basis, and may involve removing clothes and being touched. Avoid also any practitioner who seems to be making excessive claims about the treatment or who guarantees a cure. No form of treatment – conventional or complementary – is perfect, and miracles should neither be expected nor promised.

After your initial consultation, ask the following:

- Was the practitioner's conduct entirely professional?
- Did the practitioner answer any questions clearly and thoroughly?
- Were you given information to look through at your leisure?
- What is the practitioner's attitude toward any conventional medicine you may be receiving? Avoid those who suggest changing your conventional medicine without first consulting your doctor.

USEFUL ADDRESSES

There are professional associations for many of the therapies described in this encyclopedia. Readers seeking a local practitioner may contact any of the organizations listed here. Although many groups provide referrals at no cost, a few charge a fee for directories.

GENERAL ORGANIZATIONS

American Holistic Health Association
PO Box 17400
Anaheim, CA
92817–7400
Tel: (714) 779–6152
A nonprofit educational organization established to promote a holistic approach to health and well-being. The association serves as a national clearing house for information about conventional and complementary health resources, and provides a variety of free educational materials.

Office of Alternative Medicine
National Institutes of Health
PO Box 8218
Silver Spring, MD
20907–8218
Tel: (888) 644–6226
or (301) 496–4000

American Academy of Pain Management
13947 Mono Way #A
Sonora, CA
95370
Tel: (209) 533–9741
Certifies multidisciplinary practitioners in pain management. Provides information and referrals to over 6,000 practitioners who have a degree or at least two years' experience. Maintains a code of ethics and patient bill of rights.

The Upledger Institute
Suite D325
11211 Prosperity Farms Road
Palm Beach Gardens, FL
33410
Tel: (800) 233–5880
In addition to being the professional association for CranioSacral therapy, the institute also runs seminars on complementary health.

Wholistic Referral Network
1025 Central Expressway
Ste 300LB347
Plano, TX
75075
Tel: (800) 520–WELL
Provides free referrals to a wide variety of complementary health care practitioners who use a holistic approach to treat patients.

SPECIFIC ORGANIZATIONS

ACUPRESSURE
See Acupuncture

ACUPUNCTURE
American Academy of Medical Acupuncture
Suite 500
5820 Wilshire Boulevard
Los Angeles, CA
90036
Tel: (213) 937–5514
Represents medically qualified acupuncturists only, and sets standards of training, with a proficiency exam and certification.
American Association of Acupuncture and Oriental Medicine
433 Front Street
Catasaugua, PA
18032
Tel: (610) 226–1433
The largest membership organization for practitioners, it promotes public education about acupuncture and oriental medicine techniques and provides information on the therapies.
American Foundation of Traditional Chinese Medicine
505 Beach Street
San Francisco, CA
94133
Tel: (415) 776–0502
The National Commission for Certification of Acupuncturists
Suite 501
1424 16th Street NW
Washington, DC
20036
Tel: (202) 232–1404
Promotes nationally recognized standards for safe and competent acupuncture practice. Certified practitioners are designated DiplAc (NCCA).

THE ALEXANDER TECHNIQUE
North American Society of Teachers of the Alexander Technique
Suite 10
3010 Hennepin Avenue South
Minneapolis, MN
55408
Tel: (612) 824–5066
or (800) 473–0620
Ensures standards of training and publishes a directory of certified teachers.

ANTHROPOSOPHICAL MEDICINE
All anthroposophical practitioners are medically qualified doctors.
Physicians' Association for Anthroposophical Medicine
7953 California Avenue
Fair Oaks, CA
95628
Tel: (916) 966 1417

APPLIED KINESIOLOGY
Training for Applied Kinesiology is only open to those with a certain level of medical training, such as osteopaths, chiropractors, dentists and medical doctors. Worldwide postgraduate training is provided by the International College of Applied Kinesiology. Practitioners should have a certificate of "clinical competence."
International College of Applied Kinesiology
Suite 503
6405 Metcalf Avenue
Shawnee Mission, KS
66202–3929
Tel: (913) 384–5336

AROMATHERAPY
American Massage Therapy Association
Suite 100
820 Davis Street
Evanston, IL
60201–4444
Tel: (847) 864–0123
Pacific Institute of Aromatherapy
Tammy Gilman
415 Orchard
Santa Fe, NM
87501
Tel: (505) 471–5920

ART THERAPY
American Art Therapy Association
1202 Allanson Road
Mundelein, IL
60060
Tel: (847) 949–6064

ASTON-PATTERNING
The Aston Training Center
PO Box 3568
Incline Village, NV
89450
Tel: (702) 831–8228

AUDITORY INTEGRATION TRAINING
See Sound Therapy

AURA-SOMA THERAPY
c/o Trish & Will Hunter
PO Box 1688
Canyon Lake, TX
78130
Tel: (210) 935–2355

AURICULAR ACUPUNCTURE
See Acupuncture

AUTOGENIC TRAINING
There is no umbrella organization in the US for Autogenic Training, or Autogenic Therapy, as it is sometimes known. Information on any local American practitioners can, however, be obtained from:
British Association for Autogenic Training and Therapy
c/o The Royal London Homeopathic Hospital
NHS Trust
Great Ormond Street
London
WC1N 3HR
UK

AUTOSUGGESTION
See Hypnotherapy

AYURVEDA
Fully qualified Ayurvedic physicians complete a five-year degree course at Indian or Sri Lankan universities and qualify as BAMS (Batchelor of Ayurvedic Medicine and Surgery) or DAMS (Doctor of Ayurvedic Medicine and Surgery).
Ayurvedic Institute
Suite A
11311 Menaul NE
Albuquerque, NM
87112
Tel: (505) 291–9698
California College of Ayurveda
Center for Optimal Health
1117A East Main Street
Grass Valley, CA
95945
Tel: (916) 274–9100
Chopra Center for Well-Being
7630 Fay Avenue
LaJolla, CA
92037
Tel: (888) 4–CHOPRA (246772)
Educational Service of Maharishi Ayurved International
PO Box 49667
Colorado Springs, CO
80949
Tel: (800) 843–8332
Offers free referrals to 75 doctors (MD, DO, DC) nationwide who have completed a course of training and who choose to be included on the referral list.

Maharishi Ayur-Veda Health Center
1734 Jasmine Avenue
Fairfield, IA
52556
Tel: (800) 248–9050

BACH FLOWER REMEDIES
Nelson Bach USA, Ltd.
Wilmington Technology Park
100 Research Drive
Wilmington, MA
01887–4406
Tel: (800) 319–9151
The Dr. Edward Bach Centre
Mount Vernon
Sotwell
Wallingford
Oxfordshire
OX10 0PZ
UK
Maintains an international directory of practitioners, and offers advice and training.

THE BATES METHOD
The Bates Method Teachers Association
Vision Training Institute
1351 Gibson High Lands
El Cajon, CA
92021
Tel: (619) 440–5244

BIOCHEMIC TISSUE SALTS
Tissue salts and professional advice on their use can be obtained from a homeopathic pharmacy.

BIODYNAMIC MASSAGE
See Massage

BIOENERGETICS
Most practitioners are already qualified in some form of psychotherapy before training as bioenergetic therapists. The International Institute of Bioenergetic Analysis is based in New York City and there over 30 associated institutes worldwide. Some practitioners have left to form separate organizations, such as the Association of Analytical Body Psychotherapy.
The International Institute for Bioenergetic Analysis
Suite 1A
144 East 36th Street
New York, NY
10016
Tel: (212) 532–7742

BIOFEEDBACK
Finding a supervisor and equipment can be difficult, since many machines and trained operators are based in hospitals and universities. Also, people can find it difficult to reproduce at home the sensations learned in the laboratory. It may help to learn relaxation, meditation, and visualization techniques before starting biofeedback sessions.
Biofeedback Certification Institute of America
Suite 304
10200 West 44th Avenue
Wheatridge, CO
80033–2840
Tel: (303) 420–2902
Provides a national directory of certified practitioners.

BIORHYTHMS
N. Laytos CHT
PO Box 150682
San Rafael, CA
94915
Tel: (415) 458–1901
The London Biorhythm Co. Ltd.
PO Box 8390
South Kensington
London
SW7 2PT
UK

THE BOWEN TECHNIQUE
Pacific Institute of Aromatherapy
Tammy Gilman
415 Orchard
Santa Fe, NM
87501
Tel: (505) 471–5920

CHANTING
See Sound Therapy

CHAVUTTI THIRUMAL
See Ayurveda

CHELATION THERAPY
American Board of Chelation Therapy
1407 North Wells Street
Chicago, IL
60610
Tel: (800) 356–2228
American College of Advancement in Medicine
PO Box 3427
Laguna Hills, CA
92654
Tel: (714) 583–7666

CHINESE HERBALISM
American Association of Acupuncture and Oriental Medicine
433 Front Street
Catasaugua, PA
18032
Tel: (610) 226–1433
The largest membership organization for practitioners, it promotes public education about acupuncture and oriental medicine techniques and provides information on the therapies.

CHIROPRACTIC
American Chiropractic Association
1701 Clarendon Boulevard
Arlington, VA
22209
Tel: (703) 276–8800
Offers free referrals to 21,500 members. All are licensed doctors of chiropractic with over five years' postgraduate training.
Federation of Straight Chiropractors and Organizations
642 Broad Street #9
Clifton, NJ
07013
Tel: (800) 521–9856
Offers free referrals to 5,000 members. All are licensed doctors of chiropractic with over five years' postgraduate training.
International Chiropractors Association
Suite 1000
1110 North Glebe Road
Arlington, VA
22201
Tel: (800) 423–4690
Offers free referrals to over 12,000 members. All are licensed doctors of chiropractic with over five years' postgraduate training.
World Chiropractic Alliance
2950 North Dobson Road #1
Chandler, AZ
85224
Tel: (800) 347–1011
Offers free referrals to over 3,000 members. All are licensed doctors of chiropractic with over five years' postgraduate training.

CLINICAL ECOLOGY
American Academy of Environmental Medicine
Box CN 1001–8001
New Hope, PA
18938
Tel: (215) 862–4544

COLONIC HYDROTHERAPY
International Association for Colon Hydrotherapy
PO Box 461285
San Antonio, TX
78285
Tel: (210) 366–2888
American Association of Naturopathic Physicians
Suite 105
601 Valley
Seattle, WA
98109
Tel: (206) 298–0125
Maintains support and standards of practice. It also encourages research and legislative regulation of practice.

COLOR THERAPY
Bonnie Whittington
2430 Cherry Grove Street
Eugene, OR
97403
Tel: (503) 683–2127
Laura Langford-Schur
RD2 75B Sugar Loaf
Mountain Road
Chester, NY
10918

CRANIAL OSTEOPATHY
See Osteopathy

CRANIOSACRAL THERAPY
The Upledger Institute
Suite D325
11211 Prosperity Farms Road
Palm Beach Gardens, FL
33410
Tel: (561) 622–4334

CRYSTAL THERAPY
Crystal Medicine
210½ East Lake Street
Mount Shasta, CA
96067
Tel: (916) 926–1264

CYMATICS
See Sound Therapy

DANCE MOVEMENT THERAPY
American Dance Therapy Association
Suite 108
2000 Century Plaza
Columbia, MD
21044
Tel: (410) 997–4040

DO-IN
See Shiatsu

ELECTRO-ACUPUNCTURE
See Acupuncture

EUTONY
Practitioners do a four-year full-time course at a school recognized by the International Federation of Eutony.
Eutony Gerda Alexander
Monique Nagy
1203 Trevanion Street
Pittsburgh, PA
15218
Tel: (412) 371–1876
Eutony Gerda Alexander School of Quebec
c/o Ursula Stuber
1124 Coin Joli
Cap Rouge
Quebec
G1Y 2G7
Canada
Tel: (418) 651–6667

THE FELDENKRAIS METHOD
There is a part-time training course for practitioners lasting three or four years in accordance with an international training accreditation board.
The Feldenkrais Guild
PO Box 489
Albany, OR
97321–0143
Tel: (541) 926–0981
or (800) 775–2118

FENG SHUI
American Feng Shui Institute
Suite 202
108 North Ynez Avenue
Monterey Park, CA
91754
Tel: (818) 571–2757
Feng Shui Guild
PO Box 850
Boulder, CO
80306
Tel (303) 444–1548
Feng Shui Warehouse
PO Box 6689
San Diego, CA
92166
Tel: (619) 523–2158
or (800) 399–1599

FLOTATION
See General Organizations, Relaxation & Breathing, and Visualization.

GEOMANCY
See Feng Shui. Although no umbrella group exists, many practitioners have studied feng shui.

HAKOMI
Hakomi Integrated Somatic
PO Box 19438
Boulder, CO
80308
Tel: (303) 447–3290

HEALING
The Barbara Brennan School of Healing
PO Box 2005
East Hampton, NY
11937
Tel: (516) 329–0951
Ecumenical Society of Psychorientology (Holistic Faith Healing)
1407 Calle del Norte
Laredo, TX
78041
Tel: (210) 722–6391

Nurse Healers Professional Associates
1211 Locust Street
Philadelphia, PA
19107
Tel: (215) 545–8079
Offers free referrals to 1,200 members who practice Therapeutic Touch and/or other types of energy healing. Most are health care professionals.

HELLERWORK
Practitioners must train with an accredited teacher. Information on finding therapists can be obtained from:
Hellerwork International
406 Berry Street
Mount Shasta, CA
96067
Tel: (916) 926–2500
or (800) 392–3900

HOMEOPATHY
The American Institute of Homeopathy
1585 Glencoe
Denver, CO
80220
Tel: (303) 898–5477
Provides a list of all the MDs, DOs, and DDSs who have passed a written and practical competency exam.
Homeopathic Educational Services
2124 Kittredge Street
Berkeley, CA
94704
Tel: (510) 649–0294
International Foundation for Homeopathy
PO Box 7
Edmonds, WA
98020
Tel: (206) 776–4147
Offers free referrals to 124 members who practice classical homeopathy. Each has completed an IFH professional course with 120–240 hours of training, and passed an exam.
The National Center for Homeopathy
Suite 306
801 North Fairfax Street
Alexandria, VA
22314
Tel: (703) 548–7790
The largest register of members, listing over 400 members by state.

HYDROTHERAPY
American Association of Naturopathic Physicians
Suite 105
601 Valley
Seattle, WA
98109
Tel: (206) 298–0125
Maintains support and standards of practice. It also encourages research and legislative regulation of practice.

HYPNOTHERAPY
American Board of Hypnotherapy
16842 Von Karmen Avenue #475
Irvine, CA
92714
Tel: (800) 872–9996
American Council of Hypnotist Examiners
700 South Central Avenue
Glendale, CA
91204
Tel: (818) 242–5378
American Society of Clinical Hypnosis
Suite 291
2200 East Devon Avenue
Des Plaines, IL
60018
Tel: (847) 297–3317
Maintains a referral list of professionally trained and licensed practitioners.
International Medical and Dental Hypnotherapy Association
Suite 800
4110 Edgeland
Royal Oak, MI
48073
Tel: (800) 257–5467

INDIAN HEAD MASSAGE
See Ayurveda

IRIDOLOGY
Iridologists International
24360 Old Wagon Road
Escondido, CA
92027
Tel: (760) 749–2727

KAHUNA
Aloha International
PO Box 665
Kilauea, HI
96754
Tel/Fax: (808) 828–0302

KIRLIAN PHOTOGRAPHY
c/o Linda Wiggin
PO Box 1114
Provincetown, MA
02657
Tel: (508) 487–9873
Can provide further information and contacts to anyone interested in Kirlian photography.

LIGHT THERAPY
College of Syntonic Optometry
Dr. Betsy Hancock, Librarian
21 East 5th Street
Bloomsbury, PA
17815
Tel: (717) 784–2131

MAGNETIC THERAPY
Bio-Electro-Magnetics Institute
2490 West Moana Lane
Reno, NV
89509–3936
Tel: (702) 827–9099

MASSAGE
American Massage Therapy Association
Suite 100
820 Davis Street
Evanston, IL
60201–4444
Tel: (847) 864–0123
Provides information on massage and biodynamic massage.

MEDITATION
Insight Meditation Society
1030 Pleasant Street
Barre, MA
01005
Tel: (508) 355–4378
Provides workshops and retreats in mindfulness meditation throughout the country.
Maharishi Ayur-Ved Products International, Inc.
PO Box 49667
Colorado Springs, CO
80949–9667
Tel: (800) 255–8332
Offers referrals to local training centers nationwide for Transcendental Meditation.
Stress Reduction Clinic
University of Massachusetts Medical Center
55 Lake Avenue North
Worcester, MA
01655
Tel: (508) 856–1616
Conducts an eight-week program and a five-day residential program in mindfulness training and stress reduction.

THE METAMORPHIC TECHNIQUE
Practitioners need no qualification other than attending courses by the association. Information on local US practitioners can be obtained from the organization listed below, which keeps an international register of members:
UK Metamorphic Association
67 Ritherdon Road
Tooting
London
SW17 8QE
UK

MUSIC THERAPY
The National Association for Music Therapy
Suite 1000
8455 Colesville Road
Silver Spring, MD
20910
Tel: (301) 589–3300

NATUROPATHY
American Association of Naturopathic Physicians
Suite 105
601 Valley
Seattle, WA
98109
Tel: (206) 298–0125
Maintains support and standards of practice. It also encourages research and legislative regulation of practice.

NETWORK CHIROPRACTIC
Association for Network Chiropractic
444 North Main Street
Longmont, CO
80501
Tel: (303) 678–8101

NUTRITIONAL THERAPIES
American College of Advancement in Medicine
PO Box 3427
Laguna Hills, CA
92654
Tel: (714) 583–7666
The International and American Associations of Clinical Nutritionists
Suite 410
5200 Keller Springs Road
Gallup, TX
75248
Tel: (972) 250–2829

ORTHOMOLECULAR THERAPY
The International and American Associations of Clinical Nutritionists
Suite 410
5200 Keller Springs Road
Gallup, TX
75248
Tel: (972) 250–2829

OSTEOPATHY
American Academy of Osteopathy
Suite 1080
3500 DePauw Boulevard
Indianapolis, IN
46268
Tel: (317) 879–1881
American Osteopathic Association
142 East Ontario Street
Chicago, IL
60611
Tel: (312) 280–5800
The Cranial Academy
8606 Allisonville Road
Indianapolis, IN
46350
Tel: (317) 594–0411

OXYGEN/OZONE THERAPY
Europa Institute of Integrated Medicine
Suite 201
406 Avenue Paseo de Tijuana
International Border Zone
Tijuana, BC
Mexico
Tel: (909) 336–1918 (US office)

PAST LIFE THERAPY
Association for Past Life Research and Therapy
PO Box 20151
Riverside, CA
92516
Tel: (909) 784–1570

POLARITY THERAPY
It takes 18 months of part-time training to obtain the Diploma in Polarity Therapy. Practitioners are registered on the Federation of Polarity Trainings Register.

American Polarity Therapy Association
Suite 149
2888 Bluff Street
Boulder, CO
80301
Tel: (303) 545–2080
or (800) 359–5620

PSIONICS
See Radionics

PSYCHOTHERAPY & COUNSELING
American Psychological Association
750 First Street NE
Washington, DC
20002
Tel: (800) 964–2000

QIGONG
American Association of Acupuncture and Oriental Medicine
433 Front Street
Catasaugua, PA
18032
Tel: (610) 226–1433
The largest membership organization for practitioners, it promotes public education about acupuncture and oriental medicine techniques and provides information on the therapies.
American Foundation of Traditional Chinese Medicine
505 Beach Street
San Fransisco, CA
94133
Tel: (415) 776–0502
The Chi Kung School at the Body-Energy Center
PO Box 19708
Boulder, CO
80308
Tel: (303) 442–3131
East-West Academy of Healing Arts Qigong Institute
Suite 2104
450 Sutter Street
San Francisco, CA
94108
Tel: (415) 788–2227
The Healing Tao Center
PO Box 1194
Huntington, NY
11743
Tel: (516) 368–6828

RADIONICS
United States Psychotronics Organization
PO Box 22697
Louisville, KY
40252
Tel: (502) 429–6600

REFLEXOLOGY
American Academy of Reflexology
Suite B
606 East Magnolia Boulevard
Burbank, CA
91501
Tel: (818) 841–7741
International Institute of Reflexology
PO Box 12462
St. Petersburg, FL
33733
Tel: (813) 343–4811

REIKI
American Association of Acupuncture and Oriental Medicine
433 Front Street
Catasaugua, PA
18032
Tel: (610) 226–1433
The largest membership organization for practitioners, it promotes public education about acupuncture and oriental medicine techniques and provides information on the therapies.
The Center for Reiki Training
29209 Northwestern Highway #592
Southfield, MI
48034
Tel: (800) 332–8112
or (810) 948–9534

RELAXATION & BREATHING
Many complementary therapists, particularly yoga teachers and therapists, and hypnotherapists, teach relaxation and breathing techniques. A number of audiotapes are also available.
Mind/Body Medical Institute
Division of Behavioral Medicine
New England Deaconess Hospital
Boston, MA
02215
Tel: (617) 632–9525
Provides group programs for different illnesses, and has affiliated programs nationwide.
Stress Reduction Clinic
University of Massachusetts
Medical Center
55 Lake Avenue North
Worcester, MA
01655
Tel: (508) 856–1616
Conducts an eight-week program and a five-day residential program in mindfulness training and stress reduction.

ROLFING
Practitioners train over three two-month blocks of full-time study that includes anatomy, physiology, manipulation, and counseling skills. Students must have undergone personal psychotherapy and must be already qualified in other bodywork therapies, such as massage. Qualified practitioners are known as Certified Rolfers.
The Rolf Institute of Structural Integration
205 Canyon Boulevard
Boulder, CO
80302
Tel: (800) 530–8875

SHAMANISM
Foundation for Shamanic Studies
PO Box 1939
Mill Valley, CA
94942
Tel: (415) 380–8282
Offers a list of practitioners and further information.

SHEN THERAPY
Certified SHEN practitioners complete a series of modules under guidance of a teacher or "mentor."
International SHEN Therapy Association
Suite 202
3213 West Wheeler
Seattle, WA
98199
Tel: (206) 298–9468

SHIATSU
American Association of Acupuncture and Oriental Medicine
433 Front Street
Catasaugua, PA
18032
Tel: (610) 226–1433
The largest membership organization for practitioners, it promotes public education about acupuncture and oriental medicine techniques and provides information on the therapies.

Ohashi Institute, Inc.
12 West 27th Street
New York, NY
10001
Tel: (212) 684–4190
or (800) 810–4190

SILVA METHOD
The Silva Method
Silva International Inc.
1407 Calle Del Norte
Laredo, TX
78041
Tel: (956) 722–6391

SOUND THERAPY
The Institute for Music, Health, and Education
PO Box 4179
Boulder, CO
80306
Tel: (303) 443–8484
Provides information on chanting.
Sound, Listening, and Learning Center
Suite 205
2701 East Camelback
Phoenix, AZ
85016
Tel: (602) 381–0086
Provides information on Auditory Integration Training and on the Tomatis method.
Dr. Peter Manners
Bretforton Hall
Bretforton
Vale of Evesham
Worcestershire
WR1 5JA
UK
Provides information on cymatics therapy.

T'AI CHI CH'UAN
American Association of Acupuncture and Oriental Medicine
433 Front Street
Catasaugua, PA
18032
Tel: (610) 226–1433
The largest membership organization for practitioners, it promotes public education about acupuncture and oriental medicine techniques and provides information on the therapies.
American Foundation of Traditional Chinese Medicine
505 Beach Street
San Fransisco, CA
94133
Tel: (415) 776–0502
See also Qigong.

THAI MASSAGE
American Association of Acupuncture and Oriental Medicine
433 Front Street
Catasaugua, PA
18032
Tel: (610) 226–1433
The largest membership organization for practitioners, it promotes public education about acupuncture and oriental medicine techniques and provides information on the therapies.

THERAPEUTIC TOUCH
Nurse Healers Professional Associates
1211 Locust Street
Philadelphia, PA
19107
Tel: (215) 545–8079
Offers free referrals to 1,200 members who practice Therapeutic Touch and/or other types of energy healing. Most are health care professionals.

THE TOMATIS METHOD
See Sound Therapy

TOUCH FOR HEALTH
Touch for Health Kinesiology Association
Suite 201
3223 Washington Boulevard
Marina del Rey, CA
90292
Tel: (800) 466–8342
Provides information on Touch for Health, including self-help material.

TRAGERWORK
The average time to complete training and supervised practice is two years. All practitioners are re-assessed annually to ensure that their methods remain true to Dr. Trager's teaching. There are currently about 500 practitioners in the US and more than 300 elsewhere. Training is available in the US, Canada, Mexico, Europe and Australia.
The Trager Institute
21 Locust Avenue
Mill Valley, CA
94941
Tel: (415) 388–2688

VISUALIZATION
The Academy for Guided Imagery
PO Box 2070
Mill Valley, CA
94942
Tel: (800) 726–2070
See also Psychotherapy & Counseling

VOICE THERAPY
See Psychotherapy & Counseling

WESTERN HERBALISM
American Association of Naturopathic Physicians
Suite 105
601 Valley
Seattle, WA
98109
Tel: (206) 298–0125
Maintains support and standards of practice. It also encourages research and legislative regulation of practice.
American Holistic Medical Association
Suite 201
4101 Lake Boone Trail
Raleigh, NC
27607
Tel: (919) 787–5146

YOGA
American Yoga Assocation
513 South Orange Avenue
Sarasota, FL
34236
Tel: (941) 953–5859
Integral Yoga Institute
227 West 13th Street
New York, NY
10011
Tel: (212) 929–0586
International Association of Yoga Therapists
Suite A243
20 Sunnyside Avenue
Mill Valley, CA
94941-1928
Tel: (415) 332–2478
Iyengar Yoga Institute
223a Randolph Avenue
London
W9 1NL
UK
There are no formal training requirements.

ZERO BALANCING
The Zero Balancing Association
Box 1727
Capitola, CA
95010
Tel: (408) 476–0665

GLOSSARY

Words that appear in UPPER CASE type are defined elsewhere in the glossary. Page references direct you to further explanations of terms.

ACTH (adrenocorticotrophic hormone) One of the body's hormones released in response to stress. It controls levels of CORTICOSTEROIDS in the blood and is often used to treat rheumatic conditions.
Acupoint Point along a MERIDIAN at which the flow of *QI* is thought to be accessible. These points are stimulated by acupressure or by the insertion of acupuncture needles.
Acute Describes a disorder or symptom that comes on suddenly. See also CHRONIC.
Adrenal glands Two glands on the kidneys that produce EPINEPHRINE and other hormones affecting the METABOLISM.
Aerobic Designed to increase oxygen intake (when used in the context of vigorous exercise).
Allopathy Conventional system of medicine in which drugs are used to produce effects in the body that directly oppose the symptoms of illness.
Amenorrhea Absence or stopping of menstrual periods.
Amino acid Biological building block necessary to form proteins. Essential amino acids are those that the body cannot manufacture for itself and must obtain through food.
Amphetamine Highly addictive drug, used to stimulate the nervous system.
Anaerobic Not designed to increase oxygen intake (when used in the context of exercise such as stretching and weightlifting).
Anatomy Science of the structure of the body; with PHYSIOLOGY, this forms the basis of conventional medicine.
Antacid Drug that neutralizes the secretion of hydrochloric acid in the stomach.
Antibacterial Describes an ANTIBIOTIC that is active against bacteria.
Antibiotic Destroys or inhibits microorganisms.
Antibody Protein in the blood responsible for destroying invading ANTIGENS.
Anticoagulant Prevents blood clotting.
Antigen Substance that the body regards as foreign and possibly dangerous, triggering an IMMUNE RESPONSE and the production of an ANTIBODY.
Antihypertensive Reduces high blood pressure.
Antioxidant Substance capable of neutralizing FREE RADICALS (see page 37).
Asana Physical posture adopted in yoga.
Atopic Describes a disposition to various allergic reactions.
Aura Invisible energy field, believed to surround all living things.
Autoimmune disease Disorder caused by a defect in the IMMUNE SYSTEM, which fails to distinguish between substances that are "self" and those that are "nonself," and produces ANTIBODIES to destroy the body's own tissues.
Autonomic nervous system Part of the nervous system responsible for body functions that do not require conscious thought, including heart rate and breathing (see page 71).
Bacteria Group of microorganisms, all of which consist of one cell. Only a few of the many different species cause disease.
Beta-blocker Drug that helps regulate heart rhythm.
Bioflavonoid Compound that regulates the permeability of capillary walls; citrus fruits are a good source.
Biopsy Removal of a small piece of living tissue for examination in a laboratory.
Bodywork Term used to describe manipulative therapies or techniques, such as massage.
Cardiovascular Relating to the heart and all blood vessels.
Cartilage Dense and protective connective body tissue.
CAT scan (computed axial tomography) See CT SCAN (COMPUTED TOMOGRAPHY).
Central nervous system Brain and spinal cord; it receives and analyzes sensory data, then initiates a response.
Cerebrospinal fluid Clear, watery fluid that circulates around brain areas and the central canal in the spinal cord.
Chakras Energy centers on the body, according to Ayurvedic medicine, which absorb and distribute *PRANA* (see page 109).
Cholesterol Fatlike material present in blood and most tissues. High levels of cholesterol in the blood can damage the artery walls.
Chronic Describes a condition of long duration and slow changes. See also ACUTE.
Collagen Protein that helps form the body's connective tissue.
Colon Major section of the large intestine, ending at the rectum.
Corticosteroid Substance produced by the ADRENAL GLANDS that helps regulate the salt-water balance in the body.
Cortisol Hormone produced by the ADRENAL GLANDS, important for the body's defenses against inflammatory or allergic conditions.
Cranial manipulation Osteopathic technique involving the gentle manipulation of the skull bones, particularly in children (see page 81).
Cranial sutures Joints in the bones of the cranium or skull that are flexible at birth and knit together in adults (see page 81).
CT scan (computed tomography) Diagnostic technique using X rays and computers to produce a graphic cross section of the tissue being examined.
Cystoscopy Examination of the urethra and bladder with a viewing instrument that is inserted into the urethra.
Cytokine Hormonal substance that helps the IMMUNE SYSTEM combat infection.
Dantien Part of the abdomen where, according to the theory of Traditional Chinese Medicine, *QI* is said to be stored.
Demulcent Coats, soothes, and protects body surfaces such as the gastric mucous membranes.
Detoxification Process by which the body is purged of TOXINS; for example, through fasting.
Diastolic blood pressure Measurement recorded during the relaxation of the heart between beats, reflecting the resistance of all the small arteries in the body and the load against which the heart must work.
Diathermy Production of heat in the body using high-frequency electric currents; used to increase blood flow and reduce deep-seated pain, for example in rheumatic and arthritic conditions.
Digoxin Drug that increases heart muscle contractions. It is derived from foxglove.
Diuretic Stimulates urine production.
DNA (deoxyribonucleic acid) Principal molecule carrying genetic information in nearly every living organism.
ECG (electrocardiogram) Recording of the electrical activity associated with each heartbeat.
ECT (electroconvulsive therapy) Electric-shock treatment that involves passing an electrical current through the brain.
EEG (electroencephalogram) Recording of the electrical activity in different areas of the brain.
Endocrine gland Gland in the body that manufactures and releases hormones.
Endocrine system Collection of hormone-producing glands in the body.
Endorphins Morphinelike substance produced naturally by the body to relieve pain; known as the body's natural opiate.
Enema Procedure of flushing fluid through the rectum via a tube in the anus.
Enzyme Protein produced by body cells that acts as a catalyst to accelerate a biological reaction. Enzymes are essential for the healthy functioning of the body.
Epinephrine Hormone released by the ADRENAL GLANDS in response to stress, exercise, or emotions such as fear.
Ergotamine Drug that constricts blood vessels; used to treat migraines.
Essential fatty acid One of a group of unsaturated FATTY ACIDS essential for growth, which the body must obtain from the diet (see page 35).
Expectorant Stimulates coughing and helps clear phlegm from the throat and chest.
Fascia Protective tissue beneath the skin, enclosing muscles and supporting organs (see page 82).
Fatty acid Fundamental constituent of many fats and oils. Some fatty acids cannot be synthesized by the body and must be provided by the diet.
Fight-or-flight response Physiological responses to what the body sees as a threat, arousing the SYMPATHETIC NERVOUS SYSTEM and making the body more efficient in either fighting or fleeing the apparent danger.
Free radicals Natural by-products of METABOLISM; these particles are unstable and potentially dangerous since they can damage DNA and cause a range of physiological problems, from a weakened immune system to high levels of CHOLESTEROL.
Freudian psychoanalysis Theory of psychoanalysis based on Sigmund Freud's belief that the unconscious mind is profoundly motivated by the individual's primitive instincts.
Healing crisis Temporary relapse of health as a healing or treatment process takes effect in the body; for example, onset of headaches during a DETOXIFICATION program.
Heavy metals Highly dense metals, such as lead and cadmium, which can accumulate in the body; they are then classed as TOXINS.
Hippocampus Part of the LIMBIC SYSTEM in the brain linked to learning and long-term memory.
Holistic Describes an approach to treatment in which the "whole" person is taken into account rather than just specific symptoms (see page 12).
Homeostasis Processes by which the body maintains a constant internal environment despite external changes (see page 13).
Hormone replacement therapy Use of a synthetic or natural hormone to treat a hormone deficiency. Commonly refers to the replacement of estrogen hormones to treat symptoms accompanying menopause.
Hyperglycemia Excess glucose in the blood,

which can result in coma.
Hypertension Abnormally high blood pressure.
Hypoglycemia Insufficient glucose in the blood, which can result in coma.
Hypothalamus Part of the LIMBIC SYSTEM in the brain that exerts overall control over the SYMPATHETIC NERVOUS SYSTEM.
Immune response Response of the IMMUNE SYSTEM to ANTIGENS.
Immune system Body organs responsible for IMMUNITY.
Immunity Ability of the body to resist infection due to the presence of ANTIBODIES and white blood cells.
Infusion Water-based medicinal preparation in which the flowers, leaves, or stems of a plant are brewed in a similar way to tea.
Jungian analysis Psychoanalytic theory developed by Carl Gustav Jung, which stresses the notion of "archetypes" – ideas inherited from the ancient past and shared by all humanity as part of a "collective unconscious."
Kampo Japanese system of medicine adapted from Traditional Chinese Medicine.
Karma Buddhist principle of justice, linked to an individual's state of reincarnation.
Ki Japanese spelling of *QI*.
Large intestine Part of the digestive tract that absorbs water from food residue, and forms and stores feces.
Limbic system System of nerve pathways in the brain concerned with the expression of instincts, drives and emotions, and with the formation of memory patterns.
Lymph Fluid similar to blood plasma. It bathes all body tissues before being circulated into the bloodstream, and plays an important role in the IMMUNE SYSTEM.
Lymphatic system System of vessels and nodes throughout the body that carries and filters LYMPH and prevents foreign particles from entering the bloodstream.
MAOI antidepressant (monoamine oxidase inhibitor) One of the two main types of antidepressant drugs.
Melatonin Hormone secreted by the PINEAL GLAND during the hours of darkness that helps regulate the body's sleep cycles.
Meridians Energy channels that run up and down the body and are thought to transport the vital energy *QI*. Each meridian is related to either a *YIN* or *YANG* organ (see page 91).
Metabolism Collective term for chemical processes that take place in the body; the "metabolic rate" reflects the energy required to keep the body functioning when at rest.
Mother tincture Mixture of medicinal extracts, alcohol and distilled water that forms the basis of homeopathic remedies.
MRI (magnetic resonance imaging) Diagnostic technique that exposes body tissue to high-frequency radio waves; used particularly to examine the central nervous system.
Neurology Branch of medicine concerned with the nervous system, and particularly the diagnosis and treatment of its disorders.
Neuropeptide Any of several PEPTIDES found in the brain, categorized as NEUROTRANSMITTERS and sometimes hormones (see page 18).
Neurotransmitter Chemical released from nerve endings that helps transmit impulses to another nerve cell or to a muscle cell (see page 18).
Norepinephrine See EPINEPHRINE.
Nosode Homeopathic remedy devised by Samuel Hahnemann, originally made from bodily secretions and now made from many body tissues (see page 126).
Obstetric medicine Branch of medicine concerned with pregnancy, prenatal care, childbirth and postnatal care.
Occult blood Tiny quantities of blood that can only be detected microscopically or by chemical testing.
Parasympathetic nervous system Part of the AUTONOMIC NERVOUS SYSTEM that is dominant when the body is not aroused (primarily engaged in digestion and body maintenance).
Peptide A compound formed by the union of two or more AMINO ACIDS.
Peristalsis Involuntary wavelike action of muscles in certain tubular structures of the body, for example in the intestines, that causes the contents to move forward.
PET scan (positron emission tomography) Diagnostic technique in which three-dimensional images are produced, reflecting the activity of the tissues being tested.
Physiology Study of the functioning of the body, including the physical and chemical processes of cells, tissues, and organs, and their interaction.
Physiotherapy Treatment of disorders or injuries that uses physical methods, such as heat or electrical treatments, massage or manipulation, to promote healing.
Pilates A body conditioning technique that tones the muscles to increase flexibility and strength.
Pineal gland Pea-sized, cone-shaped gland in the brain that secretes the hormone MELATONIN.
Pituitary gland Gland responsible for regulating and controlling the release of hormones into the blood from other types of ENDOCRINE GLAND.
Placebo Chemically inert substance given in place of a drug, often in scientific studies (see page 17).
PMS (premenstrual syndrome) Combination of physical and emotional symptoms that occurs in women 1–2 weeks before menstruation.
Polyp Growth, usually benign, protruding from a mucous membrane.
Prana Vital "life energy" in Ayurvedic medicine, akin to *QI*.
Probiotics Friendly, disease-destroying bacteria in the digestive tract that help in the manufacture of vitamins and enzymes, so improving digestion.
Prostaglandin Drug or naturally occurring substance within the body that has several actions, such as causing muscle contractions and producing mucus in the stomach lining.
Qi "Life energy" force of Traditional Chinese Medicine that enters and can be accessed at ACUPOINTS on the body. It is said to be inherited at conception and also derived from food and air.
Radio emission therapy An umbrella term for therapies that utilize radio waves to aid healing in body tissue.
Remission Apparent disappearance or abeyance of symptoms of a disease.
Salbutamol Drug that helps to improve breathing and is used particularly in the treatment of asthma.
Saturated fat Highly concentrated fat containing FATTY ACIDS and CHOLESTEROL; usually derived from animals.
Scoliosis Curvature of the spine.
Sebum Oily secretions that reach skin around the hair follicles, help lubricate the skin, and have an ANTIBACTERIAL effect.
Serotonin Substance found particularly in the blood, intestinal wall, and CENTRAL NERVOUS SYSTEM that acts as a NEUROTRANSMITTER, relaying information across nerve endings.
Small intestine Part of the digestive tract between the stomach and large intestine.
Steroid drugs Group of drugs including CORTICOSTEROID drugs, which resemble hormones produced by the ADRENAL GLANDS, and anabolic steroids, which have an effect similar to that of the male hormones.
Streptococci BACTERIA associated with many infections, including scarlet fever.
Stressor Factor that causes stress.
Subtle body Nonphysical body that surrounds a person, according to esoteric philosophies, through which vital energy is said to flow.
Sympathetic nervous system Part of the AUTONOMIC NERVOUS SYSTEM, primarily engaged in preparing the body for action.
Systolic blood pressure Pressure created at the point of the contraction of the heart muscle.
Tanden Area in the abdomen where, according to traditional Japanese medicine, *KI* is stored.
Taoism Chinese religious system characterized by a simplicity of lifestyle and a fatalistic approach to life events.
TENS (transcutaneous electrical nerve stimulation) Stimulation of body tissue with pulses of low-voltage electricity for pain relief.
Thalamus Gray matter situated just above the brain stem; relay center for sensory information flowing into the brain, for example from the eyes.
Thrombosis Condition in which blood in a vessel becomes solid and produces a blood clot; thrombosis in an artery obstructs the flow of blood and oxygen to the tissue or organ it supplies.
Thymus Gland that forms part of the IMMUNE SYSTEM, situated behind the breastbone.
Tincture Strong preparation made by soaking a medicinal extract in alcohol and water.
Toxins Environmental poisons, and waste products produced by the body.
Trace element One of a group of minerals the body needs in minute amounts and can only obtain from food, including chromium, copper, selenium, and zinc.
Transference Technique used in psychoanalysis whereby the practitioner encourages the patient to redirect, or "transfer," feelings about a situation or person onto the practitioner, so that they can be discussed and resolved.
Trigger points Secondary points of muscle tension caused by pain from the spine and connected tissue, which feel like hard nodules when pressed.
Unsaturated fat (and polyunsaturated fat) Fat that contains FATTY ACIDS but no CHOLESTEROL.
Vasodilator Drug that causes the widening of the blood vessels and a consequent increase in blood flow; often used to lower blood pressure.
Vibrational therapies Therapies that aim to balance and strengthen the "vibrational frequencies" of the body's life force or "subtle energy," which is said to resonate through cells and organs at certain frequencies. Vibrational therapies include radionics, reiki, crystal healing, and color therapy.
Virus Smallest known type of infectious agent, capable of replication, but only within living cells.
Yin* and *yang Fundamental energies described by Traditional Chinese Medicine; all things are said to be a manifestation of *yin* or *yang* (see page 141).

BIBLIOGRAPHY

This selected listing of references is provided as a guide to those interested in learning more about the history, science, and present-day practice of complementary medicine.

GENERAL

Alexander, J.
Supertherapies (Bantam, 1996)
Benson, H.
Timeless Healing: The Power and Biology of Belief
(Simon & Schuster, 1997)
Benson, H. & Stuart, E.
The Wellness Book
(Simon & Schuster, 1992)
Brostoff, J. & Gamlin, L.
The Complete Guide to Food Allergy and Intolerance
(Crown, 1992)
The Burton Goldberg Group
Alternative Medicine: The Definitive Guide (Future Medicine Publishing, 1994)
Campbell, E.
Body, Mind, & Spirit: A Dictionary of New Age Ideas, People, Places & Terms (Charles E. Tuttle, 1994)
Carlson, K. J., Eisenstat, S. A. & Ziporyn, T.
Harvard Guide to Women's Health
(Harvard University Press, 1996)
Castleman, M.
Nature's Cures: From Acupressure & Aromatherapy to Walking & Yoga (Rodale Press, 1996)
Chopra, D.
Ageless Body, Timeless Mind: The Quantum Alternative to Growing Old (Harmony, 1993)
Collinge, W.
The American Holistic Health Association Complete Guide to Alternative Medicine
(Warner Books, 1996)
Digeronimo, T.
Chronic Pain: The Natural Way of Healing (Dell, 1995)
Ernst, E. (ed.)
Complementary Medicine: An Objective Appraisal (Butterworth Heinemann, 1996)
Fugh-Berman, A.
Alternative Medicine: What Works (Odonian Press, 1996)
Goleman, D. & Gurin, J.
Mind/Body Medicine (Consumer Reports Books, 1993)
Hirshberg, C. & Barasch, M. I.
Remarkable Recovery
(Headline, 1995)
Kastner, M.
Alternative Healing: The Complete A–Z Guide to More Than 150 Alternative Therapies
(Henry Holt, 1996)
Kusick, J.
Treasury of Natural First Aid Remedies From A–Z
(Prentice-Hall, 1994)
Linn, D.
Sacred Space (Ballantine, 1996)
Marti, J.
The Alternative Health and Medicine Encyclopedia
(Gale, 1994)
Micozzi, M. (ed.)
Fundamentals of Complementary and Alternative Medicine
(Churchill Livingstone, 1995)
Moyers, B.
Healing and the Mind
(Doubleday, 1993)
O'Connor, B.
Healing Traditions: Alternative Medicine and the Health Professions (University of Pennsylvania Press, 1995)
Ornish, D.
Dr. Dean Ornish's Program for Reversing Heart Disease
(Ballantine Books, 1990)
Ornstein, R. & Swencionis, C.
The Healing Brain: A Scientific Reader (Guilford Press, 1990)
Rankin-Box, D. (ed.)
The Nurses' Handbook of Complementary Therapies
(Churchill Livingstone, 1995)
Reader's Digest Editors
Family Guide to Natural Medicine: How to Stay Healthy the Natural Way
(Reader's Digest Assn., 1993)
Scheider, M.
Self-Healing
(Viking Penguin, 1988)
Sharma, U.
Complementary Medicine Today
(Routledge, 1991)
Smyth, A.
Complete Home Healer
(Harper San Francisco, 1995)
Stanway, A.
The New Natural Family Doctor
(North Atlantic, 1996)
University of California, Berkeley
The Wellness Encyclopedia
(Houghton Mifflin, 1991)
Watson, D.
A Dictionary of Mind and Body
(Trafalgar Square, 1996)
Weil, A.
Eight Weeks to Optimal Healing Power (Knopf, 1996)
Weil, A.
Spontaneous Healing
(Little, Brown, 1995)
Williams, R. & Williams, V.
Anger Kills (Times Books, 1993)

ACUPUNCTURE
See Traditional Chinese Medicine

ANTHROPOSOPHICAL MEDICINE
Bott, V.
Spiritual Science & the Art of Healing: Rudolf Steiner's Anthroposophical Medicine
(Inner Traditions, 1996)

APPLIED KINESIOLOGY
Holdway, A.
Kinesiology (Element, 1995)

AROMATHERAPY
Dye, J.
Aromatherapy for Women and Children (National Book Network, 1992)
Price, S.
Practical Aromatherapy
(Harper San Francisco, 1994)
Watson, F.
Aromatherapy Blends & Remedies: Over 800 Recipes for Everyday Use
(Harper San Francisco, 1996)

ART THERAPY
McNiff, S.
Art as Medicine (Shambala, 1992)

AYURVEDA
Dash, B.
Ayurvedic Cures of Common Diseases
(Hind Pocket Books, 1993)
Lad, V.
Ayurveda: The Science of Self-Healing (Lotus Light, 1990)
Morrison, J. H.
The Book of Ayurveda
(Simon & Schuster, 1995)

BACH FLOWER REMEDIES
See also Flower Remedies
Bach, E.
The Bach Flower Remedies
(Keats, 1979)
Howard, J.
Growing Up with Bach Flower Remedies (National Book Network, 1994)
Scheffer, M.
Mastering Bach Flower Therapies: A Guide to Diagnosis and Treatment (Inner Traditions, 1996)

THE BATES METHOD
Mansfield, P.
The Bates Method
(Charles E. Tuttle, 1994)

CHELATION THERAPY
Collings, J.
Beat Heart Disease without Surgery
(Harper San Francisco, 1995)

CHINESE HERBALISM
See Traditional Chinese Medicine

CHIROPRACTIC
Moore, S.
Chiropractic
(Charles E. Tuttle, 1993)

COLONIC HYDROTHERAPY
Collings, J.
Principles of Colonic Irrigation
(Harper San Francisco, 1995)

COLOR THERAPY
Sun, H.
Color Your Life
(London Bridge, 1996)
Wills, P.
Color Therapy (Element, 1993)

FENG SHUI
Craze, R. & Ling, S.
Feng Shui [For Beginners Series]
(Trafalgar Square, 1996)
Wydra, N.
Feng Shui: The Book of Cures
(Contemporary, 1996)

FLOWER REMEDIES
See also Bach Flower Remedies
Harvey, C. & Cochrane, A.
The Encyclopedia of Flower Remedies (Thorsons, 1995)
McIntyre, A.
Flower Power: Remedies for Healing Body & Soul (Henry Holt, 1996)

HEALING
Myss, C.
Anatomy of the Spirit
(Harmony, 1996)

HOMEOPATHY
Castro, M.
The Complete Homeopathy Handbook: A Guide for Everyday Health Care
(St. Martin's Press, 1991)
Lockie, A.
The Family Guide to Homeopathy
(Simon & Schuster, 1993)

Lockie, A. & Geddes, N.
The Complete Guide to Homeopathy (DK Pub., Inc., 1995)
Lockie, A. & Geddes, N.
The Women's Guide to Homeopathy (St. Martin's Press, 1994)
Ullman, D.
Homeopathic Medicine for Children and Infants (Jeremy P. Tarcher, 1992)

HYPNOTHERAPY
Caprio, F. & Berger, J.
Helping Yourself with Self-Hypnosis (Prentice-Hall, 1986)
Stiles, W.
How Hypnotherapy Can Help You: The Complementary & Alternative Method for Wellness (Kendall/Hunt, 1994)

IRIDOLOGY
Colton, J.
Iridology (Element, 1996)
Hall, D.
Iridology: How your Eyes Reveal Your Health and Personality (Keats, 1981)

KAHUNA
King, S.
Kahuna Healing (Theosophical Publishing House, 1983)

LIGHT THERAPY
Lightyears Ahead Production Staff
Lightyears Ahead: The Illustrated Guide to Full Spectrum and Colored Light MindBody Healing (Celestial Arts, 1995)

MASSAGE
Maxwell-Hudson, C.
The Complete Book of Massage (DK Pub., Inc., 1991)
Mitchell, S.
Massage (Element, 1993)
Montagu, A.
Touching: The Human Significance of the Skin (Harper & Row, 1986)

MEDITATION
Fontana, D.
The Elements of Meditation (Element, 1991)
Kabat-Zinn, J.
Full Catastrophe Living (Dell, 1990)
Kabat-Zinn, J.
Wherever You Go, There You Are: Mindfulness Meditation for Everyday Life (Hyperion, 1995)
LeShan, L.
How to Meditate (Bantam, 1984)

MUSIC THERAPY
Gardner, K.
Sounding the Inner Landscape (Element, 1997)
Garfield, L. M.
Sound Medicine: Healing with Music, Voice & Song (Celestial Arts, 1995)

NATUROPATHY
Mayell, M.
Natural First Aid (Trafalgar Square, 1996)
Murray, M. & Pizzorno, J.
Encyclopedia of Natural Medicine (Prima, 1990)
Pizzorno, J.
Total Wellness (Prima, 1996)

NUTRITIONAL THERAPIES
Davies, S. & Stewart, A.
Nutritional Medicine (Avon, 1990)
Reader's Digest Editors
Foods that Harm, Foods that Heal (Reader's Digest Association, 1996)
Werbach, M. R.
Healing through Nutrition (HarperCollins, 1994)

OSTEOPATHY
Belshaw, C.
Osteopathy: Is It For You? (Element, 1993)

PSYCHOTHERAPY & COUNSELING
Berne, E.
Games People Play (Ballantine, 1985)
Bolen, J.
The Tao of Psychology: Synchronicity & the Self (Harper San Francisco, 1982)
O'Connor, J. & McDermott, I.
NLP & Health (Harper San Francisco, 1996)
O'Connor, J. & Seymour, J.
Introducing Neuro-Linguistic Programming (Harper San Francisco, 1993)
Perls, F. S.
Gestalt Therapy Verbatim (Gestalt Journal, 1992)
Zweig, C. & Adams, J. (eds.)
Meeting the Shadow: The Hidden Power of the Dark Side of Human Nature [New Consciousness Reader Series] (Jeremy P. Tarcher, 1990)

QIGONG
See Traditional Chinese Medicine

REFLEXOLOGY
Dougans, I.
Reflexology: Foot Massage For Total Health (Element, 1997)
Gillanders, A.
Reflexology: A Step-by-Step Guide (Little, Brown, 1996)
Norman, L., with Cowan, T.
Feet First: A Guide to Foot Reflexology (Simon & Schuster, 1988)
Wills, P.
The Reflexology Manual (Inner Traditions, 1995)

RELAXATION & BREATHING
Hewitt, J.
The Complete Relaxation Book (Trafalgar Square, 1992)

SHIATSU
Cowmeadow, O.
The Art of Shiatsu (Element, 1993)
Ridolfe, R.
Shiatsu (Charles E. Tuttle, 1993)
Ridolfe, R. & Franzen, S.
Shiatsu for Women (Thorsons SF, Harper San Francisco, 1996)

T'AI CHI CH'UAN
See Traditional Chinese Medicine

THERAPEUTIC TOUCH
Krieger, D.
Accepting Your Power to Heal: The Personal Practice of Therapeutic Touch (Bear, 1993)

TRADITIONAL CHINESE MEDICINE
Bauer, C.
Acupressure for Everybody (Henry Holt, 1991)
Cohen, K.
Qigong: Chinese Energy (Ballantine, 1997)
Gascoigne, S.
The Chinese Way to Health: A Self-Help Guide to Traditional Chinese Medicine (Charles E. Tuttle, 1997)
Hicks, A.
Principles of Chinese Medicine (Harper San Francisco, 1996)
MacRitchie, J.
Chi Kung (Element, 1993)
Marcus, P.
Thorsons Introductory Guide to Acupuncture (Harper San Francisco, 1992)
McNamara, S.
Traditional Chinese Medicine (Basic, 1996)
Naeser, M.
Outline Guide to Chinese Herbal Medicines in Pill Form (Boston Chinese Medical, 1990)
Shen, P.
Massage for Pain Relief (Random House, 1996)
Tang, S. & Craze, R.
Chinese Herbal Medicine (Berkley, 1996)
Tse, M.
Qigong for Health and Vitality (St. Martin's Press, 1996)
Yan, W. & Fischer, W.
Practical Therapeutics of Traditional Chinese Medicine [J.P. Fratkin, ed.] (Paradigm, 1995)

TRAGERWORK
Trager, M.
Movement as a Way to Agelessness (Station Hill Press, 1995)

WESTERN HERBALISM
Chevallier, A.
The Encyclopedia of Medicinal Plants (DK Pub., Inc., 1996)
Hoffman, D.
The Complete Illustrated Holistic Herbal (Element, 1996)
McIntyre, A.
The Complete Women's Herbal (Henry Holt, 1995)
McIntyre, A.
Herbs for Common Ailments (Simon & Schuster, 1992)
McIntyre, A.
Herbal Medicine (Charles E. Tuttle, 1993)
Mills, S.
The Dictionary of Modern Herbalism: The Complete Guide to Herbs and Herbal Therapy (Inner Traditions, 1985)
Mills, S.
The Essential Book of Herbal Medicine (Viking Penguin, 1994)
Ody, P.
Home Herbal (DK Pub., Inc., 1995)
Rothfeld, G. & LeVert, S.
Natural Medicine for Heart Disease (Rodale Press, Inc., 1996)

YOGA
Hewitt, J.
Yoga (Random House, 1988)
Nagarathna, R., Nagendra, H. R. & Monro, R.
Yoga for Common Ailments (Simon & Schuster, 1991)
Saraawati, Swami J.
Yoga, Tantra and Meditation in Daily Life (Weiser, 1992)

INDEX

Page numbers in **bold** refer to main entries in *Key Healing Therapies*, which generally include the historical background of the therapy; its key principles and theory; evidence, research, and medical opinion on its efficacy; what happens when consulting a practitioner, with treatment examples, precautions, and case histories; and suggestions for self-help. Full details on the contents of entries in *Key Healing Therapies* and how to use them can be found on pages 50–51.

Page numbers in *italics* refer to main entries in *Treating Ailments*, which include details, causes, and symptoms of the ailment, suggestions for appropriate complementary therapies and cautions for their use, conventional approaches to and treatments for the condition, and suggestions for self-help. Full details on the contents of entries in *Treating Ailments* and how to use them can be found on pages 204–205.

A

abdominal breathing 170, 171, 172
Abrams, Albert 157
abscesses *214*
  eye (sties) *221*
  tooth 229
absent healing 105
  radionics **157**
Achilles tendon 252
acid indigestion *232*
acid reflux 232
acne *216*
acquired immunodeficiency syndrome *see* AIDS
activator (chiropractic) 72
active imagery (visualization) 178
active meditation 176
acupoints
  in acupressure 95
  in acupuncture 90, 91, 92, 93
  in auricular acupuncture 94
  in do-in 98
  in electro-acupuncture 94, 200
  in energy medicine 200
  location 90, 91, 94
  in qigong 99
  in shiatsu 96
acupressure **95**
  see also Thai massage
acupuncture **90–4**
  auricular **94**, 192
  electro-acupuncture 94, 200
  laser 94
  medical 90, 91
adaptation (stress reaction) 27
ADD (attention deficit disorder) 284
adhesive capsulitis 253
addictions *296*
additives & pesticides 36–7
addresses, practitioners' professional organizations 319–23
adenoids *280*
Ader, Robert 18
adjustments (chiropractic) 72
adrenal glands 262
aerobic exercise 40, 41, 42, 43
agni (Ayurveda) 144
agoraphobia 286
agriculture, biodynamic 125
AIDS *310–11*
ailments section, how to use *204–5*
AIT (sound therapy) 180
Alexander, Frederick Matthias 86
Alexander, Gerda 115
Alexander technique **86–7**
allergens 155, 199, 298, 299, 300, 302
allergies *298*, 308
  allergic rhinitis & hay fever *299*, 302
  anaphylaxis 302
  asthma 12, 298, *300–1*, 302
  and clinical ecology **154–5**, 299, 302
  conjunctivitis *221*
  diagnosis 155, 199, 298
  eczema & dermatitis *218*, 302
  urticaria *see* hives
  see also food allergies; food intolerances & sensitivities
alpha waves 174, 175, 190
alveoli 171, 224
Alvin, Juliette 181
Alzheimer's disease *209*
ama (Ayurveda) 144, 147
AMI (energy medicine) 200
amino acids, blood test for 199
amygdala 286
anabolic treatment (naturopathy) 120
anaerobic exercise 40, 41
analytical hypnotherapy 167
anaphylaxis & anaphylactic shock 302
anemia *248*
anger & hostility 44–5
angina pectoris *242*
animal magnetism 156
ankylosing spondylitis *261*
anma (acupressure) 95, 96
  see also shiatsu
anorexia 297
anthroposophical medicine **124–5**
anthroposophy 124
antibodies 19, 46, 298, 308
antineoplaston therapy, for cancer 307
antioxidants 37, 148, 149, 153, 305–6
anxiety *287*
  effect on immune system & health 19
  panic attacks *288*
aphthous ulcers *see* canker sores
apparatus for meridian investigation (energy medicine) 200
appetite disturbance *232*
Applied Kinesiology **196–7**
armoring (Reichian theory) 61, 89
aromatherapy **62–5**
  medical **65**
aromatograms 65
art therapy **182–3**
  in anthroposophical medicine 125
arteries 242, 243
arthritis *258–60*
  Western herbal remedies 138, 139
asanas (yoga) 108–11
Assagioli, Roberto 165
asthma 12, 298, *300–1*, 302
Aston, Judith 83
Aston-Patterning **83**
astral body (anthroposophical medicine) 124
AT *see* autogenic training
atheroma 243
atherosclerosis *243*
athlete's foot *215*
atopic eczema 218, 302
atopy 298
atria 242
attention deficit disorder (ADD) 284
auditory integration training (sound therapy) 180
auditory nerve 222
aura healing 104
Aura-Soma **190**
auras 104, 186, 201
auricle 222
auricular acupuncture **94**, 192
auriculocardiac reflex method (pulse diagnosis) 155, 192
auriculotherapy *see* auricular acupuncture
autoimmune diseases 308
  ankylosing spondylitis *261*
  Crohn's disease *234*
  multiple sclerosis *212*
  rheumatoid arthritis *260*
autogenic training (AT) **168**
autonomic nervous system 71
autosuggestion 167
Avicenna 62
awareness through movement (Feldenkrais method) 85
Ayurveda **144–7**
  chavutti thirumal **115**, 146
  diagnosis 146, 192, 193
  energy *see chakras*; *doshas*; *nadis*; *prana*
  Indian head massage **115**
  role of massage 56, 98, 115, 146, 147
  yoga **108–11**

B

B-lymphocytes 308, 309
Bach, Edward 132
Bach Flower Remedies **132–3**
back
  ankylosing spondylitis *261*
  backache *254–5*
  manipulation therapies *see* chiropractic; osteopathy
  prolapsed disk *256*
  structure 250
  Swedish/Western massage 59
bacteria, gut flora 149
bacterial infections *see* infections
bad breath *see* halitosis
balance
  problems *see* dizziness; vertigo
  role of the ear 222
balanced diet 34–7
balanitis *276*
Bandler, Richard 164
Barlow, Wilfred 86
Bates, William H. 114
Bates method **114**
baths
  aromatherapy 65
  hydrotherapy 122, 123
Bayley, Doreen 66
bed-wetting *285*
behavioral problems, children *284–5*
behavioral psychology 160
behavioral therapy (psychotherapy) 164
Bell's palsy *207*
Benor, Daniel 105
Benson, Herbert 13, 170
Berard, Guy 180
Bernard, Claude 118
Berne, Eric 165
Bhaccha, Jivaka Kumar 98
bile 233
biochemic tissue salts **131**
biochemical realm & challenges 26–7
biodynamic agriculture 125
biodynamic massage **61**
bioenergetics **89**
bioenergy 61, 157
biofeedback 18, **169**
bioflavonoids 37, 306
biomagnetic therapy *see* magnetic therapy
biorhythms **189**
Bircher-Benner, Max 152
bites & stings, first aid *317*
black box (radionics) 157
bladder 240
  problems *see* urinary system, common ailments
blood circulation *see* heart & circulation
blood pressure
  high *244–5*
  low *246*
blood tests 150, 155, 199, 298
body-armoring (Reichian theory) 61, 89
bodywork
  Bates method **114**
  bioenergetics **89**
  Bowen technique **115**
  hakomi **115**
  polarity therapy **102–3**
  SHEN therapy **115**
  Tragerwork **88**
  Zero Balancing **115**
  see also exercise therapies; manipulation therapies; massage; movement & posture reeducation therapies
boils *214*
bone marrow 308
bones 250
  cranium 81
  ear 222
  facial 225
  osteoporosis *257*
  vertebrae 250
  see also musculoskeletal system
Bonyun adjustment (chiropractic) 74
bowel, problems *see* digestion & digestive system, common ailments
Bowen technique **115**

Bowen, Tom 115
Boyesen, Gerda 61
Braid, James 166
brain & nervous system
common ailments *206–13*
effect of exercise 41
effect of visualization 178
psychoneuroimmunology 18–19
structure & functions 206
autonomic nervous system 71
brain chemistry & limbic system 286
cortex & hemispheres 175, 206
light response 188
pain response 77, 314
scent response 63
spinal cord 71, 206
brain stem 77, 206
brain wave activity
effect of biofeedback 169
effect of meditation 174, 175
BRAT diet 230
breasts
breastfeeding problems *269*
breast pain *272*
fibrocystic breast disease *272*
breath, bad *see* halitosis
breath awareness (meditation) 176
breathing
physiological process 224
problems *see* asthma; respiratory system, common ailments
relaxation & breathing **170–3**
yoga techniques (*pranayama*) 108
brief therapy (psychotherapy) 164
bright white light 188
Bristol diet 306
bronchi 171, 224
bronchioles 224
bronchitis *226*
bruises & cuts, first aid *316*
bulimia 297
burns & scalds, first aid *317*
bursae 253
bursitis *253*

C

California flower essences 132
cancer 19, 46, 47, 178, *304–7*
candidiasis *235*
see also yeast infections
canker sores *229*
capillaries 224, 242
capsulitis, adhesive 253
carbohydrates 34, 36, 152
cardiovascular endurance 40
cardiovascular problems *see* heart & circulation, common ailments
carotenoids 37
carpal tunnel syndrome *206–7*
see also repetitive strain injury
carrier oils 64, 139
catabolic treatment (naturopathy) 120
catalysts (Metamorphic technique) 69
cataracts *220*
caterpillar walk (reflexology) 68
celiac disease *235*
cells
cancerous 304
immune system 298, 308
lymphocytes (white blood cells) 308, 309, 310
macrophages (scavengers) 212
mast 298
natural killer cells, 18, 19, 47, 308, 309, 310
nerve 314
phagocytes (engulfing cells) 308
skin 214
T-cells 308, 309, 310
white blood cells 308
central fixation (eyesight) 114
cerebellum 77, 206
cerebral hemispheres 175, 178, 206
cerebrospinal fluid 81
cerebrum 206
cervical spondylosis *259*
cervicodorsal lift (osteopathy) 80
cervix 264, 269
CFS (chronic fatigue syndrome) *312–13*
Chace, Marian 112
chakras (Ayurveda)
in color therapy 186, 187, 190
in polarity therapy 102
in reiki 107
in yoga 109
challenges (Applied Kinesiology) 196, 197
change of life *see* menopause
Chang San Feng 100
chanting (sound therapy) 180
chapped skin *219*
chavutti thirumal (Ayurveda) **115**, 146
chelation therapy **157**
Chen (t'ai chi ch'uan) 100
Chen Wang Ting 100
chicken pox 217, *283*
child worships the Buddha (qigong posture) 99
childbirth & pregnancy 41, *268–9*
children
adenoids *280*
art therapy 183
atopic eczema 218
behavioral problems *284–5*
child therapy (psychotherapy) 162
colic *279*
cradle cap 219
cranial osteopathy 81
croup *279*
diaper rash *278*
dyslexia *208*
exercise 41
fevers *281*
growth & development 278
head lice *280*
infectious illnesses *281–3*
music therapy 180
teething *279*
Chinese herbalism **140–3**
Chinese Medicine, Traditional *see* Traditional Chinese Medicine
chiropractic **70–5**
McTimoney & McTimoney-Corley **75**
network spinal analysis 75
chlamydia 240, 274
Chopra, Deepak 144
chronic fatigue syndrome *312–13*
chronic (persistent) pain *314–15*
chronobiology 189
cingulate gyrus 286
circulatory system *see* heart & circulation
circumcision 276
classic migraine 210
classical homeopathy 128, 129, 130
classical induction hypnotherapy 167
claustrophobia 286
clinical ecology **154–5**
clinical psychology 160
clinical trials 16–17
cloud hands (t'ai chi ch'uan) 101
cluster migraine 210
Coca, Arthur 192
cognitive therapies (psychotherapy) 19, 164
Cohen, Nicholas 18
cold compresses
in hydrotherapy 123
in naturopathy 121
cold responders (psychological type) 45
cold sores *217*
colds & flu *see* common cold; influenza
colic *279*
colitis
mucous *see* irritable bowel syndrome
ulcerative *234*
colon 149, 230
reflexology treatment 68
colonic hydrotherapy (colonic irrigation) **157**
color illumination therapy 187
color reflection readings 187
color spine charts 187, 198
color therapy **186–7**
Aura-Soma **190**
common cold *225*
common migraine 210
complementary practitioners *see* practitioners
complex carbohydrates 34, 36
complex homeopathy 130
compresses
in Chinese herbalism 143
in hydrotherapy 123
in naturopathy 121
conductive deafness 223
conjunctiva 220
conjunctivitis *221*
constipation 149, *239*
constitutional types (homeopathy) 126, 128, 129
contact eczema or contact dermatitis 218
controlled clinical trials 16
Corbett, Margaret Darst 114
Corley, Hugh 75
cornea 150, 220
coronary arteries 242, 243
coronary artery disease *243*
cortex, brain 175, 178
Coué, Emile 167
counseling *see* psychotherapy & counseling
cradle cap 219
cramp, in muscles *250*
cranial osteopathy 81
cranial rhythmic impulse (cranial osteopathy) 81
CranioSacral therapy **81**
cranium 81
creams (herbal remedies) 137
Cretan Mediterranean diet 149, 243
CRI (cranial osteopathy) 81
Crohn's disease *234*
croup *279*
crystal therapy **133**
Culpeper, Nicholas 134
cupping (acupuncture) 92, 93
cure, laws of (homeopathy) 126
cuts & bruises, first aid *316*
cycles
biorhythmic 189
doshas (Ayurveda) 145
menstrual *see* menstruation & menstrual cycle
pain-tension 77
cymatics (sound therapy) 180
cystitis *275*
cytotoxic tests 155, 199

D

dance movement therapy **112–13**
see also eurythmy; eutony
dandruff *219*
dantien (Traditional Chinese Medicine) 92, 101
daoyin *see* do-in
deafness *223*
decoctions (herbal remedies) 137
dementia *see* Alzheimer's disease; senile dementia
dentine 229
dependency *see* addictions
depleted immune system *309*
depression *292*
effect on immune system & health 19
postnatal *269*
seasonal affective disorder (SAD) 188, *293*
dermatitis *218*
dermis 56, 214
Descartes 12–13, 158
desensitization therapy 298
in clinical ecology 155
detoxification
Ayurveda 144, 146
diet 152
naturopathy 120, 121
polarity therapy 102, 103
diabetes mellitus *263*
diagnosis 24–5, **191–201**
allergies 155, 199, 298
Ayurveda 146, 192, 193
blood tests 150, 155, 199, 298
clinical ecology 155
hara 96, 97, **194**
nutritional testing 150
Traditional Chinese Medicine 92, 97, 140, 142, 192, 193
diaper rash *278*
diaphragm 171
diaphragmatic breathing 170, 171, 172
diarrhea *238*, 278
dietary fiber 36, 151
diets
balanced 34–7
BRAT 230
Bristol 306
Cretan Mediterranean 149, 243
diet therapies 152
exclusion or elimination 150, 155, 199
Gerson therapy 152, 307

gluten-free 235
naturopathic 119, 121, 148
Ornish reversal 152, 243
polarity therapy 102, 103
Western, chemical content 36–7, 148, 151, 154, 303
see also food; nutrition
digestion & digestive system
colic *279*
common ailments *230–9*
reflexology treatment 68
structure & functions 149, 230
see also food allergies; food intolerances & sensitivities
Dioscorides 134
disk, prolapsed (slipped) *256*
distillation (essential oils) 62
diverticula 239
diverticular disease *239*
diverticulitis 239
diverticulosis 239
dizziness *208*
do-in **98**
doctrine of signatures 134
doshas (Ayurveda) 144, 145, 192, 193
double-blind trials 16
dowsing **198**
in Bach Flower Remedies **132**
in color therapy **186**
in geomancy **185**
in psionics **157**
in radionics **157**
dreaming & dreamless sleep 39
dysbiosis 148, 149, 303
dyslexia *208*
dysmenorrhea *265*
dyspepsia *see* indigestion

E

ear acupuncture *see* auricular acupuncture
earache *223*
eardrum 222
ears
acupoints 94, 192
common ailments *222–3*
glue ear *280*
structure & functions 222
eating disorders *297*
EAV (energy medicine) 200
ECGs, in biofeedback 169
eczema 143, *218*, 302
Edwards, Harry 104
EEGs 169, 175
effleurage (massage) 57
eggs (ova) 264
ejaculation, premature *295*
elbows, tennis elbow *252*
electro-acupuncture 94, 200
electro-bio photography *see* Kirlian photography
electrocardiographs, in biofeedback 169
electroencephalographs 169, 175
electromyographs, in biofeedback 169
elements *see* five elements; trace elements
elimination or exclusion diets 150, 155, 199
ELISA (enzyme-linked immuno-sorbent assay), in nutritional testing 199
EMGs, in biofeedback 169
emotional categories (Bach Flower Remedies) 132–3
emotional cycle (biorhythms) 189
emotional problems *see* psychological problems
emotional support 19, 46
emotions
effect of exercise 40, 41
mind/body interactions 12–13, 18–19
mood foods 37
negative 44–5
positive 46–7
endocrine system 18, 262
endometriosis *274*
endometrium 264
endorphins 18, 45, 56, 91, 294, 314
energy
Ayurveda *see chakras*; *doshas*; *nadis*; *prana*
bioenergy 61, 157
effect of exercise 40
energy circuits (Applied Kinesiology) 196
energy fields
geomancy 185
Therapeutic Touch 106
Zero Balancing 115
energy flow (Bowen technique) 115
energy medicine **200**
healing energy 104, 105, 106, 157
life energy 102, 103, 133
see also prana; *qi*
natural energy (SHEN therapy) 115
vibrational energy frequencies (dowsing) 198
see also vital force
enfleurage (essential oils) 62
environmental medicine *see* clinical ecology
enzyme-linked immuno-sorbent assay (ELISA), in nutritional testing 199
enzyme potentiated desensitization (clinical ecology) 155, 302
enzymes, digestive 230
epidemiological research 19
epidermis 214
epididymes 276
epiglottis 228
Epstein, Donald 75
erectile dysfunction *295*
erection, penis 276
Erickson, Milton H. 160, 166
Ericksonian hypnotherapy 167
esophagus 149, 228, 230
essential oils 62–5, 139
estrogen 264, 270
etheric body (anthroposophical medicine) 124
eurythmy 124
see also dance movement therapy
eustachian tubes 222
eutony **115**
exclusion or elimination diets 150, 155, 199
exercise 40–3
exercise therapies
dance movement therapy **112–13**
eurythmy 124
eutony **115**
polarity yoga 102, 103
qigong **99**
t'ai chi ch'uan **100–1**
yoga **108–11**
expression (essential oils) 62
external ear 222
external ear canal 222
eyeballs 220
eyes
Bates method **114**
common ailments 114, *220–1*
iridology **195**
structure & functions 114, 220

F

facet joints 254
facial bones 225
facial nerve 207
facials
aromatherapy 64
cleansing, for acne 216
facilitated subluxations (chiropractic) 75
fainting, first aid *317*
faith healing 105
fallopian tubes 264
family therapy (psychotherapy) 163
farsightedness *114*
fascia 82
fats, dietary 35
feelings *see* emotions
feet
athlete's foot *215*
massage therapies *see* metamorphic technique; reflexology
verrucae *215*
Feldenkrais, Moshe 85
Feldenkrais method **85**
feng shui **184–5**
fertilization 264
fevers, children's *281*
fiber 36, 151
fibrocystic breast disease *272*
fibroids *274*
fibromyalgia syndrome 251
fibrositis 251
fight-or-flight response
effect of autogenic training 168
effect of meditation 174
role in anxiety & stress 27, 38, 170, 171, 174, 287, 290
first aid *316–17*
homeopathic 130
sports injuries *261*
Western herbalism 139
fitness, physical 40–3
Fitzgerald, William H. 66, 67
five elements
Ayurveda 144, 145
Traditional Chinese Medicine 102, 140, 141, 184
fixations *see* subluxations
Fleiss, Wilhelm 189
flexibility 40–1
flotation therapy **177**
flower remedies & essences, Bach & California 132–3
flu *see* influenza
FMG (fibromyalgia syndrome) 251
focusing (eyesight) 114
follicle-stimulating hormone 264
follicles, hair 214
Fontaine, J. A. 157
food
digestion 149, 230
effect on mood & feelings 37, 116
food-combining 152
see also diets; nutrition
food allergies *302*
and clinical ecology 154, 192, 302
food intolerances & sensitivities 302, *303*
clinical ecology 154, 155, 192, 303
nutritional testing **199**
foreskin 276
balanitis *276*
forgetfulness *see* memory impairment
four examinations (Traditional Chinese Medicine) 92, 97, 142
fovea centralis 114
free radicals 37, 306
Freud, Anna 182
Freud, Sigmund 160, 162, 166, 182
friction (massage) 57
frontal lobe 77
frostbite *249*
frottage (massage) 57
frozen shoulder *253*
FSH (follicle-stimulating hormone) 264
Fu Hsi 184
full-spectrum light 188
functional integration 85
fungal infections *see* infections
Funk, Casimir 148
future trends, health care 20–1

G

Galen 134
gallbladder 149, 230, 233
gallstones *233*
galvanic skin response sensor (biofeedback device) 169
gas *238*
gastric ulcers 231
gastritis *231*
gastroenteritis *230*
gate control theory (pain mechanism) 91, 314
Gattefossé, René-Maurice 62
gemstones
crystal therapy **133**
gem essences 132
genital area infections *215*, *217*, 235, *273*, *276*
genital herpes *217*
geomancy **185**
geopathic stress 185, 198
Gerard, John 134
German measles *281*
Gerson, Max 152
Gerson therapy, for cancer 152, 307
Gestalt therapy (psychotherapy) 165
Ghadiali, Dinshah P. 186
gingivitis *229*
glands
adenoids 280
adrenal 262
endocrine system 262
liver 149, 230
hepatitis *233*
lymph 308
ovaries 262, 264
pancreas 149, 230, 262, 263

pineal 188, 262, 293
pituitary 262, 264
prostate 276
common ailments *277*
salivary (parotid) 282
sebaceous 216
sweat 214
testes 262, 276, 282
thymus 262, 308
thyroid 262
hypothyroidism *262*
reflexology treatment 68
glans of the penis 276
balanitis *276*
Glaser, Ronald 19
glaucoma *221*
glue ear *280*
goiter 262
Goodheart, George 196
gout *259*
gray matter 175
Green, Elmer & Alyce 169
grief *293*
Grinder, John 164
grounding (bioenergetics) 89
group therapy (psychotherapy) 162
guided imagery (visualization) 178, 179
gums, gingivitis *229*
gut flora 149

H

hacking (massage) 57
Hahnemann, Samuel 126
hair analysis **194**
hair follicles 214
hakomi **115**
halitosis *229*
hands
cloud hands (t'ai chi ch'uan) 101
Kirlian photography **201**
laying on of *see* healing
massage therapies *see* metamorphic technique; reflexology
structure 250
Swedish/Western massage 60
hara diagnosis 96, 97, **194**
hard palate 228
Hart, Roy 190
hatha yoga 108–11
Hay diet 152
hay fever *299*
Hayashi, Chujiro 107
head
cranial osteopathy 81
CranioSacral therapy **81**
Indian head massage **115**
massage therapies *see* Metamorphic technique
headaches & migraines *210–11*
shiatsu treatment 97
head lice *280*
healing **104–5**
see also radionics; reiki; Therapeutic Touch
healing crises (naturopathy) 120
healing energy 104, 105, 106, 157
health & fitness questionnaires 28–32, 42, 43
health care, future trends 20–1
healthy eating 34–7
hearing problems *see* ears, common ailments
heart & circulation
cardiovascular endurance 40
common ailments *242–9*
effect of massage 57
optimum heart rate 40
structure & functions 242
heart attack *247*
heart failure *246*
heart valve disease *246*
heartbeat, irregular *see* palpitations
heartburn *232*
heavy periods *265*
Heller, Joseph 84
Hellerwork **84**
helper T-cells 308
hemispheres, cerebral 175, 178, 206, 208
hemoglobin 248
hemorrhoids *238*
hepatitis *233*
herbal synergy (Western herbalism) 134, 135
herbalism
in Ayurveda 144, 146, 147
Chinese **140–3**
Western **134–9**
in naturopathy 119
Hering, Constantine 126
herpes virus infections *217*, 283
high blood pressure *244–5*
Hill, Adrian 182
hippocampus 63, 77, 286
Hippocrates 56, 70, 118, 126, 154, 195
hips
reflexology treatment 68
Rolfing 83
histamine 298, 299, 308
HIV infection 310
hives *216*, 302
hoarseness *see* laryngitis
holism & holistic medicine 8, 12–13, 158
in Traditional Chinese Medicine 140
homeopathy **126–30**
biochemic tissue salts **131**
homeostasis 13, 26, 27, 118, 119, 134
hook up (Tragerwork) 88
hormonal problems
acne *216*
diabetes mellitus *263*
during menopause 270–1, 294
hypothyroidism *262*
lack of sex drive *294*
obesity *263*
postnatal depression *269*
seasonal affective disorder (SAD) 188, *293*
see also reproductive system, women, common ailments
hormones 262
female reproductive system 264
psychoneuroimmunology 18–19
sex *see* estrogen; progesterone; testosterone
stress 27, 38, 56, 171, 262, 290
see also adrenaline (stress); insulin (blood sugar); melatonin (body rhythms); noradrenaline (stress); thyroxin (metabolism)
hostility & anger 44–5
hot compresses (hydrotherapy) 123
hot responders (psychological type) 45
housemaid's knee 253
Hughes, Richard 130
human immunodeficiency virus (HIV) infection 310
humanistic psychotherapy 165
humor & laughter 46–7
humors (Tibetan medicine) 157
Huxley, Aldous 114
hydrotherapy **122–3**
colonic **157**
in naturopathy 119
hyperactivity *284*
hypertension *see* high blood pressure
hyperventilation 286, *288*
hypnotherapy **166–7**
past life therapy **190**
hypotension *see* low blood pressure
hypothalamus 62, 63, 77, 188, 262
hypothyroidism *262*

I

ibn-Sina, Ali (Avicenna) 62
IBS *see* irritable bowel syndrome
IDDM (insulin-dependent diabetes mellitus) 263
IgE (immunoglobulin E) 199, 298, 303
IgG (immunoglobulin G) 199
illness, undifferentiated, compared to disease 24–5
illumination therapy 187
imbalance, causes 26–7
immune system
common ailments *309–13* *see also* allergies; autoimmune diseases
psychoneuroimmunology 18–19
structure & functions 298, 308
immunization 308
childhood infectious illnesses 278, 282, 283
immunoglobulins 199, 298
incontinence
fecal *see* diarrhea
urinary *241*
bed-wetting *285*
Indian head massage **115**
Indian medicine, traditional *see* Ayurveda
indigestion *232*
infections
childhood illnesses *281–3*
digestive system 230, 231, 233, 235, 239
ears 222, *223*, 280
eyes 221
genital area *215*, *217*, 235, *273*, *276*
herpes viruses *217*, 283
HIV 310
immune system reaction 308
infectious mononucleosis *309*
mouth & throat 228–9
nails 219
respiratory system 224–7, 279
skin 214, 215, 216, 217
urinary system 240, *275*
inferior vena cava 242
infertility
men *277*
women *266–7*
inflammatory bowel disease *see* Crohn's disease; ulcerative colitis
influenza *227*
infused oils (herbal remedies) 137
infusions (herbal remedies) 137
Ingham, Eunice 66, 67
Ingham Reflex Method of Compression Massage 66
ingrown toenails 219
inhalations, aromatherapy 65
injuries
minor, first aid *316–17*
sports *261*
insoluble fiber 36
insomnia *289*
children 284
insulin 262, 263
insulin-dependent diabetes mellitus 263
integrated medicine *see* holism & holistic medicine
intellectual cycle (biorhythms) 189
intercourse, painful sexual *294*
interference patterns (Kirlian photography) 201
intervertebral disks 256
intestines 149, 230
problems *see* digestion & digestive system, common ailments
reflexology treatment 68
intolerances, food *see* food intolerances & sensitivities
iridology **195**
iris (part of eye) 195, 220
iron-deficiency anemia 151, 248
irregular periods *265*
irritable bowel syndrome 149, *236–7*
Iscador (anthroposophical medicine) 125, 306
isopathic treatment (homeopathy) 126

J

Jacobson, Edmund 170
Janov, Arthur 165
jaundice 233
Jensen, Bernard 195
Ji Buo 140
jin shin do (acupressure) 95
jitsu (Traditional Chinese Medicine) 96
Jivaka Kumar Bhaccha 98
joints 250
ankylosing spondylitis *261*
arthritis *258–60*
bursitis *253*
facet 254
flexibility 40–1
frozen shoulder *253*
manipulation therapies *see* chiropractic; osteopathy
see also musculoskeletal system
Jung, Carl 112, 160, 162, 182
Jungian analytic psychotherapy 162

K

kahuna **115**
kapha (Ayurveda) 145, 192, 193
karma, in anthroposophical medicine 124
Katz, Richard 132

Kellogg, John 118
Kelly, George 164
Kent, James Tyler 126
keratin 214
ki see qi
kidney stones 240, *241*
kidneys 240
Kiecolt-Glaser, Janice 19
killer T-cells 308
kinesiology *see* Applied Kinesiology
Kirlian, Semyon & Valentina 201
Kirlian photography **201**
kissing disease *see* infectious mononucleosis
kits, first aid 130, 139, 316
Klein, Melanie 160, 182
kneading (massage) 57
knee, housemaid's 253
Kneipp, Father Sebastian 118, 122
knuckling (massage) 58
Krieger, Dolores 106
Kunz, Dora 106
Kurtz, Ron 115
kyo (Traditional Chinese Medicine) 96

L

Laban, Rudolf 112
labor *269*
laetrile therapy, for cancer 307
large intestine 149, 230
  colonic hydrotherapy (colonic irrigation) **157**
  reflexology treatment 68
laryngitis *229*
larynx 228
laser acupuncture 94
laughter & humor 46–7
law of potentization (homeopathy) 126, 127
law of similars (homeopathy) 126, 127
laws of cure (homeopathy) 126
laying on of hands *see* healing
legs
  sciatica *256*
  Swedish/Western massage 60
lens of the eye 114, 220
ley lines 185
LH (luteinizing hormone) 264
Li Shizhen 140
libido, loss of 294
lice, head lice *280*
life energy
  in crystal therapy 133
  in polarity therapy 102, 103
  see also chakras; *prana*; *qi*
lift (osteopathy) 79, 80
lifting (biodynamic massage) 61
ligaments 250
light therapy **188**
  in color therapy 186, 187
  psoriasis 188, 218
like cures like (homeopathy theory) 126, 127
Lilly, John C. 177
limbic system 286
Lindlahr, Henry 118
Ling, Per Henrik 56, 57
Littlejohn, John Martin 76
liver 149, 230
  hepatitis *233*
  polarity liver flush & tea 103
low blood pressure *246*
Lowen, Alexander 89
lumbar region 79
lumbar roll (chiropractic) 74
lumpy breasts *see* fibrocystic breast disease
lungs 171, 224
  problems *see* asthma; respiratory system, common ailments
luo pan compass (feng shui tool) 184
Lust, Benedict 118
luteinizing hormone 264
Luthe, Wolfgang 168
lux (light measurement) 188
lymph nodes 308
lymphatic pumping (naturopathy) 121
lymphatic system, effect of massage 57, 58, 64
lymphocytes 308, 309, 310

M

maceration (essential oils) 62
macrobiotic diet 152
macrophages 212
McTimoney & McTimoney-Corley chiropractic **75**
McTimoney, John 75
macula 221
macular degeneration *221*
magnetic therapy **156**
magnetotherapy *see* magnetic therapy
Maharishi Ayur-Ved 144
Maharishi Mahesh 144, 174
malas (Ayurveda) 144
manipulation therapies *see* chiropractic; functional integration; massage; osteopathy
Manners, Peter 180
Manning, Matthew 105
mantra meditation 176
  see also Transcendental Meditation
manual lymph drainage (massage) 58
maps
  ba-gua (feng shui) 184
  irises 195
  meridians & acupoints 90, 91, 94
  reflex points 67
marma points (Ayurveda) 146, 147
marriage counseling 163
Maslow, Abraham 160, 165
massage
  acupressure **95**
  aromatherapy **62–5**
  Aston-Patterning **83**
  in Ayurveda 56, 98, 115, 146, 147
  biodynamic **61**
  chavutti thirumal **115**, 146
  do-in **98**
  Hellerwork **84**
  Indian head massage **115**
  Ingham Reflex Method of Compression Massage 66
  kahuna **115**
  manual lymph drainage 58
  Metamorphic technique **69**
  in naturopathy 119
  in osteopathy *see* soft tissue treatment
  in polarity therapy 103
  reflexology **66–9**
  remedial 58
  Rolfing **82–3**
  shiatsu **96–7**
  Swedish/Western **56–61**
    in aromatherapy 64
  Thai **98**
mast cells 298
mastalgia 272
Matthews-Simonton, Stephanie 178
Maury, Marguerite 62
ME *see* chronic fatigue syndrome
measles *282*
  German measles *281*
median nerve 206
medical acupuncture 90, 91
medical aromatherapy **65**
medical herbalism 134
meditation **174–7**
  in qigong 99
  in t'ai chi ch'uan 100
  Tragerwork practitioners 88
megaloblastic anemia 248
megavitamin therapy *see* orthomolecular therapy
melanin 214
melatonin 188, 262, 293
membranes
  mucous 224, 225, 226
  tympanic 222
memory impairment *209*
men
  infertility *277*
  reproductive system
    common ailments *276–7*
    structure & functions 276
  sperm & sperm production 266, 276, 277
menopause *270–1*
  osteoporosis *257*
  sexual problems 294
menstruation & menstrual cycle 264
  common ailments *264–5*
mental illness, effect of brain chemistry 286
mental problems *see* psychological problems
mentastics (Tragerwork) 88
meridians
  in acupressure 95
  in *hara* diagnosis 96, 97, **194**
  meridian pulses 92, 142
  in qigong 99
  theory & location 90, 91, 94, 140
Mermet, Abbé 198
Mesmer, Franz Anton 156, 166
mesmerism 166
meta-analysis, clinical trials 16
Metamorphic technique **69**
miasms (homeopathy) 126
midbrain 206
middle ear infections 222, 223, 280
migraines *see* headaches & migraines
mind/body interactions 12–13, 18–19
mindfulness (meditation) 176
minerals
  as antioxidants 37, 305–6
  individual minerals & their actions 35, 151, 306
  orthomolecular therapy **153**
  as supplements 36, 121, 149, 151
  whole blood mineral analysis 199
minor injuries, first aid *316–17*
mirroring (dance movement therapy) 112, 113
molecular imprinting (Bach Flower Remedies) 132
mononucleosis *309*
monounsaturated fats 35
mood foods 37
MORA device (energy medicine) 200
Morell, Franz 200
Moreno, Jacob 165
morning sickness *268*
mother tincture (homeopathy) 127
motion palpation (chiropractic) 72
Motoyama, Hiroshi 200
mouth & throat
  common ailments *228–9*
  oral candidiasis 235
  structure & functions 149, 228, 230
movement & posture reeducation therapies
  Alexander technique **86–7**
  Aston-Patterning **83**
  Feldenkrais method **85**
  Hellerwork **84**
  see also exercise therapies
moxa & moxibustion (acupuncture) 92, 93
MS *see* multiple sclerosis
mucous colitis *see* irritable bowel syndrome
mucous membranes 224, 225, 226
mucus, in respiratory system 224, 225, 227, 279
multiple sclerosis *212*
mumps *282*
muscles
  Applied Kinesiology **196–7**
  cramp *250*
  diaphragm 171
  eye 220
  fascia 82
  heart 242
  muscle pain *251*
  muscle testing (clinical ecology) 155
  muscular strength & endurance 40
  pelvic floor 240
  progressive muscle relaxation 170, 173
  Psoas muscle test (chiropractic) 73
  see also musculoskeletal system
musculoskeletal system 77
  common ailments *250–61*
  effect of exercise 40–1
  manipulation therapies *see* chiropractic; functional integration; massage; osteopathy
  structure & functions 250
music therapy **181**
  see also sound therapy
myalgic encephalomyelitis *see* chronic fatigue syndrome
myocardial infarction *see* heart attack
myofascial pain 251

N

nadis (Ayurveda) 109, 115, 192
nail problems 150, *219*
natural killer cells 18, 19, 47, 308, 309, 310
natural medicine *see* naturopathy
nature cure *see* naturopathy
naturopathy **118–21**, 148
  see also hydrotherapy

Naumberg, Margaret 182
nausea & vomiting *231*
morning sickness *268*
nearsightedness 114
neck, reflexology treatment 68
needles, acupuncture 90, 92, 93
negative emotions 44–5
Nelson, Bill 200
nerve deafness 223
nerves
auditory 222
autonomic nervous system 71
facial 207
median 206
nerve cells 314
nerve fiber damage in multiple sclerosis 212
olfactory system 63
optic 220
peripheral 206, 207
spinal 71
trigeminal 207
nervous system *see* brain & nervous system
nettle rash *see* hives
network spinal analysis 75
neuralgia *207*
neuritis *see* neuropathy
neurolinguistic programming (psychotherapy) 164
neuropathy *207*
neuropeptides 18–19
neurotransmitters 18, 37, 286
NIDDM (noninsulin-dependent diabetes mellitus) 263
NLP (psychotherapy) 164
Nogier, Paul 94, 192
noninsulin-dependent diabetes mellitus 263
nonrapid eye movement sleep 39
nonspecific urethritis *240*
Nordoff, Paul 181
nosodes (homeopathic remedies) 126
NREM (nonrapid eye movement) sleep 39
nutrition
nutritional testing **199**, 150
nutritional therapies **148–52**
optimum 34–7

O

obesity *263*
object meditation 176
obsessive-compulsive disorder *288*
occlusion machine (energy medicine) 200
oils
carrier 64, 139
essential 62–5, 139
infused 137
in *shirodhara* (Ayurveda) 147
in Swedish/Western massage 58
ointments (herbal remedies) 137
olfactory system 63
oncogenes 304
open-angle glaucoma 221
optic nerve 220
optimum heart rate 40
optimum nutrition 34–7
orgasm, inability to achieve *294*
Ornish, Dean 152, 243
Ornish reversal diet 152, 243
orthomolecular therapy **153**
Osawa, George 152
ossicles 222
osteoarthritis *258*
Western herbal remedies 138, 139
see also cervical spondylosis
osteopathy **76–81**
cranial 81
in naturopathy 119
osteoporosis *257*
otosclerosis 223
Ott, John 188
ova 264
ovaries 262, 264
overbreathing 170
overflow incontinence 241
oxygen/carbon dioxide exchange 170, 171, 224, 242
oxygen/ozone therapy **157**

P

pain
backache *254–5*
breast *272*
colic *279*
during sexual intercourse *294*
menstrual *265*
muscle *251*
myofascial 251
persistent (chronic) *314–15*
sciatica *256*
teething *279*
transmission of 77, 314
pain gates 314
pain signals 77, 314
pain-tension cycle 77
palate 228
Palmer, B. J. 70, 75
Palmer, Daniel D. 70, 75
palming (Bates method) 114
palpitations *247*
PAM (sound therapy) 180
panchakarma (Ayurveda) 146, 147
pancreas 149, 230, 262, 263
panic attacks *288*
Paracelsus 134
Paré, Ambroise 56
parotid glands 282
passive concentration (autogenic training) 168
past life therapy **190**
Patanjali 108
patch tests, for allergies 298
pattern of disharmony (Traditional Chinese Medicine) 93, 142
patterns of misuse (Alexander technique) 86
Pavek, Richard R. 115
Pavlov, Ivan 164
Peczely, Ignatz von 195
pediatric osteopathy *see* cranial osteopathy
pelvic alignment (osteopathy test) 78
pelvic floor muscles 240
pelvic inflammatory disease *274*
pelvis
reflexology treatment 68
Rolfing 83
pendulum dowsing 198
penis 276
balanitis *276*
peptic ulcers *231*
periods, painful, irregular, or heavy *265*
peripheral nerves 206, 207
peristalsis 149, 236
psychoperistalsis 61
Perls, Fritz 160, 165
pernicious anemia 248
persistent (chronic) pain *314–15*
personal construct therapy (psychotherapy) 164
personal growth movement 160, 165
Pert, Candace 18–19
pesticides & additives 36–7
petrissage (massage) 57
phagocytes 308
pharynx 149, 228
phlebitis *249*
phlegm 224, 226
phobias *286*, 288
photography, diagnostic *see* iridology; Kirlian photography
physical cycle (biorhythms) 189
physical fitness 40–3
physical reeducation therapies *see* exercise therapies; movement & posture reeducation therapies
physioacoustic methodology (sound therapy) 180
physiotherapy 56
PID (pelvic inflammatory disease) *274*
piles *see* hemorrhoids
pineal gland 188, 262, 293
pink eye *see* conjunctivitis
pinna 222
Pirquet, Baron Clemens von 154
pitta (Ayurveda) 145, 192, 193
pituitary gland 262, 264
placebo controlled clinical trials 16
placebo response 13, 16, 17
plant material processing
essential oil extraction 62
for herbal remedies 135
plantar warts *see* verrucae
PMS (premenstrual syndrome) *264*
pneumonia *227*
polarity
in anthroposophical medicine 124
in polarity therapy 102
polarity liver flush & tea (polarity therapy) 103
polarity therapy **102–3**
polarity yoga 102, 103
polyunsaturated fats 35
popularity & users, complementary therapies 8–9, 14–15
positive emotions & thinking 46–7, 178, 179
post-traumatic stress disorder *288*
postnatal depression *269*
posture reeducation therapies *see* movement & posture reeducation therapies
postures
qigong 99
t'ai chi ch'uan 100, 101
yoga (*asanas*) 108–11
potentization
anthroposophical medicines 125
homeopathic remedies 126, 127
poultices, cabbage leaf 138
practitioners
finding & choosing 318
professional organizations 318
addresses 319–23
training 160–1, 318
prakriti (Ayurveda) 145
prana (Ayurveda) 98, 108, 109, 144, 192
pranayama (yoga) 108
precautions, safety 25, **52**, *204*, 318
pregnancy & childbirth 41, *268–9*
premature ejaculation *295*
premenstrual syndrome *264*
prenatal therapy *see* Metamorphic technique
Priessnitz, Vincent 122
primal therapy (psychotherapy) 165
primary dysmenorrhea 265
professional organizations
addresses 319–23
practitioners 318
progesterone 264, 270
progressive muscle relaxation 170, 173
prolapse *275*
prolapsed disk *256*
prostaglandins 314
prostate enlargement *277*
prostate gland 276
common ailments *277*
prostatitis *277*
proteins 35, 152
provocation neutralization (clinical ecology) 155, 303
Psoas muscle test (chiropractic) 73
psoriasis 188, *218*
psychoanalysis 160, 162
psychodrama 165
psychodynamic therapy 162
psychological problems 269, 286–97
childhood behavioral problems 284–5
during menopause 270
effect on health 19
and pain perception 314
see also individually by name e.g., anxiety; depression; insomnia; phobias; stress
psychological realm & challenges 26–7
psychology & psychologists 160
psychoneuroimmunology 9, 18–19
psychoperistalsis (biodynamic massage) 61
psychosexual therapy 163
psychosynthesis 165
psychotherapies
art therapy **182–3**
biodynamic massage **61**
bioenergetics **89**
dance movement therapy **112–13**
hypnotherapy **166–7**
Metamorphic technique **69**
music therapy **181**
past life therapy **190**
psychotherapy & counseling **160–5**
pulmonary artery 242
pulp, dental 229
pulse diagnosis **192**
Ayurveda 146, 192
pulse taking (Traditional Chinese Medicine) 92, 140, 142, 192
pulse tests (clinical ecology) 155, 192
punching (t'ai chi ch'uan) 101

pupil of the eye 220
Purce, Jill 180

Q

qi or *ki*
  in acupressure 95
  in acupuncture 90, 91, 92
  and diagnostic tests 192, 193, 194
  in do-in 98
  in energy medicine 200
  in feng shui 184, 185
  flow through body 90, 91, 97, 101, 140, 170
  in qigong 99
  in reiki 107
  in shiatsu 96, 97
  in t'ai chi ch'uan 100, 101
qigong **99**
  see also t'ai chi ch'uan
questionnaires
  fitness & exercise 42, 43
  hostility 44
  therapy choice **50–1**
  well-being 28–32

R

Radio Allergosorbent Test 155, 298
radionics **157**, 198
rainbow dance (qigong) 99
Randolph, Theron G. 140
randomized controlled trials 16
rapid eye movement sleep 39
rasayana (Ayurveda) 146, 147
rashes
  childhood infectious illnesses *281–3*
  diaper rash *278*
  hives *216*
  shingles *217*, 283
RAST (Radio Allergosorbent Test) 155, 298
ratings of therapies, explanation **52**, *204*
raw-foods diet 152
Raynaud's disease & Raynaud's phenomenon *249*
RDA (recommended daily allowances), dietary supplements 151, 153
realms of the body 26
  in Applied Kinesiology 196
rebirthing (psychotherapy) 165
receptive imagery (visualization) 178
receptors (nerves) 314
recommended daily allowances, dietary supplements 151, 153
rectum 149, 230
red light signals & symptoms 25, *204*
reflex points (reflexology) 66, 67
reflex recoil adjustment (chiropractic) 75
reflexology **66–9**
  vacuflex 68
regression *see* past life therapy
Reich, Wilhelm 61, 89, 112
reiki **107**
relationships & emotional support 19
relaxation & breathing **170–3**
relaxation response 13, 170
release work (chiropractic) 74
religious & spiritual beliefs 13
REM (rapid eye movement) sleep 39
remedial massage 58
remedies
  Bach Flower **132–3**
  herbal
    Ayurvedic 144, 146, 147
    Chinese 143
    Western 134–9
  homeopathic 126–30
Rentsch, Ossie 115
repertories, homeopathic 128
repetitive strain injury *252*
  see also carpal tunnel syndrome
reproductive system
  genital area infections *215, 217, 235, 273, 276*
  men
    common ailments *276–7*
    structure & functions 276
  women
    common ailments *264–7, 273–5*
    menopause *270–1*
    pregnancy & childbirth 41, *268–9*
    structure & functions 264
research & clinical trials 16–17
respiratory system
  asthma 298, *300–1*, 302
  common ailments *224–7*
  croup *279*
  structure & functions 171, 224
Reston, James 90
retina 114, 220
rheumatoid arthritis *260*
rhinitis, allergic *299*, 302
ringworm *215*
Robbins, Clive 181
Rogers, Carl 160
Rolf, Ida 82, 83
Rolfing **82–3**, 84
roof of the mouth 228
rosacea *215*
RSI (repetitive strain injury) *252*
  see also carpal tunnel syndrome
rubella *see* German measles
Ryodoraku (energy medicine) 200

S

sacro-occipital technique (cranial osteopathy) 81
SAD (seasonal affective disorder) 188, *293*
safety issues & precautions 25, **52**, *204*, 318
St. John, Robert 69
St. Pierre, Gaston 69
saliva 230
salivary glands 282
salts, Schüssler *see* biochemic tissue salts
Satir, Virginia 160
saturated fats 35
saunas (hydrotherapy) 123
scalds & burns, first aid *317*
scalp, dandruff *219*
scavenger cells 212
Scheel, John 118
Schimmel, Helmut 200
schizophrenia 153, *212*
Schultz, Johannes 168
Schüssler, Wilhelm 131
Schüssler salts *see* biochemic tissue salts
sciatica *256*
sclera 220
seawater treatments (hydrotherapy) 123
seasonal affective disorder 188, *293*
sebaceous glands 216
seborrheic eczema 218
sebum 216
secondary dysmenorrhea 265
self-healing 27
self-hypnosis 167
Selye, Hans 26–7
semicircular canals 222
seminal vesicles 276
senile dementia *209*
sensitivities, food *see* food intolerances & sensitivities
sensory deprivation chambers (flotation tanks) 177
sensory nerve endings 314
serotonin 37, 45, 188, 286, 293
sex drive, lack of *294*
sex hormones *see* estrogen; progesterone; testosterone
sexual counseling (psychotherapy) 163
sexual dysfunction 294–5
sexual intercourse, painful *294*
shaman (Ayurveda) 146
shamanism **190**
shen tao (acupressure) 95
SHEN therapy **115**
shiatsu **96–7**
  see also do-in
shingles *217*, 283
shirodhara (Ayurveda) 147
shock, first aid *317*
shodan (Ayurveda) 146
shoulders
  frozen shoulder *253*
  Swedish/Western massage 60
sickle-cell anemia 248
side roll (osteopathy) 79
sight problems *see* eyes, common ailments
signals, pain 77, 314
signatures, doctrine of 134
Silva, José 190
Silva method **190**
similars, law of (homeopathy) 126, 127
similimum (homeopathy) 130
Simonton, Carl 178
simple carbohydrates 34
sinuses 121, 225
  reflexology treatment 68
sinusitis *225*
  naturopathic treatment 121
sitz baths (hydrotherapy) 123
skin
  common ailments *214–19*
  diaper rash *278*
  sensory nerve endings 314
  structure & functions 214
skin-brushing (naturopathy) 121
skin-prick tests, for allergies 155, 298
skin temperature gauge (biofeedback device) 169
skin tests, for allergies 155, 298
Skinner, Burrhus Frederic 160
sleep 39
sleep problems
  children *284*
  insomnia *289*
slipped disk *see* prolapsed disk
small intestine 149, 230
Smith, Fritz 115
soft palate 228
soft tissue treatment (osteopathy) 77, 78, 79, 80
soluble fiber 36
solution-focused brief therapy (psychotherapy) 163
sore throat *228*
sound therapy **180**
  see also music therapy
space clearing (feng shui) 184
spas & spa towns 118, 122
spastic colon *see* irritable bowel syndrome
speech problems, stammering *285*
sperm & sperm production 266, 276, 277
spinal column 250
spinal cord 71, 206, 250
spinal nerves 71
spinal traction (chiropractic) 74
spine 71
  ankylosing spondylitis *261*
  color spine charts (color therapy) 187, 198
  CranioSacral therapy **81**
  manipulation therapies *see* chiropractic; osteopathy
  network spinal analysis 75
  Rolfing 83
  structure & functions 250
spiritual & religious beliefs 13
spiritual healing 105
  see also reiki
spiritualist healing 104–5
splashing (Bates method) 114
spleen 308
spondylitis, ankylosing *261*
spondylosis, cervical *259*
sports & exercise 40–3
sports injuries *261*
stammering *285*
steam baths (hydrotherapy) 122, 123
steam treatment
  for acne 216
  aromatherapy inhalations 65
Steiner, Rudolf 124, 182
sties *221*
Still, Andrew Taylor 76
stings & bites, first aid *317*
stomach 230
  problems *see* digestion & digestive system, common ailments
Stone, Randolph 102
stress 38, *290–1*
  adaptation to 27
  effect on immune system & health 19, 27, 171
  and food intolerances 303
  geopathic 185, 198
  and visualization techniques 179
  see also fight-or-flight response
stress hormones 27, 38, 56, 171, 262, 290
stress incontinence 241
stressors 38, 290
stroke *213*
stroking (massage) 57
structural integration *see* Rolfing
structural realm & challenges 26–7

structural subluxations (chiropractic) 75
sublingual drop tests (clinical ecology) 155
subluxations (chiropractic) 71, 75
succussion (homeopathic remedies) 127
sugars 34, 37
suggestion hypnotherapy 167
sun salutation (yoga) 111
Sun (t'ai chi ch'uan) 100
superior vena cava 242
supplements, dietary 36, 121, 149, 151
suppressor T-cells 308
Sutherland, William Garner 81
sweat glands 214
Swedish massage **56–61**
  in aromatherapy 64
swinging (Bates method) 114
Swoboda, Hermann 189
symptom picture (homeopathy) 128
symptoms, red light 25, *204*
synergy, herbal (Western herbalism) 134, 135
systematic review, clinical trials 16

T

T-cells 308, 309, 310
t'ai chi ch'uan **100–1**
Takata, Hawaio 107
Tamai Tempaku 96
tanden (Traditional Chinese Medicine) 97, 194
tapotement (massage) 57
taste buds 228
TCM *see* Traditional Chinese Medicine
teeth 228, 229
  teething *279*
  toothache *229*
Teltscher, Alfred 189
temper tantrums *285*
tendinitis *252*
tendons 250, 252
tennis elbow *252*
testes 262, 276
testosterone 262, 276, 294
tests *see* diagnosis
Thai massage **98**
thalamus 63, 77
thalassemia 248
thalassotherapy (hydrotherapy) 123
Therapeutic Touch **106**
therapies section, how to use **52–3**
therapy choice questionnaire **50–1**
therapy ratings, explanation of **52**, *204*
Thie, John 197
thighs, Swedish/Western massage 60
Thomas test (chiropractic) 73
Thomson, Samuel 134
thought in activity (Alexander technique) 87
thought-stopping (emotion management technique) 45
throat *see* mouth & throat
thrombophlebitis 249
thrush *see* candidiasis
thymus gland 262, 308
thyroid gland 262
  hypothyroidism *262*
  reflexology treatment 68
Tibetan medicine **157**
tinctures
  herbal remedies 137, 138
  mother tincture (homeopathy) 127
tinea *see* ringworm
tinnitus *222*
tissue salts *see* biochemic tissue salts
TM (Transcendental Meditation) 174, 175, 176
toenails, ingrown 219
toggle drop/recoil (chiropractic) 74, 75
Tomatis, Alfred 180
Tomatis method (sound therapy) 180
tongue 228
tongue diagnosis **193**
tonsillitis *228*
toothache *229*
Touch for Health **197**
toxins 37, 148, 149, 151, 154, 303
  ama (Ayurveda) 144
trace elements 35
trachea 171, 224
Traditional Chinese Medicine **140–1**
  acupressure **95**
  acupuncture **90–4**
  Chinese herbalism **140–3**
  feng shui **184–5**
  five elements 102, 140, 141, 184
  four examinations 92, 97, 142
  holism 140
  pulse-taking 92, 140, 142, 192
  qigong **99**
  shiatsu **96–7**
  t'ai chi ch'uan **100–1**
  tongue diagnosis 193
  vital substances 140
  yin/yang principle 90, 91, 140–1, 193
  see also meridians; *qi*
traditional Indian medicine *see* Ayurveda
Trager, Milton 88
Tragerwork (Trager psychophysical integration) **88**
training, practitioners 160–1, 318
transactional analysis (psychotherapy) 165
Transcendental Meditation 174, 175, 176
transference (psychoanalysis) 162
transpersonal therapy (psychotherapy) 165
trans-saturated fats 35
triad of health
  in Applied Kinesiology 196
  in naturopathy 119
tridosha (Ayurveda) 146
trigeminal nerve 207
trigger points (muscles) 250, 251
trigrams 90, 184
triple burner (*hara* diagnosis) 194
tryptophan 37
tsubos see acupoints
TT *see* Therapeutic Touch
tuina (acupressure) 95, 96
Turkish baths (hydrotherapy) 123
12-step program (psychotherapy) 164
tympanic membrane 222
type A behavior (psychological type) 45

U

ulcerative colitis *234*
ulcers
  mouth (aphthous) *229*
  peptic (gastric & duodenal) *231*
ultraviolet light 188
undifferentiated illnesses 24–5
unsaturated fats 35
Upledger, John 81
ureters 240
urethra 240
urethritis, nonspecific *240*
urge incontinence 241
urinary incontinence *241*
  bed-wetting *285*
urinary system
  common ailments *240–1*, *275*
  structure & functions 240
urine 240
urticaria *see* hives
users & popularity, complementary therapies 8–9, 14–15
Usui, Mikao 107
uterus 264
  fibroids *274*
  prolapse *275*
UV (ultraviolet) light 188

V

vaccination *see* immunization
vacuflex reflexology 68
vagina 264
vaginal dryness 294
vaginismus *295*
vaginitis *273*
Valnet, Jean 62, 65
valves, heart 246
vaporizers, aromatherapy 65
varicose veins *248*
vas deferens 276
vata (Ayurveda) 145, 192, 193
Vega machine & testing 150, 155, 200
vegetarian & vegan diets 152
veins 242
  varicose *248*
vena cava 242
ventricles 242
verrucae *215*
vertebrae 250, 254, 256
vertigo *208*
vibrational energy frequencies (dowsing) 198
vipassana (meditation) 176
viral infections *see* infections
vision education *see* Bates method
visual problems *see* eyes, common ailments
visualization 47, **178–9**
vital energies (Ayurveda) *see doshas*
vital force
  in dowsing 198
  in homeopathy 126, 127
  in naturopathy 118, 119
  prana 98, 108, 109, 144, 192
  in Western herbalism 134
  see also energy
vital substances (Traditional Chinese Medicine) 140
vitamins
  as antioxidants 37, 305–6
  blood vitamin analysis 199
  discovery 148
  individual vitamins & their actions 34, 151, 306
  orthomolecular therapy **153**
  as supplements 36, 121, 151
voice box 228
voice loss *see* laryngitis
voice therapy **190**
Voll, Reinhold 200
vomiting *see* nausea & vomiting
von Peczely, Ignatz 195
von Pirquet, Baron Clemens 154
vulva 264
vulvitis *273*

W

Wall, Vicky 190
warrior stretch (yoga) 110
warts *215*
water memory (homeopathic remedies) 127
water therapies *see* flotation therapy; hydrotherapy
Watson, John 160
wax, ear 222, 223
webbing pinch (reflexology) 68
Wegman, Ita 124
well-being questionnaire 28–32
Western herbalism **134–9**
Western massage **56–61**
  in aromatherapy 64
whirlpool baths (hydrotherapy) 123
white blood cells 308
white matter 175
whooping cough *283*
windpipe 224
witness (radionics) 157, 198
Wolfsohn, Alfred 190
womb *see* uterus
women
  breast problems *272*
  infertility *266–7*
  reproductive system
    common ailments *264–7*, *273–5*
    menopause *270–1*
    pregnancy & childbirth 41, *268–9*
    structure & functions 264
Woo (t'ai chi ch'uan) 100
wraps (hydrotherapy) 123
Wu (t'ai chi ch'uan) 100

Y

yang see yin/yang principle
Yang (t'ai chi ch'uan) 100
yeast infections 235, *273*
Yellow Emperor 140
Yeoman's test (chiropractic) 73
yin/yang principle 90, 91, 140–1, 193
  in macrobiotic diet 152
yoga **108–11**
  in naturopathy 119
  polarity yoga 102, 103
yoga therapy 108

Z

Zero Balancing **115**
zone therapy (reflexology) 66, 67

ACKNOWLEDGMENTS

Authors' Acknowledgments

We are enormously grateful to the many people who contributed in various ways to this book. For their professional advice, we would like to thank Penelope Best, Jill Dunley, Andrew Ferguson, Michael Copland-Griffiths, Clare Harvey, Fiona Hunter, Mark Kane, Dr. Simi Khanna, Peter Mansfield, Judith Morrison, Tuvi Orbach, Anne Palmer and Caroline Stevensen (The Royal London Homeopathic Hospital). In particular, many thanks from David to Sheelagh Taylor, Moira Jenkins, and Pamela Prentice for their help and support, and from Anne to Hilary Boyd, Debbie Cole, and Vicky Peterson for indefatigable research assistance, and to Vivienne Williams (Faculty of Health Sciences, Victoria University of Technology), Wendy Symonds, and Prue Carpenter for information on the Australasian scene. We are also grateful to Professor Edzard Ernst for permission to quote from his book *Complementary Medicine: An Objective Appraisal.*

Finally but not least, a very warm thank you to the Dorling Kindersley team, especially Stephanie Farrow, Claire Benson, Penny Warren and Christa Weil for their patience, good humor and fortitude at all times.

Publisher's Acknowledgments

Dorling Kindersley would like to thank the following for their editorial assistance: Ruth Midgley, Caroline Radula-Scott, Lesley Riley, Lorna Damms, Joy McKnight, Charlotte Evans. Many thanks to Fred and Kathie Gill for proofreading the manuscript, and to Sue Bosanko for compiling the index.

For design assistance Dorling Kindersley would like to thank Tracey Clarke and Grace Brennan, and for illustrations thanks go to John Woodcock, Roy Flooks, and Lydia Umney.

Many thanks too to Joanne Beardwell, Alison McKittrick, and Catherine Edkins for picture research; to Alistair Hughes for additional photography; to Gary Ombler for assisting Andy Crawford during photography; and to Kirsty Young, Ellen Kramer, and Sue Sian for makeup.

Dorling Kindersley are particularly grateful to the following for their expert advice and knowledge: Tracey Alderman, Beatrice Allegranti, Diana Asbridge, Judith Aston, Talia Levin Bar-Yoseph, Dr. Robert Blanks, Cyril Blau (Larkhall Green Farm), Laurena Chamlee-Cole, The Confederation of Radionic and Radiesthesia Organizations, Primrose Cooper, Jacyntha Crawley (The London Biorhythm Company Ltd.), Marnie Dobson, Agni Ecroyd, Dr. Robert Edelhauser, Dr. Donald Epstein, Simon Fielding, The Hale Clinic, The Gestalt Centre, Richard Holding, Stuart Hudson (The Oxford College of Chiropractic), Ann Gillanders, Theo Gimbel, The Goldhurst Terrace Project, Charles Hunt, Adam Jackson, Olwen Jenkins, Anne Mamok, Matthew Manning, Guy Mason, Clare Matthews, Professor Man Fong Mei (AcuMedic Foundation), David Montgomery, Garet Newell, Colin Nicholls, Katrina Patterson, Tony Pinkus (Ainsworth's Pharmacy), Jill Purce, Dr. Shelagh Smith (The National Hospital for Neurology and Neurosurgery), Aditi Silverstein, John Steele, Mike Trundley, Tyringham Naturopathic Clinic, Dr. Coralee Van Egmond, Paul Vick, Louise Walker, Dr. Lily Hua Yu.

Many thanks also to the following for their kind help in supplying equipment or materials for photography: HNE Akron, Ipswich, Suffolk; Aleph One Ltd., Cambridge; BioLab, London W1; East-West Herb Shop, London WC2; Futon Express, London NW1; Highly Sprung, London SW11; Lunn Antiques, London WC2; Magnecare, Christchurch, Dorset; Magnetic Health, London SW7; Parker Knoll Contracts, Frogmoor, Buckinghamshire; Ultramind Ltd., London EC1; VEGA Grieshaber KG, Schiltach, Germany.

Picture Credits

The publisher would like to thank the following for their kind permission to reproduce their photographs:

c=center; t=top; b=bottom; l=left; r=right; a=above

AKG, London: 18/19c, 118bl, 118bc, 160cl, 181cl; Erich Lessing 134cr; National Maritime Museum 148bc; **Allsport**: Richard Saker 179bc; **Ancient Art & Architecture**: 12bl; Ronald Sheridan 90br, 98bl, 174cra, 200tr; **Art Therapy Clients**: 182cr/crbelow/br; **Bridgeman Art Library**: Eton College, Windsor 134bl; Nasjonal Galleriet, Oslo: *The Scream* 1893 Edvard Munch, © DACS 182cl; Oriental Museum, Durham University 174bc; Spink & Son Ltd, London 108bl; **British Association for Autogenic Training and Therapy**: 168cl; **British Chiropractic Association**: 70bc; **British School of Osteopathy**: 76bc; **Carroll & Brown**: 43crbelow; **Marian Chace Foundation of the American Dance Therapy Association**: 112cl; **Jean-Loup Charmet**: 104b; **Christie's Images**: 95cl, 99cl; **Corbis/ Bettman**: UPI 178c; **CRCS Publications**: 102cl; **Mary Evans Picture Library**: 56bc, 62bc, 96cl, 122bc, 166bc/cl, 194crbelow, 198tr; **Parfumerie Fragonard**: B. Touillon 62br; **Phyllis lei Furumoto**: 107cl; **Glasgow Museum**: St. Mungo Museum of Religious Life and Art 176cl; **Goodheart, Zatkin, Hack & Associates**: 196tr; **Sally & Richard Greenhill**: 105b, 315c; **Sonia Halliday**: James Wellard 38tl; **Robert Harding Picture Library**: Rob Cousins 21tr; Simon Harris 145cl; Tom Mackie 45cr; Rainbird 12/13c; Adina Tovy 179cr; **Harvard Medical School**: Margaret Kois 170bl; **Hutchison Library**: Melanie Friend 140cr; Felix Greene 100bl; **Image Bank**: 179cbelow; Antonio M. Rosario 167br; Dag Sundberg 179c; **Images Colour Library**: 167bl; Charles Walker Collection 184cl; **Impact**: Brian Harris 145cr; Brian Rybolt 38tcl; Rajesh Vora 186cl; **The International Institute of Reflexology**: 53bl, 66bc; **The International Sivananda Yoga Vedanta Centre**: 176crbelow; **Tony Isbitt Photography**: 177br; **Bernard Jensen International**: 195tr; **Sandra Lousada**: 56cla, 57bl/bc/clbelow/cbelow, 58b/c/cr, 59bl/c/tl/tc/tr, 60tl/cl/bl/c, 61c/tl/tr/cr, 62cl, 64b/cbelow/crbelow; **The Billie Love Historical Collection**: 178bl; **Guy Mason**: 201tr/bl/br; **Natural History Photographic Agency**: John Shaw 179crbelow; **The Nordoff-Robbins Music Therapy Centre**: Chris Schwarz 181bc/cra; **Park Attwood Clinic**: Glyn Lewis 125c/br, 307br; **Powell-Cotton Museum**: 176clbelow; **Rex Features**: 105cr; **Rolf Institute**: 82cl/cr; **Science Photo Library**: Michael W. Davidson 153c; BSIP Ducloux 18bl, 26c, 27tl, 63tc; Carlos Goldin 154cbelow; Thomas Hollyman 153cla; Dr. Gopal Murti 150bl; National Library of Medicine 160bc; D. Phillips 26bl, 27tc,120bl; David Scharf 16/17c, 154c; BSIP VEM 149bl; M. I. Walker 153bc; Hattie Young 183c; **Society of Teachers of the Alexander Technique**: 86cl; **Spectrum**: 37tl, 145c, 154bc; **Frank Spooner**: Gamma, Zoja Pictures 45br; **The Rudolph Steiner House, London**: 124bc/cl; **Tony Stone Images**: J. McDermott 179br; **Chris Turner**: 26br, 27tr, 72br; **John Walmsley Photo Library**: 180bc; **Wellcome Institute Library, London**: 90bc, 126bl, 134r, 140bl, 144bl, 154cl, 192tr, 193tr, 194tr, 199tr; **Michael Wolgensinger**: 85c/b; Zefa: 16tl

Jacket: **Sandra Lousada**: front cover bc/bcl/br

Every effort has been made to trace the copyright holders of photographs. The publisher apologizes for any omissions and will amend further editions.